CORE CURRICULUM

Interdisciplinary Lactation Care

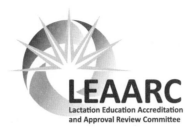

LEAARC
Lactation Education Accreditation
and Approval Review Committee

Edited by

Suzanne Hetzel Campbell, PhD, RN, IBCLC
Associate Professor
The University of British Columbia School of Nursing
Vancouver, British Columbia, Canada

Judith Lauwers, BA, IBCLC, FILCA
Executive Director
Lactation Education Accreditation and Approval Review Committee
Swedesboro, New Jersey, USA

Rebecca Mannel, MPH, IBCLC, FILCA
Clinical Assistant Professor, Department of OB/GYN
University of Oklahoma Health Sciences Center
Oklahoma City, Oklahoma, USA

Becky Spencer, PhD, RN, IBCLC
Assistant Professor
Texas Woman's University College of Nursing
Denton, Texas, USA

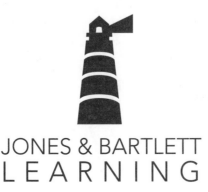

JONES & BARTLETT
LEARNING

World Headquarters
Jones & Bartlett Learning
5 Wall Street
Burlington, MA 01803
978-443-5000
info@jblearning.com
www.jblearning.com

Jones & Bartlett Learning books and products are available through most bookstores and online booksellers. To contact Jones & Bartlett Learning directly, call 800-832-0034, fax 978-443-8000, or visit our website, www.jblearning.com.

Production Credits

VP, Product Management: David D. Cella
Director of Product Management: Amanda Martin
Product Manager: Teresa Reilly
Product Assistant: Christina Freitas
Production Editor: Vanessa Richards
Marketing Communications Manager: Katie Hennessy
Product Fulfillment Manager: Wendy Kilborn
Composition: S4Carlisle Publishing Services
Cover Design: Scott Moden
Rights & Media Specialists: Wes DeShano, John Rusk
Media Development Editor: Troy Liston
Printing and Binding: McNaughton & Gunn
Cover Printing: McNaughton & Gunn

Library of Congress Cataloging-in-Publication Data

Names: Lactation Education Accreditation and Approval Review Committee,
  author. | Campbell, Suzanne Hetzel, editor. | Lauwers, Judith, 1949-
  editor. | Mannel, Rebecca, editor. | Spencer, Becky, editor.
Title: Core curriculum for interdisciplinary lactation care / Lactation
  Education Accreditation and Approval Review Committee ; edited by Suzanne
  Hetzel Campbell, Judith Lauwers, Rebecca Mannel, Becky Spencer.
Description: Burlington, Massachusetts : Jones & Bartlett Learning, [2019] |
  Includes bibliographical references and index.
Identifiers: LCCN 2018009895 | ISBN 9781284111163 (paperback)
Subjects: | MESH: Lactation--physiology | Education | Breast Feeding | Milk,
  Human--secretion | Infant Nutritional Physiological Phenomena | Curriculum
Classification: LCC QP246 | NLM WP 18 | DDC 612.6/64071--dc23
LC record available at https://lccn.loc.gov/2018009895

6048

Printed in the United States of America
22 21 20 19 18   10 9 8 7 6 5 4 3 2

Contents

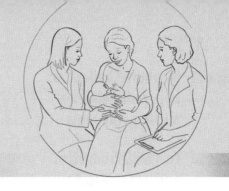

Acknowledgments

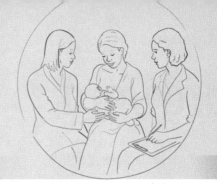

The Lactation Education Accreditation and Approval Review Committee's (LEAARC's) *Core Curriculum for Interdisciplinary Lactation Care* represents the work of scores of clinicians, researchers, and educators who have advanced the field of lactation consulting over the past 3 decades. We honor those accomplishments and recognize our peers and colleagues for inspiring us to accept the challenge of guiding the preparation of this first edition. It was a pleasure being part of such a collaboration among numerous experts throughout the world who generously shared their talents and insights into clinical practice.

Our editorial team extends our sincere gratitude to all the chapter authors whose diligence helped maintain high standards and integrity and ensured that this important resource would be relevant to clinicians, educators, and students. We extend special thanks to the team of reviewers who helped identify areas for improvement and who validated the stellar work of our chapter authors. We acknowledge Jones & Bartlett Learning staff members Teresa Reilly, Christina Freitas, Vanessa Richards, and Wes DeShano for their patience and support throughout the project. We appreciate the expert editing and guidance from our copyeditor, Jeanne Hansen, in shepherding us through the writing and editing of such an extensive text. Thank you as well to the LEAARC Board of Directors for their vision and action to ensure the lactation profession will continue to be guided by a core curriculum and for placing their trust in our editorial team to manage the process. None of us would have had the privilege to be part of this process without the mentors and guides who came before and nurtured us, the students who challenged our perspectives and rationales, and the many parents, babies, and families who taught us along the way. Finally, we thank our families for their encouragement, support, and understanding that allowed us to devote the time and focus needed to steer this text through to publication.

Suzanne Hetzel Campbell
Judith Lauwers
Rebecca Mannel
Becky Spencer

Foreword

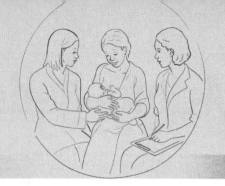

As an International Board Certified Lactation Consultant (IBCLC), physician, and educator with more than 25 years of experience with training others in lactation, I am very enthusiastic about the publication of this text. The impact it will have on the different environments in the clinical practice of human lactation will be enormous. Whether as a text for academic and professional-level human lactation courses or as a reference in the clinic, it provides evidence-based information that will undoubtedly help us expand our knowledge and assist our clients or patients in making informed decisions. This text is written following the Lactation Education Accreditation and Approval Review Committee (LEAARC) *Curriculum for Programs in Human Lactation*, which is based on the competencies that any academic program needs to offer, regardless of its setting.

My training and experience in public health have convinced me that lactation consultancy is one of the healthcare specialties in which the fundamental pillar of inter- and multidisciplinary treatment is put into practice every day. The specialists in the field who wrote this text represent a variety of professions and experiences, which further enriches the content and makes it an appropriate text to use in any academic setting. Authors and reviewers from several countries around the world give this text international relevancy because it allows the reader to apply what they have learned in different sociocultural contexts.

This text is written in gender-neutral language that avoids bias toward gender, adopting this as an important principle for lactation consultants' training and the families they serve. It also emphasizes awareness of the necessary social support and the challenges related to equity that impact breastfeeding services. I recommend without hesitation that all educators in lactation programs adopt this text, both to help design curricula and as a text for students.

I teach courses in lactation completely in Spanish. I encourage the translation of this text in the near future, to Spanish and other languages, to allow millions of readers who do not understand English to benefit from it. This will help minimize disparities and inequities around the world.

Ana M. Parrilla-Rodríguez, MD, MPH, FABM, IBCLC, FACCE
Professor
Maternal and Child Health Program, School of Public Health
University of Puerto Rico
Director Certificado Profesional en Educador en Lactancia
Academia Edupró

Contributors

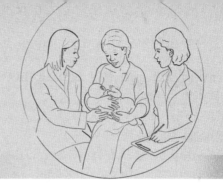

James Abbey, MD
Texas Tech Health Sciences Center Department
  of Internal Medicine
Amarillo, Texas, USA

Jonathan C. Allen, PhD, CNS
Professor, Director of Graduate Programs
Department of Food, Bioprocessing,
  and Nutrition Sciences
North Carolina State University
Raleigh, North Carolina, USA

Teresa M. Baker, MD
Associate Professor, Department of Obstetrics
  and Gynecology
Texas Tech University Health Sciences Center
Amarillo, Texas, USA

Jennifer Bañuelos, MAS
UC Davis Human Lactation Center
University of California Davis
Davis, California, USA

Jean Benedict, RN, BSN, IBCLC
Private Practice Lactation Consultant
South Lyon, Michigan, USA

Cheryl Benn, RM, IBCLC, DCur
Registered Midwife
Palmerston North, Manawatu, New Zealand

Pamela D. Berens, MD, IBCLC
Professor
University of Texas Health McGovern Medical
  School
Houston, Texas, USA

Elizabeth C. Brooks, JD, IBCLC, FILCA
Private Practice Lactation Consultant
Wyndmoor, Pennsylvania, USA

Suzanne Hetzel Campbell, PhD, RN, IBCLC
Associate Professor
The University of British Columbia School of Nursing
Vancouver, British Columbia, Canada

Virginia H. Carney, MPH, RDN, LDN, IBCLC, FILCA, FAND
Director of Clinical Nutrition Services
St. Jude Children's Research Hospital
Memphis, Tennessee, USA

Cathy Carothers, BLA, IBCLC, FILCA
Co-Director
Every Mother Inc.
Bay Springs, Mississippi, USA

Elizabeth Choi, MS, CF-SLP
Speech Language Pathologist
Lucid Speech & Language Clinic Inc.
Temecula, California, USA

Kathleen Donovan, RN, MSN, IBCLC
Lactation Consultant
Stone Springs Hospital Center
Dulles, Virginia, USA

Debi Ferrarello, MSN, MS, RN, IBCLC
Director of Parent Education and Lactation
Pennsylvania Hospital, Penn Medicine
Adjunct Professor
Drexel University
Abington, Pennsylvania, USA

April Fogleman, PhD, RD, IBCLC
Assistant Professor of Nutrition
North Carolina State University
Raleigh, North Carolina, USA

Catherine Watson Genna, BS, IBCLC
Private Practice Lactation Consultant
Woodhaven, New York, USA

Gloria A. Graham, MD
Family Medicine Physician
Clinicas de Salud del Pueblo
Coachella, California, USA

Jane Grassley, PhD, RN, IBCLC
Professor and Jody DeMeyer Endowed Chair
Boise State University
Boise, Idaho, USA

M. Karen Kerkhoff Gromada, MSN, RN, IBCLC, FILCA
Independent Consultant
Bellevue, Kentucky, USA

Laura N. Haiek, MD, MSc
Ministère de la Santé et des Services sociaux
Direction générale de la santé publique
McGill University, Department of Family Medicine
Montréal, Québec, Canada

Thomas W. Hale, RPh, PhD
Professor, Department of Pediatrics
Texas Tech University
Amarillo, Texas, USA

M. Jane Heinig, PhD, IBCLC
Executive Director, UC Davis Human Lactation
    Center
University of California Davis
Davis, California, USA

Kathleen L. Hoover, MEd, IBCLC, FILCA
Lactation Consultant, The Birth Place
Riddle Hospital
Media, Pennsylvania, USA

Vergie I. Hughes, RN, MS, IBCLC, FILCA
Program Director
Lactation Education Resources
Tracys Landing, Maryland, USA

Nina Isaac, MS, CCC-SLP, IBCLC
Speech Language Pathologist
Milk & Honey Feeding and Speech Services
Tucson, Arizona, USA

Frances Jones, RN, MSN, IBCLC
Coordinator, Lactation Services and BC Women's
    Provincial Milk Bank
British Columbia Women's Hospital
Vancouver, British Columbia, Canada

Andrea Bulera Judge, MPH, IBCLC
Clinical Instructor and Coordinator, Human
    Lactation Program
Drexel University
Philadelphia, Pennsylvania, USA

Kathleen Kendall-Tackett, PhD, IBCLC, FAPA
Clinical Professor of Nursing
University of Hawaii at Manoa
Clinical Associate Professor of Pediatrics
Texas Tech University School of Medicine
Amarillo, Texas, USA

Nekisha L. Killings, MPH, IBCLC, CLC
Lactation Consultant
Lioness Lactation
Los Angeles, California, USA

Judith Lauwers, BA, IBCLC, FILCA
Executive Director
Lactation Education Accreditation and Approval
    Review Committee
Swedesboro, New Jersey, USA

Sahira Long, MD, IBCLC, FAAP, FABM
Medical Director, Children's Health Center at
    Anacostia
Children's National Health System
Washington, DC, USA

Angela Love-Zaranka, BA, IBCLC, RLC
Founder and Director
Breastfeeding Lady LLC
Alexandria, Virginia, USA

Rebecca Mannel, MPH, IBCLC, FILCA
Clinical Assistant Professor, Department of OB/GYN
University of Oklahoma Health Sciences Center
Oklahoma City, Oklahoma, USA

Lisa Marasco, MA, IBCLC, FILCA
Clinical Lactation Consultant
Santa Barbara Public Health Department/WIC
Santa Maria, California, USA

Joan Younger Meek, MD, MS, RD, FAAP, IBCLC
Professor of Clinical Sciences
Florida State University College of Medicine
Tallahassee, Florida, USA

Anne Montgomery, MD, MBA, FAAFP, FABM, IBCLC
Program Director, Family Medicine Residency
Eisenhower Medical Center
Rancho Mirage, California, USA

Kerstin Hedberg Nyqvist, RN, PhD
Associate Professor, Department of Women's
    and Children's Health
Uppsala University
Uppsala, Sweden

Tina Revai, MN, RN, IBCLC
Co-President BC Lactation Consultants Association
Port Alberni, British Columbia, Canada

Alisa Sanders, RN, IBCLC
Clinical Director
University of Texas Health Science Center at
    Houston, Lactation Foundation
Houston, Texas, USA

Laurie K. Scherer, MS, LCPC-S
Director of Counseling and Psychological Services
St. Mary's College of Maryland
St. Mary's City, Maryland, USA

Alicia C. Simpson MS, RD, IBCLC, LD
Executive Director
Pea Pod Nutrition and Lactation Support
Atlanta, Georgia, USA

Nicola Singletary, MAT, IBCLC, PhD candidate
Department of Food, Bioprocessing and Nutrition
  Services
North Carolina State University
Raleigh, North Carolina, USA

Becky Spencer, PhD, RN, IBCLC
Assistant Professor
Texas Woman's University College of Nursing
Denton, Texas, USA

Elizabeth K. Stehel, MD, IBCLC
Associate Professor, Pediatrics
University of Texas Southwestern Medical Center
Clinical Professor, Pediatrics
Texas A&M Health Science Center
Dallas, Texas, USA

Virginia Thorley, PhD, IBCLC, FILCA
Honorary Research Fellow, School of Historical
  and Philosophical Inquiry
University of Queensland
St Lucia, Queensland, Australia

Karen Wambach, PhD, RN, IBCLC, FILCA, FAAN
Professor
University of Kansas School of Nursing
Kansas City, Kansas, USA

Amanda Watkins, PhD, RD, LDN, IBCLC
Executive Director
Global Lactation Education Associates LLC
Raleigh, North Carolina, USA

Gillian Weaver, BSc (Hons) Nutrition, RD
International Human Milk Banking Consultant
Dover, Kent, United Kingdom

Elaine Webber, DNP, PPCNP-BC, IBCLC
Assistant Clinical Professor
University of Detroit Mercy
Detroit, Michigan, USA

Michal Young, MD, FAAP, IBCLC
Associate Professor and Director, NICU
  and Newborn Nurseries
Howard University
Washington, DC, USA

Reviewers

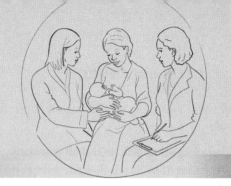

Debbie Albert, PhD, BSN, IBCLC

Denise Altman, RN, IBCLC, RLC

Lisa Amir, MBBS, MMed, PhD, IBCLC, FABM

Helen Ball, PhD

Janice Ballou, DNP, PPCNP-BC, IBCLC

Pamela D. Berens, MD, IBCLC

Glenda Dickerson, MS, RN, IBCLC

Lea Geiger, RN, BSN, IBCLC

Melanie Gingras, BScN, IBCLC

Lenore Goldfarb, PhD, IBCLC

Helen Gray, MPhil, IBCLC

Karleen Gribble, BRurSc, PhD

Jeanne Hagreen, RN, BSN, IBCLC

Alison Hazelbaker, PhD, IBCLC, FILCA, RCST

Vergie I. Hughes, RN, MS, IBCLC, FILCA

Jarold (Tom) Johnston Jr., MSN, CNM, IBCLC

Andrea Bulera Judge, MPH, IBCLC

Linda G. Leonard, RN, MSN

Joan Younger Meek, MD, MS, RD, FAAP, IBCLC

Rachel O'Leary, PGCE

Laurie Nomssen Rivers, PhD, RD, IBCLC

Attie Sandink, RN, IBCLC, CBE

Lisa Sandora, MA, CCC-SLP, IBCLC

Abigail Smetana, RN, BSN, MSN, IBCLC

Christina Smillie, MD, FAAP, IBCLC, FAB

Paige Hall Smith, MSPH, PhD

Amy Spangler, RN, MN, IBCLC

Kim Updegrove, CNM, MSN, MPH

Amanda Watkins, PhD, RD, LDN, IBCLC

Nancy Wight, MD, IBCLC, FABM, FAAP

Tracy Wilson, IBCLC, CCCE

Introduction

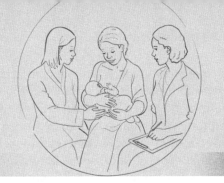

We are very excited to introduce the first edition of *Core Curriculum for Interdisciplinary Lactation Care*. The work behind this text began more than 10 years ago when the International Lactation Consultant Association (ILCA) and the International Board of Lactation Consultant Examiners (IBLCE) collaborated to establish and sponsor an organization with the purpose of developing standards for lactation education. The Lactation Education Accreditation and Approval Review Committee (LEAARC) published the *Curriculum for Programs in Human Lactation* in 2010 (with updates in 2014 and 2016), which defines the educational preparation for entry-level lactation consultants. The lactation education curriculum comprises the following topic areas: Communication and Counseling, Documentation and Communication, History Taking and Assessment, Prenatal and Perinatal Breastfeeding Support, Extended Breastfeeding Support, Problem Solving, Infant–Child Breastfeeding Challenges, Parental Breastfeeding Challenges, Public Health, Research Legislation and Policy, Professional Responsibilities and Practice, and Leadership and Teaching. Each topic area has defined core competencies, learning objectives, suggested content, and suggested skills and behaviors.

LEAARC's *Curriculum for Programs in Human Lactation* has served as the foundation for the development and review of lactation education programs worldwide. Lactation education programs that provide 90 hours of didactic education can apply to LEAARC for approval designation, and lactation education programs that provide 45 hours of didactic education can apply to LEAARC for recognized designation. Lactation education programs that are sponsored by an accredited postsecondary education institution can apply for accreditation by the Commission on Accreditation of Allied Health Education Programs (CAAHEP). LEAARC provides program evaluations and recommendations for accrediting lactation education programs to CAAHEP. The IBLCE requires that all applicants for the certification exam through Pathway 2 show evidence of completion of a comprehensive accredited lactation education program within 5 years prior to applying for the exam. The *Curriculum for Programs in Human Lactation* guides the comprehensive review and evaluation of all lactation education programs seeking approval, recognition, or accreditation.

To fully enact LEAARC's mission to "establish standards for and recognize quality in lactation education," board members recognized the need to further develop lactation education materials and resources. This new text, *Core Curriculum for Interdisciplinary Lactation Care*, exemplifies the LEAARC *Curriculum for Programs in Human Lactation*. The LEAARC Board of Directors commissioned this team of editors and an interdisciplinary team of clinical lactation experts from several countries around the world to serve as authors to develop this text. Chapters in the text received external review by experienced, internationally recognized clinicians and lactation educators. The text serves as a trustworthy source for lactation-specific information and education for students, interns, certification candidates, instructors, and clinicians—in any discipline or specialty—who provide care to breastfeeding families. We want to emphasize that the LEAARC *Curriculum for Programs in Human Lactation* and the content presented in this text are intended to provide the basic knowledge required to practice as a beginning lactation consultant. The breadth and depth of specialty lactation practice is outside the scope of this text.

Core Curriculum for Interdisciplinary Lactation Care is organized into three main sections. The *Science* section, Chapters 1–9, presents the science and biology of breastfeeding. Breast anatomy, infant anatomy related to feeding, infant behavior related to feeding, and production and biochemistry of human milk are presented with a focus on what is normal and variations of normal. Nutritional requirements and nutrition assessments for breastfeeding parents and infants are also presented. How medications, supplements, and other substances enter human milk and how to minimize infant exposure are discussed. Methods to appraise, interpret, and apply research are examined. The *Management* section, Chapters 10–24, examines specific areas related to the breastfeeding family that may impact breastfeeding and describes best practices, up-to-date research, and protocols, where available. The information in this section describes the lactation consultant's role in supporting and promoting breastfeeding and family health as part of the interprofessional team. The *Professional* section, Chapters 25–32, addresses professional aspects of working in the lactation field. The interdisciplinary nature of lactation care involves working with a team of healthcare professionals, community organizations, and governmental agencies. It involves applying communication, education, advocacy, and professional standards to improve the environment for breastfeeding outcomes. Throughout the text, the chapters feature inclusive language to represent families from diverse backgrounds and cultures, and key points to guide learning. Most chapters also contain case studies to stimulate discussions among colleagues and in classrooms, allowing application of the theoretical and clinical information to a live situation and increasing the opportunity for experiential learning.

We chose to include the term *interdisciplinary* in the title of this text to highlight the strength of having many disciplines represented within the lactation care specialty. Leading global health authorities—including, but not limited to, the World Health Organization, the U.S. Institute of Medicine, and the Interdisciplinary Association for Population Health Science—have identified the need for collaboration among teams of multidisciplinary healthcare specialists, patients, and community health workers to address the world's most pressing health concerns. This focus on interdisciplinary collaboration is a relatively new phenomenon in global health care, with an increased emphasis noted over the past 10 years. Lactation consulting has been interdisciplinary in nature from its inception as a healthcare specialty in 1985. Although the discipline has many subspecialties, we all share the same lactation knowledge base, presented in this text, that enables us to provide comprehensive care for breastfeeding families. We thoroughly enjoyed the collaborative experience with our diverse team of authors and reviewers, and we hope that you will appreciate the variety of perspectives they present within their shared expertise in lactation.

Suzanne Hetzel Campbell
Judith Lauwers
Rebecca Mannel
Becky Spencer

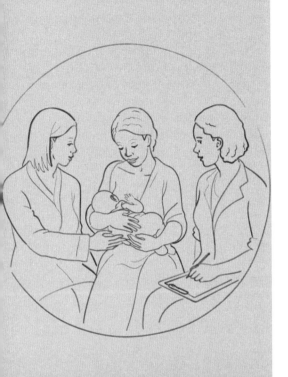

SECTION I

Science

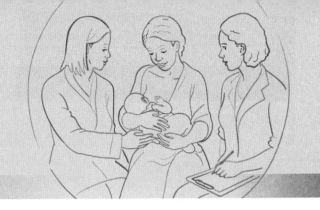

CHAPTER 1

Scientific Evidence Supporting Breastfeeding

Becky Spencer

OBJECTIVES

- Describe the current evidence for the health benefits of breastfeeding for infants.
- Describe the current evidence for the health benefits of breastfeeding for lactating parents.
- Describe the current evidence for the impact of lactation support on the initiation and duration of breastfeeding.

DEFINITIONS OF COMMONLY USED TERMS

exclusive breastfeeding When an infant receives no other food or drink except breastmilk for the first 6 months of life. Oral rehydration solutions and medicines or vitamins in liquid form are not considered other food or drink.[1]

lactation support provider Any individual who is trained, certified, or licensed to provide breastfeeding education, support, and care within the specific scope of practice defined by training, certification, or licensure.

malocclusion Misalignment of the upper and lower teeth causing an irregular bite, cross bite, or overbite. In severe cases, malocclusion can impact a person's speech or ability to eat.

meta-analysis A quantitative statistical analysis of several separate but similar studies to test the pooled data for statistical significance.

necrotizing enterocolitis (NEC) A condition that typically occurs in the 2nd to 3rd week of life in preterm, formula-fed infants; it is characterized by damage to the intestinal tract. NEC has a high rate of mortality, reaching 50 percent or more depending on the severity.

peer support Lactation support that is delivered by individuals who have common life experiences with the people they are serving.

sudden infant death syndrome (SIDS) A sudden and unexpected death, whether explained or unexplained, that occurs during infancy.

(continues)

DEFINITIONS OF COMMONLY USED TERMS *(continued)*

systematic review A detailed and strategic search strategy, evaluation, and summary of the results of available quantitative studies; provides a high level of evidence on the effectiveness of healthcare interventions.

technology-mediated support Technology platforms that are used by lactation support providers to deliver education, care, and support. Examples of technology platforms include social media sites, mobile applications, videoconferencing, and telehealth.

Any use of the term *mother*, *maternal*, or *breastfeeding* is not meant to exclude transgender or nonbinary parents who may be breastfeeding or providing human milk to their infant.

▶ Overview

The decision to breastfeed an infant is influenced by a multitude of information sources. Influences in parents' decisions include personal connections with partners, family members, and friends; connections with healthcare providers, hospitals, and clinics; and connections with social media, internet resources, and various marketing mediums in television, print, and radio. It can seem daunting to parents to sort through all the different messages about breastfeeding and differentiate valid, trustworthy, and useful information from false and misleading information. Helping parents make informed decisions about infant feeding and supporting optimal breastfeeding to meet individual goals should be the top priority of all lactation support providers.

Lactation support providers include a growing diverse interdisciplinary team of healthcare providers including physicians, nurses, midwives, registered dieticians, public health professionals, scientists, lactation consultants, peer counselors, and lay community health workers. These providers share a common commitment to promoting the health of families through breastfeeding education, care, and support. The interdisciplinary nature of lactation support is a strength, yet providing consistent messaging that is valid, trustworthy, and useful across disciplines can be challenging. The purpose of this chapter is to present the most recent evidence from scientific literature regarding the benefits of breastfeeding for infants and lactating parents. The most recent evidence demonstrating the benefits of lactation support is also presented. Providing consistent breastfeeding information using an evidence-informed foundation from all interdisciplinary perspectives will decrease contradictory messaging and increase consistent messaging to assist families in making sound infant feeding decisions. Studies cited in this chapter were conducted in low-, middle-, and high-income countries worldwide.

I. Health Benefits of Breastfeeding for Infants and Children

    A.   Breastfeeding is protective against respiratory infections.
        1.   Health benefits of breastfeeding for infants and children are reported in systematic reviews and meta-analyses of scientific literature.
        2.   In one systematic review, any breastfeeding (exclusive or partial) reduced the risk of hospitalization and mortality.[2]
        3.   Another systematic review reported that infants younger than 1 year who were exclusively breastfed for 4 months or longer had an overall reduced risk of hospitalization from lower respiratory tract infections, compared to infants who were formula fed.[3]
    B.   Breastfeeding may be associated with a reduced risk for developing asthma.
        1.   One meta-analysis of three prospective cohort studies of fair-quality evidence concluded that any breastfeeding for at least 3 months was associated with a reduced risk for asthma.[3,4]
        2.   Some evidence from cohort studies concluded that there is an increased risk of asthma and allergy with breastfeeding.[5,6]
    C.   Breastfeeding is protective against gastrointestinal infections and diarrhea.
        1.   Breastfeeding has demonstrated substantial protection against morbidity and mortality from diarrhea.[2,3,7]
        2.   Protection from diarrhea appears to be dose related, with exclusive breastfeeding providing more protection.[2]

D. Breastfeeding lowers the risk for the incidence of acute otitis media (AOM). Children who were breast-fed longer (more than 4 or 6 months, compared to less than 4 or 6 months in respective studies) had a significantly reduced risk for the incidence of AOM.[3,7,8]

E. Breastfeeding lowers the risk for the incidence of dental caries.
    1. Children who are breastfed have less risk of developing dental caries than children who are fed nonhuman milk from a bottle.[9]
    2. There is a lower risk of developing dental caries the longer children are breastfed, up to 12 months of age.[10] An increased risk of developing dental caries was associated with breastfeeding longer than 12 months. The increased risk is possibly attributed to night feedings and poor oral care after feedings in breastfed infants and toddlers.

F. Breastfeeding lowers the risk for the incidence of malocclusion.
    1. Children who were breastfed were less likely to present with malocclusions than children who were never breastfed.
    2. The longer infants were breastfed, the less likely they were to present with malocclusions.[11]

G. Breastfeeding lowers the risk for the incidence of NEC for preterm infants. In neonatal intensive care units where the parent's expressed milk or donor human milk is used with preterm infants, NEC is significantly decreased.[3,12,13]

H. Breastfeeding lowers the risk for the incidence of SIDS.
    1. Any breastfeeding is associated with a significantly reduced risk of SIDS.[3,14-16]
    2. The protective effect of breastfeeding against SIDS is strongest with exclusive breastfeeding.[15]

I. Breastfeeding lowers the risk for the incidence of developing childhood leukemia. Breastfeeding for longer than 6 months was associated with a reduced risk of acute lymphocytic leukemia.[3,17]

J. Breastfeeding may be associated with a reduced risk of obesity.
    1. Early research that explored the relationship of breastfeeding to obesity in later childhood did not account for confounding variables, selection reporting, or publication bias.[3]
    2. A systematic review found that breastfeeding was associated with decreased obesity in childhood, adolescence, and adulthood.[18] The researchers controlled for socioeconomic status, maternal body mass index, and perinatal morbidity.

K. Breastfeeding may be associated with a reduced risk of developing diabetes.
    1. A nonstatistically significant reduced risk for developing Type 2 diabetes later in life was found with infants who were ever breastfed.[18]
    2. A review of six studies concluded that breastfeeding could reduce the risk of developing Type 1 diabetes, but the retrospective nature of the studies could have introduced recall bias, which decreases the trustworthiness of the results.[3]

L. Breastfeeding may be associated with higher performance on intelligence tests in childhood and adolescence.
    1. In a meta-analysis that controlled for maternal intelligence, children who were ever breastfed scored an average of 3.4 points higher on intelligence tests than children who were never breastfed.[19]
    2. A review of eight studies that examined the association of breastfeeding and intelligence found little to no evidence for an association between breastfeeding and intelligence in later childhood.[3]

II. Health Benefits of Breastfeeding for Lactating Parents

A. Breastfeeding lowers the risk for the incidence of developing breast cancer.
    1. Multiple systematic reviews and meta-analyses show a consistent protective effect of breastfeeding against breast cancer.[3,20,21]
    2. A dose effect of breastfeeding impacts the reduction risk for breast cancer. For every 12 months of cumulative breastfeeding, the risk is reduced by 4.3 percent.[20]

B. Breastfeeding lowers the risk for the incidence of developing ovarian cancer.
    1. Multiple systematic reviews and meta-analyses show a consistent protective effect of breastfeeding against ovarian cancer.[3,20,22-24]
    2. A longer duration of breastfeeding results in a greater protective benefit. Women who breastfed for 6 months or less had a 17 percent risk reduction, compared to women who breastfed for 6 to 12 months, who had a 28 percent risk reduction.[20]

C.   Breastfeeding is associated with lactational amenorrhea, or a delay in the return of menses after birth. Exclusive breastfeeding for 6 months or longer is associated with lactational amenorrhea and increased spacing of pregnancies.[20,25,26]

D.   Breastfeeding may be associated with a reduced risk of developing Type 2 diabetes. A meta-analysis of six cohort studies demonstrated a 9 percent protection against maternal Type 2 diabetes for a 1-year increase in the total lifetime duration of breastfeeding.[27]

E.   Breastfeeding may be associated with a reduced risk of developing cardiovascular disease.

   1.   Although no systematic reviews or meta-analyses have been published, two good-quality cohort studies have demonstrated an association between breastfeeding and a reduced risk for maternal cardiovascular disease.[28,29]

   2.   Women who breastfed longer than 12 months in their lifetimes had less incidence of hypertension, diabetes, hyperlipidemia, or cardiovascular disease.[28]

   3.   In women aged 50 years or younger, never breastfeeding was associated with a higher risk for hypertension, diabetes, and obesity.[29]

III. Global Economic Impact of Breastfeeding

A.   UNICEF conducted an economic analysis of the impact of increased breastfeeding on four acute pediatric illnesses and maternal breast cancer in the United Kingdom.

   1.   The analysis was based on a moderate increase in breastfeeding, including 45 percent of women who were exclusively breastfeeding for 4 months and 75 percent of breastfeeding babies who were discharged from neonatal units. The resulting economic impact would be as follows:

      a.   A total of 3,285 fewer gastrointestinal infection related hospital admissions, resulting in £3.6 million (U.S. $5 million) saved in treatment costs annually.

      b.   A total of 5,916 fewer lower respiratory tract infection related hospital admissions, resulting in £6.7 million (U.S. $9.3 million) saved in treatment costs annually.

      c.   A total of 21,045 fewer cases of AOM healthcare provider visits, resulting in £750,000 (U.S. $1 million) saved in treatment costs annually.

      d.   A total of 361 fewer cases of NEC, resulting in more than £6 million (U.S. $8.3 million) saved in treatment costs annually.[30]

   2.   A second analysis was conducted based on a 50 percent increase in women who choose to breast-feed for up to 18 total months in their lifetimes. The resulting economic impact on the reduced incidence of breast cancer would be 865 fewer breast cancer cases, resulting in more than £21 million (U.S. $29.1 million) saved in treatment costs annually.[30]

B.   A cost analysis of suboptimal breastfeeding rates in the United States reported 3,340 additional deaths attributed to suboptimal breastfeeding.[31]

   1.   A total of 78 percent were maternal and due to myocardial infarction, breast cancer, and diabetes.

   2.   A total of 22 percent were pediatric deaths, mostly attributed to SIDS and NEC.

   3.   The total cost of premature death totaled U.S. $14.2 billion (£10.3 billion).

C.   Another cost analysis of suboptimal breastfeeding rates in the United States, with a subanalysis to examine racial disparities, reported a higher incidence of disease in the non-Hispanic black (NHB) population and the Hispanic populations in the United States.[31]

   1.   The NHB population had 1.7 times the number of excess cases of AOM, 3.3 times the number of excess cases of NEC, and 2.2 times the number of excess child deaths, compared to the non-Hispanic white (NHW) population.

   2.   The Hispanic population had 1.4 times the number of gastrointestinal infections and 1.5 times the number of excess child deaths as the NHW population.

D.   A cost analysis of suboptimal breastfeeding in Southeast Asia was based on increased breastfeeding rates to 100 percent of children exclusively breastfed to age 6 months, with continuation of some breastfeeding to age 2 years.[32]

   1.   Developmental cognitive losses were extrapolated to lost earnings income of U.S. $1.6 billion (£1.16 billion) annually.

   2.   Health expenditures increased U.S. $293.5 million (£212 million) annually.

3. A total of 1,706 maternal deaths could be averted annually with optimal breastfeeding rates.
4. A total of 3,189 cases of gastrointestinal infections are attributable to suboptimal breastfeeding rates in Southeast Asia.
5. A total of 7,528 cases of acute respiratory illness are attributable to suboptimal breastfeeding rates in Southeast Asia.

E. An estimated 823,000 lives could be saved annually in low- and middle-income countries worldwide if breastfeeding practices were optimal.[4]

▶ Key Points from This Chapter

A. Clear and consistent messaging from lactation support providers to parents about the benefits of breast-feeding will help parents make informed decisions.
B. The benefits of breastfeeding for infants, supported by systematic reviews and meta-analyses, include excellent evidence for decreased risk of respiratory infection, gastrointestinal infection, SIDS, AOM, NEC, dental caries, malocclusion, and leukemia.
C. There is moderate evidence for decreased risk of asthma, obesity, diabetes, and higher intelligence. More research is necessary.
D. The benefits of breastfeeding for parents, supported by systematic reviews and meta-analyses, include excellent evidence for decreased risk of breast cancer, ovarian cancer, and lactational amenorrhea.
E. There is moderate evidence for decreased risk of Type 2 diabetes and cardiovascular disease. More research is necessary.
F. The economic impact of suboptimal breastfeeding is significant worldwide.
G. Increasing breastfeeding to optimal levels, as defined by the World Health Organization, would have a significant impact on lives and healthcare dollars saved.[1]

🔍 CASE STUDY

You are a lactation consultant who is teaching a prenatal breastfeeding class to a group of diverse new parents and families. You ask the class participants to share what they have heard about breastfeeding from the media, friends, family, and healthcare providers. One participant states that she has read that breastfed infants have fewer ear infections, but her nephew was breastfed and had multiple ear infections. Another class participant says she heard that breastfeeding decreases a woman's chance of being diagnosed with breast cancer, but her mother breastfed four children and was recently diagnosed with breast cancer. A male participant says he was formula fed as an infant and he "turned out OK." He questions whether breastfeeding has any real impact on health.

Questions

1. How would you respectfully acknowledge the class participants' experiences that are not reflective of current research?
2. How would you use current research to address the class participant's comments about breastfeeding and the incidence of ear infections?
3. How would you use current research to address the class participant's comments about breastfeeding and the incidence of breast cancer?
4. How would you use current research to describe the overall health benefits of breastfeeding?

References

1. World Health Organization, UNICEF. *Global Strategy for Infant and Young Child Feeding.* Geneva, Switzerland: World Health Organization; 2003.
2. Horta BL, Victora CG, World Health Organization. *Short-Term Effects of Breastfeeding: A Systematic Review on the Benefits of Breastfeeding on Diarrhoea and Pneumonia Mortality.* Geneva, Switzerland: World Health Organization; 2013.
3. Ip S, Chung M, Raman G, et al. *Breastfeeding and Maternal and Infant Health Outcomes in Developed Countries: Evidence Report/ Technology Assessment No. 153.* Rockville, MD: Agency for Healthcare Research and Quality; 2007.

4. Victora CG, Bahl R, Barros AJ, et al. Breastfeeding in the 21st century: epidemiology, mechanisms, and lifelong effect. *Lancet.* 2016;387(10017):475-490.

5. Sears MR, Greene JM, Willan AR, et al. Long-term relation between breastfeeding and development of atopy and asthma in children and young adults: a longitudinal study. *Lancet.* 2002;360(9337):901-907.

6. Wegienka G, Ownby DR, Havstad S, Williams LK, Johnson CC. Breastfeeding history and childhood allergic status in a prospective birth cohort. *Ann Allergy Asthma Immunol.* 2006;97(1):78-83.

7. Duijts L, Jaddoe VW, Hofman A, Moll HA. Prolonged and exclusive breastfeeding reduces the risk of infectious diseases in infancy. *Pediatrics.* 2010;126(1):e18-e25.

8. Bowatte G, Tham R, Allen KJ, et al. Breastfeeding and childhood acute otitis media: a systematic review and meta-analysis. *Acta Paediatr.* 2015;104(S467):85-95.

9. Avila WM, Pordeus IA, Paiva SM, Martins CC. Breast and bottle feeding as risk factors for dental caries: a systematic review and meta-analysis. *PLOS One.* 2015;10(11):e0142922. doi:10.1371/journal.pone.0142922.

10. Tham R, Bowatte G, Dharmage SC, et al. Breastfeeding and the risk of dental caries: a systematic review and meta-analysis. *Acta Paediatr.* 2015;104(S467):62-84.

11. Peres KG, Cascaes AM, Nascimento GG, Victora CG. Effect of breastfeeding on malocclusions: a systematic review and meta-analysis. *Acta Paediatr.* 2015;104(S467):54-61.

12. Holman RC, Stoll BJ, Curns AT, Yorita KL, Steiner CA, Schonberger LB. Necrotising enterocolitis hospitalisations among neonates in the United States. *Paediatr Perinat Epidemiol.* 2006;20(6):498-506.

13. Quigley MA, Henderson G, Anthony MY, McGuire W. Formula milk versus donor breast milk for feeding preterm or low birth weight infants. *Cochrane Database Syst Rev.* 2007;4(4):CD002971. doi: 10.1002/14651858.CD002971.pub2.

14. Vennemann MM, Bajanowski T, Brinkmann B, et al. Does breastfeeding reduce the risk of sudden infant death syndrome? *Pediatrics.* 2009;123(3):e406-e410.

15. Hauck FR, Thompson JM, Tanabe KO, Moon RY, Vennemann MM. Breastfeeding and reduced risk of sudden infant death syndrome: a meta-analysis. *Pediatrics.* 2011;128(1):103-110.

16. Thompson JM, Tanabe K, Moon RY, et al. Duration of breastfeeding and risk of SIDS: an individual participant data meta-analysis. *Pediatrics.* 2017;140(5):e20171324. doi:10.1542/peds.2017-1324.

17. Amitay EL, Keinan-Boker L. Breastfeeding and childhood leukemia incidence: a meta-analysis and systematic review. *JAMA Pediatr.* 2015;169(6):e151025. doi:10.1001/jamapediatrics.2015.1025.

18. Horta BL, Loret de Mola C, Victora CG. Long-term consequences of breastfeeding on cholesterol, obesity, systolic blood pressure and type 2 diabetes: a systematic review and meta-analysis. *Acta Paediatr.* 2015;104(S467):30-37.

19. Horta BL, Loret de Mola C, Victora CG. Breastfeeding and intelligence: a systematic review and meta-analysis. *Acta Paediatr.* 2015;104(S467):14-19.

20. Chowdhury R, Sinha B, Sankar MJ, et al. Breastfeeding and maternal health outcomes: a systematic review and meta-analysis. *Acta Paediatr.* 2015;104(S467):96-113.

21. Collaborative Group on Hormonal Factors in Breast Cancer. Breast cancer and breastfeeding: collaborative reanalysis of individual data from 47 epidemiological studies in 30 countries, including 50 302 women with breast cancer and 96 973 women without the disease. *Lancet.* 2002;360(9328):187-195.

22. Sung HK, Ma SH, Choi JY, et al. The effect of breastfeeding duration and parity on the risk of epithelial ovarian cancer: a systematic review and meta-analysis. *J Prev Med Public Health.* 2016;49(6):349-366.

23. Li DP, Du C, Zhang ZM, et al. Breastfeeding and ovarian cancer risk: a systematic review and meta-analysis of 40 epidemiological studies. *Asian Pac J Cancer Prev.* 2014;15(12):4829-4837.

24. Luan NN, Wu QJ, Gong TT, Vogtmann E, Wang YL, Lin B. Breastfeeding and ovarian cancer risk: a meta-analysis of epidemiologic studies. *Am J Clin Nutr.* 2013;98(4):1020-1031.

25. Van der Wijden C, Manion C. Lactational amenorrhoea method for family planning. *Cochrane Database Syst Rev.* 2015;10:CD001329. doi:10.1002/14651858.CD001329.pub2.

26. Kramer MS, Kakuma R. Optimal duration of exclusive breastfeeding. *Cochrane Database Syst Rev.* 2012;8(8):CD003517. doi:10.1002/14651858 .CD003517.pub2.

27. Aune D, Norat T, Romundstad P, Vatten LJ. Breastfeeding and the maternal risk of type 2 diabetes: a systematic review and dose–response meta-analysis of cohort studies. *Nutr Metab Cardiovasc Dis.* 2014;24(2):107-115.

28. Schwarz EB, Ray RM, Stuebe AM, et al. Duration of lactation and risk factors for maternal cardiovascular disease. *Obstet Gynecol.* 2009;113(5):974-982.

29. Natland ST, Nilsen TI, Midthjell K, Andersen LF, Forsmo S. Lactation and cardiovascular risk factors in mothers in a population-based study: the HUNT study. *Int Breastfeed J.* 2012;7(1):8.

30. Renfrew MJ, Pokhrel S, Quigley M, et al. *Preventing Disease and Saving Resources: The Potential Contribution of Increasing Breastfeeding Rates in the UK.* London, England: UNICEF; 2012.

31. Bartick MC, Schwarz EB, Green BD, et al. Suboptimal breastfeeding in the United States: maternal and pediatric health outcomes and costs. *Matern Child Nutr.* 2017;13(1). doi:10.1111/mcn.12366.

32. Walters D, Horton S, Siregar AY, et al. The cost of not breastfeeding in Southeast Asia. *Health Policy Plan.* 2016;31(8):1107-1116.

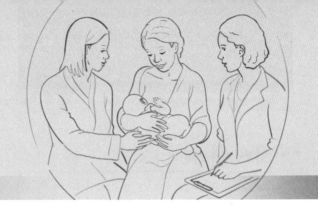

CHAPTER 2

Clinical Decision Making in Lactation Care and Support

Becky Spencer
Amanda Watkins

OBJECTIVES

- Identify the different types of research and how they are used to answer clinical questions in lactation.
- Describe basic statistical and epidemiologic concepts and how they relate to an understanding of quantitative research and apply to clinical practice.
- Describe various qualitative traditions and methodologies and issues of scientific rigor in qualitative studies.
- Apply appropriate frameworks for critiquing qualitative and quantitative research.
- Apply research findings to clinical practice in a knowledgeable and ethical manner.

DEFINITIONS OF COMMONLY USED TERMS

evidence-based practice The integration of the best available clinical evidence, clinician and provider expertise, and patient needs and preferences into a comprehensive plan of care and support.

evidence-informed practice The process by which a clinician uses knowledge and expertise to evaluate all forms of clinical evidence, patient needs and preferences, and the specific clinical presentation and circumstances to create an individualized plan of care and support.

knowledge translation "The synthesis, exchange, and application of knowledge by relevant stakeholders to accelerate the benefits of global and local innovation in strengthening health systems and improving people's health."[1(p165)]

qualitative research Scientific inquiry that seeks to interpret the meaning of life experiences, cultures, and social processes from personal perspectives predominantly through interviews and observations.[2]

quantitative research Scientific inquiry that uses precise, objective measurement and statistical analysis to describe, compare, or determine causation of interventions and effects.

systematic review A process of evaluating multiple studies of one focus area or intervention and synthesizing the results to determine the best or most evidence-supported course of action for patient care.

Any use of the term *mother*, *maternal*, or *breastfeeding* is not meant to exclude transgender or nonbinary parents who may be breastfeeding or providing human milk to their infant.

▶ Overview

Various research studies clearly demonstrate that appropriate support for breastfeeding results in increased exclusivity, incidence, and duration of breastfeeding.[3-10] This includes support from healthcare providers, professional lactation consultants, lay persons, family members, communities, employers, governments, and healthcare policy organizations. Although the research evidence is clear on the benefits of breastfeeding support, the specific interventions and activities that constitute effective breastfeeding support range from highly evidence-based research to anecdotal.

Evidence-based interventions, policies, and activities that support breastfeeding are considered best practices by all international organizations that promote and protect breastfeeding. This includes the International Lactation Consultant Association, the World Health Organization, the Academy of Breastfeeding Medicine, La Leche League International, the United Nations International Children's Emergency Fund, and Wellstart International, among many other health organizations worldwide.

Clinicians are faced with many questions regarding best practices. What constitutes evidence? How do clinicians evaluate the quality of evidence? How much evidence is necessary to define best practices? How do clinicians and support persons translate evidence into practical lactation care and support? What do clinicians do when there is no evidence for a particular practice or problem? This chapter provides guidance in finding and evaluating research about breastfeeding and how to translate evidence into interventions and practices for breastfeeding care and support.

I. Facilitating Implementation of Research into Practice

A. Evidence-based medicine and evidence-based practice (EBP) have become an expectation in health care.
   1. The movement began in the early 1970s when Professor Archie Cochrane called for patient care decisions to be based on objective evidence rather than the individual beliefs of a physician.[11]
   2. In the 1990s, evidence-based medicine was defined by three pillars: clinical evidence from systematic research, clinical expertise, and patient needs[12] (see **FIGURE 2-1**). Clinicians use information from all three pillars to create patient plans of care that should provide better outcomes than relying on clinician expertise and opinion alone.
   3. The concept of EBP is now ubiquitous in health care.
      a. Multiple models of EBP exist within multiple disciplines of health care.
      b. The Johns Hopkins Evidence-based Practice Center (JHU EPC) is one example of an EBP model to guide healthcare clinicians and providers in evaluating and implementing evidence.[13] The three main steps to EBP, as outlined by JHU EPC, include the following:
         i. Identify the clinical practice problem or question.

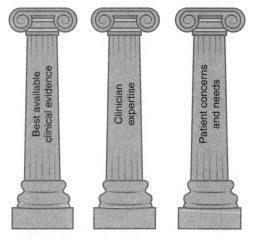

FIGURE 2-1 The three pillars of evidence-based practice.
© Becky Spencer PhD, MSN, RN, IBCLC and Amanda Watkins PhD, RD, LDN, IBCLC.

        ii.   Find and evaluate research evidence.

        iii.   Translate the evidence into clinical practice.

  4. The heaviest emphasis of EBP is on finding and evaluating clinical evidence.

     a. In EBP models, systematic reviews, meta-analyses, and randomized control trials (RCTs) are considered the highest levels of evidence for studies that test interventions.

     b. Cochrane is a British nonprofit organization that is recognized worldwide for conducting systematic reviews of RCTs.[14]

     c. The Joanna Briggs Institute (JBI) is an international nonprofit organization that conducts systematic reviews and research syntheses of all types of research. The JBI acknowledges that RCTs produce the highest level of evidence.[15]

  5. The practical application of EBP has been challenging for many healthcare disciplines across many settings. The reasons include the following:

     a. An overemphasis on RCTs as the highest level and preferred type of research evidence.[16,17]

        i.   RCTs are costly, complicated research designs that can be difficult to conduct in sociobehavioral research.[18]

        ii.   RCTs cannot be conducted when randomization to a nontreatment group is unethical (e.g., randomizing parents to a control group that will not breastfeed).

        iii. Interventions or clinical practices that have not been tested in RCTs are considered not evidence-based, or not as rigorously supported by most EBP models.

     b. By overemphasizing the EBP pillar of evidence, the pillars of clinical expertise and patient needs and concerns have been devalued in the clinical decision-making process.[17,18]

     c. Statistically significant research results from highly controlled studies may not be clinically relevant, particularly when planning and providing care for patients who have complex conditions in complex or nontraditional sociocultural living environments.[18,19]

     d. The practical application of research evidence into practice can be complicated by the local context of the clinician–patient encounter. For example, the institution where the clinician works may have organizational, political, economic, and resource constraints that are barriers to the implementation of evidence-based interventions.[16]

B. Evidence-informed practice (EIP) is an alternate model of clinical decision making.

  1. Because of the barriers and challenges with EBP, EIP models were developed from healthcare and healthcare-related disciplines, including nursing, psychology, social work, and public health because these disciplines have the following characteristics:

     a. Value a broader scope of evidence beyond RCTs.

     b. Believe that clinician experience should be elevated in the model.

     c. Understand that patients present with complex problems and have individual needs and concerns that may not be represented in highly controlled research trials.[17,19]

  2. EIP encourages the consideration of all forms of research evidence when evaluating patient care interventions.[17] One important element of the quality of each study is the selection of the appropriate method of research that fits the problem of interest.

  3. EIP values clinician intuition and clinical reasoning skills that come from day-to-day experience of working in a clinical specialty with patients.[19]

     a. Clinical expertise develops implicitly over time.

     b. Clinical experts can and should provide guidance to less-experienced clinicians.

  4. EIP values the consideration of a patient's previous experiences, values, expectations, preferences, and specific current circumstances when developing a plan of care that is equally weighted with clinician expertise and research evidence.[17]

  5. EIP encourages clinicians to consider community, cultural, and organizational contexts when developing comprehensive plans of care for patients.[16]

C. Knowledge translation (KT) is a process or plan for the actual integration of evidence into the patient's plan of care.

  1. Evidence generated from research can take up to 17 years to be implemented into clinical practice.[20]

  2. KT models were formed to address many of the barriers to evidence implementation in an effort to narrow or close the research-to-practice gap.

3. KT models include consideration of important contextual factors when implementing research, including organizational and community culture and available resources.
4. Knowledge-to-action (KTA) is one example of a KT model.[21]
    a. KTA was designed to facilitate KT by multiple stakeholder audiences, including practitioners, policy makers, patients, and the public.[22]
    b. The authors of KTA identified steps in the knowledge transfer process, including the following:
        i.   Identify the problem.
        ii.   Modify, review, and select knowledge to implement.
        iii. Adapt knowledge to local context.
        iv.   Assess barriers to knowledge use.
        v.   Select, tailor, and implement interventions.
        vi.   Monitor knowledge use.
        vii. Evaluate outcomes.
        viii. Sustain knowledge use.
    c. The KTA process is cyclical.
        i.   One step leads to the next, and the last step (sustain knowledge use) leads back to the first step (identify the problem).
        ii.   Knowledge generation, evaluation, synthesis, implementation, and evaluation comprise one continuous cycle.

II. Evaluating Scientific Evidence: Asking the Clinical Question

A. The first step in evaluating scientific evidence is to identify the clinical problem by formulating a clinical question.
    1. A spirit of inquiry, defined as "an ongoing curiosity about the best evidence to guide clinical decision making,"[23(p58)] is essential to formulating a clinical question.
    2. Lactation consultants must have both a spirit of inquiry and a work culture that supports it to fully implement EBP.[23]
B. Clinical questions can be categorized as either background or foreground.
    1. Background questions are generally broad questions that ask for general information about a clinical issue (e.g., illness, disease, condition, process, or thing).[24]
        a. These types of questions usually ask who, what, where, when, how, and why.
        b. Examples of background questions include the following:
            i.   What are the clinical manifestations of a breast abscess?
            ii. What causes inflammatory mastitis?
    2. Foreground questions tend to be specific and complex. They seek evidence to inform clinical decisions related to a specific patient (or population), intervention, or therapy.[24]
        a. The PICOT model is helpful in formulating the foreground question into a searchable query.
        b. The PICOT model includes the following five components:
            i.   P: Patient, problem, population.
            ii.   I: Intervention, prognostic factor, exposure.
            iii. C: Comparison. (For example, what is the alternative to compare with the intervention? It may be "none" or "placebo.")
            iv.   O: Outcome of interest.
            v.   T: Time involved to demonstrate outcome.
    3. The types of PICOT questions include the following[23,24]:
        a. Intervention or therapy: Determine which treatment leads to the best outcome.
        b. Etiology: Determine the greatest risk factors or causes of a condition.
        c. Diagnosis or diagnostic test: Determine the test that is most accurate and precise in diagnosing a condition.
        d. Prognosis or prediction: Determine the clinical course over time and the likely complications of a condition.
        e. Meaning: Understand the meaning of an experience for an individual, group, or community.

4. Examples of foreground questions using the PICOT model include the following:
    a. Etiology question: Are multiparous, breastfeeding women (P) who do not receive adequate sleep (C), compared to those who do receive adequate sleep (I), at higher risk for infectious mastitis (O) during the first 6 months postpartum (T)?
    b. Intervention question: In full-term, healthy infants having difficulty achieving an effective latch (P), how does the use of a nipple shield (I), compared to no intervention (i.e., no use of a nipple shield) (C), affect 3-month (T) exclusive breastfeeding rates (O)?

III. Steps to Finding Evidence

A. With lactation knowledge constantly growing, it is important to achieve and maintain a high level of information literacy.
   1. Breastfeeding families often search for information on the internet, and lactation consultants must be able to respond to this type of information in a professional way.[25]
   2. Four steps toward reaching a level of information literacy make staying current with the lactation literature manageable[25(p296)]:
      a. Define your questions in a meaningful way.
      b. Understand how to conduct a literature search.
      c. Allocate adequate time to conduct the literature search.
      d. Stay current with available information sources.
B. A literature search helps to identify clinical knowledge gaps and define the problem of interest.
   1. Define the purpose of the search (i.e., identify the clinical issue).
      a. A successful literature search depends on looking for the key issues.[25]
      b. It is important to ask searchable, answerable questions.[24]
         i. The PICOT model helps develop searchable and answerable clinical questions.
         ii. The PICOT question will guide the search and help identify the best evidence quickly and efficiently.
   2. Search for the most relevant evidence to inform clinical practice. The PICOT question helps identify keywords or phrases that may be used in your literature search.
      a. Using synonyms of main search terms can be helpful in finding the most relevant literature.
      b. Use medical subject headings (MeSH).
         i. The National Library of Medicine indexes articles according to this controlled vocabulary thesaurus.
         ii. MeSH terms describe the content of the citation.
         iii. The MeSH browser may be accessed at https://meshb.nlm.nih.gov/search.
      c. Boolean operators are simple words used as conjunctions (*and, or, not,* or *and not*) to combine or exclude keywords in a search; they are useful for narrowing a search and producing more efficient results.
   3. The sources of information include the following:
      a. Primary literature: Original research, work, or experimental results that the authors conducted themselves.
         i. This is the preferred source of literature because it is unfiltered (i.e., it has not been synthesized and evaluated by others).
         ii. Research articles that have been double-blind peer-reviewed (a critique in which the author is anonymous to the reviewer, and the reviewers are anonymous to the author) are considered to have more trustworthy information than research articles that have not been reviewed in this manner.
      b. Secondary literature: Synthesized or evaluated evidence that is derived from the primary literature. Examples of secondary literature are systematic reviews and integrative reviews that summarize multiple primary research studies.
      c. Tertiary literature: An index or database of primary and secondary sources. Examples of tertiary literature include manuals, databases, and guidebooks.

4. Research databases provide access to thousands of information sources. Some examples of common databases used in the health sciences include the following:
   a. CINAHL Plus with Full Text:
      i. The Cumulative Index to Nursing and Allied Health Literature (CINAHL) is an index for more than 4,000 journals from the fields of nursing and allied health.
      ii. More information can be found at https://health.ebsco.com/products/cinahl-plus-with-full-text.
   b. PubMed:
      i. The National Center for Biotechnology Information developed and maintains PubMed as a free resource.
      ii. PubMed comprises nearly 30 million citations for biomedical literature from MEDLINE, life science journals, and online books.
      iii. More information can be found at https://www.ncbi.nlm.nih.gov/pubmed/.
   c. PsycINFO (Ovid):
      i. PsycINFO is an index of professional and academic literature in psychology, medicine, psychiatry, nursing, sociology, education, and other areas.
      ii. More information can be found at http://www.ovid.com/site/catalog/databases/139.jsp.
   d. Cochrane Collaboration:
      i. The Cochrane database contains systematic reviews on various medical topics compiled by worldwide experts.
      ii. These reviews often rely on RCT evidence but also include studies with other research designs if they are deemed to be high quality.
      iii. This is an extremely valuable source for both systematic reviews and meta-analyses.
      iv. For more information visit www.cochrane.org.
5. There are four peer-reviewed lactation specialty journals:
   a. *Journal of Human Lactation.*
   b. *Breastfeeding Medicine.*
   c. *Clinical Lactation.*
   d. *International Breastfeeding Journal.*

IV. Steps to Evaluate Research: Quantitative Methods

A. Quantitative research is a systematic examination or inquiry of a clinical problem or question using numerical measurements. Quantitative research can be classified into one of two main categories: experimental and nonexperimental.[29]
   1. Some examples of numerical measurements include milliliters of breastmilk, weight, the score assigned on an assessment tool (e.g., Bristol Breastfeeding Assessment Tool[26] or latch, audible swallowing, type of nipple, comfort, maternal help [LATCH] tool[27]), and the score assigned on a scale or survey (e.g., Breastfeeding Self-Efficacy Scale[28]).
   2. Numerical data are collected and mathematically or statistically analyzed to describe a problem of interest, compare relationships between two or more variables of interest, or determine cause-and-effect relationships.
   3. In experimental research, researchers test an intervention or treatment by assigning some participants to receive a treatment or intervention (intervention group), while other participants receive either no treatment or intervention, or they receive a comparison or standard treatment (control or comparison group).
      a. The goal of experimental research is to determine if an intervention caused an effect in the intervention group, compared to the control group.
      b. An RCT is a type of experimental research.
         i. In RCTs participants are randomly assigned to the intervention group or the control group. Random assignment into groups protects against selection bias and confounding variables that could affect the outcome of the study; if participants are randomly assigned, the control and intervention groups should have similar characteristics.

      ii.   When intervention and control groups have similar characteristics, researchers have greater confidence that any difference in the outcome between the two groups is truly the result of the intervention.

      iii.   RCTs are considered the gold standard for testing interventions because of random assignment into study groups and the use of control groups as a comparison condition.

      iv.   In a study testing the effects of a breastfeeding education intervention for grandmothers, the participants self-selected, as opposed to being randomly assigned, to receive the education intervention or to receive general breastfeeding education brochures.[30] More grandmothers who had breastfed a child self-selected into the education intervention group, and more grandmothers who had not breastfed self-selected into the control group. The researchers wanted to measure the effect of the education intervention on breastfeeding attitudes of the grandmothers. The researchers were unable to determine if the education intervention or previous breastfeeding experience caused the difference in attitude between the intervention and control groups. Random assignment would have ensured that equal numbers of grandmothers with previous breastfeeding experience were represented in the intervention and control groups, and the effect of the education intervention on attitude could have been more reliably determined.

4.   In nonexperimental research, researchers collect data about a problem of interest without intervening or trying to manipulate a change or effect an outcome. Two main types of non-experimental research are descriptive and correlational.

    a.   The purpose of descriptive research is to observe a phenomenon of interest and collect data that provides a description of the phenomenon.

      i.   Researchers conducted a prospective cohort descriptive study examining the incidence of nipple pain, damage, and vasospasm in 360 primiparous women in Melbourne, Australia.[31] Participants completed surveys at six points over 8 weeks after birth. During the hospital stay after birth, 79 percent of women reported nipple pain. During the 8-week period after birth, 58 percent of women reported nipple damage, and 23 percent reported vasospasm. The researchers concluded that nipple pain is a common problem for new mothers in Australia.

      ii.   This study is an example of descriptive research with the outcome of describing the incidence of nipple pain, damage, and vasospasm in a population of primiparous breastfeeding women in Australia.

    b.   Correlational research designs are used to examine and describe relationships among variables. In correlational studies data are collected on variables, and statistics are used to analyze if the variables are related to each other and to what degree the variables are related.

      i.   Correlational research designs can be used when experimental designs or RCTs are unethical or not feasible.

        •   For example, if researchers want to examine the effect of breastfeeding on the incidence of ear infections in infants before 1 year of age, it would be unethical to conduct an RCT and randomly assign women to breastfeed or formula feed their infants.

        •   Researchers could conduct a retrospective correlational study in which data could be collected from medical charts. The incidence of ear infections documented from breastfed infants could be compared to nonbreastfed infants, and the relationship between breastfeeding and ear infections could be statistically analyzed.

      ii.   Correlational studies cannot be used to determine causation in the same manner as RCTs; however, strong correlations among variables provide evidence for further study.

      iii.   There are many types of correlational research designs. Several common types of correlational designs are as follows.

        •   Descriptive correlational design: Describes the variables and the relationships that occur naturally among them.

        •   Prospective cohort design: Follows a group of similar individuals over time to investigate the effects of exposure or nonexposure on future risk or disease (e.g., interviewing women in their third trimester about their social supports and confidence levels [exposures] and following them through time to see whether or not they breastfed [disease]).

- Retrospective case-control design: Follows a group of individuals backward from disease to exposure; that is, compares people with and without the disease according to their past exposure to the risk factors being studied (e.g., selecting groups of adults with and without diabetes [disease] and taking a history of their past exposure, such as breastfeeding status, eating patterns, and past engagement in physical activity to see if exposure patterns differ between the two groups).
        - Path analysis: Compares two or more causal models derived from the correlation matrix of a regression model.
   B.   Quantitative research uses statistical testing and inferential statistics to analyze data. The following information about statistics is intended to assist with understanding and evaluating data analysis in quantitative research studies.
   1.   Inferential statistics:
        a.   The study results are generalizable beyond the research sample and make statements (inferences) about the population, with realistic uncertainty about the conclusions.
        b.   For example, a study has a target population of interest from which a sample is drawn that should represent this target population.
        c.   The results should then generalize to the target population from which you took the sample (you should be able to use the data to infer information about the target population).
   2.   Dependent and independent variables:
        a.   The dependent variable (also known as the outcome variable) is the measure in which you are interested as the outcome of your research question.
        b.   The independent variables, also known as the explanatory variables, are measures used to help explain variation in the outcome measure.
        c.   In a study to examine factors influencing the duration of breastfeeding, breastfeeding duration is the outcome variable, and explanatory variables could include maternal age, ethnicity, parity, type of prenatal or postpartum counseling, and the infant's gestational age or birth weight.
   3.   Null hypothesis and alternate hypothesis:
        a.   The default setting of statistics is that there is no relationship between the explanatory and outcome variables; this is called the null hypothesis.
        b.   A researcher needs to find enough proof to reject the null hypothesis (i.e., there is no relationship or difference) and accept the alternate hypothesis (i.e., there is a relationship or difference).
   4.   The p value and the meaning of $p < .05$:
        a.   Statistical testing depends on the ideas of probability.
        b.   The p value states the probability of seeing your research result based on chance alone (i.e., assuming that the null hypothesis is correct and your result is simply part of a normal distribution of results when no relationship exists).
        c.   The notation $p < .05$ (read as "p less than point zero five") states that if the null hypothesis were correct, you would see a result like this by chance less than 5 percent of the time (.05 means .05 out of 1, or 5 out of 100, or 5 percent).
        d.   If the p value of a statistical test is less than 5 percent, you reject the null hypothesis and conclude the alternate hypothesis (i.e., there is a relationship that is statistically significant).
        e.   If a p value is less than 5 percent—for example, $p < .05, p < .01$, or $p < .001$ (less than 5 percent, 1 percent, or 0.1 percent, respectively)—conclude that there is a statistically significant finding.
        f.   If a p value is greater than 5 percent—for example, $p < .34, p < .08$, or $p < .20$ (less than 34 percent, 8 percent, or 20 percent, respectively)—it is not statistically significant (NS), so you would conclude the null hypothesis (i.e., there is no statistically significant difference or relationship).
   5.   Type I error:
        a.   A type I error occurs when the study concludes there is a statistically significant difference, even though the null hypothesis was correct at the population level.
        b.   The p value indicates the level of type I error, with $p < .05$, meaning that 5 percent of the time you could see this difference by chance alone (5 percent of the time, or 1 in 20 times, you could wrongly conclude a difference even though the null hypothesis was correct) (see **FIGURE 2-2**).

REALITY at the population level

	Null hypothesis is true (no difference)	*Alternate hypothesis is true (real difference)*
Conclude "no difference" (accept with the null hypothesis)	Correct conclusion	**Type II error**
Conclude difference exists (reject the null hypothesis and accept the alternate hypothesis)	**Type I error**	Correct conclusion

Results based on your research project (label to the left of the rows)

FIGURE 2-2 Type I and type II errors.

6. Type II error:
   a. A type II error occurs when a study concludes that there is no difference (i.e., concluding that the null hypothesis is correct), even though there really is a difference at the population level (see Figure 2-2).
   b. A type II error may occur when the sample size (N) of a study is small.
   c. For studies that conclude the difference is NS, ensure that the power of the study is sufficient to find a difference if it truly exists. One possible hint is that the p value is larger than .05; therefore, it is NS, but the value is very close (such as $p = .07$).
7. Power of a study:
   a. Power refers to how likely you are to find a real difference, if it exists, given the sample size.
   b. Good studies are designed with a power of at least 80 percent.
   c. Statistical calculations prior to the study can ensure adequate power, so there is less chance of committing a type II error.
8. Statistical significance versus clinical significance:
   a. A study can show statistically significant results, but because of very large sample sizes there may be only a small difference.
   b. Practitioners must decide whether the difference is clinically significant; that is, whether it has any clinical impact.
   c. In a research study involving a very large number of women, a new drug (costing twice as much as a standard drug already in use) increases milk production by a small but statistically significant amount of 1 milliliter per 24 hours (1 mL/24 h). This statistic is probably not clinically significant to justify the extra cost. Alternatively, if this drug increased a woman's milk production by a substantial amount (50 mL/24 h, for example), it may be both clinically and statistically significant.

C. Statistical tests:
   1. Statistical tests indicate whether there is enough proof to reject the null hypothesis and conclude the alternate hypothesis. If $p < .05$, reject the null hypothesis and accept the alternate hypothesis (that a statistically significant relationship or difference exists).
   2. The type of statistical test chosen depends on the type of data you are analyzing. **TABLE 2-1** describes several commonly used statistical tests.
   3. Parametric tests assume the data are normally distributed, whereas nonparametric tests do not assume this (e.g., nonparametric tests can be used for skewed distributions of continuous data).
   4. Statistical tests can show associations among variables, but this does not necessarily mean causation (i.e., that one caused the other).

D. Basic epidemiological terms are used to determine risk.
   1. Relative risks:
      a. Relative risks (RR) are statistics used to compare the risk or odds of disease for groups that are exposed or unexposed to something. **TABLE 2-2** shows examples of RR.
      b. RR compares the probability of getting the disease (or experiencing the condition) in the exposed group versus in the unexposed group.

TABLE 2-1 Common Statistical Tests with Examples

Statistical Test	Type of Data	Test Statistic	Example	What You Would Conclude
T-test (Student's t-test)	Compares the means of two different groups. Outcome variable: continuous data. Explanatory variable: categorical data (two groups).	t	Is there a difference in the mean birth weight of male and female full-term newborns? Males: 3,692 g (95% CI 3,648–3,726). Females: 3,557 g (95% CI 3,512–3,502). $t = 4.18$, 809 df, two-tailed, $p < .001$.	Yes because $p < .05$ (p is much less, at .001). Male newborns have a higher average birth weight, compared to females.
Paired t-test	Compares two different measures of the same person. Outcome variable: continuous data. Explanatory variable: categorical data (one group measured twice).	t	Is the hospital discharge weight of a full-term newborn less than the birth weight? Mean birth weight 3629 g. Mean discharge weight 3443 g. Mean difference: –186 g (95% CI –179 to –194 g), paired t-test $t = -48.5$, df 771, one-tailed, $p < .00001$	Yes because $p < .05$. There is a weight loss of full-term newborns that is probably somewhere between 179 and 194 g. This is called a "one-tailed" test because it has a directional hypothesis ("less") rather than just a difference (is there any difference). A one-tailed test has more power.
Analysis of variance (ANOVA)	Compares the means of more than two groups (are the group means different or similar?). Outcome variable: continuous data. Explanatory variable: categorical data (several groups). Note: If you find $p < .5$, a subsequent statistical test (such as a Duncan's multiple range test or Tukey's multiple comparison test) must be done to find out which of the groups differ.	f	Is there a difference in birth weight for those full-term newborns who are exclusively breastfed, exclusively formula fed, or partially breastfed while in hospital? Means of groups: Formula-fed 3,588 g; Partial 3,648 g; Exclusively breastfed 3,618 g. ANOVA test: $f = 0.71$, df 2,810; $p = 0.49$, NS)	No because $p > .05$ (the p value is greater than .05 or 5%). $P = 0.49$. The notation "NS" is often used for "not statistically significant." Thus, we would stay with the null hypothesis, i.e., conclude that there is no evidence to show that differences in birth weight of full-term newborns are predictors of type of feeding in hospital.

Nonparametric equivalents of the preceding tests are used when the outcome measure is ordinal data or when there is a breech in the assumptions of continuous data (such as skewed data or other nonnormally distributed continuous data). Nonparametric tests compare medians rather than means.

Instead of the parametric t-test, use the nonparametric Mann–Whitney U test.

Instead of the paired t-test, use the Wilcoxon test.

Instead of ANOVA, use the Kruskal–Wallis test.

Statistical Test	Type of Data	Test Statistic	Example	What You Would Conclude
Chi-square test	Compares proportions (are the proportions in two or more groups different?). Explanatory and outcome variables are categorical data. Usually data are displayed in the form of a table (called a contingency table).	X^2	Are primiparous women more likely to experience a cesarean birth than multiparous women? $n = 807$ (287 primiparous, 520 multiparous). 60 primiparous and 55 multiparous women had cesarean births. $X^2 = 16.1$, df 1, $p < .0001$.	Yes because $p < 0.5$. Primiparous women were twice as likely as multiparous women (20.9% versus 10.6%) to experience cesarean birth.

Alternatives to chi-square test:
- Fisher's exact test: For small counts.
- McNemar's test: Paired data (i.e., two categorical measures of the same person).

Statistical Test	Type of Data	Test Statistic	Example	What You Would Conclude
Correlation (Pearson correlation)	Looks at the relationship between two continuous variables (you measure two different things about the same person over many people) and asks if it is a linear relationship. Correlation coefficients have values between −1 (strong negative relationship, with one number getting larger as the other gets smaller) and +1 (strong positive relationship, with one number getting larger as the other gets larger), with 0 meaning no relationship (the null hypothesis). The amount of variation explained by this relationship is equal to the square of the correlation coefficient, r.	r	Is there a correlation between healthy, full-term newborn birth weight and the percentage of weight loss in the hospital? $r = 0.128$, df 773; $r < 0.0004$.	Yes because the correlation is positive (i.e., the higher the birth weight, the higher the weight loss). However, this relationship does not explain much of the variation ($r^2 = 0.016$, or 1.6% of the total variation).

The nonparametric equivalent of the Pearson correlation is the Spearman rank-order correlation coefficient (Spearman's correlation), which is used for continuous data that is nonnormal, or ordinal data.

(continues)

TABLE 2-1 Common Statistical Tests with Examples   *(continued)*

Statistical Test	Type of Data	Test Statistic	Example	What You Would Conclude
Multiple regression	Looks at the unique contribution of several explanatory variables on a continuous outcome measure. Explanatory variables can be continuous or categorical. Multiple regressions produce an equation of how each explanatory variable uniquely contributes to the outcome variable.	F, t	What are the predictors of birth weight of full-term newborns? Birth weight (grams) = −2,065 + 142 (gestational age in weeks) − 114 (female) + 142 (multiparous) + 129 (cesarean birth). Model: $f = 38.5$; df 4,798; $p < .0001$, $r^2 = 0.16$. Each explanatory variable was significant ($p < .05$).	This model explains 16% of the variation in birth weight ($r^2 = 0.16$) and shows the unique contribution of each explanatory variable. You can calculate the mean birth weight of a newborn from the equation. Example: For a male baby (male coded as 1, female as coded as 0 in the equation) born at 40 weeks to a multiparous (coded as 1) mother vaginally (coded as 0), the predicted mean birth weight = −2,065 + 142 (40) − 114 (0) + 142 (1) + 129 (0) = 3,757 g.
Logistic regression	Looks at the unique contribution of several explanatory variables on a dichotomous categorical outcome variable (e.g., yes–no, alive–dead, breastfed–not). Explanatory variables can be continuous or categorical. Odds ratios (OR) show the unique contribution of each explanatory variable on the outcome.	X^2	What factors are associated with a breastfed baby being exclusively breastfed (this is a yes–no measure) while in the hospital? Explanatory variables include parity, sex of newborn, high birth weight (> 4,000 g) or not, type of delivery (cesarean or not), and use of a spinal epidural or not during delivery. $n = 696$, model $p < .001$, $r^2 = 0.05$; parity ($p = .71$, NS); sex ($p = .20$, NS); type of delivery ($p < .0005$, OR = 0.42); epidural ($p < .02$, OR = 0.63); normal birth weight ($p < .02$, OR = 1.6).	Parity and the sex of the newborn are not statistically significant factors associated with exclusive breastfeeding. Statistically significant factors ($p < .05$) include cesarean delivery and having an epidural; they both reduce the chance of being exclusively breastfed (the OR is less than 1); having a normal birth weight significantly increases the chance of being exclusively breastfed.

Note: CI is confidence interval; df is degrees of freedom.

c. RR is an intuitive measure. An RR of 2 means the exposed group has twice the risk of the unexposed group.

d. In Table 2-2, the RR of being supplemented if the baby has a high birth weight is calculated by taking the probability of getting the disease (e.g., being supplemented) in the exposed (e.g., high birth weight) versus in the unexposed (e.g., normal weight) groups. For high birth weight, 67 of 142 babies were supplemented, for a probability of .472. For normal weight, 204 of 558 babies were supplemented, for a probability of .366. In other words, 47.2 percent of high birth weight and 36.6 percent of normal birth weight babies were supplemented. So, RR = (67 ÷ 142 divided by 204 ÷ 558) = (0.472 ÷ 0.366) = 1.29. This means the risk of supplementation for high birth weight babies was 1.29 times the risk for normal birth weight babies; you could also say that the risk of supplementation was 29 percent higher for high birth weight compared to normal birth weight babies.

TABLE 2-2 Is the Risk of Being Supplemented Associated with a Full-Term Breastfed Newborn's[a] Birth Weight?			
	Supplemented (diseased)	**Exclusively breastfed (not diseased)**	**Total**
High birth weight (exposed)	67 (47.2%)	75	142
Normal birth weight (not exposed)	204 (36.6%)	354	558
			700

Note: Chi-square = 5.38, 1 df, *p* < .25 (because the *p* value is less than .05, it means there is a statistically significant association between high birth weight and supplementation).
[a]The full-term breastfed newborns in hospital were exclusively breastfed or supplemented.

2. Odds ratio:
    a. OR compares the odds of getting a disease in the exposed group versus in the unexposed group.
    b. An OR is a calculation of the number of times an event happens divided by the number of times it did not happen.
    c. In Table 2-2, the odds of being supplemented for high birth weight is $67 \div 75$, or 0.893; the odds of being supplemented for normal birth weight babies is $204 \div 354$, or 0.576. The OR is the odds of getting the disease for the exposed group, compared to the unexposed group, or $0.893 \div 0.576 = 1.55$.
    d. OR is a much more complex idea and does not translate as intuitively as RR. Sometimes people use the word *likelihood* to describe OR. For example, the likelihood of supplementation is 1.55 times greater for the high birth weight babies, compared to normal birth weight babies. That does not translate as intuitively as RR (see the previous example).
3. For both RR and OR, 1 means there is the same risk, greater than 1 (> 1) means a greater risk, and less than 1 (< 1) means a smaller risk.
    a. RR and OR are often shown with 95 percent CI. If the 95 percent CI includes 1, it is NS, and we conclude that the exposure has no significant effect on the risk of disease.
    b. For example, RR = 1.4 (95 percent CI 1.3–1.5). From this example, conclude that there is a statistically significantly higher risk of disease in the exposed group because the RR is greater than 1, and the 95 percent CI does not include 1. If RR is 1.2 (95 percent CI 0.9–1.5, NS), it is NS because the 95 percent CI includes 1, so you can conclude that there is no statistically significant increase in the risk of disease. When RR = 0.5 (95 percent CI 0.3–0.7), conclude that there is a statistically significantly lower risk of disease in the exposed group because the RR is less than 1 and the 95 percent CI does not include 1.
    c. RR and OR are very close numerically only if the prevalence of disease is small; that is, less than 10 percent.[32]
    d. Certain types of statistical analyses (such as logistic regression) and study designs (such as case-control studies) produce OR values rather than RR. Be very careful of the interpretation of OR when the outcome is not a rare event (i.e., more than 10 percent).
4. Various other measures are used in epidemiologic studies, such as risk difference, attributable risk (exposed), and population-attributable risk (see **TABLE 2-3**).
    a. The number needed to treat (NNT) is usually used to describe a positive intervention, such as a pharmaceutical or program intervention.
    b. NNT is calculated by $1 \div RD$ (see Table 2-3).
    c. NNT answers the question, "How many people would you need to treat to see the effect?"
    d. Example: In a longitudinal study on infant feeding and its relationship to Type 2 diabetes, it was found that 10 percent of adults who had been exclusively breastfed and 17 percent of adults who had been exclusively formula fed had adult Type 2 diabetes. The RD is $17\% - 10\% = 7\%$ (or 0.07 as a fraction of 1 rather than a percentage). NNT = $(1 \div 0.07) = 14$, meaning that 14 babies must be exclusively breastfed to prevent one case of adult Type 2 diabetes.

TABLE 2-3 Epidemiologic Concepts, Meanings, and Examples

Measure	Other Names	What This Means	Example	Interpreting the Example
Relative risk (RR)	Risk ratio Rate ratio	Comparing two groups. What risk for disease has the exposed group compared to the unexposed group?	Of breastfed full-term newborns ($n = 700$), 47.2% of high birth weight babies were supplemented, but only 36.6% of other newborns were supplemented. RR = 1.29 (OR = 1.55)	A high birth weight newborn was 1.29 times (29%) more likely to be supplemented, compared to a normal birth weight newborn. Note that the OR similarly shows that there is a greater chance, or odds of (OR = 1.55), but it is not as intuitive as RR. OR and RR are very close only if the outcome is rare.
Risk difference (RD)	Rate difference Absolute risk reduction	What is the excess risk of disease for individuals who have the exposure compared to those who do not?	Of breastfed full-term newborns ($n = 700$), 47.2% of high birth weight babies were supplemented, but only 36.6% of other newborns were supplemented. RD = 0.472 − 0.366 = 0.106 (or 10.6% difference)	10.6% more babies were supplemented in the high birth weight group. This gives an idea of how large the true difference is. Note: You can have a large RR and a very small RD. For example, if only 1% of high birth weight babies and 0.78% of the others were supplemented, the RR would still be 1.29, but the RD is a very small amount (i.e., 1% − 0.78% = 0.22%).
Attributable risk (exposed)	Attributable fraction exposed, (or proportion exposed, or risk percent exposed)	Among those "exposed" to the risk factor, what proportion of "disease" resulted because of being exposed?	Attributable risk (exposed) = (RR − 1) ÷ RR = (1.29-1) ÷ 1.29 = 0.225 or 22.5%	Among those having the risk factor of high birth weight, .225 or 22.5% of them were supplemented because of this risk factor. In other words, some of these babies would have been supplemented just because supplementation also occurred in the nonrisk (nonhigh birth weight) babies. Thus, 22.5% of the high birth weight babies were supplemented due to being high birth weight.
Population attributable risk	Etiologic fraction, population attributable fraction, population attributable proportion, population attributable risk percent	Among the WHOLE population, what proportion of the disease cases resulted because of being exposed?	Population attributable risk = P (RR − 1) ÷ [P (RR − 1) + 1] = .203 (1.29 - 1) ÷ [.203 (1.29 − 1) + 1] = .056 or 5.6% To calculate population attributable risk, you need to know the overall proportion of high birth weight (P) in your population. In Table 2-2, P, which is 142 of the 700 babies, or 20.3%.	Of all the supplemented newborns (both high birth weight and normal birth weight), 5.6% of them were supplemented because they were "exposed" (because they were of high birth weight).

V. Steps to Evaluate Research: Qualitative Methods

A. Qualitative research is a method of inquiry used by a variety of disciplines, including sociology, anthropology, and various health sciences. Each of these disciplines has a specific area of interest or domain.

B. Qualitative researchers seek to develop a comprehensive understanding of human behavior and the ways in which individuals create meaning in their lives.

   1. Qualitative methodologies provide a means of exploring the depth, richness, and complexity of human phenomena.

   2. The researcher becomes the instrument used to collect data through interviews and observations from key informants, known as participants or respondents. These key informants have special knowledge about the phenomena under study and often help the researcher locate information or individuals (informants) to interview.

C. The following discusses philosophical assumptions of qualitative research.

   1. Multiple constructed realities:

      a. Reality is based on perception and is different for each person.

      b. The qualitative researcher must consider multiple perspectives to fully understand a phenomenon.

   2. Subject–object interaction:

      a. The researcher and participant interact to influence each other.

      b. The participant has personal knowledge about the phenomenon of interest. This knowledge may be unwritten and unspoken and includes personal beliefs and attitudes (called tacit knowledge).

   3. Simultaneous mutual shaping:

      a. One goal in *quantitative* research is to determine cause and effect among variables. In *qualitative* research there is no attempt to determine causality; rather the goal is to form plausible explanations from detailed observations.

      b. The researcher, when using qualitative methods, does not try to show that one thing causes another; the researcher is instead interested in understanding a phenomenon.

   4. Value-bound inquiry:

      a. The values, perspectives, and assumptions of the qualitative researcher influence the data collection and data analysis in qualitative research.

      b. Bracketing is a technique used by qualitative researchers to identify and acknowledge personal bias and values. Bracketing assists qualitative researchers to position their values and biases both alongside and in conjunction with the inquiry.

D. Qualitative research traditions include the following.

   1. Each type of qualitative method has a philosophy that guides the research questions asked, the observations made, and the data interpretation. Domain refers to the focus of study, such as delineating health or understanding illness and the medium, so to speak, where that is examined—through the culture or one's lived experience. Research tradition refers to the methodology and historical underpinnings of the research.

   2. Examples by type of research are provided as follows, recognizing that many qualitative methods come from disciplines that are often within the social, behavioral, and health sciences.

      a. Anthropology:

         i.   Domain: Culture.

         ii. Research tradition: Ethnography, ethnoscience.

         iii. Example: "Families, Markets, and Medicalization: The Role of Paid Support for Childbirth and Breastfeeding."[33] An ethnographic approach was used to explore why certain aspects of maternity support are provided by the commercial market.

      b. Philosophy:

         i.   Domain: Lived experience.

         ii. Research tradition: Phenomenology, hermeneutics.

         iii. Example: "'I Had One Job and That Was to Make Milk': Mothers' Experiences Expressing Milk for Their Very-Low-Birth-Weight Infants."[34] The purpose of this study was to describe mothers' experiences in expressing milk for their very low birth weight infants in a neonatal intensive care unit (NICU).

      c.   Sociology:
         i.   Domain: Social settings.
         ii.   Research tradition: Grounded theory methods.
         iii.   Example: "Remote Lactation Consultation: A Qualitative Study of Maternal Response to Experience and Recommendations."[35] Using a grounded theory approach, the aim of this study was to describe the maternal experience of lactation consultation by using videoconferencing technology, compared to standard care.

      d.   Sociolinguistics:
         i.   Domain: Human communication.
         ii.   Research tradition: Narrative analysis, discourse analysis.
         iii.   Example: "The Experience of Nursing Women with Breastfeeding Support: A Qualitative Inquiry."[36] In this study, the authors explore breastfeeding mothers' experiences with help, advice, and support for breastfeeding.

      e.   Historical research:
         i.   Domain: Past events, behavior.
         ii.   Research tradition: Historical.
         iii.   Example: "Breastfeeding in America: A History of Influencing Factors."[37] This study is a review and analysis of historical influencing factors related to infant feeding practices in America.

E.   The following describes characteristics of qualitative research:
   1.   Setting: Natural settings are appropriate for conducting the investigation.
   2.   Researcher is the instrument: The researcher gathers data through interviews and observations rather than using survey tools, measurement instruments, or observation checklists (pen and paper measures).
   3.   Shared meaning: Qualitative researchers use tacit knowledge to understand the world of the informants.
   4.   Data collection: Often (but not exclusively) uses qualitative data and methods.
      a.   Deals with narrative (words).
      b.   Interpretative–phenomenological research is an approach that aims to offer insights into how a given individual, in a specific context, makes sense of an identified phenomenon.
   5.   Purposive sampling: Participants are selected for the study based on their knowledge about the phenomena of interest.
   6.   Inductive data analysis: Putting pieces together to make a whole.
   7.   Emergent research design: The research design emerges during the study.
   8.   Tentative application: Generalizability is not a goal of qualitative research, so qualitative researchers do not make broad applications of the study findings.
   9.   Focus-determined boundaries: The qualitative researcher sets boundaries to the inquiry based on the research question, perceptions of the participants, setting, and values.

F.   The following methods are the most commonly used interpretative methodologies, differentiated by methodologies of qualitative research:
   1.   Method is selected according to the nature of the problem and what is known about the phenomenon being studied. Basic qualitative description:
      a.   Generic form of qualitative research.
      b.   Offers a topical, thematic summary or survey of events.
      c.   Least interpreted of qualitative descriptions.
      d.   Example: "Informal Human Milk Sharing: A Qualitative Exploration of the Attitudes and Experiences of Mothers."[38] The purpose of this study was to explore the experiences of and attitudes toward human milk sharing among mothers with experience of human milk feeding and breast pump use.
   2.   Phenomenology:
      a.   Focus is on the discovery of meaning of people's lived experience.
      b.   Goal is to describe fully the lived experience and the perceptions to which it gives rise.
      c.   Source of data is in-depth conversations.
      d.   Steps in the process include bracketing, intuiting, analyzing, and describing.
         i.   Bracketing: Researcher is aware of preconceived thoughts and opinions about the phenomena of interest.

        ii.   Intuiting: Researcher is open to the meaning of the phenomena from the participants' perspectives.

        iii.   Analyzing: Researcher identifies the structure of the phenomena under study.

        iv.   Describing: Researcher represents a perspective or interpretation of the phenomena.

   e.   Example: "Attitudes and Expectations in the Intergenerational Transmission of Breastfeeding: A Phenomenological Study."[39] The purpose of this study was to explore, based on their experiences with breastfeeding, the objectives and positioning of women today with respect to their role as future grandmothers.

3.   Ethnography:

   a.   Goal is to describe and interpret cultural behavior.

   b.   Culture is inferred from the group's words, actions, and artifacts.

   c.   Assumption is that cultures guide the way people structure their experience.

   d.   Seeks an emic (insider) perspective of the culture.

   e.   Sources of data include participant observations, in-depth interviews with key informants, records, charts, physical evidence, photographs, and video recordings.

   f.   Steps in the process include description, analysis, and interpretation.

   g.   Example: "Providing Mother's Own Milk in the Context of the NICU: A Paradoxical Experience."[40] The aim of this study was to understand the experience of mothers of hospitalized very preterm infants related to their daily pumping routine during a NICU stay.

4.   Grounded theory:

   a.   Best identifies and analyzes complex processes.

   b.   Generates theory from data. Theory is grounded in and connected to the data.

   c.   Goal is to generate comprehensive explanations of phenomena that are grounded in reality.

   d.   Data collection, data analysis, and sampling occur simultaneously.

        i.   Sources of data: In-depth interviews (occasionally observations).

        ii.   Steps: Constant comparison, categories, core category, and basic social process.

   e.   Example: "Expanding the Supply of Pasteurized Donor Milk: Understanding Why Peer-to-Peer Milk Sharers in the United States Do Not Donate to Milk Banks."[41] The purpose of this grounded theory study was to explore how lactating women with a surplus of milk come to the decision to share their milk with a peer rather than donate to a milk bank.

G.   The following describes the phases in qualitative design:

1.   Qualitative methodologies use a flexible rather than a linear approach.

   a.   Identify the problem or phenomenon of interest:

        i.   The phenomenon of interest may be broad or focused.

        ii.   Qualitative studies do not use hypotheses.

   b.   Conduct a literature review.

   c.   Address ethical issues. This is more of a concern than in quantitative methodologies because of the close relationship between the researcher and the participants.

   d.   Gaining entry (access to setting or participants the researcher is interested in).

   e.   Focused exploration:

        i.   Data collection and data analysis occur simultaneously in an iterative fashion.

        ii.   Data analysis after data saturation, which occurs during data collection when no new information is obtained during interviews or participant observation (the point of saturation). At this point, there is redundancy in the information.

   f.   Confirmation and closure occur when the researchers have identified themes that are representative of the problem or phenomena of interest.

        i.   Exiting the setting.

        ii.   Ensuring trustworthiness; this is similar to reliability and validity in quantitative research. When a study is trustworthy, the reader is reassured that the findings accurately reflect the viewpoints and experiences of the participants.

   g.   Dissemination:

        i.   Dissemination of research findings is critical as a means for sharing new knowledge.

        ii.   This may occur through a variety of venues, such as oral or poster presentations at relevant conferences or through publication in professional journals or books.

      iii.   Findings may be shared with the community and other populations who may be interested in the findings.

2.   Sampling in qualitative research is how researchers identify participants for their studies.

   a.   Type of sample:

      i.   Purposive: Seek participants who have knowledge about the phenomena and can share that information.

      ii.   Convenience: May be referred to as a volunteer sample and can be used when the researcher needs potential participants to come forward. However, this is not the preferred sampling method for qualitative research because a convenience sample may not provide the researcher with the rich data needed to understand the phenomenon.

      iii.   Maximum variation sampling: Involves intentionally selecting participants who have a wide variation of dimensions specific to the phenomenon of interest.

      iv.   Snowball sampling: Asking participants to refer other participants who have knowledge of the phenomenon being investigated.

      v.   Theoretical: Select participants based on ongoing analysis to ensure adequacy and accuracy of the emerging categories, themes, or theory.

   b.   Interview or observe people who have experience. This should be done at the informant's convenience because of time commitments.

   c.   Data and theoretical saturation are used to decide when to stop sampling.

3.   Types of data in qualitative research:

   a.   Interviews:

      i.   Researchers use semistructured, open-ended questions.

      ii.   One or two topics are examined in detail.

      iii.   Interviewers follow the participant's lead in formulating further questions; the researcher avoids asking leading questions.

      iv.   Interviewers are sensitive to language.

      v.   Interviewers check to make sure they have an accurate reflection of the participant's response to questions.

      vi.   As interviews progress, researchers may add additional questions.

   b.   Types of questions asked in interviews:

      i.   Behaviors or experiences of participants.

      ii.   Opinions or beliefs of participants.

      iii.   Feelings of participants.

      iv.   Knowledge of participants.

      v.   Sensory experiences of participants.

      vi.   Background or demographics of participants.

   c.   Background or demographics:

      i.   A means of describing, through observations, the ways in which people construct their reality.

      ii.   A means of describing, through observations, the activities and interactions of a setting.

      iii.   Data are recorded as field notes.

4.   Steps in participant observation:

   a.   Gaining entry (permission to conduct the study).

   b.   Researcher introduction and explanation of study purpose.

   c.   Develop trust and a cooperative relationship with participants by being unobtrusive, honest, and unassuming.

   d.   Observe physical space, participants, activities, objects, events, time sequencing, and feelings.

5.   Document review; this may include a review of written records, such as diaries, letters, newspapers, meeting minutes, and legal documents.

6.   Artifacts, which may include an analysis of items made or used by the culture, such as feeding vessels or feeding utensils.

7.   Data analysis:

   a.   Data analysis begins when the researcher begins to collect data.

   b.   Data analysis is an iterative process (a repeated cycle of operations).

      i.   Data analysis guides further data collection, sampling, and analysis.

      ii.   Data analysis begins with the process of comparison and the development of category schemes. Data can then be coded according to correspondence with the various categories.

    c.   The product is a rich, thick description (a very thorough description of the setting, interactions, and features of the phenomena).

    d.   Computer software programs (HyperRESEARCH, ATLAS.ti, NVivo, and others) are available for organizing and managing qualitative data.

8.   Trustworthiness:

    a.   The researcher must persuade readers that the findings accurately reflect the experiences and viewpoints of the participants.

    b.   Rigor or trustworthiness in qualitative research ensures that data collection and analysis are truthful.

    c.   Trustworthiness in qualitative research is similar to reliability and validity in quantitative research.

9.   Credibility:

    a.   Techniques are employed that make it more likely that credible findings and interpretations will be produced.

    b.   Prolonged engagement in the setting should be long enough to learn the culture, develop trust, and minimize misinformation.

    c.   Persistent observation is used to identify characteristics and elements in the situation that are most relevant to the problem.

    d.   Triangulation involves the use of corroborating evidence to draw conclusions about the phenomena. Triangulation allows for a multidimensional perspective of the phenomena of interest and can enhance the credibility of a study. Triangulation refers to the use of multiple and different data sources, data collection methods, investigators, and theories.

10.   Peer debriefing occurs when researchers expose themselves to a disinterested peer to keep the inquirer honest, test the working hypotheses, and test the next step in the methodological design.

    a.   Negative case analysis is when the researcher looks for disconfirming data (i.e., data that challenge the researcher's understanding of the phenomena) in both past and future observations or interviews. Analyzing disconfirming data provides new understanding about the emerging conceptualization.

    b.   Member checks are when data and beginning interpretations are confirmed by study participants.

11.   Dependability:

    a.   The stability of qualitative data over time and conditions is evaluated.

    b.   An inquiry audit, a scrutiny of the data collection, and analysis by an external reviewer ensure dependability.

12.   Confirmability:

    a.   Confirmability refers to the objectivity of the data. Inquiry audits are used to ensure confirmability.

    b.   The researcher demonstrates confirmability with a well-developed audit trail, including materials that are consistently and conscientiously recorded and organized throughout the research. Demonstrating the data collection and analysis strategies in a recorded fashion allows an independent auditor to use the same data and come to similar conclusions.

13.   Transferability:

    a.   Transferability refers to the extent to which the researcher has provided a thorough description of the phenomenon (thick description).

    b.   The researcher is responsible for providing a thick description that makes transferability judgments possible on the part of the potential appliers.

14.   Ethical concerns:

    a.   The same ethical principles for quantitative methods apply to qualitative methods. Given the nature of qualitative methods, the implementation of these principles throughout the research process may be different.

    b.   Ethical concerns include issues of harm, consent, deception, privacy, and confidentiality of data.

    c.   Prior to data collection, a designated board (e.g., institutional review board, behavioral research ethics boards, or human subjects review committee) must provide an ethics review and grant approval, and permission must be obtained from the data collection site.

    d.   Consent is ongoing in qualitative studies.

e. Anonymity must be preserved.
   i. Anonymity requires more than changing persons' names; as many identifiers as possible must be removed.
   ii. Report demographic characteristics as group data.
   iii. Change the names of institutions, cities, suburbs, and so forth.
f. Participants have the following rights:
   i. To be fully informed of the study's purpose.
   ii. To be aware of the time required and amount of involvement for participation.
   iii. To confidentiality and anonymity.
   iv. To ask questions of the investigator.
   v. To refuse to participate without negative ramifications.
   vi. To refuse to answer any questions.
   vii. To withdraw from the study at any time.
   viii. To know what to expect during the research process.
   ix. To know what information is being obtained about them.
   x. To know who will have access to the information.
   xi. To know how the information will be used.
   xii. To receive a copy of the findings, if desired.

VI. Critique of Qualitative and Quantitative Research

A. Hierarchy of evidence refers to a ranking of different types of research methods with respect to identifying the most valid and reliable evidence to guide practice.
   1. The first step in critiquing research is to determine the type and level of each study being evaluated.
   2. EBP relies heavily on classifying different types of research into levels of evidence. The results of studies that are considered higher-level evidence are graded above study results that are classified as lower-level evidence.
   3. There are many models of levels of evidence. The JHU EPC divides levels of evidence into three main categories (see **FIGURE 2-3**):[13]
      a. Level 1: Experimental research, RCTs, systematic reviews, meta-analyses, mixed methods studies with RCTs.

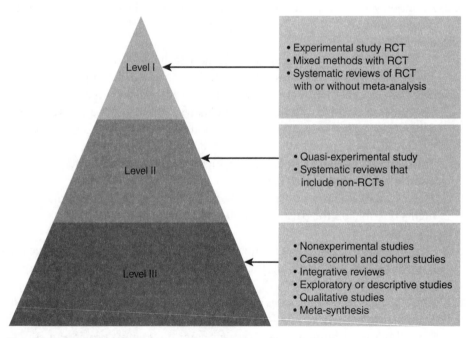

FIGURE 2-3 Hierarchy of types of evidence.

Abbreviation: RCT, randomized control trial.

Data from Dearholt S, Dang D. *Johns Hopkins Nursing Evidence-Based Practice: Models and Guidelines.* 3rd ed. Indianapolis, IN: Sigma Theta Tau; 2017.[13] © Becky Spencer PhD, MSN, RN, IBCLC and Amanda Watkins PhD, RD, LDN, IBCLC.

   b. Level 2: Quasi-experimental studies, systematic reviews of quasi-experimental studies, mixed methods studies with quasi-experimental studies.
   c. Level 3: Nonexperimental studies, case control and cohort studies, integrative reviews, exploratory or descriptive studies, qualitative studies, and metasyntheses of qualitative studies.
4. Alternate approaches to the hierarchy of evidence in sociobehavioral breastfeeding research include the following:
   a. Given that RCTs are not always practical or possible when studying clinical interventions, particularly sociobehavioral interventions, all types of evidence should be used when evaluating interventions.[42-44]
      i. For example, a recent Cochrane Review evaluated the impact of antenatal breastfeeding education on increasing breastfeeding duration.[45] Only RCTs were included in the analysis of evidence. The authors concluded that no conclusive evidence exists to support antenatal breastfeeding education because no statistically significant difference was found between control groups (no antenatal breastfeeding education or routine care) and experimental groups (antenatal breastfeeding education) with regard to breastfeeding initiation, exclusivity, or duration. The authors called for better-quality RCTs to evaluate the effectiveness and adverse effects of antenatal breastfeeding education.
      ii. Most clinicians agree that antenatal breastfeeding education is extremely beneficial to new parents. Other research methods may be more appropriate to evaluate the benefits and effectiveness of antenatal breastfeeding education (e.g., qualitative or case control methods).
   b. The Family Resource Information, Education, and Network Development Service (FRIENDS) created a unique interpretation of EBP, EIP, and KT used to evaluate interventions and program effectiveness for child abuse prevention.[46]
      i. In the FRIENDS model, evidence-based interventions and programs are considered well supported or supported based on the amount, levels, and quality of research evidence.
      ii. In the FRIENDS model, evidence-informed interventions and programs are considered to be promising or emerging if the practices are new or innovative, but they are less supported in research literature.
      iii. Interventions and programs fall on a continuum of EIP to EBP.
      iv. To fall within the EIP–EBP continuum, an intervention or program must be clearly defined; be generally accepted by clinicians and patients; have been shown to do no harm or have low risk of harm; have established research results or be in the process of study or evaluation.
      v. **FIGURE 2-4** is an adaptation of the FRIENDS EIP–EBP continuum to assist with clinical decision making in lactation care and support.

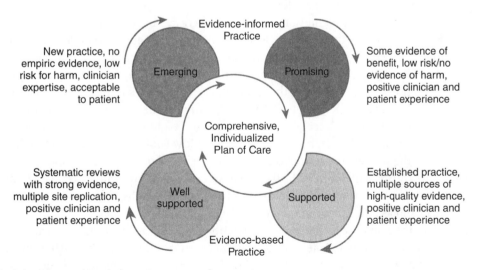

FIGURE 2-4 Clinical decision making in lactation care and support.

Data from FRIENDS National Resource Center. Evidence-based practice in CBCAP. FRIENDS website. https://www.friendsnrc.org/evidence-based-practice-in-cbcap. Published 2017. Accessed October 10, 2017.[46] © Becky Spencer PhD, MSN, RN, IBCLC and Amanda Watkins PhD, RD, LDN, IBCLC.

        vi.   Lactation support interventions can be categorized as emerging, promising, supported, or well supported based on the amount, quality, and levels of support.

       vii.   Priorities for interventions or practices that need more research can be justified with emerging or promising categorization.

      viii.   The continuum allows for practices to move from one category to the next with increased supportive evidence and positive clinician and patient experience.

       ix.   All levels of evidence can be considered when evaluating interventions or practices.

       x.   Clinician expertise and patient experience are equally valued when planning comprehensive, individualized care.

B.   Quantitative research critiques require a systematic approach and can be done using the following guidelines:

   1.   Critical appraisal of research is an essential tool in selecting the current best practice as a lactation consultant.

   2.   A systematic and objective method of evaluating the strengths and limitations of the research being reviewed should be employed.

   3.   Guidelines for critiquing a quantitative research study include four components that influence the believability (i.e., credibility and integrity) of the research.

      a.   Is the article well written and organized in a logical manner?

      b.   Do the researcher's academic and professional qualifications demonstrate expertise in the particular field?

      c.   Does the title clearly and accurately convey what the research is about?

      d.   Does the abstract succinctly describe the purpose of the paper, why the research was undertaken, and the sample, findings, conclusions, and recommendations?

   4.   Twelve components influence the robustness of the research.[47]

      a.   Does the researcher adequately state the purpose of the study (i.e., research problem)?

      b.   Does the article follow the steps of the research process in a logical manner? It should flow from the introduction, to the purpose, literature review, theoretical framework, research question, methodology, data analysis, findings, and conclusion.

      c.   Is the literature review logically organized, relevant, and current? Are primary sources used?

      d.   Has an appropriate conceptual or theoretical framework been identified and adequately described and integrated into the study?

      e.   Have research aims and objectives, a research question, and a hypothesis been identified? Are they clearly stated and congruent with the information presented in the literature review?

      f.   Have the number of participants, their characteristics, and the selection process been described? Was it a probability or nonprobability sample? Are inclusion and exclusion criteria adequately described? Were payments made to participants?

      g.   Were the ethical procedures used to protect participants from harm and to protect their autonomy and confidentiality clearly explained? Was ethical permission granted for the study? Did participants provide informed consent?

      h.   Are the operational definitions (i.e., terms, theories, and concepts) for the study clearly defined?

      i.   Has the research design been clearly identified? Is it appropriate for answering the research question? Have the survey instruments been tested for reliability and validity?

         i.   Reliability: How reproducible are the results? Example: Weighing a baby on a scale several times should give you the same (or similar) results if the scale is reliable.

         ii.   Validity: How close to the truth are the results? Example: How close is a scale to the true weight? A scale can give a similar weight several times (reliable), but it could be consistently weighing too high or too low (not valid). The data would be valid only if the scale were calibrated to a particular standard and then produced consistent results.

      j.   Were the steps involved in the data analysis explained? Were all data considered? Are the results relevant to the research questions? Do the tables, graphs, and figures accurately portray the data and aid the reader in understanding the analysis?

      k.   Have the results been interpreted in relation to the research question and aims? Have the results been discussed with reference to the research question, hypothesis (if applicable), and theoretical or conceptual frameworks? Are the recommendations and conclusions the researchers make supported by the data analysis?

      l.   Are all materials (books, journals, and other media) cited in the article accurately referenced?

C.   A qualitative research critique also requires a systematic review approach.
    1.   Qualitative and quantitative studies differ in their approach to research.
        a.   Although a critical analysis of a qualitative study involves an in-depth review of how each step of the research was undertaken, it necessitates a different approach due to the philosophical underpinnings of the various qualitative research methods.[48]
        b.   Qualitative research is subjective and is often regarded as more difficult to critique.[48]
    2.   The guidelines for critiquing a qualitative research study are as follows[48]:
        a.   Four components influence the believability of research:
            i.   Is the article logically organized and well written?
            ii.   What are the researcher's academic and professional qualifications?
            iii.   Is the title of the article clear, concise, and accurate?
            iv.   Does the abstract include the essential components of the research (i.e., research problem, sample, methodology, findings, and recommendations)?
        b.   Twelve components influence the robustness of the research:
            i.   Is the phenomenon of interest clearly identified? Is the research question congruent with the phenomenon of interest?
            ii.   Does the researcher clearly state the importance of undertaking the study and how it will add to the extant literature?
            iii.   Has a thorough and objective literature review been undertaken? Does the literature review support the philosophical underpinnings of the study?
            iv.   If a conceptual or theoretical framework was identified, was it adequately described, and is it appropriate?
            v.   Has the philosophical approach and the rationale for its selection been explained?
            vi.   What sampling method was chosen, and was it appropriate? How did the researcher determine if the sample size was adequate (e.g., no new emerging themes were found)?
            vii.   Was the research conducted ethically? Participants should give informed consent, their anonymity should be protected, and they should be protected from harm. They should fully understand the purpose of the study and how their contributions will be used. Proper institutional review board approval should be in place.
            viii.   Were the data gathering methods and data analysis described, and were they appropriate? Was data saturation achieved?
            ix.   Were measures taken to ensure trustworthiness of the data (e.g., were credibility, dependability, transferability, and goodness discussed)?
            x.   Are the findings situated within the context of the study and presented appropriately? Did the researcher address the purpose of the study?
            xi.   Are the implications of the findings identified? Are the conclusions appropriate given the findings that were reported? What recommendations were made for how the research findings could be developed?
            xii.   Were all sources used in the preparation of the article accurately referenced?
D.   The following section outlines resources for quantitative and qualitative research critique.
    1.   Enhancing the QUAlity and Transparency Of health Research (EQUATOR) is an international initiative that promotes transparent and accurate reporting and wider use of comprehensive reporting guidelines in published research literature.[49]
    2.   The EQUATOR website (http://www.equator-network.org/) is a clearinghouse that contains guidelines for reporting research results from specific types of quantitative and qualitative studies. The published guidelines can also be used as a guide for evaluating research studies. Some of the most common guidelines are as follows:
        a.   Consolidated Standards of Reporting Trials (CONSORT):
            i.   The CONSORT 2010 Statement is an evidence-based set of guidelines for reporting randomized trials in a standardized manner.
            ii.   It comprises a 25-item checklist and a flow diagram, which offer a standard way for authors to report how the trial was designed, analyzed, and interpreted, and to illustrate the flow of participants through each stage of the randomized trial.[50]
            iii.   The checklist and flow diagram may be downloaded from http://www.consort-statement.org.

    b. Strengthening the Reporting of Observational Studies in Epidemiology (STROBE):

        i. Minimum reporting guidelines are provided for observational studies in epidemiology (i.e., cohort studies, case-control studies, and cross-sectional studies).[49,51]

        ii. The six available STROBE checklists may be downloaded from https://www.strobe-statement.org/index.php?id=available-checklists.

    c. Preferred Reporting Items for Systematic Reviews and Meta-Analyses (PRISMA):

        i. The PRISMA Statement is an evidence-based set of guidelines that details the minimum set of items for reporting in systematic reviews and meta-analyses. Although PRISMA focuses on the reporting of reviews evaluating randomized trials, it may also be used as a standard for reporting reviews of other types of research (e.g., evaluations of interventions).

        ii. It consists of a 27-item checklist and a four-phase flow diagram.

        iii. The PRISMA Statement, checklist, and flow diagram may be downloaded from http://www.prisma-statement.org.

    d. Consolidated Criteria for Reporting Qualitative Research (COREQ):

        i. COREQ is a 32-item checklist that helps authors in the compendious reporting of qualitative studies (i.e., in-depth interviews and focus groups).[52]

        ii. The full text article with checklist items and description may be downloaded from https://academic.oup.com/intqhc/article/19/6/349/1791966.

    e. Case Report Guidelines (CARE):

        i. CARE provides comprehensive reporting guidelines for case reports.[53]

        ii. The 13-item checklist may be downloaded from http://www.care-statement.org/resources/checklist.

    f. Standards for Quality Improvement Reporting Excellence (SQUIRE):

        i. SQUIRE underscores the importance of reporting three key components to improve the quality, value, and safety of health care.[54]

        ii. Key components to report include the use of theory in planning, implementing, and evaluating quality improvement work and the context in which the work and intervention study were done.[54]

        iii. The 18-item checklist may be downloaded from http://www.equator-network.org/reporting-guidelines/squire/.

E. Evaluating research involves questioning the presence of bias that could have impacted the results of the study in ways that the researcher either did not disclose or was not aware of. Uncovering bias in research is an intuitive process. The following information describes different types of bias and how to evaluate for bias.

  1. Many different types of bias can affect the results of research.

    a. Bias occurs when systematic error is introduced at any point during the research process.

    b. Examining the human elements of the research process allows us to minimize the potential impact that bias has in lactation research.

  2. Researcher bias[29]:

    a. Researcher bias occurs when the researcher intentionally or unintentionally influences the results to portray a certain outcome.

    b. Some bias arises when researchers select participants that are more likely to produce the desired results (sampling bias) or when researchers use participants' information to confirm their hypothesis (confirmation bias).

    c. Culture bias can be introduced when assumptions about participants' motivations and influences are based on the researcher's personal cultural experiences.

    d. Question bias[29]:

        i. The order of questions can introduce bias; one question can influence answers to subsequent questions (question-order bias). To minimize bias, ask general questions before specific questions and positive questions before negative questions.

        ii. Assuming relationships between a feeling and a behavior can introduce bias. Rather than elaborating on a participant's answer, ask questions that use the participant's language.

  3. Respondent bias[29]:

    a. Some participants tend to agree to all the questions in the questionnaire (acquiescence bias), leading to untruthful reporting or contradictory responses.

b.   Others may provide socially desirable answers to sensitive questions. Breastfeeding is a health-related behavior that may elicit socially desirable answers by some participants. Careful consideration should be given to how the questions are phrased, the order of the questions, and the manner in which they are administered. Using a computer to administer a survey may help invoke neutrality.
c.   Demand bias occurs when participants unconsciously change their behavior to meet the expectations of the research. Therefore, it is best, to the extent possible, to blind the participant to the hypothesis being tested.
d.   Participants' feelings and opinions about the organization sponsoring the research may also bias their answers.
4.   Publication bias[29]:
a.   The way in which the results are disseminated in the literature can create bias.
b.   Most commonly, publication bias occurs because research that produces significant results tends to be reported more often than research in which the null hypothesis is upheld.
c.   The extent to which commercial entities (e.g., formula manufacturers and pharmaceutical companies) publicize favorable findings, while burying some research, is not known.
d.   When publication bias is present, meta-analyses and systematic reviews are impacted; findings will not be based on a representative sample of the available evidence.

▶ Key Points from This Chapter

A.   EBP, EIP, and KT are all important models for planning comprehensive breastfeeding care and support: (1) EBP models are predominantly focused on finding and evaluating evidence; (2) EIP models balance the three pillars of evidence, clinician expertise, and patient needs and values when planning care and support; and (3) KT provides guidance with the process of implementing EBP and EIP.
B.   The Clinical Decision Making in Lactation Care and Support Model can be used to differentiate lactation care and support interventions into emerging, promising, supported, and well-supported practices.
C.   The Clinical Decision Making in Lactation Care and Support Model can be used to help clinicians use all forms of evidence when evaluating lactation support interventions.
D.   The Clinical Decision Making in Lactation Care and Support Model can be used to integrate clinician experience and patient concerns and needs when planning comprehensive, individualized lactation care.

🔍 CASE STUDY

Monica, a lactation consultant with 2 years of experience working for a Women, Infants, and Children (WIC) Supplemental Nutrition clinic in the United States, is performing a breastfeeding consult with Maria, who is currently breastfeeding her first child, Robert. Robert was born preterm at 32 weeks and spent 4 weeks in the NICU. Maria has been expressing milk with an electric breast pump, and the expressed milk is fed to Robert by bottle. Maria and Robert are home now, and Maria would like to feed Robert at the breast. Monica has tried several times to help Robert latch, each time unsuccessfully. Monica heard that other lactation consultants suggest the use of nipple shields to help an infant transition from the bottle to the breast for feeding, but she does not have experience using nipple shields. Monica also remembers learning in lactation education classes that using nipple shields could result in decreased milk production.

Questions
1. Where should Monica go to learn about the use of nipple shields?
2. What other sources of information can Monica access about the use of nipple shields?
3. What tools could Monica use to evaluate research evidence about nipple shields?
4. Write a clinical question to guide your evaluation of the use of nipple shields.
5. What evidence can you find about the use of nipple shields?
6. What is your assessment of the evidence on nipple shield use?
7. Is the practice of using nipple shields with infants born prematurely an emerging, promising, supported, or well-supported practice?

References

1. Straus SE, Tetroe J, Graham I. Defining knowledge translation. *Can Med Assoc J.* 2009;181(3-4):165-168.
2. Grove SK, Burns N, Gray J. *The Practice of Nursing Research: Appraisal, Synthesis, and Generation of Evidence.* St. Louis, MO: Elsevier Health Sciences; 2012.
3. Sinha B, Chowdhury R, Sankar MJ, et al. Interventions to improve breastfeeding outcomes: a systematic review and meta-analysis. *Acta Paediatr.* 2015;104(S467):114-134.
4. Renfrew MJ, McCormick FM, Wade A, Quinn B, Dowswell T. Support for healthy breastfeeding mothers with healthy term babies. *Cochrane Database Syst Rev.* 2012;5:CD001141. doi:10.1002/14651858.CD001141.pub4.
5. McFadden A, Gavine A, Renfrew MJ, et al. Support for healthy breastfeeding mothers with healthy term babies. *Cochrane Database Syst Rev.* 2017;2:CD001141. doi:10.1002/14651858.CD001141.pub5.
6. Haroon S, Das JK, Salam RA, Imdad A, Bhutta ZA. Breastfeeding promotion interventions and breastfeeding practices: a systematic review. *BMC Public Health.* 2013;13(3):S20.
7. Demirtas B. Strategies to support breastfeeding: a review. *Intl Nurs Rev.* 2012;59(4):474-481.
8. Sipsma HL, Jones KL, Cole-Lewis H. Breastfeeding among adolescent mothers: a systematic review of interventions from high-income countries. *J Hum Lactation.* 2015;31(2):221-229.
9. Bibbins-Domingo K, Grossman DC, Curry SJ, et al. Primary care interventions to support breastfeeding: US Preventive Services Task Force recommendation statement. *JAMA.* 2016;316(16):1688-1693.
10. Feldman-Winter L. Evidence-based interventions to support breastfeeding. *Pediatr Clin.* 2013;60(1):169-187.
11. Cochrane AL. *Effectiveness and Efficiency: Random Reflections on Health Services.* London, England: Nuffield Provincial Hospitals Trust; 1972.
12. Sackett DL, Rosenberg WM, Gray JM, Haynes RB, Richardson WS. Evidence based medicine: what it is and what it isn't. *BMJ.* 1992;312(7023):71-72.
13. Dearholt S, Dang D. *Johns Hopkins Nursing Evidence-Based Practice: Models and Guidelines.* 3rd ed. Indianapolis, IN: Sigma Theta Tau; 2017.
14. Cochrane. About us. Cochrane website. http://www.cochrane.org/about-us. Published 2017. Accessed October 10, 2017.
15. Joanna Briggs Institute. About us. Joanna Briggs Institute website. http://joannabriggs.org/about.html. Published 2017. Accessed October 10, 2017.
16. Shlonsky A, Mildon R. Methodological pluralism in the age of evidence-informed practice and policy. *Scand J Soc Med.* 2014;42(suppl):18-27.
17. Epstein I. Promoting harmony where there is commonly conflict: evidence-informed practice as an integrative strategy. *Soc Work Health Care.* 2009;48(3):216-231.
18. Greenhalgh T, Howick J, Maskrey N. Evidence based medicine: a movement in crisis? *BMJ.* 2014;348:3725.
19. Nevo I, Slonim-Nevo V. The myth of evidence-based practice: towards evidence-informed practice. *Br J Soc Work.* 2011;41(6):1176-1197.
20. Green L, Ottoson J, García C, Hiatt R. Diffusion theory and knowledge dissemination, utilization, and integration in public health. *Annu Rev Public Health.* 2009;30:151-174.
21. Ward V, House A, Hamer S. Developing a framework for transferring knowledge into action: a thematic analysis of the literature. *J Health Serv Res Policy.* 2009;14(3):156-164.
22. Sudsawad P. *Knowledge Translation: Introduction to Models, Strategies, and Measures.* Austin, TX: Southwest Educational Development Laboratory, National Center for the Dissemination of Disability Research; 2007.
23. Stillwell SB, Fineout-Overholt E, Melnyk BM, Williamson KM. Asking the clinical question: a key step in evidence-based practice. *Am J Nurs.* 2010;110(3):58-61.
24. Fineout-Overholt E, Stillwell SB. Asking compelling clinical questions. In: Melnyk BM, Fineout-Overholt E, eds. *Evidence-Based Practice in Nursing and Healthcare:A Guide to Best Practice.* 3rd ed. Philadelphia, PA: Wolters Kluwer Health; 2015:24-39.
25. Bartels EM. How to perform a systematic search. *Best Pract Res Clin Rheumatol.* 2013;27:295-306.
26. Ingram J, Johnson D, Copeland M, Churchill C, Taylor H. The development of a new breast feeding assessment tool and the relationship with breast feeding self-efficacy. *Midwifery.* 2015;31(1):132-137.
27. Jensen D, Wallace S, Kelsay P. LATCH: a breastfeeding charting system and documentation tool. *J Obstet Gynecol Neonatal Nurs.* 1994;23(1):27-32.
28. Dennis CL. The breastfeeding self-efficacy scale: psychometric assessment of the short form. *J Obstet Gynecol Neonatal Nurs.* 2003;32(6):734-744.
29. Polit DF, Beck CT. *Nursing Research: Generating and Assessing Evidence for Nursing Practice.* 10th ed. Philadelphia, PA: Williams & Wilkins; 2016.
30. Grassley JS, Spencer BS, Law B. A grandmothers' tea: evaluation of a breastfeeding support intervention. *J Perinat Educ.* 2012;21(2):80-89.
31. Buck ML, Amir LH, Cullinane M, Donath SM, CASTLE Study Team. Nipple pain, damage, and vasospasm in the first 8 weeks postpartum. *Breastfeeding Med.* 2014;9(2):56-62.
32. Zhang J. What's the relative risk? A method of correcting the odds ratio in cohort studies of common outcomes. *JAMA.* 1998;280:1690-1691.
33. Torres JMC. Families, markets, and medicalization: the role of paid support for childbirth and breastfeeding. *Qual Health Res.* 2015;25(7):899-911.
34. Bower K, Burnette T, Lewis D, Wright C, Kavanagh K. "I had one job and that was to make milk": mothers' experiences expressing milk for their very-low-birth-weight infants. *J Hum Lactation.* 2017;33(1):188-194.
35. Habibi MF, Nicklas J, Spence M, Hedberg S, Magnuson E, Kavanagh KF. Remote lactation consultation: a qualitative study of maternal response to experience and recommendations. *J Hum Lactation.* 2012;28(2):211-217.
36. Chaput KH, Adair CE, Nettel-Aguirre A, Musto R, Tough SC. The experience of nursing women with breastfeeding support: a qualitative inquiry. *CAMJ Open.* 2015;3(3):E305-E309.

37. Thulier DD. Breastfeeding in America: a history of influencing factors. *J Hum Lactation.* 2009;25(1):85-94.
38. O'Sullivan EJ, Geraghty SR, Rasmussen KM. Informal human milk sharing: a qualitative exploration of the attitudes and experiences of mothers. *J Hum Lactation.* 2016;32(3):416-424.
39. Vazquez RR, Losa-Iglesias ME, Corral-Liria I, Jimenez-Fernandez R, Becerro-de-Bengoa-Vallejo R. Attitudes and expectations in the intergenerational transmission of breastfeeding: a phenomenological study. *J Hum Lactation.* 2017;33(3):588-594.
40. Hurst N, Engebretson J, Mahoney JS. Providing mother's own milk in the context of the NICU: a paradoxical experience. *J Hum Lactation.* 2013;29(3):366-373.
41. Perrin MT, Goodell LS, Fogleman A, Pettus H, Bodenheimer AL, Palmquist AE. Expanding the supply of pasteurized donor milk: understanding why peer-to-peer milk sharers in the United States do not donate to milk banks. *J Hum Lactation.* 2016;32(2):229-237.
42. Rosner AL. Evidence-based medicine: revisiting the pyramid of priorities. *J Bodyw Mov Ther.* 2012;16(1):42-49.
43. Gugiu PC. Hierarchy of evidence and appraisal of limitations (HEAL) grading system. *Eval Program Plann.* 2015;48:149-159.
44. La Caze A. Evidence-based medicine can't be.... *Soc Epistemol.* 2008;22(4):353-370.
45. Lumbiganon P, Martis R, Laopaiboon M, Festin MR, Ho JJ, Hakimi M. Antenatal breastfeeding education for increasing breastfeeding duration. *Cochrane Database Syst Rev.* 2016;12:CD006425. doi:10.1002/14651858.CD006425.pub4.
46. FRIENDS National Resource Center. Evidence-based practice in CBCAP. FRIENDS website. https://www.friendsnrc.org/evidence-based-practice-in-cbcap. Published 2017. Accessed October 10, 2017.
47. Coughlan M, Cronin P, Ryan F. Step-by-step guide to critiquing resarch. Part 1: quantitative research. *Br J Nurs.* 2007;16(11):658-663.
48. Ryan F, Coughlan M, Cronin P. Step-by-step guide to critiquing research. Part 2: qualitative research. *Br J Nurs.* 2007;16(12):738-744.
49. EQUATOR Network. Enhancing the quality and transparency of health research. EQUATOR Network website. https://www.equator-network.org/. Published 2017. Accessed December 5, 2017.
50. CONSORT. Welcome to the CONSORT website. CONSORT website. http://www.consort-statement.org/. Accessed December 5, 2017.
51. von Elm E, Altman D, Egger M, Pocock S, Gotzsche P, Vandenbroucke J. The strengthening the reporting of observational studies in epidemiology (STROBE) statement: guidelines for reporting observational studies. EQUATOR Network website. http://www.equator-network.org/reporting-guidelines/strobe/. Published 2007. Accessed December 5, 2017.
52. Tong A, Sainsbury P, Craig J. Consolidated criteria for reporting qualitative research (COREQ): a 32-item checklist for interviews and focus groups. *Intl J Qual Health Care.* 2007;19(6):349-357.
53. Gagnier J, Kienle G, Altman D, Moher D, Sox H, Riley D; CARE Group. The CARE guidelines: consensus-based clinical case report guideline development. *J Clin Epidemiol.* 2014;67(1):46-51.
54. Ogrinc G, Davies L, Goodman D, Batalden P, Davidoff F, Stevens D. SQUIRE 2.0: standards for quality improvement reporting excellence: revised publication guidelines from a detailed consensus process. *J Am Coll Surg.* 2016;222(3):317-323.

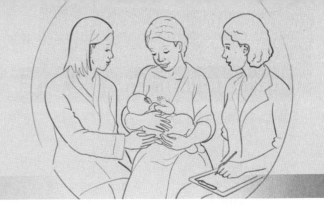

CHAPTER 3

Infant Anatomy and Physiology for Feeding

Nina Isaac
Elizabeth Choi

OBJECTIVES

- Describe and assess infant orofacial structures and identify abnormal presentations.
- Identify infant reflexes related to feeding and describe abnormal presentations.
- Describe infant motor functions for sucking and swallowing.

DEFINITIONS OF COMMONLY USED TERMS

ankyloglossia A condition involving an atypically short, thick, or tight frenulum that tethers the bottom of the tongue to the floor of the mouth, restricting the range of motion of the tongue.

cleft Abnormal fissure or opening resulting from failure of fusion during embryonic development; used in this chapter to describe cleft lip or palate.

dysphagia Swallowing disorder characterized by difficulties swallowing foods or liquids.

dysrhythmic Having an irregular rhythm.

frenectomy Resection of the lingual frenulum to improve tongue movement.

frenotomy Release of the tongue by revising the lingual frenulum with scissors.

frenulum A small fold of tissue that helps secure or restrict the movement of a semimobile body part. Frenula can be found throughout the body, but in the oral cavity, it is located under the tongue and between the upper lip and gums (maxillary gingiva) medially.

hypertonia A condition of muscle rigidity or too much (increased) muscle tone.

hypotonia A condition of muscle flaccidity or decreased muscle tone.

macroglossia An abnormally large tongue.

micrognathia A condition of having a smaller than normal lower jaw.

(continues)

Any use of the term *mother, maternal,* or *breastfeeding* is not meant to exclude transgender or nonbinary parents who may be breastfeeding or providing human milk to their infant.

▶ Overview

This chapter provides an overview of the structures and functions of an infant's face and mouth, with an emphasis on their roles in the process of breastfeeding. It outlines typical and atypical presentations of anatomy and function and their impact on feeding-related behaviors. Infant reflexes and the suck–swallow–breathe pattern that is integral to infant feeding are also discussed to provide a comprehensive understanding of infant anatomy and physiology.

I. Oral Assessment of the Infant

A. An oral assessment of the breastfeeding infant begins following global assessments of the infant's tone and color, state, behavior, symmetry, and respiration.
B. The oral assessment focuses on the following elements:
    1. Observation of the infant's orofacial anatomy.
    2. Identification of deviations in infant oral anatomy and consideration of how those deviations may contribute to dysfunctional or poor feeding behaviors.
    3. Observation of the infant's feeding reflexes and identification of abnormal presentations.
    4. Observation of the effectiveness of feeding (i.e., suck–swallow–breathe coordination).
    5. Observation of the "fit" between the infant's mouth and the nipple.

II. Anatomy of the Infant's Oral Cavity

A. Feeding, respiration, dentition, and speech are influenced by the anatomy of the mouth. Feeding is further affected by the tone and functioning of the muscles of the face, neck, and trunk.
    1. Some aspects of infant orofacial structure and function vary from typical presentations as a result of various factors, including prematurity, minor injuries (e.g., traumatic birth process), congenital malformation, neurological deficits, and illness.
    2. Variations or abnormalities in the orofacial structure or function can negatively affect breastfeeding. The presence of risk factors indicates the need for a more focused assessment, and they increase the potential need for lactation support.[1,2]
B. The lips assist the tongue in drawing in the nipple and stabilizing it in the mouth.[2]
    1. Typically, lips are intact with no evidence of a cleft; they appear mobile, well defined, and expressive. A bow-shaped upper lip with a well-defined philtrum generally indicates a typical presentation.
    2. The lips remain in a neutral position (neither retracted nor overly flanged) and seal smoothly around the breast during breastfeeding.
    3. Abnormal presentations include the following:
        a. Hypotonic (abnormally low muscle tone) lips:
            i. Hypotonia or weakness, often due to prematurity, neuromuscular deficits, or illness, may result in a weakened ability to maintain a lip seal around the breast. This may impact the

amount of suction the infant can generate and increase the work of feeding, contributing to milk loss and fatigue as feedings progress.

   b. Hypertonic (abnormally high muscle tone) lips or overuse of lips:
      i. Hypertonic lips, or even a reliance on increased lip activity to hold the breast in the mouth, may reflect a neurological abnormality or injury of the tongue, jaws, or facial nerves.[3]
      ii. Increased lip activity while breastfeeding may be compensatory due to muscular weakness in the cheeks, jaw, or tongue, or reduced lingual or labial mobility secondary to a tight labial frenulum or ankyloglossia (i.e., tongue-tie).
      iii. Restricted lip movement may be sensory in nature (i.e., hypo- or hypersensitive).[4]
   c. Tethered maxillary frenulum, commonly referred to as an *upper* or *superior* labial frenulum (tightness or thickness in the band of tissue that attaches the upper lip to the upper gum):
      i. This is classified as a minor midline congenital defect. A tight or thick labial frenulum exhibiting low-lying attachment with restriction may affect dentition (e.g., may create a diastema, or gap, between the front teeth) and increase the risk of dental caries.[5]
      ii. If the maxillary frenulum is nonelastic and restricts labial movement, it may contribute to lip *curling*, reduced mobility, or a poor seal during breastfeeding. This may add to latch difficulties, causing friction trauma to the nipples and potentially reducing the overall transfer of milk.[5-8] Research in this area is limited but ongoing.
      iii. Treatment may be warranted if restriction is noted along with apparent breastfeeding or dental difficulties and the cause of the restriction is determined to be from the tethered labial frenulum. If a restriction is present with no apparent dental or breastfeeding difficulties, treatment is most likely not warranted.[5-8]
   d. Cleft lip (a fissure or opening, in the upper lip that may extend into the nose; may be unilateral or bilateral):
      i. A cleft lip is a congenital midline defect that is generally repaired in the first few months of life.
      ii. It is the second most-common birth defect in the United States.[9]
      iii. Cleft lip often does not significantly interfere with breastfeeding[10] when proper support and assistance with optimal positioning are provided.

4. Assess the lips to observe for shape and positioning during feedings.
   a. Properly position the infant and observe for the presence of a possible tight maxillary frenulum by gently lifting the upper lip. Observe for blanching of the frenulum, attachment of the frenulum at the gum line, and overall tension (i.e., reduced lip movement).[6]
   b. Apply gentle digital pressure against the lips; there should be some resistance.
   c. Observe an entire feeding to determine whether the infant can seal the lips smoothly around the breast and maintain the seal during feeding without evidence of early fatigue.
      i. Listen for breaks in the seal while the infant feeds. Abnormal tongue movements and abnormally wide jaw excursions can cause breaks in the lip seal. Although these factors do not directly involve the lips, they can affect the lip seal.
      ii. Observe for lip retraction and lip tremors.
      iii. Observe for leaking milk (during breast and alternative feeding).
   d. Assess for other events related to the lips.
      i. Observe the infant while crying for signs of neonatal asymmetric crying facies, which is a relatively common condition (1 per 160 live births) that is marked by asymmetrical lip movement seen when the infant cries.[11]
      ii. Determine if sucking blisters are present. Sucking blisters are believed to be caused by friction resulting from retracted lips during breastfeeding or by a tight maxillary frenulum that restricts upper lip mobility. Blisters may also be secondary to other causes, such as a tight lingual frenulum (tongue-tie) or hypertonia.

5. Methods of assisting when the feeding problem results from structural abnormalities or abnormal tone of the lips include the following:
   a. Provide firm pressure stimulus (i.e., tapping) on the lips prior to feeding to improve tone and strengthen the lip seal.[12]

  b. Insert a clean finger or a round, somewhat firm pacifier, then partially pull it out of the infant's mouth to induce the infant to pull it back. This resistance training exercise may lead to improved strength in the lips and other oral musculature, which may facilitate improved breastfeeding.

  c. Observe the infant for stress cues when engaging in these activities (see Chapter 4, *Normal Infant Behavior*). Discontinue attempts when the infant becomes fatigued or distressed so the experience stays positive.

  d. When a cleft lip is present, teach the parent to use a finger or shape the breast tissue to seal the cleft.

   i. If the infant prefers one breast over the other, guide the parent to slide the infant to the other breast without repositioning the infant. Use pillows for support as needed.

   ii. Communicate with cleft lip and palate teams to facilitate support for breastfeeding.

   iii. Share research that documents the fact that postoperative breastfeeding after cleft lip repair is safe and results in better weight gain than bottle feeding.[13]

  e. If the upper lip is observed to curl or tuck under during feeding, demonstrate to the parent how to use a fingertip to gently flip out the baby's upper lip to improve the seal on the breast. The parent can manually return the lip to the neutral position as often as needed, especially if lip retraction causes nipple pain or reduces the seal on the breast.

  f. If a tight labial frenulum appears to require a release to facilitate breastfeeding, provide referrals to appropriate specialists for evaluation.

  g. Reassure parents that feeding skills typically improve with maturity and growth. Pumping or hand expression may be necessary to maintain milk production during this time.

  h. Provide a referral to a speech-language pathologist or occupational therapist who specializes in infant feeding and has additional knowledge about breastfeeding and lactation. The feeding therapist can provide an assessment and remediation as needed for difficulties that are unresolved or fall outside the lactation consultant's scope of practice.

C. The buccal pads, or subcutaneous fat deposits in the cheeks, help provide structural support for an infant's oral and pharyngeal activity.[1,2]

 1. Low facial tone or poorly developed buccal pads, due to prematurity or low birth weight, can result in difficulty creating or sustaining adequate levels of suction for feeding.

 2. Abnormal presentations of the cheeks include hypotonia and thin cheeks.

  a. Facial hypotonia can contribute to decreased cheek stability due to decreased resistance against pressure, which can further hinder the seal on the breast.

  b. Thin cheeks (i.e., underdeveloped buccal fat pads or musculature) can contribute to decreased cheek stability due to increased intraoral space. As a result, the infant must create a greater vacuum to generate and sustain suction, further increasing the work of feeding. The infant can become fatigued before the feeding is complete.

 3. An assessment of the cheeks includes the following[2,14]:

  a. Assess the buccal pads in the cheeks by placing a gloved finger inside the infant's mouth and placing a thumb on the outside of the cheek to sense the thickness of the fat pads. In babies with thin cheeks, the finger and thumb almost touch.

  b. Observe the shape of the cheeks at rest and during feeding.

   i. Look for deep creases under the infant's eyes; these are a marker for thin cheeks.

   ii. If the cheeks are weak, thin, or unstable, they will collapse while the baby sucks. Identify any cheek collapsing by looking for dimples.

  c. Observe the overall efficiency of the feeding and signs of fatigue, such as reduced active sucking and swallowing or early discontinuation of feeding, such as falling asleep early during the feeding.

  d. Early discontinuation of feeds secondary to fatigue is a risk factor for poor infant intake and poor stimulation of milk production. Test weights, or weighted feeds, with an appropriate digital scale can be useful, when conducted properly, to help reveal the entire breastfeeding picture.[15,16]

 4. Methods of assisting when feeding problems or slow growth result from thin cheeks, reduced cheek strength, or low facial muscle tone include the following:

  a. Use the Dancer hold to provide external cheek support during feeding. Teach parents how to support the breast while supporting the infant's jaw and cheeks during feeding to improve stability.[16] (See Chapter 24, *Breastfeeding Devices and Topical Treatments*, for information about the Dancer hold.)

    b.   Closely monitor the infant's weight gain and overall growth. Provide supplementary feedings as necessary, ideally with expressed milk, to improve infant growth. As the fat pads develop in the cheeks, the cheek stability may improve, which can lead to an improvement in breastfeeding skills and infant growth.

D.   The jaw provides stability for movements of the tongue, lips, and cheeks.[2,13,16,17]

    1.   Normal jaw movements are neither too wide nor too narrow during feeding, and they are smooth and graded.

    2.   Preterm infants often exhibit jaw instability due to immature or underdeveloped muscles and hypotonia.

    3.   Abnormal presentations of the jaw include the following:

        a.   Micrognathia (abnormally small lower jaw) and retrognathia (abnormally receding lower jaw) can be familial. They are associated with chromosomal disorders or can result from intrauterine positioning that prevents the jaw from growing larger or moving forward (as in certain breech presentations).

            i.   Some degree of mandibular retrognathia is characteristic in infants. Dramatic forward growth usually occurs during the first few months of life.[18]

            ii.   Severe micrognathia or retrognathia positions the tongue posteriorly, where it can obstruct the airway, as in Pierre Robin sequence.[19]

            iii.   A receding jaw can contribute to nipple pain, nipple damage, or latch difficulties. Tipping the infant's head back in a slightly extended position may bring the chin closer to the breast and help attain a more comfortable latch.

            iv.   Jaw asymmetry contributes to poor jaw function and unstable feeding, including difficulty or inability to breastfeed. It can be caused by birth trauma, congenital or acquired torticollis, injury, paralysis, breech position, or structural deformity.[20] Note how the face of the infant in **FIGURE 3-1** droops to the right. Jaw asymmetry and low facial tone can contribute to inefficient feeding and failure to thrive.

        b.   In abnormally wide jaw excursions, poor grading of the jaw movements can cause breaks in the seal formed at the breast, resulting in loss of suction and increased work of feeding that can affect overall milk intake.

        c.   Infants may clench their jaws to manage rapid milk flow; however, jaw clenching can also be a sign of hypertonia or weakness in a different area (e.g., poor tongue or lip function). Jaw clenching can contribute to nipple pain and damage.

    4.   An assessment of the jaws should include the following:

        a.   Observe for asymmetry.

        b.   Identify micrognathia or retrognathia.

        c.   Observe breastfeeding to identify jaw grading, clenching, or tremors.

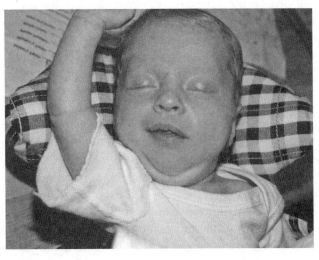

FIGURE 3-1 Facial asymmetry and low facial tone.

   d.   Insert a gloved pinkie finger in the corner of the infant's mouth between the posterior gum
         pads.
         i.   Count the number of reflexive bites (chews) elicited.
         ii.   The infant should respond with approximately 10 little chews on each side.
         iii. Observe for difficulty producing these reflexive bites or for infant stress cues during this
               assessment.
         iv.   Weakness of the jaw is revealed by an inability to perform the activity.[17]
   5.   Methods of assisting when a feeding problem relates to abnormalities, weakness, or injury involving
        the jaws include the following:
        a.   Provide external jaw support with a finger placed under the bony part of the lower jaw to control
              and stabilize the distance of jaw excursions while breastfeeding.
        b.   Work carefully to identify feeding positions that emphasize postural stability.
              i.   Hip flexion and stabilization of the infant's trunk facilitates stable feeding.[21]
              ii.   Position the infant carefully and maintain head extension as a strategy to bring the lower
                    jaw closer to the breast.
        c.   Exercise the jaws several times a day, using the same assessment method described previously
              to elicit an increased number of reflexive bites. Avoid stressing the infant.
        d.   Refer the infant for physical therapy or bodywork (e.g., chiropractic care, craniosacral therapy,
              myofascial release) if issues relating to abnormal muscular tension impinge on jaw activity.
        e.   Refer the infant for speech or occupational therapy for assessment and remediation as needed
              for feeding difficulties that do not resolve with intervention or fall outside the lactation con-
              sultant's scope of practice.
E.   The tongue helps the lips draw the nipple into the oral cavity, sealing the cavity to maintain suction. It
     also forms a central groove that provides a channel to organize the bolus of milk for safe swallowing, and
     it aids suck–swallow–breathe coordination.[2,17,22,23]
     1.   The neonatal tongue typically presents with less fat and soft tissue than an adult tongue. Its muscu-
          lature also differs from that of the adult tongue in ways that appear to be specialized for suckling.
     2.   Many professionals who work with infants believe the position of the tongue at rest and while feeding
          shapes the structures in the mouth, particularly the hard palate, which may further impact dentition
          and speech.[24] Additional research is needed in this area.
     3.   As part of the suckling cycle, tongue movement in conjunction with mandible oscillation generates
          adequate negative intraoral pressure in the oral cavity while the peristaltic or wave-like movements
          of the posterior portion of the tongue aid in coordinating swallowing and breathing.[22,25-27]
          a.   The tongue must be able to elevate freely and to compress and elongate the nipple against the
                hard palate so that with each subsequent lowering of the tongue, an adequate enlargement of
                the oral cavity generates negative pressure.[22]
          b.   The tongue tip extends over the lower gum ridge, providing a degree of padding during breast-
                feeding that helps protect the nipples while allowing the infant to compress the areola. The
                tongue must also extend, draw in the nipple, and stabilize it against the palate.
     4.   When the tongue moves improperly, the infant may not be able to maintain an optimal seal on the
          breast and often cannot suck, swallow, and breathe in a coordinated, efficient manner.
          a.   The work of feeding increases in such cases, putting the infant at risk for early discontin-
                uation of feedings and limited intake, secondary to inefficient or uncoordinated feeding
                and fatigue.
          b.   Limitations in the mobility or strength of the tongue require the infant to use compensatory
                activities (e.g., jaw clenching or lip retraction) to feed, which often damage the nipples.
     5.   Abnormal presentations of the tongue include the following:
          a.   Ankyloglossia, or tongue-tie, is a congenital midline anomaly in which the lingual frenulum,
                a membrane extending from the floor of the mouth to the underside of the tongue, is tight or
                thick and limits the tongue's range of motion.[28,29]
                i.   In tongue-ties with anterior attachment, there is typically a heart-shaped indented appear-
                      ance to the tongue tip at rest or with extension. Tongue-ties with posterior attachment
                      can be more difficult to visualize; they may also interfere with breastfeeding if they affect
                      tongue mobility and range of motion.[6,30-32]

ii. The incidence of ankyloglossia ranges from 0.02 to 10.7 percent of infants, occurring more commonly in males.[31] It is theorized that the incidence would be higher if studies included posterior tongue-ties, but this claim has not been substantiated.

iii. Typically, ankyloglossia is an isolated anatomic variation and can run in families. Current discussions exist regarding the potential connection between ankyloglossia and specific gene mutations, but additional research is needed.

iv. Ankyloglossia appears with increased frequency in association with various congenital syndromes and other midline defects.[28,33]

v. Approximately 50 percent of infants diagnosed with ankyloglossia can breastfeed without difficulty.[31] In other cases, ankyloglossia may negatively impact comfort during breastfeeding. Ankyloglossia may decrease milk transfer, which can then impact milk production and the infant's milk intake and growth.[6,32,34,35]

vi. Either frenotomy (simple release achieved by revising the lingual frenulum) or frenectomy (resection of the tongue) may be curative by changing the latching abilities and sucking dynamics of the breastfeeding infant.[6,36] There are currently no in-depth studies comparing outcomes using various techniques.

- Frenotomy is often performed without anesthesia as an in-office procedure and has a high satisfaction rate and few complications.[37,38]
- Laser frenectomy is a simple in-office procedure that is performed with or without local anesthesia. This technique is commonly utilized by pediatricians, otolaryngologists, and dentists. It is considered a safe alternative to scissors,[6] with more predictable results and fewer postoperative complications.[36]

b. A bunched or retracted tongue can be caused by a traumatic birth process, tightness and asymmetries (e.g., torticollis), ankyloglossia, hypertonia, and the early introduction of bottles for some infants.

c. Tongue protrusion may result from abnormal tongue development such as macroglossia (an abnormally large tongue) or hypotonia (as in Down syndrome, or trisomy 21). Tongue protrusion contributes to poor coordination of sucking and swallowing.

d. Tongue-tip elevation is an adaptive compensatory behavior that can make latching to the breast frustrating and difficult. It is often seen in babies who were born prematurely, experienced birth trauma, or present with hypotonia, ankyloglossia, or respiratory involvement. This behavior may be associated with airway protection, increased work of breathing, or increased respiratory rate, especially in the preterm infant.[39,40]

e. Tongue asymmetry can result from injury (e.g., forceps trauma resulting in damage to the nerves controlling the tongue)[3] or central nervous system involvement (e.g., cerebral palsy). Tongue asymmetry may also be associated with syndromic conditions, and it can be seen in infants with torticollis secondary to positioning in utero or a traumatic birth process.

6. An assessment of the tongue should consider the following:

a. Sometimes a poor infant head position during feeding negatively influences the tongue position. Correct the positioning at the breast before evaluating the tongue during feeding.

b. While the infant is breastfeeding, gently pull the breast away from the cheek and observe the corners of the lips. While breastfeeding, the tongue is visibly cupped at the corners of the mouth, helping the lips form a seal to preserve suction.

c. Listen for breaks in the seal, which cause clicking or smacking sounds.

i. A weak tongue or a tongue with reduced mobility (such as tongue-tie) can interfere with maintaining a seal at the breast; however, a typical infant who is struggling with rapid milk flow may deliberately break the seal at the breast.

ii. In a compromised infant, clicking or smacking sounds often mean the tongue has lost contact with the breast (e.g., intermittent loss of suction). A visual assessment of the tongue shape and position at rest, or when the infant is crying, may provide additional information regarding tongue-tie and other abnormal presentations.

d. Examine the tongue's function using gentle pressure of a clean, gloved fingertip to the surface of the tongue at the midsection.

i. There should be some resistance to gentle pressure, and the examiner should sense the tongue pressing up against the finger.

      ii.   The insertion of a finger and the gentle placement of a finger pad against the roof of the mouth should elicit sealing and sucking. Sense whether the tongue extends and cups around the finger, with an anterior-to-posterior peristaltic, rhythmic movement of the tongue.

     e.   With the baby's mouth open wide, observe the elevation of the tongue past the midline of the mouth; it is ideal to observe when the baby is crying. A limited elevation suggests possible ankyloglossia, even without visualization of an overtly anteriorly attached lingual frenulum.[30]

     f.   Observe the tongue extension by tapping the tongue tip or by rubbing the bottom gums to elicit tongue protrusion. Some infants may even imitate tongue extension. Notice whether the infant can extend the tongue beyond the gum, and ideally the lower lip line. An inhibition of extension may suggest ankyloglossia.

     g.   Observe tongue lateralization by providing a stimulus to the left and right bottom gums. The tongue should lateralize toward the examiner's finger as it moves from side to side. Limited lateralization, or twisting of the tongue with lateralization, may suggest ankyloglossia.

   7.   Methods of assisting when a feeding problem results from dysfunction or anomalies of the tongue include the following:

     a.   Specific oral motor exercises, such as resistance training with a finger or pacifier, may be appropriate depending on the presentation of symptoms and the infant's response to exercises.

     b.   Short, frequent feedings provide recovery time if the infant exhibits fatigue during feedings or if feedings are prolonged.

     c.   Positioning the infant with the head in extension brings the lower jaw close in to the breast. Reducing the distance that a short or restricted tongue must reach to extend over the lower gum ridge can help protect the nipples from trauma and help the infant to more readily access the breast.

     d.   Inform the parent of ways to treat sore or damaged nipples (e.g., topical treatment to heal damage and help avoid infection).

     e.   Refer the infant to a specialist for evaluation to release ankyloglossia. Appropriate specialists include pediatricians, family practice doctors, pediatric otolaryngologists, or pediatric dentists.

     f.   It may be appropriate to refer the infant to a speech or occupational therapist specializing in infant feeding. This professional can facilitate improved function if the tongue is weak, uncoordinated, or dysfunctional secondary to injury, paralysis, a genetic condition, or if the infant is recovering from a frenotomy or frenectomy and improvements are not seen with traditional interventions.

     g.   Reassure the parents that although some infants exhibit immediate improvements in feeding skills following tongue-tie revisions, other infants require longer recovery times.

     h.   Supplement feedings with expressed milk if needed to stabilize infant growth and protect milk production as long as necessary.

F.   The infant's hard and soft palate play an integral role in effective milk transfer.[2,41-46]

   1.   The hard palate assists with positioning and stability of the nipple within the mouth.

     a.   The hard palate should be intact with no evidence of a cleft. Its slope should be moderate and smooth, approximating the shape of the tongue.

     b.   Small, round, white cysts (Epstein pearls; see **FIGURE 3-2**) are often observed along the ridge of the hard palate and occasionally along the gums, where they may resemble teeth. Although they are sometimes mistaken for oral thrush, these cysts are benign, resolve around 2 months of age, and do not interfere with feeding.[25]

   2.   The soft palate creates the posterior seal of the oral cavity in conjunction with the tongue, allowing suction to occur.

     a.   The soft palate should elevate during swallowing.

     b.   The soft palate is composed of tissues and muscles with an intact uvula projecting from the back of the roof of the mouth.

   3.   The shape of the palate can be influenced by hereditary and genetic factors or may result from circumstances that prevent typical shaping of the hard palate during gestation.

     a.   A high-arched, grooved, or bubble-shaped hard palate can make it difficult for the infant to properly position the nipple and to compress it with the tongue. **FIGURE 3-3** shows an infant

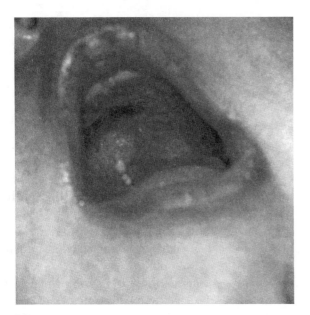

FIGURE 3-2 Epstein pearls on the palate (sometimes mistaken for thrush).

Reproduced with permission from Wilson-Clay B, Hoover K. *The Breastfeeding Atlas*. Austin, TX: LactNews Press; 2008.

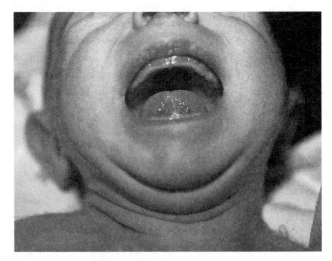

FIGURE 3-3 Bubble palate (note limited tongue elevation).

Reproduced with permission from Wilson-Clay B, Hoover K. *The Breastfeeding Atlas*. Austin, TX: LactNews Press; 2008.

after a frenotomy to revise an anteriorly attached lingual frenulum. However, the infant still demonstrates limited ability to elevate the tongue to the upper gum ridge.[30] Note the bubble shape of the hard palate that may have resulted from ankyloglossia. Many professionals believe that the palate is shaped in utero while the infant is learning to suck and swallow; thus, if an infant presents with reduced lingual mobility, the result may be a higher, arched bubble-shaped palate. Research supporting this theory is lacking, and it may be correlative rather than causative in nature.

    b.   Long periods of intubation, or syndromic conditions such as Down or Turner syndrome, can create grooves in the hard palate that may contribute to the higher incidence of breastfeeding problems in these infant populations.[47]

4.   A cleft palate is a congenital midline defect resulting from incomplete fusion of orofacial structures in utero.

    a.   Clefts of the hard and soft palates exhibit the following characteristics:

        i.   Clefts can be unilateral or bilateral and are classified as partial or incomplete, or complete. They can involve the hard palate, soft palate, or both.

        ii.   A partial or incomplete cleft is isolated.

        iii.   A complete cleft extends from the upper lip to the soft palate and may also involve the nose.

    b.   Regardless of the size, clefts of the hard or soft palate make it difficult or impossible for the infant to breastfeed.

        i.   The infant is unable to seal the oral cavity to generate suction, which negatively affects milk transfer.

        ii.   Some infants with wide palatal clefts exhibit additional swallowing problems due to atypical tongue movements because the palatal back guard is absent.[47]

        iii.   An infant with a cleft may feed constantly and often sleep at the breast.

    c.   Submucosal clefts are defects in the closure of the hard palate shelves.

        i.   They are difficult to identify due to a layer of tissue that has grown over the cleft.

        ii.   Possible indicators of a submucosal cleft include a bifid (or forked) uvula, absent or notched posterior nasal spine, a zona pellucida (or blue zone), and a paranasal bulge (i.e., transverse bony ridge alongside the nose).

5.   A weak or dysfunctional soft palate presents feeding challenges.

    a.   Generalized hypotonia resulting from prematurity, structural differences, neurologic involvement, or a syndromic condition can negatively impact soft palate function.

        b.   Velopharyngeal dysfunction, an inability to close the nasal cavity from the oral cavity due to abnormalities in the anatomy or movement of oral structures, may adversely affect swallowing coordination and quality of feeding.

        c.   Poor infant stamina can influence the function of the soft palate. As the infant tires and loses muscle control, coordination of the soft palate may become disorganized and further affect the suck–swallow–breathe pattern.

   6.   Assessment of the hard and soft palates includes the following:

        a.   A family history of cleft lip or cleft palate should cue the lactation consultant to carefully examine the palate.

        b.   A visual assessment of the palate should identify intact structures and the presence of a well-formed uvula. A bifid or absent uvula indicates possible abnormal formation of the soft palate.

        c.   Gently slide a gloved fingertip along the hard palate, starting just behind the upper gum ridge. Assess the slope of the hard palate for bony prominences, clefts, or abnormally prominent rugae (ridges).

        d.   Observe an entire feeding and elicit information regarding nasal regurgitation, which may indicate a weak soft palate seal or, more rarely, the presence of a submucosal cleft.[48]

   7.   Methods of assisting when a feeding problem results from abnormalities of the hard or soft palates are as follows:

        a.   Breastfeeding an infant with a cleft palate is possible and should be encouraged when feasible. However, in most situations, exclusive breastfeeding is not likely due to the infant's inability to obtain a closed seal, which significantly impacts the ability to effectively access milk from the breast.

        b.   Clefts of the soft and hard palates are typically not surgically corrected until at least 10 months of age. A palatal obturator is a prosthetic device that may be used to assist with breast or bottle feeding prior to surgical revision; however, it is not routinely used, especially in developing countries. There is conflicting evidence to support the use of palatal obturators to improve feeding efficiency.[46,49,50]

        c.   Help the parent with suggestions to assist with feedings.

            i.   Upright positions, such as the seated straddle, may be effective.

           ii.   Demonstrate chin support to stabilize the latch.

          iii.   Teach the use of rhythmic breast compressions for expressing milk into the infant's mouth.

        d.   If an infant with a cleft palate is exclusively or primarily breastfeeding, the overall growth should be closely monitored. Weighted feeds using an accurate scale should be included in assessments to ensure adequate intake.

        e.   Ideally, supplement feedings with expressed milk or banked milk. The incidence of chronic otitis media, a risk for infants with cleft defects, is increased when infants are not fed human milk.[13,51]

        f.   Protect milk production by establishing an appropriate pumping schedule.

        g.   If necessary, help the parent experiment to find an alternative method of feeding that is effective and does not stress the infant.

            i.   Specially designed bottles for infants with cleft palates, typically bottles with one-way valves, are often used in addition to or in place of the breast. They allow the infant to solely use compression to access milk in the absence of creating a seal.

           ii.   Teach the parent to observe the infant for stress cues to prevent the development of feeding aversions.[52]

          iii.   A gastrostomy tube (G-tube), in addition to oral feedings at the breast or with a specialty bottle, may be necessary in certain cases when oral feeding is either not possible or not sufficient for growth. Oral feeding and G-tubes are not mutually exclusive.

        h.   Provide referrals to appropriate specialists, including cleft palate teams and speech pathologists.

  G.   Occlusion of nasal passages can interfere with effective breastfeeding.[2,12,14,53]

    1.   Although infants are typically nose breathers, they can switch to mouth breathing if the nasal passages are occluded. If nasal breathing is impaired, the infant will present with difficulty breastfeeding, and may even resist feeding, because breathing is prioritized.

2. Abnormal presentations of the nasal passages are as follows:
    a. Nasal congestion, in the absence of respiratory illness, can reveal dried accumulations of milk that were nasally regurgitated during feedings.
    b. A deviated nasal septum may impact breathing while feeding.[54]
    c. Rarely, abnormally small nasal openings are observed. Choanal atresia is a congenital condition in which the openings of one or both of the nasal cavities are partially or completely blocked by a bony or membranous occlusion.
    d. Facial bruising (e.g., resulting from birth trauma or instrument-assisted delivery) can cause swelling of the nose and impair breathing.
3. Assessments of the nasal passages should include the following:
    a. The nasal passages should be visually assessed if the infant's breathing sounds congested or if the infant struggles, pulls away, or gasps while feeding.
    b. Elicit information from the parent about the birth process, instrument-assisted delivery, bruising, nasal regurgitation, recent illnesses, and so forth.
4. Methods to assist an infant with feeding problems related to the nasal passages include the following:
    a. Baby-strength saline nose drops or breastmilk can help clear the nasal passages. Note that bulb syringes used to extract nasal debris can inadvertently increase internal swelling.
    b. Employ external pacing methods during feedings as needed to protect respiratory and physiological stability.
    c. Refer the infant to a primary medical care provider or pediatric otolaryngologist for further assessment if a problem related to the nasal passages interferes with feeding.

III. Oral Reflexes

A. The infant's reflexes provide important information regarding the infant's sensory, motor, and neurological status.[55]
    1. When assessing an infant's neurobehavioral responses, it is important to take note of the infant's state of arousal.
    2. Closely observe for any indicators of stress, including hiccupping, sneezing, mottling of skin, and behaviors that are often used for self-regulation (e.g., eye aversion or changing to a lower state of arousal). If an infant exhibits these behaviors or physiological changes secondary to stress, it is important to slow or cease the examination and allow adequate recovery time.[56]
B. Adaptive reflexes assist the infant with facilitating feedings.
    1. The rooting reflex[2] is elicited when the infant's lips or cheek are touched or stroked. The infant's head turns toward the stimulus and the mouth opens (gape response). Rooting helps the infant locate the nipple.
        a. This reflex appears at 32 weeks' gestation; it typically integrates between 4 to 6 months but may persist longer in breastfed infants.
        b. An absent or diminished rooting reflex can signal poor tactile receptivity or poor neural integration.
        c. A hypersensitive or hyperactive rooting reflex can interfere with latching.
    2. The sucking reflex is elicited with a light touch of the nipple or a finger to the infant's lips or tongue, resulting in the complex movements of the suckle.
        a. This reflex appears between 15 and 18 weeks' gestation; it fully integrates between 6 and 12 months.
        b. It is categorized into two modes: nutritive sucking and nonnutritive sucking.[57]
        c. Nutritive sucking is organized into a series of sucking bursts and pauses and occurs solely with the presence of oral fluid.
            i. The sucking rate is slower during nutritive sucking than during nonnutritive sucking to allow coordination of breathing and swallowing.
            ii. The breathing rate increases during pauses that occur between sucking bursts.[2,12,17,27]
                *   Infants with a weak or immature suck are not able to sustain long sucking bursts (e.g., 10 sucks per burst),[17,58] but this can be secondary to respiratory compromise.
                *   Short sucking bursts due to prematurity often normalize with maturation occurring at about 36 to 38 weeks,[17] but they may persist past 40 weeks in some preterm newborns. Sucking problems secondary to other factors may endure longer and be more difficult to resolve.

d.   Nonnutritive sucking is characterized by fast, shallow sucks and a typical ratio of six to eight sucks to one swallow. Nonnutritive sucking occurs for reasons other than feeding.

    i.   It stimulates the milk ejection reflex (MER).

    ii.   It regulates the physiological state and helps the infant to self-soothe.

    iii.   It increases peristalsis of the gastrointestinal tract and enhances secretion of digestive fluids.

    iv.   It helps to manage pain and to reduce the risk of sudden infant death syndrome.[12,17,55,59-62]

    v.   The American Academy of Pediatrics currently recommends delaying the use of pacifiers until breastfeeding is firmly established.[63]

e.   Absent or diminished sucking may indicate central nervous system immaturity or maldevelopment (e.g., various trisomies), prematurity, delayed maturation, prenatal central nervous system insults (e.g., drugs in labor, asphyxia or hypoxia, or trauma), or systemic congenital problems (e.g., cardiovascular abnormalities, sepsis, or infant hypothyroidism).[64]

f.   A weak suck may indicate central nervous system abnormalities associated with hypotonia, genetic conditions such as Down syndrome, abnormalities of the muscles resulting in weak oral musculature, or, rarely, conditions such as medullary lesions, myasthenia gravis, or botulism.[64]

    i.   A weak suck may also be present in a sleepy, ill, malnourished, or jaundiced infant and has also been seen in babies with tongue-tie.

    ii.   An infant with a weak suck may provide inadequate breast stimulation, increasing the risk of rapid, early down regulation of milk production.[65]

    iii.   Close monitoring of infant growth is required for infants with a weak suck. They may need supplemental feedings with an alternate feeding method, preferably with expressed milk.

g.   A disorganized suck is characterized by an immature pattern of short sucking bursts (i.e., 3 to 5 sucks) with varying pauses between each burst.[55] A dysrhythmic and uncoordinated suck may be present.

h.   A dysfunctional suck is characterized by unusual or inconsistent movements while sucking.[55]

3.   The swallowing reflex is elicited by a bolus of fluid contacting the sensory receptors of the soft palate, tongue, and back of the mouth.

a.   The swallowing reflex plays a role in the regulation of amniotic fluid volume and composition, regulation of solutes from the fetal environment, and maturation of the fetal gastrointestinal tract.[66]

b.   The reflex appears between 9 and 14 weeks' gestation and persists into adulthood.

4.   The tongue thrust reflex occurs when the tongue moves down and forward in anticipation of grasping the breast and drawing it into the mouth. It appears at 28 weeks' gestation and typically integrates by 6 months of age.

C.   Protective reflexes help prevent choking and aspiration.

1.   The gag reflex is elicited in the newborn at the mid- to posterior tongue and is the first line of defense to help prevent choking.

a.   It appears at 18 weeks' gestation and persists into adulthood.

b.   A gentle exam with a gloved finger can identify a hyperactive gag reflex (i.e., triggered by shallow oral stimulation).

    i.   A hyperactive gag reflex may indicate immaturity.

    ii.   Constant activation of the gag reflex due to invasive procedures can create oral and feeding aversion.

    iii.   Some infants with a hyperactive gag reflex may require speech or occupational therapy to facilitate acceptance of objects in the mouth.

2.   The cough reflex protects the airway from aspiration of liquids.

a.   Research indicates that this reflex is often not observed at birth as it is only seen in 25 percent of preterm infants and 25 to 50 percent of term infants at birth. 90 percent of newborns exhibited a fully functioning cough reflex by 1 to 2 months of age.[67,68]

    i.   A delayed cough reflex can contribute to an increased risk of penetration (to the level of the vocal folds) or aspiration (past the vocal folds and into the airway) of liquids.

    ii.   Silent aspiration (i.e., aspiration of fluids without coughing) can occur in immature infants.[69]

    b.   Coughing during feeding may be in response to the penetration or aspiration of fluids.

        i.   To date, there is no scientific evidence that attributes increased lung damage to aspiration of small amounts of human milk.

        ii.   Intermittent coughing while breastfeeding is considered normal for many typically developing infants, especially toward the beginning of feedings and when milk ejection is fast.

D.   Other newborn behaviors and reflexes persist up to 6 months of age.

    1.   The stepping reflex is a response used to crawl to the breast.[70]

    2.   The palmar grasp reflex is the closing and grasping of fingers in response to stimulus to the palm. It is typically fully integrated by 5 to 6 months of age.

    3.   The moro response (startle reflex) is the extension of arms, legs, and fingers in response to being startled or a feeling of falling. It is typically fully integrated by 3 to 6 months of age.

    4.   Predictable hand movements are used to stimulate, move, and shape the breast.[71,72]

IV. Suckling Cycle

A.   Recent studies regarding the biomechanics of breastfeeding suggest that effective breastfeeding involves a cycling motion of the mandible and the anterior portion of the tongue; rhythmic peristaltic movement of the posterior portion of the tongue; and milk ejection (see **FIGURE 3-4A** and **FIGURE 3-4B**).[22,26,27,73]

    1.   Downward movement of the posterior portion of the tongue increases negative intraoral pressure (i.e., increases vacuum).

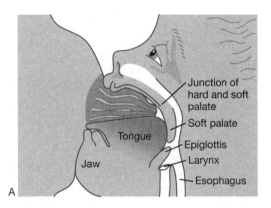

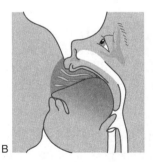
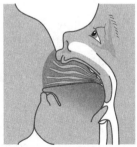
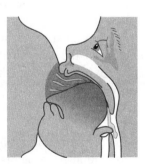

FIGURE 3-4 A. Cross-section of infant latch at the breast with optimal nipple placement 6 to 8 mm from the hard and soft palate junction. **B.** (1) Tongue up: A baseline vacuum is applied. The nipple is compressed and elongated. No milk is evident as the tongue is in contact with the palate. (2) Tongue down: In the first half of the suck cycle the nipple expands and moves closer to the hard and soft palate junction and milk flows into the oral cavity as vacuum strength increases. (3) Tongue up: In the second half of the suck cycle the nipple is compressed again and milk is moved beyond the soft palate to the pharynx as vacuum decreases.

A. Reproduced from Lauwers J, Swisher A. *Counseling the Nursing Mother: A Lactation Consultant's Guide*. 6th ed. Burlington, MA: Jones and Bartlett Learning; 2016. Courtesy of Rebecca Glover, RN, RM, IBCLC.

2. Peristaltic movements, which are visible along the midline of the tongue via 3-D ultrasound imaging, aid in the coordination of swallowing and breathing.
3. Effective breastfeeding is achieved by the combined contributions of both intraoral pressure cycles (i.e., alternating positive and negative pressure changes) and peristaltic tongue movements.

B. The suckling cycle is characterized by the following mechanics:
1. The infant draws the nipple into the mouth by means of a vacuum. The vacuum places the nipple in the optimal position (6 to 8 mm from the hard and soft palate junction) for removing milk from the breast and clearing it from the oral cavity.
2. The lips and cheeks facilitate the formation of a seal and the creation of negative pressure in the oral cavity, while the jaw provides a stable base for the movements of other structures, including the tongue, lips, and cheeks.
3. The tongue is drawn downward along with the soft palate, evenly expanding the nipple and increasing the diameter of the nipple duct, moving the nipple closer to the hard and soft palate junction and increasing the vacuum. As a result of this process along with milk ejection, milk flows into the infant's oral cavity, completing the first half of the suck cycle.
4. A combination of mandibular movements, undulations of the tongue, and decreased vacuum in the oral cavity channels the milk bolus posteriorly and triggers the swallow reflex. Simultaneously, the soft palate elevates and makes contact with the posterior pharyngeal wall to seal the nasal passages and allow the milk bolus to be swallowed, completing the second half of the suck cycle.
5. The tongue then remains in contact with the palate until the beginning of the next suck cycle.

V. Coordination of the Suck–Swallow–Breathe Triad

A. The feeding evaluation must consider all three aspects of suck–swallow–breathe coordination.
1. Sucking, swallowing, and breathing are functionally and anatomically interrelated, with overlapping functions of cranial nerves and structures.
2. Dysrhythmic sucking and poor coordination of the suck–swallow–breathe cycle are common, even in term infants during the first few days of life.[58]
3. Current research suggests that the suck–swallow–breathe cycle is highly variable during breastfeeding so the infant can rapidly adapt to changing milk flow rates during milk ejection.[73]
4. Newborn oral and pharyngeal anatomy differs from adult anatomy in that it allows close proximity among the base of the tongue, the soft palate, and the epiglottis; this is protective in nature and is believed to allow for maturation of suck–swallow–breathe coordination.
5. The evaluation of feedings in compromised infants should include observation of the entire feeding to permit identification of fatigue, loss of rhythm, evidence of respiratory distress, and color changes.[2,12,55] The infant's behavioral state should be noted, including deep sleep, quiet alert, active sleep, active alert, drowsiness, crying, and indeterminate states.[53]

B. Suck–swallow–breathe components[65-79]
1. Optimal coordination of the suck–swallow–breathe cycle has been described as a 1:1:1 ratio; however, much of the research has involved bottle-feeding infants. Suck–swallow–breathe coordination matures in infants so that the pattern in the first week of life differs from the patterns that present between 2 and 4 weeks of age. This is characterized by a decreased number of swallows during prolonged respiratory pauses.
2. Sucking
    a. In breastfed infants, the number of sucks varies throughout a breastfeeding session in relation to a number of factors, including milk ejection, milk flow, milk production, and individual infant abilities.
    b. Nonnutritive sucking has been observed more often at the beginning and end of feedings, while bursts of nutritive sucking occur more often at the beginning and middle of a breastfeeding session.
3. Swallowing
    a. The process of swallowing consists of three main phases:
        i. Oral (preparatory and transport): Milk is removed from the breast, and the bolus is propelled toward the back of the oral cavity.

ii.   Pharyngeal: After the swallow is triggered, a series of complex and protective mechanisms occurs resulting in the following: excursion of the hyoid bone and larynx, inversion of the epiglottis over the airway, adduction (i.e., coming together) of the vocal folds, and propulsion of the bolus into the pharyngeal space. Of note, infant anatomy and physiology greatly differ from adult anatomy and physiology due to proportional differences in infants so that oropharyngeal structures are closer in proximity. This is believed to be ultimately protective in nature as the infant is learning to effectively coordinate the suck-swallow-breathe cycle. Breathing ceases for approximately 0.5 seconds while the bolus is directed toward the esophagus and away from the airway.

iii.   Esophageal: The bolus then travels down the esophagus toward the stomach.

b.   In infants younger than 3 months of age, drooling is associated with weak swallow control (even of the infant's own saliva) or can reveal pharyngeal or esophageal obstruction.[25]

c.   Abnormalities of the tongue and palate, and discoordination of sucking, swallowing, and breathing, can increase the risk of dysphagia (i.e., difficulty swallowing) and aspiration.

i.   Dysphagia can result in poor weight gain and aversive feeding responses.

ii.   Dysphagia is often seen in infants who are diagnosed with reflux.

4.   Breathing

a.   Most full-term infants swallow in coordination with inhalation and exhalation, taking adequate respiratory pauses between sucking bursts.

b.   Preterm infants are more likely to swallow mid-inhalation, increasing the risk of oxygen desaturation, bradycardia, and laryngeal penetration or aspiration.[73,75]

C.   Observe feedings for the following indicators of poor feeding quality:

1.   Respiratory noises:

a.   Stridor is a raspy respiratory noise heard on inhalation, exhalation, or both. It is caused by narrowing, floppiness, or obstruction of the airway.

b.   Wheezing is a high-pitched noise that occurs most often during exhalation, typically as a result of airway constriction. It can be secondary to inflammation or reactive airway disease.

2.   Apnea: Apnea is prolonged periodic breath holding while attempting to manage swallows.[69]

3.   Fatigue: An infant may fall asleep too soon during a feeding due to stress or other causes that inhibit the ability to manage the work of feeding. Research has shown that energy expenditure is typically lower when breastfeeding than when bottle feeding.[76-82]

4.   Poor intake: Weighted feeds on reliable scales are critical when assessing the intake of an unstable feeder.[83,84]

5.   Poor growth:

a.   An infant's weight loss of 10 percent by the 5th day after birth and a failure to promptly recover the birth weight are markers for suboptimal infant feeding behavior and indicate the need for evaluation.[85]

b.   Recent studies have highlighted the association between excess weight loss in breastfed infants and maternal intrapartum fluid balance.[86,87] Intrapartum fluid administration may result in an inaccurate baseline birth weight.[87] Further research into this association is ongoing.

6.   Feeding aversion: A feeding aversion can result from aspiration, respiratory compromise, choking, reflux, or sensory-based factors.[17] It can also result from negative oral experiences, such as medical procedures and stressful feedings.

▶ Key Points from This Chapter

A.   International Board Certified Lactation Consultants need to have a strong foundation on the basics of typical infant oral anatomy and physiology to identify when abnormal presentations occur and negatively impact breastfeeding.

B.   International Board Certified Lactation Consultants should also have a solid understanding of the following:

1.   Typical presentations of newborn reflexes and their relation to feeding

2.   Major components of the suckling cycle as part of the breastfeeding process

3.   Major components of suck–swallow–breathe coordination

4.   Indicators of poor-quality feeding

🔍 *CASE STUDY*

Diana brought twins Patricia and Ryan to be seen following an unremarkable pregnancy and vaginal birth (Ryan was born breech) at full term. APGAR scores were within normal limits and there were no other issues or concerns. The twins were discharged from the hospital exclusively breastfed. Collection of case and developmental history revealed that the twins' mother had successfully breastfed her first daughter past 2 years of age without latch or breastfeeding difficulties, weight gain concerns, or milk supply issues.

Breastfeeding reportedly continued to go well, without supplemental bottles or pacifiers, but breastfeeding was always painful and latch issues persisted. Diana was breastfeeding the twins on demand, often throughout the day and when they woke at night, without limiting how often they breastfed or how long they were at the breast. Around 4 months of age, weight gain began to slow. Between 6 and 9 months of age, Patricia gained only 6 oz, while Ryan gained only 12 oz, and they both exhibited difficulty transitioning to solids. At 9 months, Patricia pushed food out with her tongue when offered, and Ryan also gagged, coughed, and choked on larger and lumpier food textures. The pediatrician recommended formula supplementation. Diana did not want to supplement with formula and both infants would not bottle-feed.

At 9 months of age, the twins were referred by the pediatrician to a Speech-Language Pathologist who was also an International Board Certified Lactation Consultant for concerns related to slow weight gain and persistent breastfeeding challenges. The oral structures of both infants were examined. Patricia presented with a high, arched palate, while Ryan presented with a bubble-shaped palate and retrognathic chin. Both infants presented with Type 3 posterior ankyloglossia (tongue-tie) along with low-lying, thick, and restrictive maxillary frenulum. On examination, the infants' father was also observed to present with a posterior tongue-tie (PTT) and maxillary tie (note that diagnosing ankyloglossia and maxillary restrictions are within the scope of practice of a Speech-Language Pathologist [CCC-SLP]. Although it is not within the scope of practice of a lactation consultant, a lactation consultant can note oral assessment findings and observations and make recommendations for referral to a healthcare provider who is qualified to diagnose.)

Latch, breastfeeding efficiency, and milk transfer were then assessed. The twins both presented with a shallow latch and narrow gape on the breast. They slipped off the breast intermittently throughout feeding and both visibly and audibly lost suction multiple times. Feedings were prolonged and appeared inefficient as exhibited by reduced milk transfer. Diana reported that feedings were somewhat painful but manageable.

All observations were shared with the parents and referring pediatrician, and the following plan of care was provided:

- Recommendation for a consult with a specialist for assessment of both lingual and labial frenula to determine if frenotomy was warranted.
- Encouragement to Diana to continue to breastfeed babies on demand.
- Encouragement to Diana to continue to offer solids, particularly more mashable, easy-to-manage foods instead of foods with more challenging textures, especially for Ryan who appeared at risk for aspiration and/or choking.
- Recommendation to begin feeding therapy for continued management of breastfeeding, transition to solids, weight gain, and development for both babies.

Maxillary and lingual frenectomies were performed on both twins at 9.5 months of age by a pediatrician specializing in frenectomies. Within 1 month post-frenectomies, both infants gained over 2 lbs each. By 14 months of age, Patricia gained 4.4 lbs and was in the 14th percentile for weight (compared to 1st percentile on initial evaluation), and Ryan gained 6.8 lbs and was in the 31st percentile for weight (compared to 0 percentile on initial evaluation) (see **FIGURE 3-5A** and **FIGURE 3-5B**). Diana no longer felt nipple pain within days post-procedure. Observations revealed that both infants' latch appeared to improve almost immediately, with increased ability to maintain latch and improved gape and seal. Feedings were more efficient overall with milk transfer within normal range. In terms of solid foods, Patricia no longer pushed food out with her tongue and transitioned to solids with 1–2 additional feeding therapy sessions needed. Patricia was then discharged from feeding therapy with no further need for intervention. Ryan continued to improve with solids post-frenectomy, exhibiting significantly less gagging, coughing, and choking with solids. Both babies continued to breastfeed past 2 years of age.

Questions
1. What concerns within the infants' overall histories indicated a need for consult with a lactation consultant?
2. What major signs within feeding behaviors (breastfeeding and solids) indicated concerns for ankyloglossia?
3. What observations within the oral examinations supported those concerns?
4. What additional thoughts or recommendations do you have in addition to the ones listed?

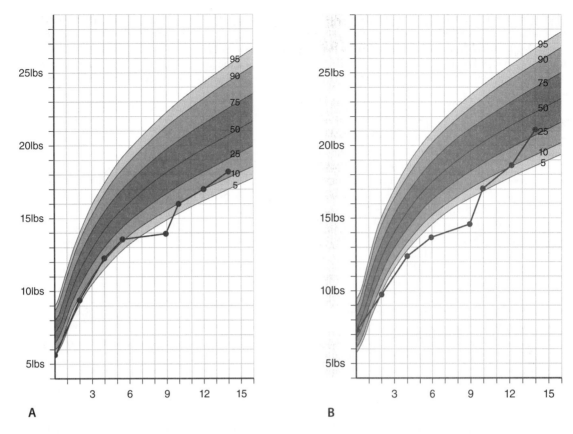

FIGURE 3-5 A. Growth trajectory for Patricia. **B.** Growth trajectory for Ryan.

Data from World Health Organization. The WHO child growth standards. http://www.who.int/childgrowth/standards/en/. Accessed January 9, 2018.[88]

References

1. Genna CW. *Supporting Sucking Skills in Breastfeeding Infants*. 3rd ed. Burlington, MA: Jones & Bartlett Learning; 2017.
2. Wolf L, Glass R. *Feeding and Swallowing Disorders in Infancy*. Tucson, AZ: Therapy Skill Builders; 1992.
3. Smith JD, Crumley RL, Harker LA. Facial paralysis in the newborn. *J Otolaryngol Head Neck Surg*. 1981;89:1021-1024.
4. Morris SE, Klein MD. *Pre-Feeding Skills*. 2nd ed. San Antonio, TX: Therapy Skill Builders; 2000.
5. Kotlow LA. Diagnosing and understanding the maxillary lip-tie (superior labial, the maxillary labial frenum) as it relates to breastfeeding. *J Hum Lactation*. 2013;29(4):458-464.
6. Ghaheri BA, Cole M, Fausel SC, Chuop M, Mace JC. Breastfeeding improvement following tongue-tie and lip-tie release: a prospective cohort study. *Laryngoscope*. 2016;127(5):1217-1223.
7. Benoiton L, Morgan M, Baguley K. Management of posterior ankyloglossia and upper lip ties in a tertiary otolaryngology outpatient clinic. *Int J Pediatr Otorhinolaryngol*. 2016;88:13-16.
8. Pransky SM, Lago D, Hong P. Breastfeeding difficulties and oral cavity anomalies: the influence of posterior ankyloglossia and upper-lip ties. *Int J Pediatr Otorhinolaryngol*. 2015;79:1714-1717.
9. Parker SE, Mai CT, Canfield MA, et al. Updated national birth prevalence estimates for selected birth defects in the United States, 2004–2006. *Birth Defects Res A Clin Mol Teratol*. 2010; 88(12):1008-1016.
10. Garcez LW, Giugliani ERJ. Population-based study on the practice of breastfeeding in children born with cleft lip and palate. *Cleft Palate Craniofac J*. 2005;42(6):687-693.
11. Sapin SO, Miller AA, Bass HN. Neonatal asymmetric crying facies: a new look at an old problem. *Clin Pediatr (Phila)*. 2005;44(2):109-119.
12. Alper BS, Manno CJ. Dysphagia in infants and children with oral-motor deficits: assessment and management. *Semin Speech Lang*. 1996;17(4):283-310.
13. Reilly S, Reid J, Skeat J, Cahir P, Mei C, Bunik, Academy of Breastfeeding Medicine. ABM clinical protocol # 17: guidelines for breastfeeding infants with cleft lip, cleft palate, or cleft lip and palate, revision 2013. *Breastfeed Med*. 2013;8:349-353.
14. Wilson-Clay B. *External Pacing Techniques: Protecting Respiratory Stability during Feeding* [independent study module]. Amarillo, TX: Pharmasoft Publishing; 2005.
15. Wolf L, Glass R. The Goldilocks problem: milk flow that is not too fast, not too slow, but just right. In: Genna CW, ed. *Supporting Sucking Skills in Breastfeeding Infants*. 2nd ed. Burlington, MA: Jones & Bartlett Learning; 2013:149-170.

16. Thomas J, Marinelli KA, Academy of Breastfeeding Medicine. ABM clinical protocol # 16: breastfeeding the hypotonic infant, revision 2016. *Breastfeed Med*. 2016;11:271-276.

17. Palmer MM, Crawley K, Blanco IA. Neonatal oral-motor assessment scale: a reliability study. *J Perinatol*. 1993;13(1):28-35.

18. Coquerelle M, Prados-Frutos JC, Benazzi S, et al. Infant growth patterns of the mandible in modern humans: a closer exploration of the developmental interactions between the symphyseal bone, the teeth, and the suprahyoid and tongue muscle insertion sites. *J Anat*. 2013;222(2):178-192.

19. Bull MJ, Givan DC, Sadove AM, Bixler D, Hearn D. Improved outcome in Pierre Robin sequence: effect of multidisciplinary evaluation and management. *Pediatrics*. 1990;86(2):294-301.

20. Wall V, Glass R. Mandibular asymmetry and breastfeeding problems: experience from 11 cases. *J Hum Lactation*. 2006;22(3):328-334.

21. Redstone F, West JF. The importance of postural control for feeding. *Pediatr Nurs*. 2004;30(2):97-100.

22. Elad E, Kozlovsky P, Blum O, et al. Biomechanics of milk extraction during breast-feeding. *Proc Natl Acad Sci USA*. 2014;111(14):5230-5235.

23. Iskander A, Sanders I. Morphological comparison between neonatal and adult human tongues. *Ann Otol Rhinol Laryngol*. 2003;112(9):768-776.

24. Hohoff A, Rabe H, Ehmer U, Harms E. Palatal development of preterm and low birthweight infants compared to term infants—what do we know? Part I: the palate of the term newborn. *Head Face Med*. 2005;1:8.

25. Wambach K, Riordan J. *Breastfeeding and Human Lactation*. 4th ed. Burlington, MA: Jones & Bartlett Learning; 2014.

26. Burton P, Deng J, McDonald D, Fewtrell MS. Real-time 3D ultrasound imaging of infant tongue movements during breast-feeding. *Early Hum Dev*. 2013;89(9):635-641.

27. Geddes DT, Sakalidis VS, Hepworth AR, et al. Tongue movement and intra-oral vacuum of term infants during breastfeeding and feeding from an experimental teat that released milk under vacuum only. *Early Hum Dev*. 2012;88(6):443-449.

28. Lalakea ML, Messner AH. Ankyloglossia: does it matter? *Pediatr Clin North Am*. 2003;50(2):381-397.

29. Messner AH, Lalakea ML, Aby J, Macmahon J, Bair E. Ankyloglossia: incidence and associated feeding difficulties. *Arch Otolaryngol Head Neck Surg*. 2000;126(1):36-39.

30. Coryllos E, Genna CW, Salloum A. Congenital tongue-tie and its impact on breastfeeding. In: American Academy of Pediatrics Section on Breastfeeding. *Breastfeeding: Best for Baby and Mother*. 2004;1-6.

31. Hong P, Lago D, Seargeant J, Pellman L, Magit AE, Pransky SM. Defining ankyloglossia: a case series of anterior and posterior tongue ties. *Int J Pediatr Otorhinolaryngol*. 2010;74(9):1003-1006.

32. Power RF, Murphy JF. Tongue-tie and frenotomy in infants with breastfeeding difficulties: achieving a balance. *Arch Dis Child*. 2015;100(5):489-494.

33. Ricke LA, Baker NJ, Madlon-Kay DJ, DeFor TA. Newborn tongue-tie: prevalence and effect on breast-feeding. *J Am Board Fam Pract*. 2005;18(1):1-7.

34. Ballard JL, Auer CE, Khoury JC. Ankyloglossia: assessment, incidence, and effect of frenuloplasty on the breastfeeding dyad. *Pediatrics*. 2004;110(5):e63.

35. Forlenza GP, Paradise Black NM, McNamara EG, Sullivan SE. Ankyloglossia, exclusive breastfeeding, and failure to thrive. *Pediatrics*. 2010;126(6):e1500-e1504.

36. Junqueira MA, Cunha NNO, Costa e Silva LL, et al. Surgical techniques for the treatment of ankyloglossia in children: a case series. *J Appl Oral Sci*. 2014;22(3):241-248.

37. Amir LH, James JP, Beatty J. Review of tongue-tie release at a tertiary maternity hospital. *J Paediatr Child Health*. 2005;41(5-6):243-245.

38. Buryk M, Bloom D, Shope T. Efficacy of neonatal release of ankyloglossia: a randomized trial. *Pediatrics*. 2011;128(2):280-288.

39. Ludwig SM. Oral feeding and the late preterm infant. *Newborn Infant Nurs Rev*. 2007;7(2):72-75.

40. Shaker C. Question about tongue tip elevation in the preterm infant. Pediatric Feeding News website. http://pediatricfeedingnews.com/question-about-tongue-tip-elevation-in-the-preterm-infant-by-catherine-shaker-msccc-slp-bcs-s/. Published August 3, 2014. Accessed June 1, 2017.

41. ACPA Family Services. Cleft and craniofacial educational materials. American Cleft Palate-Craniofacial Association website. http://cleftline.org/what_we_do/publications. Accessed November 13, 2017.

42. Bessell A, Hooper L, Shaw WC, Reilly S, Reid J, Glenny A-M. Feeding interventions for growth and development in infants with cleft lip, cleft palate, or cleft lip and palate. *Cochrane Database Syst Rev*. 2011;16(2):CD003315. doi:10.1002/14651858.CD003315.pub3.

43. Goldman AS. The immune system of human milk: antimicrobial, anti-inflammatory and immunomodulating properties. *Pediatr Infect Dis J*. 1993;12(8):664-671.

44. Paradise JL, Elster BA, Tan L. Evidence in infants with cleft palate that breast milk protects against otitis media. *Pediatrics*. 1994;94(6):853-860.

45. Snyder JB. Bubble palate and failure to thrive: a case report. *J Hum Lactation*. 1997;13(2):139-143.

46. Turner L, Jacobsen C, Humenczuk M, Singhal VK, Moore D, Bell H. The effects of lactation education and a prosthetic obturator appliance on feeding efficiency in infants with cleft lip and palate. *Cleft Palate Craniofac J*. 2001;38(5):519-524.

47. Lawrence RA, Lawrence RM. *Breastfeeding: A Guide for the Medical Profession*. 7th ed. Maryland Heights, MO: Mosby/Elsevier; 2011.

48. Eshete M, Camison L, Abate F, et al. Congenital palatal fistula associated with submucous cleft palate. *Plast Reconstr Surg Glob Open*. 2016;4(2):e613.

49. Masarei AG, Wade A, Mars M, Sommerlad BC, Sell D. A randomized control trial investigating the effect of presurgical orthopedics on feeding in infants with cleft lip and/or palate. *Cleft Palate Craniofac J*. 2007;44(2):182-193.

50. Tomita Y, Kuroda S, Nakanishi H, Tanaka E. Severity of alveolar cleft affects prognosis of infant orthopedics in complete unilateral cleft lip and palate: three-dimensional evaluation from cheiloplasty to palatoplasty. *J Craniofac Surg*. 2010;21(5):1503-1507.

51. Abrahams SW, Labbok MH. Breastfeeding and otitis media: a review of recent evidence. *Curr Allergy Asthma Rep*. 2011;11(6):508-512.

52. Abadie V, André A, Zaouche A, Thouvenin B, Baujat G, Schmitz J. Early feeding resistance: a possible consequence of neonatal oro-oesophageal dyskinesia. *Acta Paediatr*. 2001;90(7):738-745.

53. Bosma J. Structure and function of the infant oral and pharyngeal mechanisms. In: Wilson J, ed. *Oral-Motor Function and Dysfunction in Children*. Chapel Hill, NC: University of North Carolina at Chapel Hill; 1977:33-38.

54. Pooniya V, Pandey N. A novel approach to treatment of symptomatic deviated nasal septum in a newborn baby. *Int J Pediatr Otorhinolaryngology Extra.* 2012;7(3):147-8.

55. Harding C, Frank L, Botting N, Hilari K. Assessment and management of infant feeding. *Infant.* 2015;11(3):85-89.

56. Brown N, Spittle A. Neurobehavioral evaluation in the preterm and term infant. *Curr Pediatr Rev.* 2014;10(1):65-72.

57. Mizuno K, Ueda A. Changes in sucking performance from nonnutritive sucking to nutritive sucking during breast- and bottle-feeding. *Pediatr Res.* 2006;59(5):728-731.

58. Bamford O, Taciak V, Gewolb IH. The relationship between rhythmic swallowing and breathing during suckle feeding in term neonates. *Pediatr Res.* 1992;31(6):619-624.

59. Gray L, Miller LW, Philipp BL, Blass EM. Breastfeeding is analgesic in healthy newborns. *Pediatrics.* 2002;109(4):590-593.

60. Hauck FR, Herman SM, Donovan M, et al. Sleep environment and the risk of sudden infant death syndrome in an urban population: the Chicago infant mortality study. *Pediatrics.* 2003;111(5):1207-1214.

61. Kahn A, Groswasser J, Franco P, et al. Sudden infant deaths: stress, arousal and SIDS. *Early Hum Dev.* 2003;75:S147-S166.

62. Premji SS, Paes B. Gastrointestinal function and growth in premature infants: is non-nutritive sucking vital? *J Perinatol.* 2000;20(1):46-53.

63. AAP Task Force on Sudden Infant Death Syndrome. SIDS and other sleep-related infant deaths: updated 2016 recommendations for a safe infant sleeping environment. *Pediatrics.* 2016;138(5):e20162938.

64. McBride MC, Danner SC. Sucking disorders in neurologically impaired infants: assessment and facilitation of breastfeeding. *Clin Perinatol.* 1987;14(1):109-130.

65. Kent JC, Mitoulas L, Cox DB, Owens RA, Hartmann PE. Breast volume and milk production during extended lactation in women. *Exp Physiol.* 1999;84(2):435-447.

66. Ross MG, Nijland MJ. Fetal swallowing: relation to amniotic fluid regulation. *Clin Obstet Gynecol.* 1997;40(2):352-365.

67. Arvedson JC. *Interpretation of Videofluoroscopic Swallow Studies of Infants and Children: A Study Guide to Improve Diagnostic Skills and Treatment Planning.* Gaylord, MI: Northern Speech Services; 2006.

68. Thach BT. Maturation of cough and other reflexes that protect the fetal and neonatal airway. *Pulm Pharm & Therapeutics.* 2007;20(4):365-70.

69. Law-Morstatt L, Judd DM, Snyder P, Baier RJ, Dhanireddy R. Pacing as a treatment technique for transitional sucking patterns. *J Perinatol.* 2003;23(6):483-488.

70. Colson SD, Meek JH, Hawdon JM. Optimal positions for the release of primitive neonatal reflexes stimulating breastfeeding. *Early Hum Dev.* 2008;84(7):441-449.

71. Matthiesen AS, Ransjö-Arvidson AB, Nissen E, Uvnäs-Moberg K. Postpartum maternal oxytocin release by newborns: effects of infant hand massage and sucking. *Birth.* 2001;28(1):13-19.

72. Genna CW, Barak D. Facilitating autonomous infant hand use during breastfeeding. *Clin Lact.* 2010;1(1):15-20.

73. Sakalidis VS, Geddes DT. Suck-swallow-breathe dynamics in breastfed infants. *J Hum Lactation.* 2016;32(2):201-211.

74. Kelly BN, Huckabee M-L, Jones RD, Frampton CM. The first year of human life: coordinating respiration and nutritive swallowing. *Dysphagia.* 2007;22(1):37-43.

75. Lau C. Development of infant oral feeding skills: what do we know? *Am J Clin Nutr.* 2016;103(2):616S-621S.

76. Barbas KH, Kelleher DK. Breastfeeding success among infants with congenital heart disease. *Pediatr Nurs.* 2004;30(4):285-289.

77. Berger I, Weintraub V, Dollberg S, Kopolovitz R, Mandel D. Energy expenditure for breastfeeding and bottle-feeding preterm infants. *Pediatrics.* 2009;124(6):e1149-e1152.

78. Blaymore Bier JA, Ferguson AE, Morales Y, Liebling JA, Oh W, Vohr BR. Breastfeeding infants who were extremely low birth weight. *Pediatrics.* 1997;100(6):E3.

79. Chapman DJ, Berger RD, Weintraub I, Dollberg V, Kopolovitz S, Mandel D. Building the evidence base: preterm infants' energy expenditure after breastfeeding versus bottle-feeding. *J Human Lactation.* 2009;124:e1149-e1152.

80. Chen CH. The effect of breast- and bottle-feeding on oxygen saturation and body temperature in preterm infants. *J Hum Lactation.* 2000;16(1):21-27.

81. Jadcherla SR, Vijayapal AS, Leuthner S. Feeding abilities in neonates with congenital heart disease: a retrospective study. *J Perinatol.* 2009;29(2):112-118.

82. Lubetzky R, Vaisman N, Mimouni FB, Dollberg S. Energy expenditure in human milk- versus formula-fed preterm infants. *J Pediatr.* 2003;143(6):750-753.

83. Sachs M, Oddie S. Breastfeeding—weighing in the balance: reappraising the role of weighing babies in the early days. *MIDIRS Midwifery Digest.* 2002;12(3):296-300.

84. Scanlon KS, Alexander MP, Serdula MK, Davis MK, Bowman BA. Assessment of infant feeding: the validity of measuring milk intake. *Nutr Rev.* 2002;60(8):235-251.

85. Kellams A, Harrel C, Omage S, Gregory C, Rosen-Carole C, Academy of Breastfeeding Medicine. ABM clinical protocol# 3: supplementary feedings in the healthy term breastfed neonate, revised 2017. *Breastfeed Med.* 2017;2:188-198.

86. Chantry CJ, Nommsen-Rivers LA, Peerson JM, Cohen RJ, Dewey KG. Excess weight loss in first-born breastfed newborns relates to maternal intrapartum fluid balance. *Pediatrics.* 2011;127(1):e171-e179.

87. Noel-Weiss J, Woodend AK, Peterson WE, Gibb W, Groll DL. An observational study of associations among maternal fluids during parturition, neonatal output, and breastfed newborn weight loss. *Int Breastfeed J.* 2011;6:9.

88. World Health Organization. The WHO child growth standards. http://www.who.int/childgrowth/standards/en/. Accessed January 9, 2018.

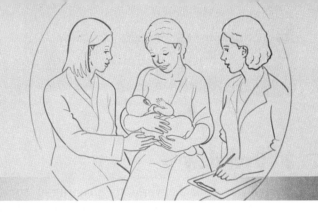

CHAPTER 4

Normal Infant Behavior

M. Jane Heinig
Jennifer Bañuelos

OBJECTIVES

- Explain how infant behavior may influence infant-feeding decisions.
- Describe the six infant states.
- Differentiate infant cues.
- List the reasons why infants may cry.
- Describe infant sleep patterns.

DEFINITIONS OF COMMONLY USED TERMS

active alert A state of frequent body and facial movements, irregular breathing, and open eyes.
active sleep A state of rapid eye movement, body and facial twitches, and irregular breathing.
crying A state of jerky movements, facial color changes, muscle tension, and rapid breathing.
disengagement cues Cues to communicate when the infant wants a change in activity, circumstances, or environment.
drowsy A state of variable body movement, irregular breathing, glazed eyes, and delayed reaction time.
engagement cues Cues to communicate the infant's desire to interact, play, or feed.
feeding cues Cues that communicate the infant's hunger.
infant behavioral states A group of behaviors that occur together, including degree and nature of body movement, eye movement, respirations, and responsiveness.
quiet alert A state of little body movement, open eyes, and steady, regular breathing.
quiet sleep A state of very little body or facial movement except occasional bursts of sucking.
regulation, entrainment, structure, touch (REST) An intervention associated with reduced daily crying and parental stress during early infancy.
repetition to soothe Interventions such as stroking, rocking, or speaking softly to infants using the same repeated words or phrases used to calm infants.
self-soothing behaviors Bringing hands to mouth and sucking.
sudden unexplained infant death (SUID) The sudden death of an infant less than 1 year of age that cannot be explained after a thorough investigation has occurred.

▶ Overview

In many areas of the world, the majority of women initiate breastfeeding, but the duration and exclusivity of breastfeeding remain low.[1-12] Although many factors influence infant-feeding decisions, perceived insufficient milk is reported to be one of the most common reasons for supplementing or weaning healthy breastfed infants.[13-17] Despite education about clinical indicators of sufficient milk production, parents of healthy, thriving infants may be convinced that their infants are not satisfied by their milk alone because of their infants' behaviors (such as crying and waking).[18-22] A misunderstanding of infants' broader cues may lead to feeding practices that are not responsive to the infants' needs, and these practices may increase the infants' risk for childhood obesity.[23,24] Given how frequently women report that their infants are not satisfied by their milk,[15,16,25-27] lactation consultants can be better prepared to promote and support exclusive breastfeeding when they are familiar with normal infant behavior. Lactation consultants can use education about normal baby behavior to help parents develop realistic expectations about parenting newborns and prevent unnecessary weaning.

I. The Six Infant Behavioral States

An infant state is indicated by a group of behaviors that occur together, including degree and nature of body movement, eye movement, respirations, and responsiveness.[28] Understanding infants' states and how and why infants move through these states can help lactation consultants engage parents who are seeking answers to questions about their infants' behavior and development.

A. There are six defined infant behavioral states.
   1. Crying infants have jerky movements, facial color changes, muscle tension, and rapid breathing. Newborns do not shed tears; infants' tear ducts typically are blocked until they are between 2 and 4 months of age. Initially, crying infants may not be responsive to caregiver efforts to calm them. Caregivers need to be reassured that it takes time to calm crying infants.[26,29]
   2. Infants in an active alert state have moderate to frequent body and facial movements, irregular breathing, and open eyes. They are sometimes fussy and sensitive to stimuli in the environment. The active alert state is common before feeding.[28]
   3. Infants in a quiet alert state have little body movement; their eyes are open and they have steady, regular breathing. Infants in the quiet alert state are highly responsive, and this is the best state for interaction and play with caregivers. It is challenging for young infants to maintain this state and, consequently, they may tire quickly.[28]
   4. Drowsy infants have variable body movement, irregular breathing, glazed eyes, and delayed reaction time. They may open and close their eyes. Typically, drowsy infants have limited interest in interaction.[28]
   5. Active sleep is characterized by rapid eye movement, body and facial twitches, and irregular breathing. Infants dream during active sleep, and they can be awakened easily while dreaming.[30,31]
   6. Quiet sleep results in very little body or facial movement except occasional bursts of sucking. Infants in quiet sleep may startle with movement or loud noises but typically do not wake. The baby's respirations are regular, and the body is relaxed. Infants in deep sleep may be difficult to wake.[30,31]
B. Infants gain increasing ability to regulate their behavioral states over the first few months of life.
   1. Newborns are challenged by a limited ability to shut out environmental stimuli (called habituation). Although some infants are born with more capacity to self-regulate their states, young infants' states are less predictable than those of older infants.[32]
   2. As soon as they are able to, infants may use a variety of self-soothing behaviors, including bringing their hands to their mouths, sucking, and providing cues to caregivers. However, the fact that infants attempt to console themselves does not imply that they should be left to cry. Rather, parents should allow their infants' efforts to self-soothe but step in quickly with consoling behaviors as soon as it is clear that the baby's self-soothing behaviors are not effective.[32,33]

3. Caregiver actions can assist with infants' efforts to regulate and change behavioral states.[32,33]
   a. Parents can be taught to use different positions, touch, or sounds to wake a sleepy infant; this approach is called *variety to waken*.[32] This process can take a significant amount of time with very sleepy babies, particularly those who are sleepy as a result of stress during birth or exposure to medications.
   b. Infants who are overstimulated or distressed respond well to sustained, low-level, repetitive stimulation. Interventions such as stroking, rocking, or speaking softly to infants using the same repeated words or phrases can be used to calm them; this approach is called *repetition to soothe*.[32] It may take several minutes to calm a crying infant who is very upset or very young.

II. Infant Communication

A. Infants use simple cues to communicate their needs to caregivers.
   1. Infants use engagement cues to communicate their desire to interact, play, or feed. Examples of these cues include open eyes; looking intently at the caregiver's face; following objects, voices, and faces with their eyes; relaxed face; smooth body movements; smiling; and feeding cues.[34]
   2. Infants use disengagement cues to communicate when they want a change in activity, circumstances, or environment. For example, infants often give disengagement cues such as turning or arching away when they are overwhelmed by an interaction. Other examples of disengagement cues include pushing away, crying, stiff hands and arms, grimacing, yawning, or falling asleep.[34]
   3. Infants use multiple cues at the same time to indicate important needs such as hunger or satiation.
      a. Newborns who are hungry demonstrate feeding cues, including clenching their fingers and fists over their chest and tummy, flexing their arms and legs, mouthing or rooting, quickening their breathing, and making sucking noises and motions.[35-37]
      b. Healthy, thriving infants who are full may extend their arms and legs, turn or push away from the breast, arch their back, slow (decrease) or stop sucking, or fall asleep.[36,38] If these behaviors are seen early during feeding or in an infant who is not gaining enough weight, a further evaluation of milk transfer is necessary.
      c. Although feeding cues are apparent almost immediately after birth in healthy full-term infants, these cues are modified both by caregiver responsiveness and over time as the infant's motor control and communication skills improve.[36] When caregivers are not responsive to feeding cues or these cues are overridden, infants' abilities to self-regulate intake may be compromised, resulting in poor growth or greater risk for obesity.[39]
   4. Although parents' brains are wired to be responsive to their infants' cues, these cues are nonspecific.[33] Parents may need to investigate the reasons behind the cues to determine how best to meet the baby's needs. When cues are not addressed promptly, infants may escalate the cue to obtain or redirect caregiver attention.[28] For example, overstimulated infants may first turn their faces away from interactions with excited siblings. If the child continues to engage the infant, the infant may escalate the cue by twisting away, arching away, or starting to cry.
B. Crying is an important way for infants to communicate their needs.
   1. Crying is a common and normal part of infancy. Infants use crying as a powerful way to communicate their distress[40] and to drive caregiver activity.[41,42] There is enormous variation in crying behavior from baby to baby, and even from day to day for each baby. Therefore, it is not possible to determine the amount or duration of normal crying during infancy.[40]
   2. Infants cry for many reasons, although caregivers may believe that infants cry predominantly because of hunger.[20,43] This belief may result in weaning from the breast if parents believe that crying indicates their infant is not satisfied by breast milk.[15,21,26]
      a. Infants cry when they are uncomfortable (e.g., if they have a wet or dirty diaper, are too hot or too cold, need to be burped, or are sick or hungry).
      b. They may cry when they need a change in their environment (e.g., when they are overstimulated by too much noise or too many new faces).
      c. Crying infants may need quiet time, to be close to their parents, or a break from stimulation.

3. If parents respond quickly and effectively to infant cues, crying may be minimized, thereby reducing related parent stress.[32,40]

   a. Parental concerns about infant crying may result in a significant burden on the healthcare system, leading to approximately 20 percent of pediatric consultations in the first 3 months of life.[44]

   b. Anticipatory guidance for new parents about infant crying may reduce associated healthcare costs. In a recent study, education about normal patterns of infant crying significantly reduced unnecessary emergency department visits for crying complaints.[45]

4. In the past, excessive crying was referred to as colic.

   a. The classification of crying as excessive is highly subjective and related to parents' cultural norms, their expectations of how infants should behave, and the characteristics of the infant.[40,44,46]

   b. Self-efficacy may play a mediating role in both the amount of infant crying and parents' response to excessive crying.[47]

   c. The subjective nature of the classification has contributed to a wide range of prevalence estimates for excessive crying, ranging from 14 to 30 percent among infants in the first 12 weeks.[44] Many researchers use the terms *persistent crying* or *problem crying* to describe daily inconsolable crying.[26,48,49]

5. Persistent crying is rarely associated with an organic cause,[26] and the evidence related to the effectiveness of treatment regimens is sparse and inconsistent.[50]

   a. Persistent crying is one of the most frequent reasons why parents seek medical care. In extreme cases, it may be associated with dysfunctional patterns of interactions with caregivers, maternal depression, or child abuse.[40,42,44,51]

   b. Although gastrointestinal distress is most often ascribed by caregivers as the cause of persistent crying, objective evidence does not support this association in the majority of cases. Multiple biopsychosocial factors are likely involved.[40,44,50,52]

   c. Although many interventions for excessive crying have been suggested and tested, the complex nature of the etiology surrounding persistent crying precludes the identification of a one-size-fits-all approach.[44]

6. Repetitive, sustained stimuli may be used to reduce crying.[32]

   a. When infants continue to cry despite parents' efforts to address the immediate issue (such as a wet diaper, hunger, or fatigue), the use of repetition to soothe, such as rocking, singing, or stroking, may reduce the infant's level of stimulation and calm the infant.[32]

   b. Carrying a crying infant is particularly effective for calming the infant. It potentially taps into neurophysiologic responses typically found in mammalian species.[53]

   c. An extensive intervention called regulation, entrainment, structure, touch (REST) has been associated with reduced daily crying and reduced parental stress during the early infancy period.[49]

III. Infant Sleep

A. Researchers have described two primary sleep states: active sleep (also called light sleep) and quiet sleep (also called deep sleep).

   1. Active sleep:

      a. Dreaming occurs during active sleep, resulting in rapid eye movement, body and facial twitches, and irregular breathing.[32,54]

      b. During active sleep, blood flow to the brain is increased and neural cells are stimulated, contributing to brain growth and development.[30,31]

      c. Infants are easily awakened during active sleep periods.[30,55] The ability to awaken easily is considered important for babies' health and safety, given that an inability to rouse a baby may be associated with sudden unexpected infant death (SUID).[56]

   2. Quiet sleep (nonactive):

      a. During quiet sleep, infants exhibit little body or facial movement other than short bursts of sucking and startle responses. Their breathing is regular,[54] and they are more difficult to rouse than infants in light sleep.[55]

        b.   During quiet sleep, most infants sleep deeply and can resist environmental stimuli. This restorative state is important for accruing the energy required for interacting and feeding when the infant awakens.[28,31] Quiet sleep also plays a role in memory development.[57]

B.   Infants have several types of sleep patterns.

    1.   Newborns sleep an average of 16 to 17 hours, and older infants sleep about 13 to 14 hours, per 24-hour period.[55,58]

        a.   Initially, newborns may wake with each cycle, or every 1 to 3 hours.[31] This frequency of waking may surprise and concern parents of healthy newborns.

        b.   When assessing the quality of their infants' sleep, many parents overemphasize the frequency of waking to be one of the most important indicators and are unaware of age-appropriate sleep patterns.[58]

    2.   Infants' sleep cycles differ from those of adults, and the cycles change as infants get older.

        a.   Adult sleep cycles are 90 to 110 minutes long, whereas infant sleep cycles are about 60 minutes long.[31,54] When adults first transition to sleep, they go through multiple stages of nonrapid eye movement (NREM) sleep into deep sleep, transitioning periodically into rapid eye movement (REM) sleep and back to deep sleep over the course of a night.[30,31,59]

        b.   Newborn sleep stages are described more simply as active, indeterminate, or nonactive. Newborns enter active sleep (which includes dreaming and REM), and after about 20 to 30 minutes, they transition into nonactive sleep.[30,31] During periods of active sleep, infants' small and large muscles may twitch and move because motor activity is not inhibited in early infancy, as it is in older children and adults during REM sleep.[31]

        c.   Between age 3 and 5 months, infants begin sleep in quiet (nonactive) sleep, as adults do, and night waking decreases.[31,54] The sleep states become more consistent, and the percentage of total sleep spent in quiet sleep increases from 50 percent in newborns, to 60 percent in infants aged 3–5 months, to 70–75 percent at 1 year of age.[30,31,54]

    3.   Although infants' physiology contributes to individual variation in the duration of sleep,[60] their typical longest stretch of sleep increases with age. The following averages may be useful as a guideline, but parents should be cautioned against trying to influence their infants' natural sleeping patterns to meet an arbitrary norm.[60]

        a.   By 2 to 6 weeks of age, most infants sleep 2 to 4 hours at one time. At approximately 6 to 8 weeks of age, infants' sleep becomes more concentrated during the nighttime because they are more awake during the day.[30,59,61]

        b.   By 3 months of age, infants' sleep–wake periods consolidate, and their circadian rhythms follow the light–dark cycle as circadian-driven hormones, such as cortisol and melatonin, become endogenously produced.[30,58,61] Infants are able to sleep about 4 to 5 hours at one time, and typically the longest stretch is during the nighttime.[59,62]

        c.   By 6 months of age, babies may be able to sleep up to 6 or 8 hours at one time.[59,62,63] In one study, 90 percent of 6-month-old infants "slept regularly through the night" (defined as sleeping 6 hours without waking but not necessarily every night).[64(p97)] In another study of the same age group, 53 percent of 6-month olds were sleeping 8 hours for a minium of 5 out of 6 nights.[63] Sleeping and waking patterns may change again among older infants.

    4.   There are several benefits of periodic waking.

        a.   Night waking may be essential to young infants' health.[65]

            i.   An infant's ability to arouse during sleep is important to signal parents about unmet needs, such as hunger, discomfort, or temperature control.

            ii.   As infants get older, they typically require less adult intervention at night because, when they are physiologically ready to do so, they develop the ability to return to sleep after waking.[60,62]

        b.   Very young infants who have long periods of quiet sleep are at greater risk for SUID, possibly because their arousal thresholds increase with time spent in quiet sleep.[60,65]

        c.   Night waking is beneficial for breastfeeding parents because nighttime feedings help build and maintain milk production, reduce the risk of hormone-related cancers,[66] and delay menstruation.[67]

    5.   Infants with unexplained frequent waking should be referred to an appropriate medical professional.

        a.   The following infant-related conditions may affect infants' abilities to maintain sleep states:

            i.   In infants with physical immaturity, such as prematurity, a lack of brain maturation influences infant sleep states and patterns. Preterm infants sleep more total hours than term infants do, but they wake more often and have shorter sustained bouts of sleep. Preterm infants are more likely than term infants to have a limited ability to control and maintain active and quiet sleep states.[32,68]

    ii.   Ineffective or poor feeding may result in lower intakes and shorter intervals between feedings. A feeding assessment should be considered when parents report excessive infant waking. Also, infants need to be in an alert state to feed effectively. A lack of alertness during feedings can lead to difficulty with infants' coordination of sucking, swallowing, and breathing, which are needed to feed effectively.[32]

    iii.   Discomfort caused by symptoms of common illnesses, such as congestion or pain from an ear infection, or minor injuries may cause an infant to wake more often than expected. The sleep disturbance may continue until the illness or injury is resolved.[69,70]

  b.   The following external factors also influence infant sleep states:

    i.   The increase in stimulation from having a television on, or other interruptions in the room where the infant sleeps, may cause increased arousals, especially during active sleep phases. Some infants are more sensitive to lights and sounds. These infants must expend needed energy trying to shut out external stimuli during sleep.[28,60,71]

    ii.   A breastfeeding parent's caffeine intake can disrupt the infant's sleep. The transfer of caffeine to milk is low, but caffeine accumulates in the infant because of the infant's limited ability to metabolize it.[72] Six to eight cups of caffeinated beverages per day have been linked to infant hyperactivity and short sleep duration.[73]

C.   Feeding impacts infants' sleep.

  1.   Many studies of infant sleep lack information related to feeding method,[58] rely on the parents' reports rather than objective measurements,[58,62] include only small numbers of infants, or have inconsistent definitions of the duration or timing of the term *nighttime*.[55,74]

  2.   The question of whether breastfed or formula-fed infants wake more often is controversial, and studies have yielded mixed results.

    a.   Infant feeding may influence the pattern of infants' sleep cycles. Breastfed infants have more active sleep and, therefore, are more likely to wake if they are uncomfortable or need parental assistance. One study reported that breastfed infants were more likely to wake in active sleep than formula-fed infants at 2 to 3 months of age.[65]

    b.   Several studies report no differences between breastfeeding and formula-feeding groups with regard to night waking, self-soothing, or sleep duration.

      i.   No significant differences were reported in studies that collected parents' reports of total infant sleep[75,76] or night awakenings[77,78] by feeding method.

      ii.   No difference was found between formula-fed and breastfed infants in nighttime waking at 3 months, as measured by infrared video recordings,[79] or in sleep period length at 2–4 weeks, 2–3 months, and 5–6 months in a study that used polysomnography.[65]

    c.   Other studies reported differences in night waking and total sleep duration by feeding method.[80-82]

      i.   One study reported that breastfed infants between the ages of 2 weeks and 4 months showed more total sleep but shorter stretches of sleep than formula-fed infants. In addition, formula-fed infants cried more frequently in the evenings and at night, suggesting increased awakenings for parental assistance.[82]

      ii.   Another study reported that awakenings in breastfed infants at 1 and 3 months of age remained consistent, whereas awakenings of formula-fed infants dropped at 3 months of age.[80]

  3.   Studies indicate little or no difference in the parent's sleep, whether infants are breastfed or formula fed.

    a.   Some studies found that breastfeeding mothers got more total sleep than mothers who fed formula to their infants.[83-85]

      i.   One study found that although there was no difference in self-reported sleep duration, direct observations indicated that mothers who exclusively breastfed their infants slept 45 to 47 minutes longer at night than those who supplemented with formula.[83]

      ii.   The same study reported that at 1 month postpartum, mothers who were exclusively breastfeeding slept about 30 minutes more at night than formula-feeding mothers but there were no differences in daytime sleep, sleep fragmentation, or subjective disturbances between groups.[83]

   b. Other studies indicate no difference in parental sleep or fatigue by feeding method.[86-88]

     i. One study found that breastfeeding and formula-feeding mothers had comparable total sleep times, but breastfeeding mothers were awake longer during the night.[87]

     ii. Another study reported that there was no difference in maternal postpartum fatigue by feeding method at 4 and 16 weeks postpartum.[88]

  4. Parents may assume that adding cereal to feedings will increase infant sleep;[43,89-92] however, research does not support this belief.

   a. Two thirds of the mothers (44 breastfeeding and 33 formula feeding) in a small study thought that adding cereal to their infants' feeding would increase their sleep duration. However, the intervention showed no significant difference in sleep duration, number of night wakings (midnight to 5 a.m.), or minutes awake during the night (midnight to 5 a.m.) among infants who were fed rice cereal at night, compared to the control group (no cereal at night).[93]

   b. Another study indicates that cereal added to bottles of formula or human milk did not influence sleep patterns. At 7 weeks of age, infants who were not given cereal were more likely to sleep 8 hours at night.[75]

▶ Key Points from This Chapter

A. Parents of healthy, thriving infants may be convinced that their infants are not satisfied by their milk alone because of their infants' behaviors (such as crying and waking).

B. Lactation consultants can use an understanding of infants' states to engage parents who seek answers to questions about their infants' behavior and development.

C. Infants who are overstimulated or distressed respond well to sustained, low-level, repetitive stimulation.

D. Infants use engagement cues to communicate their desire to interact, play, or feed and disengagement cues to communicate when they want a change in activity, circumstances, or environment.

E. Active and quiet sleep are important for infants' development.

F. Infants are easily awakened during active sleep periods. The ability to awaken easily is considered important for babies' health and safety.

🔍 CASE STUDY

You are working with the mother of 6-day old Katrina. Katrina's mother Alanna fed her first child formula, but has chosen to breastfeed Katrina. Her pediatric follow-up (day 4) showed that Katrina had lost less than 3 percent of birthweight and was within normal limits on all assessments. However, Katrina is fussy almost every afternoon and Alanna is feeling frustrated, saying "I just don't have enough milk to keep her happy. My first child was on the bottle and that was fine. This is too much. I don't know how people do this."

Questions
1. What information does Alanna need to know about Katrina's behavior?
2. Why do you think Katrina is crying frequently in the afternoon?
3. How will you start the conversation with Alanna?
4. How will you share information with Alanna about Katrina's behavior?

References

1. Agboado G, Michel E, Jackson E, Verma A. Factors associated with breastfeeding cessation in nursing mothers in a peer support programme in eastern Lancashire. *BMC Pediatr.* 2010;10:3.
2. Al-Hreashy F, Tamim H, Eldemerdash A, et al. Patterns of breastfeeding practice during the first 6 months of life in Saudi Arabia. *Saudi Med J.* 2008;29(3):427-431.
3. Chalmers B, Levitt C, Heaman M, O'Brien B, Sauve R, Kaczorowski J. Breastfeeding rates and hospital breastfeeding practices in Canada: a national survey of women. *Birth.* 2009;36(2):122-132.
4. Cramton R, Zain-Ul-Abideen M, Whalen B. Optimizing successful breastfeeding in the newborn. *Curr Opinion Pediatr.* 2009;21(3):386-396.
5. Dashti M, Scott J, Edwards C, Al-Sughayer M. Determinants of breastfeeding initiation among mothers in Kuwait. *Int Breastfeeding J.* 2010;5:7.

6. Gill S. Breastfeeding by Hispanic women. *J Obstet Gynecol Neonatal Nurs*. 2009;8(2):244-252.

7. Hauck Y, Fenwick J, Dhaliwal S, Butt J. A western Australian survey of breastfeeding initiation, prevalence and early cessation patterns. *Maternal Child Health J*. 2011;15(2):260-268.

8. Henninger M, Irving S, Naleway A, et al. Predictors of breastfeeding initiation and maintenance in an integrated healthcare setting. *J Hum Lactation*. 2017;33(2):256-266.

9. Ryan A, Zhou W. Lower breastfeeding rates persist among the special supplemental nutrition program for women, infants, and children participants, 1978-2003. *Pediatrics*. 2006;117(4):1136-1146.

10. Thomson J, Tussing-Humphreys L, Goodman M, Landry A, Olender S. Low rate of initiation and short duration of breastfeeding in a maternal and infant home visiting project targeting rural, southern, African American women. *Int Breastfeeding J*. 2017;12:15.

11. Walker M. International breastfeeding initiatives and their relevance to the current state of breastfeeding in the United States. *J Midwifery Womens Health*. 2007;52(6):549-555.

12. Wallenborn J, Ihongbe T, Rozario S, Masho S. Knowledge of breastfeeding recommendations and breastfeeding duration: a survival analysis on infant feeding practices II. *Breastfeeding Med*. 2017;12:156-162.

13. Balogun O, Dagvadorj A, Anigo K, Ota E, Sasaki S. Factors influencing breastfeeding exclusivity during the first 6 months of life in developing countries: a quantitative and qualitative systematic review. *Maternal Child Nutr*. 2015;11(4):433-451.

14. Bunik M, Shobe P, Kempe A, et al. Are 2 weeks of daily breastfeeding support insufficient to overcome the influences of formula? *Academic Pediatr*. 2010;10(1):21-28.

15. Galipeau R, Dumas L, Lepage M. Perception of not having enough milk and actual milk production of first-time breastfeeding mothers: is there a difference? *Breastfeeding Med*. 2017;12:210-217.

16. Gatti L. Maternal perceptions of insufficient milk supply in breastfeeding. *J Nurs Scholarship*. 2008;40(4):355-363.

17. Kent J, Gardner H, Geddes D. Breastmilk production in the first 4 weeks after birth of term infants. *Nutrients*. 2016;8(12):756.

18. Donath S, Amir L. Breastfeeding and the introduction of solids in Australian infants: data from the 2001 national health survey. *Aust N Z J Public Health*. 2005;29(2):171-175.

19. Grummer-Strawn L, Scanlon K, Fein S. Infant feeding and feeding transitions during the first year of life. *Pediatrics*. 2008;122(suppl 2):S36-S42.

20. Heinig M, Follett J, Ishii K, Kavanagh-Prochaska K, Cohen R, Panchula J. Barriers to compliance with infant-feeding recommendations among low-income women. *J Hum Lactation*. 2006;22(1):27-38.

21. Jacknowitz A, Novillo D, Tiehen L. Special supplemental nutrition program for women, infants, and children and infant feeding practices. *Pediatrics*. 2007;119(2):281-289.

22. Pierro J, Abulaimoun B, Roth P, Blau J. Factors associated with supplemental formula feeding of breastfeeding infants during postpartum hospital stay. *Breastfeeding Med*. 2016;11:196-202.

23. Birch L. Learning to eat: behavioral and psychological aspects. *Nestle Nutr Institute Workshop Series*. 2016;85:125-134.

24. McNally J, Hugh-Jones S, Caton S, Vereijken C, Weenen H, Hetherington M. Communicating hunger and satiation in the first 2 years of life: a systematic review. *Maternal Child Nutr*. 2016;12(2):205-228.

25. Gross R, Fierman A, Messito M, et al. Maternal perceptions of infant hunger, satiety, and pressuring feeding styles in an urban Latina WIC population. *Academic Pediatr*. 2010;10(1):29-35.

26. Hiscock H. The crying baby. *Aust Fam Physician*. 2006;35(9):680.

27. Hodges E, Hughes S, Hopkinson J, Fisher J. Maternal decisions about the initiation and termination of infant feeding. *Appetite*. 2008;50(2-3):333-339.

28. Nugent J. *Understanding Newborn Behavior & Early Relationships: The Newborn Behavioral Observations (NBO) System Handbook*. Baltimore, MD: Brookes Pub; 2007.

29. Howard C, Lanphear N, Lanphear B, Eberly S, Lawrence R. Parental responses to infant crying and colic: the effect on breastfeeding duration. *Breastfeeding Med*. 2006;1(3):146-155.

30. Peirano P, Algarín C, Uauy R. Sleep-wake states and their regulatory mechanisms throughout early human development. *J Pediatr*. 2003;143(suppl 4):S70-S79.

31. Bathory E, Tomopoulos S. Sleep regulation, physiology and development, sleep duration and patterns, and sleep hygiene in infants, toddlers, and preschool-age children. *Curr Problems Pediatr Adolesc Health Care*. 2017;47(2):29-42.

32. Barnard K. Keys to developing early parent–child relationships. In: Lester B, Sparrow J, ed. *Nurturing Children and Families*. Malden, MA: Blackwell Publishing; 2010:53-63.

33. Young K, Parsons C, Stark E, Stein A, Kringelbach M. Understanding the human parental brain: a critical role of the orbitofrontal cortex. *Soc Neurosci*. 2013;8(6):525-543.

34. White C, Simon M, Bryan A. Using evidence to educate birthing center nursing staff about infant states, cues, and behaviors. *MCN. Am J Maternal Child Nurs*. 2002;27(5):294-298.

35. Hetherington M. Understanding infant eating behaviour—lessons learned from observation. *Physiol Behav*. 2017;176:117-124.

36. Hodges E, Wasser H, Colgan B, Bentley M. Development of feeding cues during infancy and toddlerhood. *MCN. Am J Maternal Child Nurs*. 2016;41(4):244-251.

37. Rochat P, Hespos SJ. Differential rooting response by neonates: evidence for an early sense of self. *Early Dev Parenting*. 1997;6:105-112.

38. Pridham K, Knight C, Stephenson G. Mothers' working models of infant feeding: description and influencing factors. *J Adv Nurs*. 1989;14(12):1051-1061.

39. DiSantis K, Hodges E, Johnson S, Fisher J. The role of responsive feeding in overweight during infancy and toddlerhood: a systematic review. *Int J Obes*. 2011;35(4):480-492.

40. Evanoo G. Infant crying: a clinical conundrum. *J Pediatr Health Care*. 2007;21(5):333-338.

41. Crockenberg S. Infant irritability, mother responsiveness, and social support influences on the security of infant-mother attachment. *Child Dev*. 1981;52(3):857-865.

42. Kurth E, Spichiger E, Cignacco E, et al. Predictors of crying problems in the early postpartum period. *J Obstet Gynecol Neonatal Nurs.* 2010;39(3):250-262.

43. Harrison M, Brodribb W, Hepworth J. A qualitative systematic review of maternal infant feeding practices in transitioning from milk feeds to family foods. *Maternal Child Nutr.* 2017;13(2). [Epub ahead of print]. doi: 10.1111/mcn.12360.

44. Halpern R, Coelho R. Excessive crying in infants. *Jornal De Pediatria.* 2016;92(3 suppl 1):S40-S45.

45. Barr R, Rajabali F, Aragon M, Colbourne M, Brant R. Education about crying in normal infants is associated with a reduction in pediatric emergency room visits for crying complaints. *J Dev Behav Pediatr: JDBP.* 2015;36(4):252-257.

46. Leavitt A. Infant crying: expectations and parental response. In: Barr R, St. James-Roberts I, eds. *New Evidence on Unexplained Early Infant Crying: Its Origins, Nature, and Management.* Langhorne, PA: Johnson and Johnson Pediatric Institute; 2001:43-50.

47. Bolten M, Fink N, Stadler C. Maternal self-efficacy reduces the impact of prenatal stress on infant's crying behavior. *J Pediatr.* 2012;161(1):104-109.

48. Douglas P, Hiscock H. The unsettled baby: crying out for an integrated, multidisciplinary primary care approach. *Med J Aust.* 2010;193(9):533-536.

49. Keefe M, Kajrlsen K, Lobo M, Kotzer A, Dudley W. Reducing parenting stress in families with irritable infants. *Nurs Res.* 2006;55(3): 198-205.

50. Biagioli E, Tarasco V, Lingua C, Moja L, Savino F. Pain-relieving agents for infantile colic. *Cochrane Database Syst Rev.* 2016;9:CD009999. doi: 10.1002/14651858.CD009999.pub2.

51. Kurth E, Kennedy H, Spichiger E, Hösli I, Stutz E. Crying babies, tired mothers: what do we know? A systematic review. *Midwifery.* 2011;27(2):187-194.

52. Chua C, Setlik J, Niklas V. Emergency department triage of the "incessantly crying" baby. *Pediatr Ann.* 2016;45(11):e394-e398.

53. Esposito G, Setoh P, Yoshida S, Kuroda K. The calming effect of maternal carrying in different mammalian species. *Frontiers Psychol.* 2015;6:445.

54. Heraghty J, Hilliard T, Henderson A, Fleming P. The physiology of sleep in infants. *Arch Dis Child.* 2008;93(11):982-985.

55. Rosen LA. Infant sleep and feeding. *J Obstet Gynecol Neonatal Nurs.* 2008;37(6):706-714.

56. American Academy of Pediatrics. The changing concept of sudden infant death syndrome: diagnostic coding shifts, controversies regarding the sleeping environment, and new variables to consider in reducing risk. *Pediatrics* [serial online]. 2005;116(5):1245-1255.

57. Graven S, Browne J. Sleep and brain development: the critical role of sleep in fetal and early neonatal brain development. *Newborn Infant Nurs Rev.* 2008;8(4):173-179.

58. Galland B, Taylor B, Elder D, Herbison P. Normal sleep patterns in infants and children: a systematic review of observational studies. *Sleep Med Rev.* 2012;16(3):213-222.

59. Coons S, Guilleminault C. Development of consolidated sleep and wakeful periods in relation to the day/night cycle in infancy. *Dev Med Child Neurol.* 1984;26(2):169-176.

60. Whittingham K, Douglas P. Optimizing parent-infant sleep from birth to 6 months: a new paradigm. *Infant Ment Health J.* 2014;35(6):614-623.

61. Jenni O, LeBourgeois M. Understanding sleep-wake behavior and sleep disorders in children: the value of a model. *Curr Opinion Psychiatry.* 2006;19(3):282-287.

62. Goodlin-Jones B, Burnham M, Gaylor E, Anders T. Night waking, sleep-wake organization, and self-soothing in the first year of life. *J Dev Behav Pediatr.* 2001;22(4):226-233.

63. Henderson J, France K, Owens J, Blampied N. Sleeping through the night: the consolidation of self-regulated sleep across the first year of life. *Pediatrics.* 2010;126(5):e1081-e1087.

64. Adams S, Jones D, Esmail A, Mitchell E. What affects the age of first sleeping through the night? *J Paediatr Child Health.* 2004;40(3): 96-101.

65. Horne R, Parslow P, Ferens D, Watts A, Adamson T. Comparison of evoked arousability in breast and formula fed infants. *Arch Dis Childhood.* 2004;89(1):22-25.

66. Heinig M, Dewey K. Health effects of breast feeding for mothers: a critical review. *Nutr Res Rev.* 1997;10(1):35-56.

67. Heinig M, Nommsen-Rivers L, Peerson J, Dewey K. Factors related to duration of postpartum amenorrhoea among USA women with prolonged lactation. *J Biosoc Sci.* 1994;26(4):517-527.

68. Trachtenbarg D, Golemon T. Care of the premature infant: part I. Monitoring growth and development. *Am Fam Physician.* 1998;57(9):2123-2130.

69. Sadeh A, Anders T. Infant sleep problems: origins, assessment, interventions. *Infant Ment Health J.* 1993;14(1):17-34.

70. Tirosh E, Scher A, Sadeh A, Jaffe M, Rubin A, Lavie P. The effects of illness on sleep behaviour in infants. *Eur J Pediatr.* 1993;152(1):15-17.

71. Field T. Infant sleep problems and interventions: a review. *Infant Behav Dev.* 2017;47:40-53.

72. Hale T, Rowe H. *Medications and Mothers' Milk 2017.* New York, NY: Springer Publishing Company; 2016.

73. Lawrence R, Lawrence R. *Breastfeeding: A Guide for the Medical Professional.* Maryland Heights, MO: Elsevier Mosby; 2010.

74. Figueiredo B, Dias C, Pinto T, Field T. Infant sleep-wake behaviors at two weeks, three and six months. *Infant Behav Dev.* 2016;44:169-178.

75. Macknin M, Medendorp S, Maier M. Infant sleep and bedtime cereal. *Am J Dis Children.* 1989;143(9):1066-1068.

76. Quillin S. Infant and mother sleep patterns during 4th postpartum week. *Issues Compr Pediatr Nurs.* 1997;20(2):115-123.

77. Alley J, Rogers C. Sleep patterns of breast-fed and nonbreast-fed infants. *Pediatr Nurs.* 1986;12(5):349-351.

78. Anders T, Halpern L, Hua J. Sleeping through the night: a developmental perspective. *Pediatrics.* 1992;90(4):554-560.

79. St James-Roberts I, Roberts M, Hovish K, Owen C. Video evidence that London infants can resettle themselves back to sleep after waking in the night, as well as sleep for long periods, by 3 months of age. *J Dev Behav Pediatr.* 2015;36(5):324-329.

80. Ball H. Breastfeeding, bed-sharing, and infant sleep. *Birth.* 2003;30(3):181-188.

81. Elias M, Nicolson N, Bora C, Johnston J. Sleep/wake patterns of breast-fed infants in the first 2 years of life. *Pediatrics.* 1986;77(3):322-329.

82. Lee K. Crying and behavior pattern in breast- and formula-fed infants. *Early Hum Dev.* 2000;58(2):133-140.

83. Doan T, Gardiner A, Gay C, Lee K. Breast-feeding increases sleep duration of new parents. *J Perinat Neonatal Nurs.* 2007;21(3):200-206.

84. Doan T, Gay C, Kennedy H, Newman J, Lee K. Nighttime breastfeeding behavior is associated with more nocturnal sleep among first-time mothers at one month postpartum. *J Clin Sleep Med.* 2014;10(3):313-319.

85. Kendall-Tackett K, Cong Z, Hale T. The effect of feeding method on sleep duration, maternal well-being, and postpartum depression. *Clin Lactation.* 2011;2(2):22-26.

86. Brown A, Harries V. Infant sleep and night feeding patterns during later infancy: association with breastfeeding frequency, daytime complementary food intake, and infant weight. *Breastfeeding Med.* 2015;10(5):246-252.

87. Gay C, Lee K, Lee S. Sleep patterns and fatigue in new mothers and fathers. *Biol Res Nurs.* 2004;5(4):311-318.

88. Tobback E, Behaeghel K, Hanoulle I, et al. Comparison of subjective sleep and fatigue in breast- and bottle-feeding mothers. *Midwifery.* 2017;47:22-27.

89. Clayton H, Li R, Perrine C, Scanlon K. Prevalence and reasons for introducing infants early to solid foods: variations by milk feeding type. *Pediatrics.* 2013;131(4):e1108-e1114.

90. Crocetti M, Dudas R, Krugman S. Parental beliefs and practices regarding early introduction of solid foods to their children. *Clin Pediatr.* 2004;43(6):541-547.

91. Horodynski M, Olson B, Arndt M, Brophy-Herb H, Shirer K, Shemanski R. Low-income mothers' decisions regarding when and why to introduce solid foods to their infants: influencing factors. *J Community Health Nurs.* 2007;24(2):101-118.

92. Redsell S, Atkinson P, Nathan D, Siriwardena A, Swift J, Glazebrook C. Parents' beliefs about appropriate infant size, growth and feeding behaviour: implications for the prevention of childhood obesity. *BMC Public Health.* 2010;10:711.

93. Keane V, Charney E, Straus J, Roberts K. Do solids help baby sleep through the night? *Am J Dis Child.* 1988;142(4):404-405.

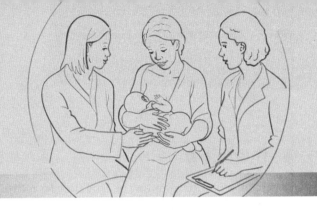

CHAPTER 5

Lactation Pharmacology

Thomas W. Hale
James Abbey
Teresa M. Baker

OBJECTIVES

- Describe the principles of drug entry into human milk.
- Identify the factors of drug transfer from maternal circulation to breastmilk.
- Describe the calculations that help predict drug exposure to infants.
- Predict the risk of medication to the infant.
- Identify the toxicity of a drug to the infant.
- Describe the clinical implications of drug excretion during lactation.
- Describe the steps to minimize medication exposure to infants.
- Describe the monitoring of an infant with potential drug exposures.
- Describe galactogogues that stimulate milk production.
- Describe recreational and illegal substance use as it relates to breastfeeding.
- Describe topical use of medications on the breast.

DEFINITIONS OF COMMONLY USED TERMS

acid–base dissociation constant (pKa) Factor that determines the likelihood of a drug being trapped in the milk compartment, called ion trapping.
bioavailability A measure of how much medication reaches the plasma.
dalton Unit used in expressing the molecular weight of proteins, equivalent to atomic mass unit.
diffusion Transfer of molecules of a substance between the plasma compartment and the milk compartment.
lipid solubility Capability of a substance to dissolve in lipids, fats, or oils.
milk-to-plasma ratio Tool to evaluate the relative concentration of medication in the plasma compared to the milk compartment.
protein binding Degree to which a drug binds to the proteins within blood plasma. The less bound a drug is, the more efficiently it can traverse cell membranes or diffuse.

Any use of the term *mother*, *maternal*, or *breastfeeding* is not meant to exclude transgender or nonbinary parents who may be breastfeeding or providing human milk to their infant.

▶ Overview

Although our understanding of drug transfer into human milk has advanced over the past 20 years, it is still rather obscure. While we understand some of the basic requirements for medication transfer into milk, we are still unable to adequately predict with certainty how much of a drug is likely to transfer into this compartment. Of the several published kinetic modeling systems, most are highly sophisticated and predict milk levels rather poorly. Thus, we are still dependent on rare clinical trials to accurately determine the level of a drug in milk. Unfortunately, far fewer than 30 percent of drugs currently marketed have been studied in relation to breastfeeding. While the U.S. Food and Drug Administration (FDA) is increasing pressure on pharmaceutical firms to do breastfeeding studies on new drugs, many older drugs have still not been studied in breastfeeding mothers.

The most difficult task is to understand and predict the overall safety of a medication that might transfer into milk. In essence, the question is how the infant will respond to the dose of medication found in the milk. Thus, the level of evidence needed to declare a medication safe is often not attainable. Most drugs are generally considered compatible with breastfeeding, although we are unable to predict the safety, with certainty, of some drugs. This chapter reviews the science behind lactation pharmacology, describes the process of risk assessment as it applies to infant drug exposure, and provides the reader with the proper tools to evaluate a drug.

The use of medications in breastfeeding mothers is often complicated in encounters with attending physicians. The prescribing provider has different priorities and makes the argument that a new medication is necessary to the health of the parent. If the physician does not properly address the issue of breastfeeding safety, the mother may be forced to seek outside counsel and ultimately have to decide whether the benefits of the drug outweigh the importance of breastfeeding. In other words, if it is assumed that the drug is both hazardous and necessary, the question becomes whether the breastfeeding benefit to the baby exceeds the drug exposure risk to the baby. There is not always an adequate answer for this conundrum.

I. Kinetics of Drug Entry into Human Milk

A. The amount of drug excreted into milk depends on a number of factors. Drugs enter the milk primarily by diffusion, driven by equilibrium forces between the maternal plasma compartment and the maternal milk compartment.[1]

   1. Medications enter the milk by transferring from the maternal plasma, through the capillary walls, past the alveolar epithelium, and into the milk compartment.[2]
   2. During the first 4 days postpartum, large gaps exist among alveolar cells (see **FIGURE 5-1**).
   3. These gaps might permit enhanced drug entry into milk during the colostral period, while the absolute amount of the drug in the milk might still be quite low.
   4. After 4 to 6 days, the alveolar cells enlarge, shutting off many of the intercellular gaps, and the amount of drug entry into the milk is reduced.
   5. Because the alveolar epithelium has rather tight junctions, most drugs must dissolve through the bilayer membranes of the alveolar cells before they can enter the milk.
   6. It is difficult for most medications to dissolve through the bilayer lipid membranes, particularly for drugs that are ionic or polar.
   7. The more lipid soluble a drug is, the greater its capability to penetrate into the milk.
   8. Drugs that are active in the central nervous system generally attain higher levels in the milk compartment because their chemistry is ideal for entry. Ideal physicochemistry includes higher lipid solubility, smaller molecular weight, and higher plasma levels.
   9. Drugs in the maternal plasma compartment are in complete equilibrium with the milk compartment. There might be more or less in the milk compartment, but they are still in equilibrium.

B. The chemistry of drug transfer into human milk is largely a function of the chemical structure of the drug.[1]

   1. Lipid solubility is a factor in the drug's transfer into the milk. In general, the more lipid soluble a drug is, the greater the likelihood it will penetrate the alveolar compartment. However, many lipid-soluble

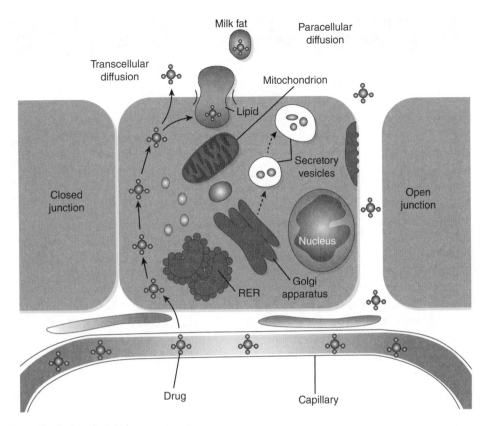

FIGURE 5-1 Alveolar cells during first 4 days postpartum.

      drugs have high volumes of distribution, which generally means they will be sequestered in peripheral compartments, such as adipose tissue, brain, and other lipid-rich compartments. This may actually reduce drug levels in milk because the drug is removed from the plasma compartment and deposited in the peripheral compartment, and thus the drug is shunted away from the milk compartment.

2. The acid–base dissociation constant (pKa) of a drug determines its likelihood of being trapped in the milk compartment, which is called ion trapping. Drugs with a pKa higher than 7.2 may be trapped in the alveolar milk and be unable to exit successfully. This is rarely important clinically.[2]

3. The molecular size of the drug largely determines its transfer into human milk. Without exception, the higher the molecular weight of the drug, the less enters the milk compartment. Drugs greater than 800 daltons have great difficulty attaining clinically relevant levels in milk. In essence, they simply leak into milk through pores that are open due to the loss of a lactocyte or through gaps between cells. Drugs that have large molecular sizes (25,000–200,000 daltons) are virtually excluded from milk in clinically relevant amounts. This includes drugs such as heparin, insulin, interferons, low-molecular-weight heparins, most new biological drugs, and many more.

4. All drugs must attain certain levels in the plasma compartment before they can enter the milk. At present, we know of no other way for drugs to enter milk without first transferring from the plasma. Thus, if a drug does not produce clinically relevant levels in the plasma, it is unlikely to be present in the milk.

5. The volume of distribution of a drug determines its ability to stay in the plasma compartment. Drugs with high volume of distribution are easily transferred out of the plasma to other deep compartments, such as adipose tissue, muscle, and brain.

6. Drugs with high protein binding are largely sequestered in the plasma and have great difficulty entering the milk. Nonsteroidal anti-inflammatory drugs (NSAIDs) are classic examples, with greater than 95 percent protein binding and low levels in milk. Warfarin, with more than 99 percent binding in the plasma compartment, is unable to enter milk at all.

7. The bioavailability of a medication is a measure of how much medication reaches the plasma. Some drugs are destroyed in the gastrointestinal (GI) tract (e.g., proteins, peptides, and aminoglycosides).

BOX 5-1 Relative Infant Dose

$$RID = \frac{Dose.infant\left[\dfrac{mg/kg}{day}\right]}{Dose.mother\left[\dfrac{mg/kg}{day}\right]}$$

Dose.infant = dose in infant per day
Dose.parent = dose in mother per day

Others are not absorbed in the small intestine (e.g., vancomycin). Some are significantly metabolized in the gut wall (e.g., domperidone). Regardless, the lower the bioavailability of the drug, the less is transferred into milk. Thus, we prefer drugs with low oral bioavailability.

8. In general, drugs with longer half-lives may build up in the milk production simply because their presence in the plasma is extended, leaving more time for some of the drug to enter the milk.

C. The milk-to-plasma ratio is a useful tool to evaluate the relative concentration of medication in the plasma, compared to the parental milk compartment.

1. Drugs with a high milk-to-plasma ratio enter milk easily, while drugs with low milk-to-plasma ratios are less able to enter the milk compartment.

2. In the case where a medication has a high milk-to-plasma ratio (e.g., 5) and an extremely low maternal plasma level, then five times a very low level is still very low (e.g., bupropion).

3. Unless a great deal is known about the plasma level, the milk-to-plasma ratio might give the clinician the wrong impression. It is therefore recommended that the milk-to-plasma ratio not be used clinically.

D. The relative infant dose (RID) is perhaps the most important clinical parameter to determine the safety of a drug entering the milk.

1. To calculate the actual dose (D_{inf}) received by the infant, you must know the actual concentration of medication in the milk and the volume of milk that is transferred.

   a. Published studies of many drugs provide the peak concentration (C_{max}) or the average concentration (C_{av}) for the drug.

   b. More recent studies[2] calculate the area under the curve value for the medication or C_{ave}. This methodology accurately estimates the average daily intake by the infant and is much more accurate than the C_{max} estimates.

2. Ultimately, the simplest method for determining the safety of a medication is to relate the weight-normalized dose to that used during therapy in infants where specific data is available. For example, if the normal dose of a drug that an infant would receive is 10 mg/kg/day, and the infant is receiving 1 mg/kg/day via milk, then you can estimate that the dose is 10 percent of the clinical dose.

3. The volume of milk ingested is highly variable and depends on the age of the infant and the extent to which the infant is exclusively breastfed. Many clinicians use 150 mL/kg/day to estimate the amount of milk ingested by the infant. However, the most useful and accurate measure of exposure is to calculate the RID (see **BOX 5-1**).

4. This value is generally expressed as a percentage of the maternal dose. It provides a standardized method of relating the infant's dose to the maternal dose. One recommendation for full-term infants is that an RID of greater than 10 percent should be the theoretical level of concern for most medications.[3] Nevertheless, the 10 percent level of concern is relative, and each situation should be evaluated individually according to the overall toxicity of the medication.

5. In preterm infants, this level of concern may require lowering the dose appropriately, depending on the medication. It should always be remembered that many neonates may have been exposed in utero and that in utero exposure may be an order of magnitude greater than that received through the milk. Thus, infants who were exposed in utero to methadone go through significant withdrawal upon delivery, even with breastfeeding.

II. Maternal Factors That Affect Drug Transfer

A. Determine the dose of medication by considering the postpartum interval.
1. At 2 to 4 days postpartum, the dose the infant receives is minimal because the volume of colostrum is minimal (30 to 60 mL/day).
2. If the infant is 2 weeks to 6 months old, the clinical dose of the drug may be significant because the volume of milk is high. Thus, more caution is required in infants during this stage of development.
3. At 12 or more months postpartum, the volume of milk is much lower, so the amount of the drug transferred to the infant is lower.
4. As the infant matures, the ability to metabolize and excrete medications increases. The infant's metabolism becomes highly functional at 9 to 12 months, and infants can adequately handle small loads of drugs through milk.
B. The maternal dose of drug can vary enormously. If the maternal dose is excessively high, use caution in recommending breastfeeding.
C. Drugs with sustained release formulations change the overall plasma half-life of the drug. More caution is recommended with these formulations because plasma and milk levels may be higher and sustained over longer periods, and the clinical dose transferred to the infant may be higher.
D. Dosing intervals of various medications can provide relatively high plasma levels as the drug is absorbed and reaches a peak in the plasma.
1. Breastfeeding at the peak may produce higher milk levels.
2. In these situations, and for drugs with a short half-life, it may be possible to breastfeed, take the medication, and avoid breastfeeding at the peak.
3. This strategy is ideal for drugs such as penicillin antibiotics, isoniazid, and hundreds of other drugs with a short half-life (1 to 4 hours). It generally will not work for drugs with a half-life longer than 4 hours.
E. The oral bioavailability of the drug largely determines the plasma levels and the overall risk to the breastfed infant. Determine whether the dose of medication is actually absorbed orally.
F. Many topical preparations are not absorbed transcutaneously, and pose no problem.
G. Many oral preparations are poorly absorbed from the GI tract, so the plasma levels are significantly lower. These drugs are often not a problem.
H. Hair dyes, most topical creams, drugs such as vancomycin, and dozens of other drugs are poorly absorbed orally and pose little risk to a breastfed infant.
I. Most new biological drugs, such as those used in Crohn's disease, ulcerative colitis, and other syndromes, are monoclonal antibodies (IgG) and thus are more than 150,000 daltons in size. Due to their size, they have consistently been found to produce low milk levels. Further, they are unlikely to be absorbed orally in the GI tract due to the many proteases that break down proteins.
J. Most asthma medications are inhaled; therefore, the level of medication in the plasma level is virtually nil, and it will not likely appear in the milk. Almost all inhaled medications are designed to deliver the drug directly to the pulmonary tissues, and most of these medications are designed to not be absorbed orally or taken up by the liver on the first pass.

III. Predicting Risks of Medications to the Infant

A. Risk factors for an infant depend on several factors.
1. An infant's metabolic status determines the risk of a negative drug effect.
a. Low risk: Generally older infants (6 to 18 months) who can metabolize and handle drugs efficiently
b. Moderate risk: Infants younger than 4 months who have additional risk factors, such as complications from delivery, GI anomalies, hepatitis, or other metabolic problems
c. High risk: Unstable neonates, preterm infants, or infants with poor renal function
2. Compare the milk dose with existing pediatric dosing.

3. If the milk levels are known, compare the normal oral dose used in the infant with that transferred via milk. This assessment will provide insight into the risk posed by the level of drug in the milk.

4. Assess if the medication is orally absorbed by the infant. If not, the risk is minimal.

B. Medications with local GI effects can impact the breastfeeding infant.

    1. Local effects in the GI tract have been known for many years.

        a. Changes in gut flora and diarrhea have been reported following the use of antibiotics. Generally, this is self-limiting and is not a major problem.

        b. The chronic use of various anticholinergic drugs (e.g., amitriptyline and atropine) and opiates could induce severe constipation. Similar effects are found in adults who use these and other constipating drugs.

    2. Breastfeeding should proceed with caution following the use of highly potent or toxic drugs.

        a. In general, the higher the toxicity of the drug, the greater the risk with breastfeeding.

        b. Breastfeeding in mothers using anticancer, antimetabolite, and other highly noxious drugs should follow guidelines for pumping and discarding contaminated milk for five to seven half-lives.[1] This milk cannot be saved, stored, or fed to an infant.

C. Radioactive drugs should be closely evaluated prior to using milk that is contaminated with these substances.

    1. Radioactive iodine (I-131) transfers readily into human milk (approximately 27 percent of the maternal dose).[4] Individuals who are planning treatment with this isotope should discontinue breastfeeding and cease lactation prior to its use to prevent high radiation exposure to breast tissues.

    2. Close contact with infants or adults should be avoided for up to 10 days after treatment. Additionally, I-131 is highly dangerous to infants, and precautions are mandatory if it is used during breastfeeding.

    3. Other isotopes, such as technetium-99, can be used relatively safely.

        a. Although some agencies may not recommend interrupting breastfeeding, technetium-99 has a brief half-life of only 6 hours.

        b. In most cases it is possible to interrupt breastfeeding and use expressed milk for a brief period. Therefore, the recommendation to withhold breastfeeding for 24 hours is a conservative option.

        c. Pumped milk can be stored for 2 to 4 days and used later because the radioisotope will have completely decayed by then and poses no risk.

    4. Other radioisotopes may pose some hazard. The InfantRisk Center at Texas Tech University (http://www.infantrisk.com/) can provide recommendations and describe known hazards posed by other radioisotopes.

D. Radiocontrast agents used in CT scans pose little risk to breastfed infants.

    1. These agents consist of covalently bound iodine molecules, which are largely unable to decouple from the main carrier molecule; thus, the drug is rapidly cleared from the maternal plasma compartment. As a group, radiocontrast agents are virtually unabsorbed after oral administration (less than 0.1 percent).

        a. Many of these contrast agents have a brief half-life of 1 to 2 hours, and the estimated dose ingested by the infant is negligible.[5] They can even be used intravenously in infants.

        b. Although most package inserts suggest that an infant be removed from breastfeeding for 24 hours, no untoward effects have been reported with these products in breastfed infants.[5]

    2. The iodine in these chemical radiocontrast agents is transported in limited amounts to human milk and poses little or no risk to a breastfed infant. The amount of free iodine may be enough to alter a thyroid scan.

    3. Gadolinium-containing radiocontrast agents used in MRIs do not readily transfer into human milk[5] (gadolinium is a heavy metal). However, there has been recent concern that a gadolinium ion can decouple from these contrast agents and build up in the brain of adults. At present, we do not know if this produces untoward complications in humans or if it enhances the transfer of gadolinium agents into human milk. In one recent study, no gadolinium deposition occurred in children after repeated exposure to gadolinium-containing radiocontrast agents.[6]

E. Drugs with limited oral bioavailability may or may not be used in breastfeeding infants. Some drugs (e.g., doxorubicin and methotrexate) that are sequestered in the GI tract of the infant could pose severe hazards. Thus, breastfeeding following the use of noxious, particularly anticancer, drugs is not recommended until they have been eliminated from the maternal circulation.

IV. Clinical Implications of Drug Excretion during Lactation

A. The clinical implications of excreting common drugs during lactation include the following:
1. Acetaminophen: Acetaminophen is approved for use in infants, so there is little concern about the use of this product during lactation. Monitor that the dose is not too high or prolonged. Avoid breastfeeding with excessively high or prolonged dosing.
2. Aspirin: In low doses, aspirin poses little risk to a breastfed infant. A brief waiting period of 2 hours would likely remove any risk, although this is probably unnecessary. Recent data suggests that doses of 81 mg and even 325 mg are not detectable in human milk immediately following their use.[7] Aspirin is removed from the portal circulation in the gut by the liver before it reaches systemic levels.
3. Ibuprofen: The RID is very low.[8] The delivered drug is far below the FDA recommended dose that can be directly given to infants.
4. Celecoxib: The RID is low in short-term use, but chronic use may be problematic.[9]
5. Diphenhydramine: This antihistamine is used for allergic conditions. It is also used as a sleep aid and as an antiemetic agent to prevent motion sickness.
    a. Small but unreported levels are thought to be secreted into milk. Following an intramuscular (IM) dose of 100 mg, drug levels in milk were undetectable in two individuals, and they ranged from 42 to 100 µg/L in two subjects.[10] Although these levels are low, this sedating antihistamine should be used only for a short duration during lactation.
    b. Nonsedating antihistamines are generally preferred.
    c. There are anecdotal reports that diphenhydramine suppresses milk production. There are no data to support this theory.

B. The clinical implications of vaccine excretion during lactation include the following:
1. As a general rule, vaccines are safe while breastfeeding.
2. The yellow fever vaccine is not recommended for use while breastfeeding. However, according to Centers for Disease Control and Prevention recommendations, all persons aged 9 months and older who travel to or live in areas of high yellow fever transmission should be vaccinated. In addition, it is preferable to avoid vaccinating during lactation when infants are less than 9 months old. However, if travel is unavoidable to an endemic area or an area where the risk of exposure to the yellow fever virus is high, the potential benefits of the vaccine outweigh the potential risks, and immunization should be considered.[11]

C. The clinical implications of antibiotic and antiviral drug excretion during lactation include the following:
1. Tetracyclines:
    a. The transfer rate of tetracycline antibiotics is very low; however, its absorption may be significant over time.
    b. The short-term use of these compounds for up to 3 weeks is permissible and suitable for the treatment of various infections.
    c. Long-term use, such as for acne, is not recommended during lactation due to the possibility of dental staining in the infant and reduced linear growth rate.
2. Acyclovir:
    a. Acyclovir is used to treat herpes simplex virus infections, varicella zoster, and other viral infections.
    b. There is almost no percutaneous absorption following topical application, and the plasma levels are undetectable. Therefore, there is no risk in breastfeeding unless the herpetic lesion is on the breast and comes into direct contact with the infant.
    c. Acyclovir levels in milk are reported to be 0.6 to 4.1 times the maternal plasma levels.[12] The maximum ingested doses were calculated to be 1,500 µg/day, assuming a 750 mL milk intake.
    d. An additional study measured milk levels following maternal intake of 200 mg five times daily, and the average milk concentration was 1.06 mg/L.[13]
3. Penicillins:
    a. Many penicillins have been studied, and are proven to be safe during lactation. Six mothers taking amoxicillin 1 gram orally were studied, and the levels in milk were 0.68 to 1.3 mg/L. This amount is less than 0.5 percent of a typical infant dose of amoxicillin.[14]

    b.   Ampicillin has been well studied and found to have a RID of 0.2 to 0.5 percent, with the highest reported milk level of 1.02 mg/L in a patient receiving 700 mg three times daily. Ampicillin is commonly used in neonates with no pediatric concerns.[15]

    c.   It is believed that penicillins can be safely used while breastfeeding.

4.   Cephalosporins:

    a.   Cephalexin is a commonly used first-generation cephalosporin antibiotic.

    b.   Only minimal concentrations are secreted into human milk. Following a 1 gram maternal oral dose, milk levels at 1, 2, 3, 4, and 5 hours were 0.20, 0.28, 0.39, 0.50, and 0.47 mg/L, respectively.[14] These levels are too low to be clinically relevant.

    c.   Cefotetan is a third-generation cephalosporin that is poorly absorbed orally and is typically used IM or intravenously (IV). The drug is distributed into human milk in very low concentrations with an RID of 0.02 to 0.03 percent.[16]

    d.   The cephalosporins have been used in breastfeeding without any safety concerns.

5.   Fluoroquinolones:

    a.   Studies of the new fluoroquinolones suggest that ofloxacin (and its derivatives) concentrations in milk are probably lowest.

    b.   Ciprofloxacin concentrations in human milk vary over a wide range but are generally quite low (2.1 to 2.6 percent).[17,18]

    c.   Ciprofloxacin use in pediatrics has increased in recent years, and numerous studies indicate little risk from exposure.

6.   Metronidazole:

    a.   Following an oral dose of 400 mg three times daily, the maximum concentration in milk was reported as 15.5 mg/L.[19] The reported RIDs were moderate, approximating 10 to 13 percent of the maternal dose.

    b.   Some reports suggest that a metallic taste is imparted to the milk.

    c.   High oral doses, such as 2 g for the treatment of trichomoniasis, may produce high milk levels. At this dose, a brief interruption of breastfeeding is recommended for 12 to 24 hours.

7.   Macrolides:

    a.   New data suggests that the use of erythromycin early in the postnatal period increases the risk of hypertrophic pyloric stenosis.[20]

    b.   For this reason, azithromycin or clarithromycin are the preferred choices during the postnatal period.

8.   Fluconazole:

    a.   A significant transfer (RID = 12 percent) into the milk has been proven safe and is far less than clinical doses that are commonly prescribed for infants.

    b.   Although there is some risk of elevated liver enzymes, none have been reported following exposure to fluconazole in milk.

9.   Antifungals:

    a.   Topical antifungals, such as nystatin or miconazole, are often used to treat candidiasis and are considered safe as long as minimal amounts are applied to limit oral absorption by the infant.

    b.   Clotrimazole has been implicated in contact dermatitis and should be avoided if possible.[21]

D.   The clinical implications of selective serotonin reuptake inhibitor (SSRI) excretion during lactation include the following:

1.   Antidepressant therapy in breastfeeding women is strongly recommended for maternal depression. Interestingly, this is the drug class that is most often studied in lactation. Clinical studies of sertraline and paroxetine clearly suggest that the transfer of these agents into milk is quite minimal.[22,23]

2.   Neonatal withdrawal symptoms are commonly reported in 30 percent or less of infants exposed to certain SSRIs during pregnancy. Early postnatal symptoms consist of poor adaptation, irritability, jitteriness, and poor gaze control in neonates exposed to paroxetine, sertraline, and, less so, fluoxetine.

3.   In contrast to transfer across the placenta, the SSRI levels in milk are very low, and uptake by the infant is even lower. There is strong evidence of safety while using this family of drugs during breastfeeding.[22,24,25]

E. The clinical implications of anticoagulant medication excretion during lactation include the following:
 1. Warfarin:
   a. Warfarin is highly protein bound, and very little is secreted into human milk.
   b. In one study, two patients were anticoagulated with warfarin. No warfarin was detected in the infants' serum, and no changes in coagulation were detected.[26]
   c. In another study of 13 mothers using warfarin, less than 0.08 μmol/L was detected in milk, and no warfarin was detected in the infants' plasma.[27]
   d. Supplementation with vitamin K will negate any small amount of warfarin that a breastfed infant might receive.
 2. Enoxaparin:
   a. Enoxaparin is a low-molecular-weight heparin used for anticoagulation.
   b. In one study of 12 women using 20 to 40 mg daily, no change in anti-Xa level was noted in any of the 12 breastfed infants.[28]
F. The clinical implications of antiseizure medication excretion during lactation include the following:
 1. Lamotrigine:
   a. Lamotrigine is an anticonvulsant used as an antiseizure medication.
   b. In a study of nine breastfeeding mothers at 3 weeks postpartum, the median milk-to-plasma ratio was 0.61, and the breastfed infants maintained lamotrigine concentrations of approximately 30 percent of the maternal plasma level.[29] There is one case report of an infant with severe apnea.[30] The mother was receiving 850 mg/day and breastfeeding. Lamotrigine is extensively used in seizure and bipolar disorders during lactation, with little or no reported complications. If low to moderate doses are used, it has proven safe to use while breastfeeding.[31]
 2. Valproic acid (VPA):
   a. VPA is a popular anticonvulsant used for seizure management.
   b. In one study of 16 patients receiving 300 to 2,400 mg/day, VPA concentrations ranged from 0.4 to 3.9 mg/L. The milk-to-plasma ratio was 0.05 in the study participants.[32]
   c. Most experts agree that the amount of VPA that transfers into milk is very low and that this drug can be used safely while breastfeeding.
   d. However, VPA is a known teratogen, and its use should be restricted in women who may become pregnant or those who are breastfeeding and may become pregnant. If VPA is used, effective birth control is mandatory.
   e. Some VPA will transfer into human milk and could reduce neurobehavioral development in the breastfed infant.[33] Due to the availability of numerous effective anticonvulsants, the use of VPA in breastfeeding women is not recommended unless all other options have been ruled out.
 3. Topiramate (used as an anticonvulsant):
   a. In one study of two women receiving 150 to 200 mg/day at 3 weeks postpartum, the concentration of topiramate in milk averaged 7.9 μM.[34] The absolute infant dose was 0.1 to 0.7 mg/kg/day. The plasma concentrations in the two infants were 1.4 and 1.6 μM, which was 10 to 20 percent of the mothers' plasma level.
   b. Infants should be closely monitored for sedation. Occasional blood level monitoring is recommended.
G. The clinical implications of antihypertensive medication excretion during lactation include the following:
 1. Calcium channel blockers:
   a. Nifedipine is a commonly used antihypertensive.
     i. There are two studies that indicate nifedipine is transferred into human milk in very low levels. Both published studies agree that the level transferred into human milk is of no clinical consequence to infants.
     ii. One study measured milk levels following doses ranging from 10 to 30 mg three times daily. The highest concentration in milk was 53.35 μg/L, measured at 1 hour after a 30 mg dose.[35]
     iii. Another study followed concentrations of nifedipine in human milk 1 to 8 hours after 10 mg doses. The levels varied from less than 1 to 10.3 μg/L in 6 of 11 patients.[36]

b.   Nicardipine has been studied in breastfeeding mothers, and the RID was estimated to be 0.07 percent.[37]

c.   Calcium channel blockers are considered safe for use in breastfeeding.

2.   Beta-blockers:

a.   Labetalol is a selective beta-blocker often used as an antihypertensive. In one study of three women receiving 600 to 1,200 mg/day, the peak concentrations of labetalol in milk were 129, 223, and 662 µg/L, respectively.[38]

b.   Metoprolol is a cardioselective beta-1 blocker used as an antihypertensive. In a study of three women at 4 to 6 months postpartum who were receiving 100 mg twice daily, the peak concentration of metoprolol ranged from 0.38 to 2.58 µmol/L.[38] The RID is approximately 1.4 percent.[39]

c.   Propranolol is a beta-blocker used for hypertension and migraine headaches. In general, the parental plasma levels are very low. One study of three patients revealed that the average milk concentration was 35.4 µg/L after multiple doses.[40]

d.   Atenolol and acebutolol are the only beta-blockers that require caution. Case reports describe infants with cyanosis and bradycardia when their mothers were being treated with these two beta-blockers.[41]

3.   ACE inhibitors:

a.   Captopril is an ACE inhibitor that is used as an antihypertensive. In a report of 12 women treated with 100 mg three times daily, the milk levels were 4.7 µg/L at 3.8 hours after a dose.[42]

b.   Lisinopril is commonly used as an antihypertensive, but there is no breastfeeding data for this drug.

c.   The concern for this class of drugs is the theoretic risk of an extremely preterm infant being exposed to these medications. In pregnancy, ACE inhibitors are avoided due to known fetotoxic effects. Because the kidney does not fully mature until after birth, there is some concern about potential renal effects of ACE inhibitor exposure through milk in a preterm infant, although this is a theoretical risk.

4.   Diuretics:

a.   Furosemide is a potent loop diuretic with a 3 hour half-life. It is used extensively in the immediate postpartum period as an antihypertensive and to help remove excess intravascular volume. It is used frequently in neonates in intensive care units and in pediatrics. It has very low oral bioavailability in neonates. Furosemide levels in milk have not been reported.

b.   Hydrochlorothiazide is a thiazide diuretic that is often used postpartum for volume control and for hypertension. In one study, a mother received 50 mg every morning, and her milk levels were 25 percent of her plasma levels. This means the infant would receive approximately 50 µg/day, which is not clinically significant.[43]

H.   The clinical implications of pain management drug excretion during lactation include the following:

1.   Hydrocodone is a narcotic analgesic. Its active metabolite is hydromorphone.

a.   Hydrocodone is very effective for the relief of postpartum and postoperative pain, and it is commonly used.

b.   In a recent study, hydrocodone and hydromorphone levels were measured in 125 milk samples obtained from 30 women receiving 0.14 to 0.21 mg/kg/day. The authors concluded that a fully breastfed infant would receive about 2.4 percent of the maternal hydrocodone dose.[44]

c.   Milk samples in two of the studied women were very high, with a hydromorphone-to-hydrocodone ratio of 2.8 and 3.1. It is possible that these women metabolized the drug faster, so the risks of opiate exposure to their infants were higher.

d.   Overall, it is recommended that hydrocodone is safe if used for short time frames and less than 30 mg daily.

2.   Codeine is a mild opiate analgesic, and its metabolite is morphine (approximately 7 percent).

a.   The amount of codeine secreted into milk is low.

b.   Four cases of neonatal apnea have been reported following maternal administration of 60 mg of codeine every 4 to 6 hours.[45]

        c.   An infant death has been reported following maternal use of codeine. The genotype of this mother indicated that she was an ultrarapid metabolizer of codeine.[46]

        d.   Caution should be used with codeine. Numerous national drug advisory groups around the world, including the FDA, have recommended that it no longer be used during lactation.

   3.   Morphine is a potent analgesic.

        a.   In a group of five lactating women, the highest morphine concentration in milk following two epidural doses was only 82 μg/L at 30 minutes.[47] The highest milk level following 15 mg IV or IM administration was only 0.5 mg/L, and it dropped to almost 0.01 mg/L in 4 hours.

        b.   In another study of women receiving morphine via patient-controlled analgesia (PCA) pump for 12 to 48 hours postpartum, the concentration of morphine in milk ranged from 50 to 60 μg/L.[48]

        c.   The oral bioavailability of morphine is low because it is rapidly cleared by the liver; however, the clearance of morphine is slower in an infant less than 1 month old.

        d.   Morphine can be safely used for short time frames and if the infant is monitored for signs of increased sedation or poor feeding.

   4.   Hydromorphone is a potent semisynthetic narcotic analgesic that is approximately 7 to 10 times more potent than morphine, but it is used in equivalently lower doses.

        a.   In a group of eight women who received 2 mg of intranasal hydromorphone, the milk levels ranged from about 6 μg/L at 1 to 1.5 hours to 0.2 μg/L at 24 hours (estimated from a graph). The observed milk-to-plasma ratio averaged 2.56, and the half-life of hydromorphone in milk was 10.5 hours. The authors of this study estimated an RID of 0.67 percent.[49]

        b.   If a maternal dose were 4 mg of hydromorphone every 6 hours, the infant would ingest about 0.002 mg/kg/day, or 2.2 μg of the 4 mg taken.[49] This is significantly less than the clinical oral dose recommended for infants and children with pain (0.03 to 0.06 mg/kg/dose every 4 hours as needed).

   5.   Tramadol is used as an analgesic and closely resembles opiates but has a reduced addictive potential.

        a.   In a study of 75 mothers who received 100 mg every 6 hours after cesarean section, milk samples were taken on days 2 to 4 postpartum in transitional milk. The estimated absolute and relative infant doses were 112 μg/kg/day and 30 μg/kg/day for rac-tramadol and its desmethyl metabolite. No significant issues arose with infants exposed to these doses in breastmilk.[50]

        b.   Although the FDA no longer recommends this drug during lactation, there are no reported complications in any breastfed infant.

I.   The clinical implications of excreting drugs of abuse during lactation include the following:

   1.   Alcohol:

        a.   The consumption of ethanol has been shown to inhibit oxytocin release and decrease milk delivery to the infant.[51]

        b.   An average-sized woman will metabolize a standard drink (14 g pure ethanol) in about 2 hours. Thus, a waiting period of 2 hours per drink consumed is recommended.[52]

   2.   Tobacco:

        a.   Studies show a linear relationship among smoking in the breastfeeding parent, nicotine levels in the milk, and urine cotinine (nicotine's main metabolite) levels in the breastfed infant.

        b.   Second-hand smoke can contribute to otitis media, respiratory tract infections, sudden infant death syndrome, and asthma in the infant.

   3.   Marijuana or cannabis:

        a.   Research is limited concerning the concentration of marijuana in milk. The milk levels are reportedly low, but the milk-to-plasma ratio has been reported as high.

        b.   Thus far, no study has demonstrated measurable clinical effects in infants exposed to marijuana.

        c.   Significant evidence has begun to emerge suggesting that exposure to THC in pregnancy, or chronic use in adolescence and early adulthood, may result in changes to the endocannabinoid system in the brain, which regulates mood, reward, and goal-directed behavior.

      d.   Adverse neurobehavioral effects have not yet been demonstrated in infants exposed to THC. Mothers who deliver infants who are drug-screen positive should be advised to discontinue the use of cannabis, but they should be permitted to continue breastfeeding.

      e.   Current studies are underway that may alter these recommendations. Unpublished data from our laboratories suggest that the RID for smoked marijuana is approximately 2.4 percent.

   4. Opiate drugs:

      a.   Opiate medications are commonly used in breastfeeding mothers, but these drugs must be used with caution because respiratory depression can occur with high doses.

      b.   Morphine is generally considered the best choice because it is poorly absorbed in infants.

      c.   Opiate derivatives, such as heroin, fentanyl, sufentanil, and meperidine, should be avoided when used at high doses in abusive situations.

   5. Cocaine:

      a.   There are no available data on the transfer of cocaine into human milk.

      b.   Due to its chemistry, cocaine levels in milk may be excessive, and users should avoid using cocaine while breastfeeding.

      c.   Studies with exact estimates of cocaine transmission into breastmilk have not been reported due to the difficulty of determining maternal dose and timing of milk samples. However, case reports demonstrating transmission of this drug and its metabolites into milk do exist.

      d.   In the first case, a mother reported using 0.5 g of cocaine intranasally over 4 hours, and she breastfed her infant five times during this period.[53] The infant became irritable; had vomiting, diarrhea, and dilated pupils; and had difficulty focusing on the mother's face. On examination, the infant was tremulous, irritable, tachycardiac, tachypneic, and hypertensive with an increased startling response. The infant's pupils were dilated with a poor response to light, and the reflexes were increased.

      e.   A waiting period of 24 hours, following the use of cocaine is recommended, during which milk is pumped and discarded.[1]

      f.   Drug screens will remain positive for more than 5 days after the use of this drug.

J. The clinical implications of biological drug excretion during lactation include the following:

   1. Many new biological drugs are, in most cases, derived from the human immune globulin IgG_1, although some are derived from IgG_4. These drugs are used to treat syndromes such as multiple sclerosis, arthritis, Crohn's disease, ulcerative colitis, and cancer in a new era of using immune therapy to combat disease.

   2. All these drugs consist of a specially modified IgG molecule, which on average weighs about 150,000 daltons. These compounds leak into milk at low levels through random gaps in the alveolar apparatus.

   3. At present, numerous studies suggest that milk levels are exceedingly low and that any of the drug that is present in milk is probably not orally absorbed because the molecules are rapidly denatured by gastrointestinal proteases.[54-56]

   4. It currently appears that the benefits of breastfeeding and enhanced maternal health greatly outweigh any potential side effects from this class of medications.

V. Galactagogues That Stimulate Milk Production

A. Herbal drugs:

   1. Fenugreek is the most commonly used herb for increasing milk production.

   2. There is little hard evidence that herbal preparations may increase milk production. The most recent placebo-controlled study published as an abstract in 2011 suggested that fenugreek had no effect on either prolactin levels or milk volume.[57] This study included 26 mothers of preterm infants that took 1,725 mg fenugreek three times a day for 3 weeks.

   3. Although no adverse effects are noted, herbal products are not controlled by the FDA, so the quality and consistency of products are unknown and may put the mother or infant at risk of unknown adverse effects.

   4. Fenugreek is not recommended to improve milk production.

B. Domperidone:
   1. Numerous studies over the past 30 years have documented that domperidone is a major galactagogue.
   2. Formerly introduced as a gastrokinetic drug, domperidone stimulates prolactin production to a major degree. As such, in women who are hypoprolactinemic while breastfeeding, it will increase milk synthesis and production rapidly and efficiently.
   3. More than a dozen studies have clearly documented that domperidone will increase milk production in some women.[58-64]
      a. This occurs only if prolactin levels are low (less than 79 ng/mL). It will not work when prolactin levels are high. Thus, determining the prolactin level is a major requirement before instituting therapy with this drug.
      b. Patients should be advised to breastfeed, then after 2 hours a plasma sample should be taken to determine the prolactin level. At 2 hours, the peak will have been avoided, and the trough level will be present in the plasma. If this level is low (10 to 50 ng/mL), domperidone will probably increase milk production significantly.
   4. Following prolonged therapy, a withdrawal period is recommended in most cases to prevent a precipitous drop in prolactin levels. In a recent study to determine the effect of domperidone withdrawal on subsequent milk production kinetics, 25 women who initially received domperidone (20 mg four times daily) were gently withdrawn stepwise over a period of 2 to 4 weeks, from 20 mg four times daily, to 10 mg four times daily, to nil.[65] In the study, 23 of 25 cases (93 percent) reported no significant increase in formula use after stopping domperidone. Normal infant growth was reported in all cases.
   5. Domperidone is known in some rare cases to induce arrhythmias.[66,67] This occurs primarily in older males and in individuals who are proarrhythmic. Do not use domperidone at doses higher than 20 mg three times daily. As the dose escalates, the risk of arrhythmias increases.
C. Metoclopramide:
   1. Metoclopramide, a dopamine receptor blocker, has multiple functions and is primarily used for increasing the tone of the lower esophageal sphincter in patients who have gastroesophageal reflux. It is sometimes used during lactation to stimulate prolactin release from the pituitary gland and enhance milk production.[68,69]
   2. Although metoclopramide is well known to increase the release of prolactin, similar to domperidone, it is fraught with side effects, such as depression, although some patients have used it successfully for months. The FDA has warned that therapy longer than 3 months may be associated with tardive dyskinesia and extrapyramidal symptoms. The exposure should be limited to no more than 1 month.
   3. The general recommendation is to taper the dose. One possible regimen is to decrease the dose by 10 mg per week.

▸ Key Points from This Chapter

A. During the colostral period, the transfer of drugs into milk is higher. However, the total dose transferred is lower because of the limited volume of colostrum during the first few days.
B. Medications enter the milk compartment only from the mother's blood. If the drug is not absorbed into the plasma compartment, it does not enter the milk compartment.
C. Although all drugs enter milk, most drugs enter at clinically insignificant levels. Determine the levels in milk, the Relative Infant Dose (RID), and the lactation risk category.
D. Recommend discontinuing breastfeeding if the drug poses a major risk to the infant. This includes high doses of sedative drugs, opiate narcotics, radioactive agents, anticancer drugs, and other noxious drugs.
E. Be cautious of high vitamin doses. Do not use high doses of iodine. Advise moderation in the use of any drug.
F. Keep breastfeeding parents healthy to avoid the need for medicinal treatment. Make sure they take care of their health, both mental and physical. If a health condition requires treatment, carefully choose the drugs to treat it.

🔍 *CASE STUDY*

A 31-year-old mother delivered vaginally at 28 weeks' gestation due to preterm labor and bleeding and a presumed placental abruption. The infant weighed 850 grams, had Apgar scores of 5 and 8, and a pH of 7.1. At delivery, the infant was intubated and transferred to the neonatal intensive care unit (NICU). A review of the prenatal records indicated a history of chronic back pain since a car accident 3 years before. At delivery, the mother was reportedly using 130 mg oxycodone daily, 600 mg gabapentin three times daily, and cyclobenzaprine 10 mg three times daily for chronic pain syndrome. The mother was stable in the recovery room and requested to breastfeed.

The mother's oxycodone dose is exceedingly high, and the gabapentin and cyclobenzaprine doses are at the highest levels. The infant will undoubtedly go through withdrawal over the next few days. It is likely that the amount of these agents in the milk is sufficient to allay the severity of withdrawal, but only to a limited degree. New data suggest that adding gabapentin or pregabalin to opiate therapy greatly exaggerates withdrawal symptoms in infants.

The fact that this infant was placed in the NICU is beneficial because respiratory function, blood pressure, and other biological functions can be closely monitored by the NICU staff, both during withdrawal and before discharge to home while breastfeeding continues. It is possible that this infant can be fed expressed milk or can breastfeed later, with the recommendation that the maternal doses of these medications be reduced significantly over the ensuing weeks. Had this infant been born at full term and not admitted to the NICU, breastfeeding after hospital discharge would require continued monitoring at home.

Questions

1. If the mother had undergone general anesthesia for an emergent cesarean section, and the medications used on induction included propofol and succinylcholine, at what time postprocedure would it be safe for her to breastfeed?
2. If the mother had a seizure in the recovery room and was placed on a magnesium infusion for seizure prophylaxis, would it be safe for her to breastfeed the infant?
3. What if the mother developed acute shortness of breast/chest pain during her postpartum course and there was concern for a pulmonary embolism? She undergoes a CT angiogram with IV contrast to rule out pulmonary embolism. Is there any contraindication to breastfeeding with contrast agents?
4. What if a urine toxicology screen was sent on the mother to rule out illicit drug use and the urine toxicology indicated use of cannabis products? Would marijuana use change your counseling on breastfeeding safety?

References

1. Hale TW, Rowe HE. *Medications and Mothers' Milk.* 17th ed. New York, NY: Springer Publishing; 2017.
2. Hale T, Hartmann PE. *Textbook of Human Lactation.* Vol 1. Amarillo, TX: Hale Publishing LP; 2007.
3. Bennett P. *Drugs and Human Lactation.* Vol 1. 2nd ed. New York, NY: Elsevier; 1996.
4. Robinson PS, Barker P, Campbell A, Henson P, Surveyor I, Young PR. Iodine-131 in breast milk following therapy for thyroid carcinoma. *J Nucl Med.* 1994;35(11):1797-1801.
5. Webb JA, Thomsen HS, Morcos SK, Members of Contrast Media Safety Committee of European Society of Urogenital R. The use of iodinated and gadolinium contrast media during pregnancy and lactation. *Eur Radiol.* 2005;15(6):1234-1240.
6. Tibussek D, Rademacher C, Caspers J, et al. Gadolinium brain deposition after macrocyclic gadolinium administration: a pediatric case-control study. *Radiology.* 2017;285:223-230.
7. Datta P, Rewers-Felkins K, Kallem RR, Baker T, Hale TW. Transfer of low dose aspirin into human milk. *J Hum Lactation.* 2017;33(2):296-299.
8. Walter K, Dilger C. Ibuprofen in human milk. *Br J Clin Pharmacol.* 1997;44(2):211-212.
9. Hale TW, McDonald R, Boger J. Transfer of celecoxib into human milk. *J Hum Lactation.* 2004;20(4):397-403.
10. Rindi V. La eliminazione degli antistaminici di sintesi con il latte e l'azione latto-goga de questi. *Riv Ital Ginecol.* 1951;34:147-157.
11. Staples JE, Gershman M, Fischer M. Yellow fever vaccine: recommendations of the Advisory Committee on Immunization Practices (ACIP). *MMWR Recomm Rep.* 2010;59(Rr-7):1-27.
12. Lau RJ, Emery MG, Galinsky RE. Unexpected accumulation of acyclovir in breast milk with estimation of infant exposure. *Obstet Gynecol.* 1987;69(3 pt 2):468-471.
13. Meyer LJ, de Miranda P, Sheth N, Spruance S. Acyclovir in human breast milk. *Am J Obstet Gynecol.* 1988;158(3 pt 1):586-588.
14. Kafetzis DA, Siafas CA, Georgakopoulos PA, Papadatos CJ. Passage of cephalosporins and amoxicillin into the breast milk. *Acta Paediatr Scand.* 1981;70(3):285-288.
15. Branebjerg PE, Heisterberg L. Blood and milk concentrations of ampicillin in mothers treated with pivampicillin and in their infants. *J Perinat Med.* 1987;15(6):555-558.
16. Novelli A. The penetration of intramuscular cefotetan disodium into human esta-vascular fluid and maternal milk secretion. *Chemoterapia.* 1983;11(5):337-342.
17. Cover DL, Mueller BA. Ciprofloxacin penetration into human breast milk: a case report. *DICP.* 1990;24(7-8):703-704.

18. Gardner DK, Gabbe SG, Harter C. Simultaneous concentrations of ciprofloxacin in breast milk and in serum in mother and breast-fed infant. *Clin Pharm.* 1992;11(4):352-354.

19. Passmore CM, McElnay JC, Rainey EA, D'Arcy PF. Metronidazole excretion in human milk and its effect on the suckling neonate. *Br J Clin Pharmacol.* 1988;26(1):45-51.

20. Murchison L, De Coppi P, Eaton S. Post-natal erythromycin exposure and risk of infantile hypertrophic pyloric stenosis: a systematic review and meta-analysis. *Pediatr Surg Int.* 2016;32(12):1147-1152.

21. Abhinav C, Mahajan VK, Mehta KS, Chauhan PS. Allergic contact dermatitis due to clotrimazole with cross-reaction to miconazole. *Indian J Dermatol Venereol Leprol.* 2015;81(1):80-82.

22. Stowe ZN, Owens MJ, Landry JC, et al. Sertraline and desmethylsertraline in human breast milk and nursing infants. *Am J Psychiatry.* 1997;154(9):1255-1260.

23. Stowe ZN, Cohen LS, Hostetter A, Ritchie JC, Owens MJ, Nemeroff CB. Paroxetine in human breast milk and nursing infants. *Am J Psychiatry.* 2000;157(2):185-189.

24. Altshuler LL, Burt VK, McMullen M, Hendrick V. Breastfeeding and sertraline: a 24-hour analysis. *J Clin Psychiatry.* 1995;56(6):243-245.

25. Kendall-Tackett K, Hale TW. The use of antidepressants in pregnant and breastfeeding women: a review of recent studies. *J Hum Lactation.* 2010;26(2):187-195.

26. McKenna R, Cole ER, Vasan U. Is warfarin sodium contraindicated in the lactating mother? *J Pediatr.* 1983;103(2):325-327.

27. Orme ML, Lewis PJ, de Swiet M, et al. May mothers given warfarin breast-feed their infants? *Br Med J.* 1977;1(6076):1564-1565.

28. Guillonneau M, de Crepy A, Aufrant C, Hurtaud-Roux MF, Jacqz-Aigrain E. Breast-feeding is possible in case of maternal treatment with enoxaparin. *Arch Pediatr.* 1996;3(5):513-514.

29. Ohman I, Vitols S, Tomson T. Lamotrigine in pregnancy: pharmacokinetics during delivery, in the neonate, and during lactation. *Epilepsia.* 2000;41(6):709-713.

30. Nordmo E, Aronsen L, Wasland K, Smabrekke L, Vorren S. Severe apnea in an infant exposed to lamotrigine in breast milk. *Ann Pharmacother.* 2009;43(11):1893-1897.

31. Veiby G, Engelsen BA, Gilhus NE. Early child development and exposure to antiepileptic drugs prenatally and through breastfeeding: a prospective cohort study on children of women with epilepsy. *JAMA Neurol.* 2013;70(11):1367-1374.

32. von Unruh GE FW, Hoffmann F, Niesen M. Valporic acid in breast milk: how much is really there? *Ther Drug Monit.* 1984;6(3):272-276.

33. Gentile S. Risks of neurobehavioral teratogenicity associated with prenatal exposure to valproate monotherapy: a systematic review with regulatory repercussions. *CNS Spectr.* 2014;19(4):305-315.

34. Ohman I, Vitols S, Luef G, Soderfeldt B, Tomson T. Topiramate kinetics during delivery, lactation, and in the neonate: preliminary observations. *Epilepsia.* 2002;43(10):1157-1160.

35. Manninen AK, Juhakoski A. Nifedipine concentrations in maternal and umbilical serum, amniotic fluid, breast milk and urine of mothers and offspring. *Int J Clin Pharmacol Res.* 1991;11(5):231-236.

36. Ehrenkranz RA, Ackerman BA, Hulse JD. Nifedipine transfer into human milk. *J Pediatr.* 1989; 114(3):478-480.

37. Jarreau P BC, Gukkonneau M, Jacqz-Aigrain E. Excretion of nicardipine in human milk. 2000;4(1):28-30.

38. Lunell NO, Kulas J, Rane A. Transfer of labetalol into amniotic fluid and breast milk in lactating women. *Eur J Clin Pharmacol.* 1985;28(5):597-599.

39. Liedholm H, Melander A, Bitzen PO, et al. Accumulation of atenolol and metoprolol in human breast milk. *Eur J Clin Pharmacol.* 1981;20(3):229-231.

40. Smith MT, Livingstone I, Hooper WD, Eadie MJ, Triggs EJ. Propranolol, propranolol glucuronide, and naphthoxylactic acid in breast milk and plasma. *Ther Drug Monit.* 1983;5(1):87-93.

41. Schimmel MS, Eidelman AI, Wilschanski MA, Shaw D Jr, Ogilvie RJ, Koren G. Toxic effects of atenolol consumed during breast feeding. *J Pediatr.* 1989;114(3):476-478.

42. Devlin RG, Fleiss PM. Captopril in human blood and breast milk. *J Clin Pharmacol.* 1981;21(2):110-113.

43. Miller ME, Cohn RD, Burghart PH. Hydrochlorothiazide disposition in a mother and her breast-fed infant. *J Pediatr.* 1982;101(5):789-791.

44. Sauberan JB, Anderson PO, Lane JR, et al. Breast milk hydrocodone and hydromorphone levels in mothers using hydrocodone for postpartum pain. *Obstet Gynecol.* 2011;117(3):611-617.

45. Davis JM, Bhutani VK, Bongiovanni AM. Neonatal apnea and maternal codeine use. *Ped Res.* 1985;19(4):170A.

46. Koren G, Cairns J, Chitayat D, Gaedigk A, Leeder SJ. Pharmacogenetics of morphine poisoning in a breastfed neonate of a codeine-prescribed mother. *Lancet.* 2006;368(9536):704.

47. Feilberg VL, Rosenborg D, Broen Christensen C, Mogensen JV. Excretion of morphine in human breast milk. *Acta Anaesthesiol Scand.* 1989;33(5):426-428.

48. Wittels B, Scott DT, Sinatra RS. Exogenous opioids in human breast milk and acute neonatal neurobehavior: a preliminary study. *Anesthesiology.* 1990;73(5):864-869.

49. Edwards JE, Rudy AC, Wermeling DP, Desai N, McNamara PJ. Hydromorphone transfer into breast milk after intranasal administration. *Pharmacotherapy.* 2003;23(2):153-158.

50. Ilett KF, Paech MJ, Page-Sharp M, et al. Use of a sparse sampling study design to assess transfer of tramadol and its O-desmethyl metabolite into transitional breast milk. *Br J Clin Pharmacol.* 2008;65(5):661-666.

51. Mennella JA, Beauchamp GK. Maternal diet alters the sensory qualities of human milk and the nursling's behavior. *Pediatrics.* 1991;88(4):737-744.

52. Ho E, Collantes A, Kapur BM, Moretti M, Koren G. Alcohol and breast feeding: calculation of time to zero level in milk. *Biol Neonate.* 2001;80(3):219-222.

53. Chasnoff IJ, Douglas LE, Squires L. Cocaine intoxication in a breast-fed infant. *Pediatrics.* 1987;80:836-838.

54. Keeling S, Wolbink GJ. Measuring multiple etanercept levels in the breast milk of a nursing mother with rheumatoid arthritis. *J Rheumatol.* 2010;37(7):1551.

55. Murashima A, Watanabe N, Ozawa N, Saito H, Yamaguchi K. Etanercept during pregnancy and lactation in a patient with rheumatoid arthritis: drug levels in maternal serum, cord blood, breast milk and the infant's serum. *Ann Rheum Dis.* 2009;68(11):1793-1794.

56. Forger F, Matthias T, Oppermann M, Ostensen M, Helmke K. Infliximab in breast milk. *Lupus.* 2004;13(9):753.

57. Reeder C, Legrand A, O'Conner-Von S. The effect of fenugreek on milk production and prolactin levels in mothers of premature infants [abstract]. *J Hum Lactation.* 2011;27:74.

58. Campbell-Yeo ML, Allen AC, Joseph KS, et al. Effect of domperidone on the composition of preterm human breast milk. *Pediatrics.* 2010;125(1):e107-e114.

59. da Silva OP, Knoppert DC, Angelini MM, Forret PA. Effect of domperidone on milk production in mothers of premature newborns: a randomized, double-blind, placebo-controlled trial. *CMAJ.* 2001;164(1):17-21.

60. Hofmeyr GJ, van Iddekinge B. Domperidone and lactation. *Lancet.* 1983;1(8325):647.

61. Hofmeyr GJ, Van Iddekinge B, Blott JA. Domperidone: secretion in breast milk and effect on puerperal prolactin levels. *Br J Obstet Gynaecol.* 1985;92(2):141-144.

62. Knoppert DC, Page A, Warren J, et al. The effect of two different domperidone doses on maternal milk production. *J Hum Lactation.* 2013;29(1):38-44.

63. Livingstone V, Stanchera B, Stringer J. The effect of withdrawing domperidone on formula supplementation. *Breastfeed Med.* 2007;2:178.

64. Wan EW, Davey K, Page-Sharp M, Hartmann PE, Simmer K, Ilett KF. Dose-effect study of domperidone as a galactagogue in preterm mothers with insufficient milk supply, and its transfer into milk. *Br J Clin Pharmacol.* 2008;66(2):283-289.

65. Livingstone V, Blaga Stancheva L, Stringer J. The effect of withdrawing domperidone on formula supplementation. *Breastfeed Med.* 2007;2:178.

66. Doggrell SA, Hancox JC. Cardiac safety concerns for domperidone, an antiemetic and prokinetic, and galactogogue medicine. *Expert Opin Drug Saf.* 2014 ;13(1):131-138. doi:10.1517/14740338.2014.851193.

67. Paul C, Zénut M, Dorut A, et al. Use of domperidone as a galactagogue drug: a systematic review of the benefit-risk ratio. *J Hum Lactation.* 2015;31(1):57-63. doi:10.1177/0890334414561265.

68. Kauppila A, Arvela P, Koivisto M, Kivinen S, Ylikorkala O, Pelkonen O. Metoclopramide and breast feeding: transfer into milk and the newborn. *Eur J Clin Pharmacol.* 1983;25(6):819-823.

69. Budd SC, Erdman SH, Long DM, Trombley SK, Udall JN Jr. Improved lactation with metoclopramide. A case report. *Clin Pediatr (Phila).* 1993;32(1):53-57.

Additional Resources

InfantRisk Center. http://www.infantrisk.com.

Motherisk. Pregnancy and Breastfeeding Safety Guide. http://www.motherisk.org/women/contactUs.jsp.

National Institutes of Health. LactMed: A Toxnet Database. https://toxnet.nlm.nih.gov/newtoxnet/lactmed.htm.

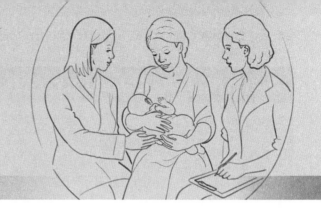

CHAPTER 6

Breast Anatomy and Milk Production

Gloria A. Graham
Anne Montgomery

OBJECTIVES

- Describe breast development and structures of the breast.
- Characterize anatomic and structural changes of the breast during pregnancy.
- Assess the breast to determine if changes are consistent with adequate function in lactation.
- Assess milk production.
- Compare autocrine and structural changes of the breast during pregnancy.
- Explain neuroendocrine control of milk ejection.
- Describe lactogenesis, including the process of involution.
- Describe the process of milk synthesis, including autocrine (local) control and the feedback inhibitor of lactation.

DEFINITIONS OF COMMONLY USED TERMS

alveoli The milk-producing components of the breast.
apoptosis The death of cells that occurs as a normal and controlled part of an organism's growth or development.
areola The circular, dark-pigmented area that surrounds the nipple.
Cooper's ligaments Connective tissue in the breast that helps maintain structural integrity. They are named for Astley Cooper, who first described them in 1840.
feedback inhibitor of lactation A small active whey protein that is synthesized by the lactocytes and accumulates in the alveolar lumen.
galactopoiesis The maintenance of milk production.
involution The removal of milk-producing cells after weaning by apoptosis.
lactocytes Specialized epithelial cells that line the interior of the alveolus.

(continues)

lactogenesis The process of cellular changes in glandular tissue in the breast whereby mammary epithelial cells are converted from a nonsecretory state (milk producing) to a secretory state (milk producing).

lactogenesis I Differentiation of alveolar epithelial cells into lactocytes that secrete colostrum.

lactogenesis II The onset of copious milk production that begins 32 to 96 hours after birth.

mammogenesis The development of mammary glands and breast structures from birth through puberty, pregnancy, and lactation.

Montgomery glands Sebaceous glands in the areola surrounding the nipple that make oily secretions to keep the areola and the nipple lubricated and protected.

myoepithelial cells Cells that encase the alveoli and contract in response to oxytocin to eject milk into ductules.

parenchyma The functional tissue of an organ as distinguished from the connective and supporting tissue.

Poland syndrome Unilateral hypoplasia of the breast combined with hypoplasia of the thorax and pectoral muscles.

prolactin receptor sites Sites in the lactocytes that allow prolactin to be absorbed from the blood and enter into the alveoli to stimulate milk production

Sheehan syndrome A pituitary infarct caused by severe postpartum hemorrhage.

tail of Spence Mammary glandular tissue that projects into the axillary region.

Any use of the term *mother*, *maternal*, or *breastfeeding* is not meant to exclude transgender or nonbinary parents who may be breastfeeding or providing human milk to their infant.

▶ Overview

The breast, or mammary gland, is a remarkable endocrine organ that experiences growth, differentiation, and lactation in response to a complex interplay of hormones and stimulation. The breast, which is the only organ that is not fully developed at birth, provides both nutrition and nurturing. Mammogenesis, which is the development of the mammary gland and related structures within the breast, occurs throughout fetal, adolescent, and adult life. It is a time of growth, functional differentiation, and regression.

The hormonal environment during pregnancy finishes preparing the breasts to assume the role of nourishing the infant following birth. After delivery, a profound change occurs in the hormonal milieu, enabling an elaborate system of neuroendocrine feedback to produce and deliver milk of a changing volume and composition to meet the needs and stores of the infant as he or she grows and develops. The breasts are capable of full lactation from about 16 weeks of pregnancy onward. Milk does not "come in" because it is already present before delivery, during lactogenesis I, in the form of colostrum.

Milk production is under endocrine or hormonal control before delivery of the placenta and changes to autocrine (or local) control during lactogenesis II. Abundant production is suppressed during pregnancy by inhibiting hormones until placental delivery, when the change in hormonal checks and balances followed by the stimulus of infant suckling signal the breasts to produce copious amounts of milk. Primary factors (e.g., maternal health) and secondary factors (e.g., mismanagement of early breastfeeding) can affect this robust but critical and carefully programmed physiologic process. The lactation consultant benefits from a familiarity with the cascade of events and its influence on lactation.

I. Breast Development

A.   Breast development undergoes many changes during the embryonic and neonatal stages.
1.   Weeks 3 to 4: A primitive milk streak forms and runs bilaterally from the axilla to the groin.
2.   Weeks 4 to 5: The milk streak becomes a mammary milk ridge or galactic band. Paired breasts develop from this line of glandular tissue.
3.   Weeks 7 to 8: Thickening and inward growth into the chest wall continues.
4.   Weeks 12 to 16: Specialized cells differentiate into the smooth muscle of nipples and areolas.
  a.   Epithelial cells develop into mammary buds.
  b.   Epithelial branches form to eventually become alveoli.

5.   Weeks 15 to 25: Shallow epithelial depressions (mammary pits) begin to form, which represent future secretory alveoli.
     a.   The inversion of 8 to 15 strips that will become the lactiferous ducts and their branches form an opening into the mammary pit.
     b.   The mammary pit becomes elevated, forming the nipple and areola.
     c.   An inverted nipple results when the pit fails to elevate.
6.   After 32 weeks: A lumen (canal) forms in each part of the branching system.
7.   Near term: 15 to 25 mammary ducts form the fetal mammary gland.
8.   Neonate: Galactorrhea (also called witches' milk) begins, which is the secretion of colostral-like fluid from neonatal mammary tissue resulting from the influence of maternal hormones.

B.   Breast development continues through puberty.
1.   Breast growth keeps pace with general physical growth.
2.   The growth of the breast parenchyma (i.e., functional parts of the breast) produces ducts, lobes, alveoli, and surrounding fat pads.
3.   The onset of menses at age 10 to 12 years continues breast development.
     a.   Primary and secondary ducts grow and divide.
     b.   Terminal end buds form, which later become alveoli (small sacs where milk is secreted) in the mature female breast.
     c.   Proliferation and active growth of ductal tissue takes place during each menstrual cycle and continues to about age 35 years.

C.   Complete development of mammary function occurs only in pregnancy.
1.   The breast size increases, the skin appears thinner, and the veins become more prominent.
2.   The areola diameter increases,[1] the Montgomery glands enlarge, and the nipple pigment darkens.

D.   Anomalies in breast development may result from some illnesses, chemotherapy, therapeutic radiation to the chest, chest surgery, or injuries to the chest.

E.   Programmed apoptosis (cell death) that occurs at the end of lactation has been suggested as one theory for lower breast cancer rates in women who have breastfed.[2]

II. General Anatomy of a Mature Breast

A.   The exterior breast is located in the superficial fascia (fibrous tissue beneath the skin) between the second rib and the sixth intercostal space. (See **FIGURE 6-1**.)
1.   Mammary glandular tissue that projects into the axillary region is called tail of Spence.
     a.   It is distinguished from supernumerary tissue because it connects to the duct system.
     b.   This potential area can also be affected by mastitis.
2.   The skin surface contains the nipple, areola, and Montgomery glands.
3.   Although breast size may indicate milk storage potential,[3,4] size is not related to functional capacity. Fat composition of the breast gives it its size and shape.

B.   The nipple areola complex provides a target for the newborn to latch and feed. (See **FIGURE 6-2**.)
1.   The nipple is a conical elevation located slightly below the center of the areola.
     a.   The average diameter of a nipple is 1.6 cm; the average length is 0.7 cm.[5]
     b.   Smooth muscle fibers function as a closure mechanism to keep milk from continuously leaking from the nipple.
     c.   The nipple is densely innervated with sensory nerve endings.
     d.   Longitudinal inner muscles and outer circular and radial muscles make the nipple erect when contracted.
     e.   Venostasis slows the blood flow and decreases the surface area.
     f.   The nipple becomes smaller, firmer, and more prominent to help the infant latch.
2.   The areola is a circular, dark-pigmented area that surrounds the nipple.
     a.   The average diameter is 6.4 cm.[5]
     b.   It is constructed of smooth muscle and collagenous, elastic, connective tissue fibers in a radial and circular arrangement.
     c.   An increase in melanin deposits during pregnancy causes darkening to occur, which is usually accompanied by enlargement.

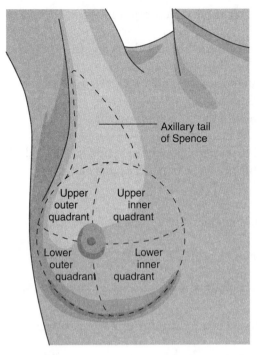

FIGURE 6-1 Breast quadrants and axillary tail of Spence.

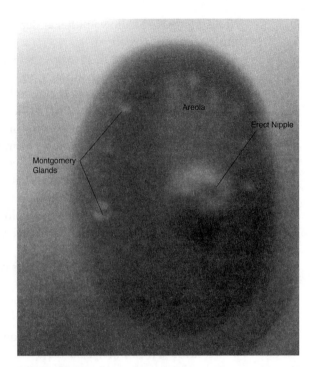

FIGURE 6-2 Nipple areolar complex.

  d. Montgomery tubercles are located around the areola.
    i. They contain ductal openings of sebaceous and lactiferous glands and sweat glands.
    ii. The tubercles enlarge during pregnancy.
    iii. They secrete a substance that lubricates and protects the nipples.
    iv. The secretions produce a scent to help the infant locate the nipple.[6,7]
 C. The parenchyma constitutes the functional parts of the breast (see **FIGURE 6-3**).
  1. Alveoli (also called acini) are the basic components of the mature mammary gland.
   a. Alveoli are the milk-producing units in the breast (see **FIGURE 6-4**).
    i. Lactocytes, which are specialized epithelial cells that line the interior of the alveolus, absorb nutrients, immunoglobulin, and hormones from the bloodstream to compose milk.
    ii. Prolactin receptor sites in the lactocytes allow prolactin to be absorbed from the blood and enter into the alveoli to stimulate milk production.
   b. Myoepithelial cells encase the alveoli and contract in response to oxytocin to eject milk into ductules.
  2. Lobes are clusters of lobules that are filled with alveoli. The breast contains 15 to 25 lobes that carry milk through the ductules from the alveoli to the nipple.
   a. Each lobe contains from 10 to 100 alveoli in an intricate system of ductules that branch out from the lobes and converge into lactiferous ducts behind the nipple.
   b. Ultrasound imaging shows the connections between the lobes.[8]
   c. Ducts branch very close to the nipple. They widen temporarily in response to milk ejection and then narrow when the duct is drained.[9,10]
   d. Milk that is not removed flows backward up the collecting ducts.
  3. Lactiferous ducts lead to openings in the nipple. Each nipple has 4 to 18 openings; there is an average of 9 openings.[11]
 D. Stroma, the supporting tissues of the breast, include connective tissue, fat tissue, blood vessels, nerves, and lymphatics.
  1. Cooper's ligaments run vertically through the breast and attach the deep layer of subcutaneous tissue to the dermis layer of the skin.

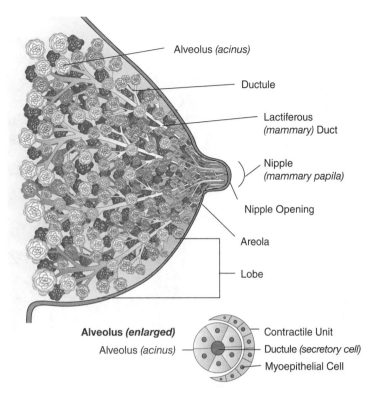

FIGURE 6-3 Structure of a lactating breast.

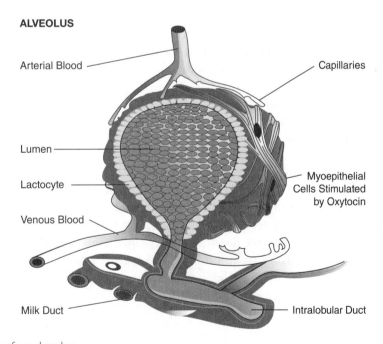

FIGURE 6-4 Cross section of an alveolus.

Reproduced from Riordan J, Wambach K. *Breastfeeding and Human Lactation*. 4th ed. Sudbury, MA: Jones and Bartlett; 2010.

2. The breast is highly vascular (see **FIGURE 6-5**).
    a. The internal mammary artery supplies 60 percent of the blood in the breast.
    b. The lateral thoracic artery supplies 30 percent of the blood in the breast.
    c. Blood vessels within the breast enlarge with an increase in progesterone.

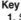

Key
1. Subclavian artery
2. Superior thoracic artery
3. Internal thoracic artery
4. Major pectoralis muscle
5. Perforating branches of the internal mammary artery
6. Arterial plexus around areola
7. Intercostal arteries
8. Pectoral branches of the lateral thoracic artery
9. Circumflex scapular artery
10. Minor pectoralis muscle
11. Subscapular artery
12. Lateral thoracic artery
13. Pectoral branch of the thoracoacromial artery
14. Axillary artery
15. Deltoid branch of the thoracoacromial artery

FIGURE 6-5 Arterial blood supply to the breast.

     d.   Surges of estrogen stimulate duct growth.
     e.   Surges of progesterone cause glandular tissue to expand.
  3.   The lymphatic system collects excess fluids from tissue spaces, bacteria, and cast-off cell parts. It drains mainly to the axillary lymph nodes (see **FIGURE 6-6**).
  4.   Breast innervation derives mainly from branches of the fourth intercostal nerve which is the primary nerve that affects lactation due to its importance in the endocrine loop that involves oxytocin and prolactin (see **FIGURE 6-7**).
     a.   The supply of nerves to the innermost areas of the breast is sparse.
     b.   The fourth intercostal nerve penetrates the posterior aspect of the breast.
        i.   It supplies the greatest amount of sensation to the areola, at the four o'clock position on the left breast and at the eight o'clock position on the right breast.
       ii.   It becomes more superficial as it reaches the areola, where it divides into five branches.
      iii.   The lowermost branch penetrates the areola at the five o'clock position on the left breast and at the seven o'clock position on the right breast.
      iv.   Trauma to this nerve might result in some loss of sensation in the breast. If the lowermost branch is severed, the nipple and areola might lose sensation.
       v.   Aberrant sensory or autonomic nerve distributions in the nipple–areola complex could affect the milk ejection reflex and the secretion of prolactin and oxytocin. Breast augmentation or reduction surgery may sever or cause nerve trauma affecting such a reflex.

III. Variations in Breast Anatomy

  A.   Breasts vary in size, shape, color, and placement on the chest wall (see **TABLE 6-1** and **FIGURE 6-8**).
    1.   The weight of the breast increases through pregnancy and lactation:
     a.   Nonpregnant woman: Mature breast weighs about 200 g.
     b.   Pregnancy near term: Breast weighs between 400 and 600 g.
     c.   Lactation: Breast can weigh 600 to 800 g.
    2.   Asymmetry is common; the left breast is often larger than the right breast.[12]

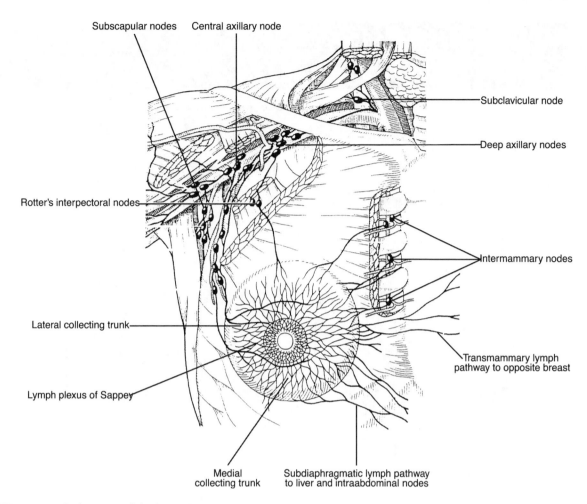

FIGURE 6-6 Lymph drainage of the breast.

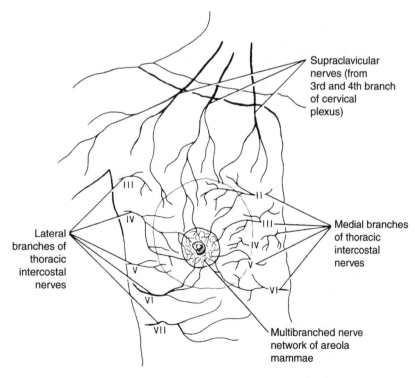

FIGURE 6-7 Innervation of the breast.

TABLE 6-1 Breast Types Classified by Physical Characteristics

Breast Type	Physical Characteristics
Type 1	Round breasts, normal lower, medial, and lateral quadrants
Type 2	Hypoplasia of the lower medial quadrant
Type 3	Hypoplasia of the lower medial and lateral quadrants
Type 4	Severe constrictions, minimal breast base

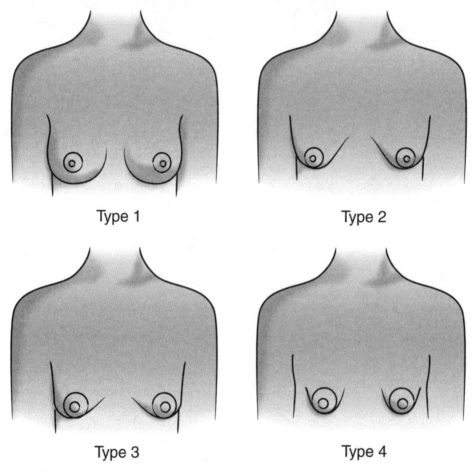

FIGURE 6-8 Breast classifications.

Reproduced from Huggins K, Petok ES, Mireles O. Markers of lactation insufficiency. In: Auerbach KG, ed. *Current Issues in Clinical Lactation*. Sudbury, MA: Jones and Bartlett: 2000:25-35.[17] Used with permission of Kathleen Huggins.

B.   Breast malformations include the following:
1.   Polythelia is the presence of extra nipples.
   a.   An accessory or supernumerary nipple develops along the milk line between the axilla and the groin.[13,14]
   b.   It is often prominent during pregnancy and lactation.
   c.   It may be associated with renal or other organ system anomalies and should be investigated if it is seen in a newborn.[15]
2.   Polymastia is the presence of extra breast tissue. Accessory glandular tissues can lactate and undergo malignant changes.[5]
3.   Hyperthelia describes a nipple without accompanying mammary tissue.
4.   Hypertrophy describes an abnormally large breast.
5.   Hypomastia describes an abnormally small breast.
6.   Hyperplasia is the overdevelopment of the breast; hyperplastic breast.

7. Hypoplasia is insufficient glandular tissue.[16]
    a. Hypoplasia results in a tubular or tuberous shape because of the lack of glandular tissue.
    b. The breasts may have large areolas.
    c. The breasts are frequently asymmetric and widely spaced.
    d. This condition may present an increased risk for insufficient milk production.[17]
    e. Unilateral hypoplasia of the breast combined with hypoplasia of the thorax and pectoral muscles is known as Poland syndrome.
C. Nipple variations include the following (see **TABLE 6-2**):
    1. Restricted protractility
        a. The nipple should evert and become protractile when compressed or stimulated.
        b. The incidence of poor protractility in primigravida women ranges from 10 to 35 percent.[18-21]

TABLE 6-2 Five Basic Types of Nipples		
Type of Nipple	**Before Stimulation**	**After Stimulation**
Common nipple: The majority of parents have what is referred to as a common nipple. It protrudes slightly when at rest and becomes erect and more graspable when stimulated. A baby has no trouble finding and grasping this nipple and can pull in a large amount of breast tissue and stretch it to the roof of the mouth.		
Flat or short-shanked nipple: A flat nipple may be soft and pliable and have the ability to form ridges so it can mold to the infant's mouth without a problem. A flat nipple may have a short shank that makes it more difficult to form ridges and for the baby to find and grasp. In response to stimulation, this nipple may remain unchanged, or it may retract with compression. A slight movement inward or outward may be present, but it is not enough to help the baby find and initially grasp the breast on center. This nipple may benefit from the use of a syringe to increase its protractility.		
Pseudo-inverted nipple: A pseudo-inverted nipple may appear inverted, but it becomes erect after compression or stimulation. This nipple needs no correction and presents no grasping problems.		
Retracted nipple: A retracted nipple is the most common type of inverted nipple. Initially, this nipple appears to be graspable. However, it retracts on stimulation, making attachment difficult. This nipple responds well to techniques that increase nipple protrusion.		
Inverted nipple: A truly inverted nipple is retracted both at rest and when stimulated. This nipple is very uncommon and is more difficult for the baby to grasp. All techniques used to enhance the protractility of breast tissue can be used to improve attachment. Even if the nipple remains retracted, the baby should be able to latch on if the parent helps form the breast into the baby's mouth.		

     c. Protractility improves during pregnancy. The effect on latch is minimal when the baby has a large mouthful of breast tissue.

     d. Nipple inversion occurs in about 3 percent of women and is usually bilateral.[22]

          i. A truly inverted nipple remains inverted when it is compressed or stimulated, which is also called the pinch test.

          ii. A pseudo-inverted nipple appears inverted but everts when compressed or stimulated.

          iii. A short-shanked nipple appears everted but retracts when compressed or stimulated.

  2. Other nipple variations

     a. Bulbous: Large nipple that may be difficult for a baby to grasp and achieve a successful latch.

     b. Dimpled: Increases the risk for maceration because the nipple is enveloped by the areola.

     c. Bifurcated: A single nipple that is separated by a slit into 2 or more sections.

     d. Double or multiple nipples close together.

     e. Skin tag: A small benign skin growth that may appear on the breast or nipple. Skin tags are more prevalent during pregnancy.

  3. Nipple piercings, studs, and bars

     a. Nipple piercings generally do not affect milk production.[23]

     b. Nipple piercing can contribute to maternal discomfort, poor latch, altered milk flow during feeding, and increased milk leakage.

     c. Wearing jewelry on the nipple during feeding could put the infant at risk of aspiration and to injuries of the gums, soft palate, and tongue.

     d. Nipple jewelry should be removed before breastfeeding.

IV. Mammogenesis: Prenatal Breast Development

A. Final preparation for lactation occurs during pregnancy.

  1. Early in the first trimester, mammary epithelial cells proliferate, ductal sprouting and branching begin, and lobular proliferation occurs.

  2. Ducts proliferate into the fatty pad, and the ductal end buds differentiate into alveoli.

  3. Increases occur in mammary blood flow, interstitial water, and electrolyte concentrations.

  4. Mammary blood vessels increase their luminal diameters and form new capillaries around the lobules.

  5. During the last trimester, secretory cells fill with fat droplets, and the alveoli are distended with colostrum.

  6. Mammary cells become competent to secrete milk proteins at midpregnancy, but they are kept in check by high circulating levels of steroids, particularly progesterone.

  7. Most milk products that are secreted during pregnancy find their way back into the plasma via the leaky junctions (spaces between the mammary alveolar cells).

B. Hormonal changes influence prenatal breast changes.

  1. Lactogenesis is hormonally driven by the endocrine control system.

  2. Human placental lactogen, prolactin, and human chorionic gonadotropin accelerate growth.

  3. A form of estrogen called 17 beta-estradiol is required for mammary growth and epithelial proliferation during pregnancy.

  4. Glucocorticoids enhance formation of the lobules during pregnancy.

  5. Estrogen increases during pregnancy and stimulates ductal sprouting.

  6. Prolactin is necessary for complete growth of the gland.[24]

     a. It is secreted by the anterior pituitary gland.

     b. It stimulates prolactin receptor sites for the initiation of milk secretion located on the alveolar cell surfaces.

     c. Prolactin levels rise throughout pregnancy and during sleep.[25]

     d. Prolactin is prevented from exerting its positive influence on milk secretion during pregnancy by the elevated levels of circulating progesterone.

     e. Prolactin-inhibiting factor (PIF) is secreted by the hypothalamus to negatively control prolactin's effects in response to fatigue, depression, or stress. Dopamine is an example of PIF.

7. Progesterone increases during pregnancy.
   a. It stimulates lobuloalveolar growth while suppressing secretory activity.
   b. It sensitizes mammary cells to the effects of insulin and growth factors.
   c. Progesterone may be involved in the final preparation of the glandular tissue for copious milk production (lactogenesis II).

V. Lactogenesis I or Secretory Differentiation

A. Lactogenesis I is the beginning of secretory cellular activity and milk production.
B. It occurs at about the 16th prenatal week.[26]
C. It is the stage at which the breast is first capable of synthesizing unique milk components. Human placental lactogen and growth factors are thought to be responsible.[27]
D. Thyroid hormones increase the responsiveness of mammary cells to prolactin and can improve lactation performance.
E. The main reproductive hormones that are necessary for secretory differentiation include estrogen, progesterone, placental lactogen, and prolactin.
F. Supportive metabolic hormones include glucocorticoids such as cortisol, insulin, thyroid–parathyroid hormone, and growth hormone.[28]
G. The antepartum secretion, or colostrum, shows a gradually increasing presence of lactose, casein, and alpha-lactalbumin.
H. Colostrum (early milk) is available to the infant at birth. In addition, an increase in the concentrations of two immunoprotective proteins in colostrum, secretory immunoglobulin A and lactoferrin, occurs after delivery.

VI. Lactogenesis II or Secretory Activation

A. Lactogenesis II is the onset of copious milk secretion.
   1. It occurs between 30 and 72 hours following delivery of the placenta.
   2. Women typically begin feeling breast fullness around 50 to 72 hours after birth.[5]
   3. Initially under endocrine control, it is now under autocrine, or local, control. Lactogenesis I is completely dependent on hormonal changes (endocrine) that occur during pregnancy. Lactogenesis II is maintained by stimulation of the nipple and regular milk removal from the breast (autocrine).[29-31]
B. Placental expulsion following delivery precipitates an abrupt decline in levels of human placental lactogen, estrogen, and progesterone.
   1. Progesterone is a prolactin inhibitor and the decline in progesterone levels is thought to be the initiating event for lactogenesis II.
   2. This decline in progesterone acts in the presence of a lactogenic complex of hormones, including prolactin, insulin, and cortisol, for full secretory activation.[32]
   3. Changes in milk composition occur, including a sharp rise in citrate and alpha-lactalbumin.
C. The risk factors for delayed onset of lactation include the following:
   1. Fluid volume overload in labor.[33,34]
   2. Cesarean section[35] or stressful vaginal birth with long stage 2 labor.[36]
   3. Maternal health status:
      a. Type 1 diabetes mellitus: May cause a temporary imbalance in the amount of insulin required for glucose homeostasis, which is a requirement for the initiation of lactation.[37]
      b. Obesity.[38,39]
      c. History of reduction mammoplasty.
      d. Hypoplasia (insufficient mammary tissue), polycystic ovarian syndrome, infertility,[5] and thyroid dysfunction.
   4. Any maternal illness or situation interfering with early milk removal,[36] including Sheehan syndrome, which is a pituitary infarct caused by severe postpartum hemorrhage.
   5. Parity: Primiparas are at increased risk of delayed lactogenesis.[40]
   6. Retained placental fragments.

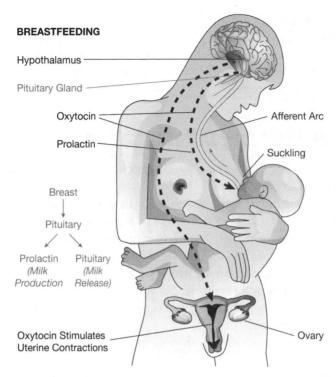

BREASTFEEDING

Hypothalamus

Pituitary Gland

Oxytocin

Prolactin

Afferent Arc

Suckling

Breast
↓
Pituitary
↙ ↘
Prolactin   Pituitary
(Milk   (Milk
Production)   Release)

Oxytocin Stimulates
Uterine Contractions

Ovary

FIGURE 6-9 Neuroendocrine reflex arc.

    D.   Prolactin levels increase sharply after placenta delivery and rise and fall with the frequency, intensity, and duration of nipple stimulation.

        1.   Prolactin levels fall about 50 percent in the first week postpartum. Prolactin has been detected in mature milk up to 40 weeks postpartum.[5] In addition, there is a prolactin circadian rhythm, with prolactin release being higher at night, surging in response to the baby's suckling or with manual or mechanical milk removal.

        2.   Frequent feeding in early lactation stimulates the development of prolactin receptor sites in the mammary gland. The theory is that the controlling factor in milk production is the number of prolactin receptor sites, not the amount of prolactin in circulating blood.[5] However, a recent small study showed an increase in milk volume with administration of recombinant prolactin.[41]

        3.   Lactogenesis II occurs earlier if the parent has breastfed before, possibly because of the increased number of prolactin receptor sites.[42]

        4.   In birth parents who are not breastfeeding, prolactin drops to prepregnancy levels at 2 weeks postpartum.

        5.   Although prolactin is necessary for milk secretion, its levels are not directly related to the volume of milk produced; that is, prolactin becomes permissive in its function.

        6.   Prolactin release occurs only in response to direct stimulation of the nipple and areola in a neuro-hormonal feedback pathway (see **FIGURE 6-9**). This autocrine control is responsible for the next stage of milk production, lactogenesis III.

VII. Lactogenesis III or Galactopoiesis

    A.   The stage of mature milk production (also known as galactopoiesis), which is defined as later than 9 days after birth to the beginning of involution,[43] is the maintenance phase of lactation. It is dependent on autocrine, or local, control.

    B.   Milk synthesis is controlled by two mechanisms (see **FIGURE 6-10**).

        1.   Feedback inhibitor of lactation (FIL) is described as a small active whey protein that is synthesized by the lactocytes and accumulates in the alveolar lumen.[44]

            a.   The role of FIL appears to be to moderate milk synthesis locally, based on the fullness of the breast.

            b.   The rate of milk synthesis slows when milk accumulates in the breast because more FIL is present in the milk, which initiates this chemical feedback loop.

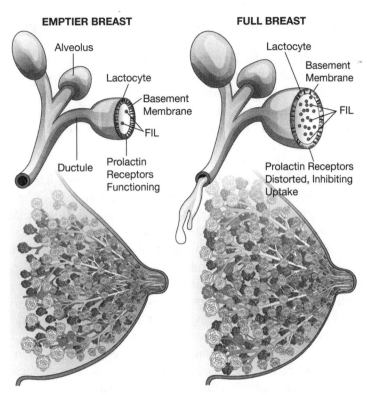

EMPTIER BREAST

FULL BREAST

FIGURE 6-10 Milk synthesis control: feedback inhibitor of lactation and prolactin receptor theory.
Courtesy of Lactation Education Resources.

    c.   The rate of milk synthesis speeds up when milk is removed from the breast and less FIL is present.

    d.   Frequent and complete milk removal will, theoretically, result in greater milk production.

    e.   Recent research suggests that FIL is not solely responsible for autocrine control of milk production at the cellular level. Several bioactive factors have been found to influence autocrine control of milk production in non-human mammalian studies including β1-integrin, α-Lactalbumin, transforming growth factor β, insulin-like growth factor-binding protein 5, and lactoferrin.[45]

2.   Prolactin receptor theory suggests a local mechanism that regulates the rate of milk synthesis, involving prolactin receptors in the basement membrane of the alveoli that lactocytes are attached to.

    a.   As milk accumulates in the breast, the shape of the lactocyte is distorted and prolactin cannot bind to its receptor, creating an inhibitory effect on the level of milk production.[46,47]

    b.   Prolactin uptake is inhibited by alveolar distension, which down regulates milk synthesis.[48]

VIII. Involution: Apoptosis of Secretory Cells

A.   Involution occurs when the milk-producing system in the breast is no longer being used, which results in secretory epithelial apoptosis, or cell death.[49]

B.   Complete involution typically occurs approximately 40 days after complete cessation of breastfeeding.

C.   Involution depends on the type of weaning process, whether it is abrupt or gradual.

D.   Anecdotally, parents report that the longer they are actively producing milk, the longer it takes for milk production to completely cease.

IX. Milk Production and Synthesis

A.   Milk production is affected by many factors.

    1.   The volume of milk removed from the breast at a feeding or during expression is correlated to the needs of the baby, an elegant example of supply and demand.

    2.   Studies show an increased sensitivity of prolactin receptors in multiparous women, which can affect overall milk production.[42]

3. Maternal conditions such as breast hypoplasia, obesity, disease, and metabolism rate can affect milk production.

4. Maternal medications, specifically prolactin-inhibiting factors (also known as dopamine agonists) such as bromocriptine and ergotamine, can inhibit prolactin secretion.[5]

B. Milk is stored in the alveoli and in small ducts adjacent to the cells that secrete milk. This storage compresses and flattens the cells.

1. The storage capacity of breasts varies greatly among individuals. The measured storage capacity of a breast increases with breast size.

2. Cells that line both the alveoli and the smaller ductules appear to be capable of secreting milk.

C. The rate of milk synthesis is the rate at which newly manufactured milk accumulates within the breast.

1. The degree to which milk is removed signals the amount of milk to be made for the next feeding. Milk synthesis responds to the varying amount of residual milk remaining in the breast after a feeding (FIL factor; see Figure 6-10).

2. The degree of fullness in a breast and the rate of short-term synthesis are inversely related.[50-53]

3. There is wide variability in the rate of milk synthesis, ranging from 17 to 33 mL per hour.[54,55]

4. Local, or autocrine, control regulates short-term milk synthesis.

5. Milk synthesis is controlled independently in each breast.

6. Small breasts are capable of secreting as much milk over a 24-hour period as large breasts.[11]

D. Milk synthesis occurs in the lactocyte (or secretory epithelial cell) after the uptake of substrates from the blood that are necessary for milk production.[48] Five pathways are involved in milk synthesis.[51]

1. Pathway I: Protein secretion, with the most important proteins synthesized by the mammary cell being casein, lactoferrin, alpha-lactalbumin, and lysozyme.

2. Pathway II: Lactose secretion.

3. Pathway III: Milk fat synthesis.

4. Pathway IV: Monovalent ion secretion into milk includes sodium, potassium, and chloride.

5. Pathway V: Plasma protein secretion, where plasma immunoglobulin A binds to the mammary alveolar cell and is released into the milk; it is involved in disease protection.

E. Milk release, also referred to as milk ejection reflex or the letdown reflex, results from stimulation of sensory neurons and the release of oxytocin.

1. Direct stimulation by the infant to sensory neurons in the areola initiates a neuroendocrine arc to the posterior pituitary to release oxytocin into the bloodstream (see Figure 6-10).

   a. Impulses from the cerebral cortex, ears, and eyes can also elicit the release of oxytocin through exteroceptive stimuli (such as hearing a baby cry).[24]

   b. Some parents feel the milk ejection reflex as increased pressure or tingling within the breast or as shooting pains, whereas some parents never feel the milk ejection reflex.

   c. The response to oxytocin release from the posterior pituitary includes the following:

      i. For the first few days after birth, breastfeeding will be accompanied by uterine cramping. Also known as afterbirth pains (Figure 6-10) the cramping is especially felt by multiparous women.

      ii. Oxytocin release might also elicit increased thirst, a warm or flushed feeling, increased heat from the breasts, or a feeling of sleepiness or calmness.

   d. Milk ejection signs include milk dripping from the breast and when the baby begins audibly swallowing milk (when the rapid pattern of two sucks per second decreases to one suck or so per second with swallowing).

   e. The milk ejection reflex serves to increase the intraductal mammary pressure and to maintain it at levels that are sufficient to overcome resistance to the outflow of milk from the breast.

   f. The amount of milk transferred by the infant is correlated to the number of milk ejections per feeding and is independent of the amount of time spent at the breast.[9]

2. Oxytocin causes a contraction of the myoepithelial cells surrounding the alveoli, forcing milk into the collecting ducts of the breast.

   a. A simultaneous and closed secretion of oxytocin occurs in brain regions of the lactating parent.[54-57]

      i. Has a calming, analgesic affect.

      ii. Lowers maternal blood pressure.

      iii.   Decreases cortisol levels, decreases anxiety and aggressive behavior.
      iv.   Permeates the areas of the brain associated with parenting and bonding behaviors.
  b. Nipple stimulation causes oxytocin release of brief 3 to 4 second pulsatile bursts into the bloodstream every 5 to 15 minutes.[36]
  c. Variable and intermittent bursts of oxytocin are also seen from stimuli before breastfeeding and mechanical stimulation from a breast pump.[60]
  d. Oxytocin causes shortening of the ducts without constricting them, thus increasing milk pressure.[36]
  e. Oxytocin secretion can be inhibited by pain, fatigue, anxiety, or stress[5,61]; alcohol[62]; and certain labor practices because induction or augmentation of labor with synthetic oxytocin has been found to interfere with the release of endogenous oxytocin.[63,64]

▸ Key Points from This Chapter

A.   Complete development of mammary function occurs only in pregnancy.
B.   Alveoli are the basic components of the mature mammary gland; within them lactocytes absorb nutrients, immunoglobulins, and hormones from the blood to compose milk.
C.   A cluster of alveoli form lobules which form lobes. Lobes cluster together and milk flows through ductules which converge into lactiferous ducts which lead into openings in the nipple.
D.   Prolactin stimulates milk production.
E.   Oxytocin release triggers milk ejection or letdown.
F.   17 beta-estradiol is required for mammary growth and epithelial proliferation during pregnancy.
G.   The elevated levels of progesterone during pregnancy prevent prolactin from influencing milk production.
H.   Initiation of lactogenesis II is caused by the abrupt drop in progesterone.
I.   Rate of milk synthesis slows when milk accumulates in the breast because more FIL is present in the milk.

🔍 CASE STUDY

Tanya is 24 hours post cesarean section with her first baby, Cameron. Cameron was born at 39 weeks. The indication for cesarean section was breech presentation. Cameron is healthy and weighed 8 pounds 9 ounces (3383 g) at birth. Skin-to-skin contact did not occur at birth. Cameron's first attempt at breastfeeding was 4 hours after birth, followed by 3 subsequent feedings at breast with sustained latch and audible swallowing. You are the lactation consultant at the hospital and Tanya requests your assistance with the next feeding. Tanya expresses concern about having no milk and fears that Cameron is not getting any milk.

Questions
1. How would you address Tanya's concerns?
2. How would you explain the process of lactogenesis I and II to Tanya?
3. What health history questions would you ask regarding Tanya's breast development before and during pregnancy?
4. How would you assess Tanya's breasts?
5. What breast assessment findings would be concerning?
6. What physical signs of lactogenesis II would you explain to Tanya?
7. What recommendations would you give to Tanya regarding practices that will support lactogenesis II?

References

1. Hytten FE. Clinical and chemical studies in human lactation-IX. *BMJ.* 1954;18:1447-1452.
2. Shema L, Ore L, Ben-Shachar M, Haj M, Linn S. The association between breastfeeding and breast cancer occurrence among Israeli Jewish women: a case control study. *J Cancer Res Clin Oncol.* 2007;133(8):539-546.
3. Daly S, Hartmann P. Infant demand and milk supply. Part 1: infant demand and milk production in lactating women. *J Hum Lactation.* 1995;11:21-26.
4. Hartmann PE, Owns RA, Cox DB. Establishing lactation. Breast development and control of milk synthesis. *Food Nutr Bull.* 1996;17:1-10.

5. Wambach K, Riordan J. *Breastfeeding and Human Lactation.* 5th ed. Burlington, MA: Jones & Bartlett Learning; 2016.
6. Doucet S, Soussignan R, Sagot P, Schaal B. The secretion of areolar (Montgomery's) glands from lactating women elicits selective, unconditional responses in neonates. *PLOS One.* 2009;4:e7579. doi: 10.1371/journal.pone.0007579.
7. Schaal B, Doucet S, Sagot P, Hertling E, Soussignan R. Human breast areolae as scent organs: morphological data and possible involvement in maternal-neonatal coadaptation. *Dev Psychobiology.* 2006;48:100-110.
8. Geddes D. Inside the lactating breast: the latest anatomy research. *J Midwifery Womens Health.* 2007;52:556-563.
9. Ramsay D, Kent J, Owens R, Hartmann P. Ultrasound imaging of milk ejection in the breast of lactating women. *Pediatrics.* 2004;113:361-367.
10. Ramsay D, Mitoulas L, Kent J, Larsson M, Hartmann P. The use of ultrasound to characterize milk ejection in women using an electric breast pump. *J Hum Lactation.* 2005;21:421-428.
11. Ramsay DT, Kent JC, Hartmann RA, Hartmann PE. Anatomy of the lactating human breast redefined with ultrasound imaging. *J Anat.* 2005;206:525-534.
12. Losken A, Fishman I, Denson D, Moyer H, Carlson G. An objective evaluation of breast symmetry and shape differences using 3-dimensional images. *Ann Plast Surg.* 2005;55:571-575.
13. Schmidt H. Supernumerary nipples: prevalence, size, sex and side predilection—a prospective clinical study. *Eur J Pediatr.* 1998;157:821-823.
14. Velanovich V. Ectopic breast tissue, supernumerary breasts, and supernumerary nipples. *South Med J.* 1995;88:903-906.
15. Berman M, Davis G. Lactation from axillary breast tissue in the absence of a supernumerary nipple. A case report. *J Reprod Med.* 1994;39:657-659.
16. McGuire E, Rowan M. PCOS, breast hypoplasia and low milk supply: a case study. *Breastfeeding Rev.* 2015;23:29-32.
17. Huggins K, Petok ES, Mireles O. Markers of lactation insufficiency. In: Auerbach KG, ed. *Current Issues in Clinical Lactation.* Sudbury, MA: Jones and Bartlett; 2000:25-35.
18. Alexander JM, Grant AM, Campbell MJ. Randomised controlled trial of breast shells and Hoffman's exercises for inverted and non-protractile nipples. *BMJ.* 1992;18:1030-1032.
19. Blaikley J, Clarke S, MacKeith R, Ogden KM. Breast-feeding: factors affecting success. *BJOG.* 1953;60:657-669.
20. Hytten FE, Baird D. The development of the nipple in pregnancy. *Lancet.* 1958;271:1201-1204.
21. Waller H. The early failure of breastfeeding. *Arch Dis Child.* 1946;21;1-12.
22. Park H, Yoon C, Kim H. The prevalence of congenital inverted nipple. *Aesthetic Plast Surg.* 1999;23:144-146.
23. Holbrook J, Minocha J, Laumann A. Body piercing: complications and prevention of health risks. *Am J Clin Dermatol.* 2012;13:1-17.
24. Uvnäs-Moberg K, Widström A, Werner S, Matthiesen A, Winberg J. Oxytocin and prolactin levels in breast-feeding women. Correlation with milk yield and duration of breast-feeding. *Acta Obstet Gynecol Scand.* 1990;69:301-306.
25. Cregan M, Mitoulas L, Hartmann P. Milk prolactin, feed volume and duration between feeds in women breastfeeding their full-term infants over a 24 h period. *Exp Physiol.* 2002;87:207-214.
26. Lawrence RA, Lawrence RM. *Breastfeeding: A Guide for the Medical Professional.* 8th ed. Philadelphia, PA: Elsevier Health Sciences; 2015.
27. Buhimschi C. Endocrinology of lactation. *Obstet Gynecol Clin North Am.* 2004;31:963-979.
28. Hurst N. Recognizing and treating delayed or failed lactogenesis II. *J Midwifery Womens Health.* 2007;52:588-594.
29. De Coopman J. Breastfeeding after pituitary resection: support for a theory of autocrine control of milk supply? *J Hum Lactation.* 1993;9:35-40.
30. Wilde C, Addey C, Boddy L, Peaker M. Autocrine regulation of milk secretion by a protein in milk. *Biochem J.* 1995;305:51-58.
31. Wilde CJ, Prentice A, Peaker M. Breast-feeding: matching supply with demand in human lactation. *Proc Nutr Soc.* 1995;54:401-406.
32. Pang W, Hartmann P. Initiation of human lactation: secretory differentiation and secretory activation. *J Mammary Gland Biol Neoplasia.* 2007;12:211-221.
33. Cotterman K. Reverse pressure softening: a simple tool to prepare areola for easier latching during engorgement. *J Hum Lactation.* 2004;20:227-237.
34. Lauwers J, Swisher A. *Counseling the Nursing Mother.* 6th ed. Burlington, MA: Jones & Bartlett Learning; 2016.
35. Dewey K, Nommsen-Rivers L, Heinig M, Cohen R. Risk factors for suboptimal infant breastfeeding behavior, delayed onset of lactation, and excess neonatal weight loss. *Pediatrics.* 2003;112:607-619.
36. Neville M, Morton J. Physiology and endocrine changes underlying human lactogenesis II. *J Nutr.* 2001;131(11):3005S-3008S.
37. Oliveira A, Cunha C, Penha-Silva N, Abdallah V, Jorge P. Interference of the blood glucose control in the transition between phases I and II of lactogenesis in patients with type 1 diabetes mellitus. *Arq Bras Endocrinol Metabol.* 2008;52:473-481.
38. Nommsen-Rivers LA, Chantry CJ, Peerson JM, Cohen RJ, Dewey KG. Delayed onset of lactogenesis among first-time mothers is related to maternal obesity and factors associated with ineffective breastfeeding. *Am J Clin Nutr.* 2010;92:574-584.
39. Rasmussen K, Kjolhede C. Prepregnant overweight and obesity diminish the prolactin response to suckling in the first week postpartum. *Pediatrics.* 2004;113(5):e465-e471.
40. Scott J, Binns C, Oddy W. Predictors of delayed onset of lactation. *Maternal Child Nutr.* 2007;3:186-193.
41. Powe C, Puopolo K, Welt C, et al. Effects of recombinant human prolactin on breast milk composition. *Pediatrics.* 2011;127:e359-e366.
42. Zuppa AA, Tornesello A, Papacci P, et al. Relationship between maternal parity, basal prolactin levels and neonatal breast milk intake. *Neonatology.* 1988;5:144-147.
43. Uvnäs-Moberg K, Eriksson M. Breastfeeding: physiological, endocrine and behavioural adaptations caused by oxytocin and local neurogenic activity in the nipple and mammary gland. *Acta Paediatrica.* 1996;85:525-530.
44. Wilde CJ, Calvert DT, Daly A, Peaker M. The effect of goat milk fractions on synthesis of milk constituents by rabbit mammary explants and on milk yield in vivo. Evidence for autocrine control of milk secretion. *Biochemical J.* 1987;242(1):285-288.
45. Weaver SR, Hernandez LL. Autocrine-paracrine regulation of the mammary gland. *J Dairy Science.* 2016;99(1):842-853.
46. van Veldhuizen-Staas C. Overabundant milk supply: an alternative way to intervene by full drainage and block feeding. *Int Breastfeed J.* 2007;2:11.

47. Zoubiane G, Valentijn A, Streuli C, et al. A role for the cytoskeleton in prolactin-dependent mammary epithelial cell differentiation. *J Cell Sci.* 2004;117:271-280.
48. Hale TW, Hartmann PE. *Hale and Hartmann's Textbook of Human Lactation.* New York, NY: Springer; 2007.
49. Watson CJ. Key stages in mammary gland development-involution: apoptosis and tissue remodelling that convert the mammary gland from milk factory to a quiescent organ. *Breast Cancer Res.* 2006;8:203.
50. Daly SE, Kent JC, Huynh DQ, et al. The determination of short-term breast volume changes and the rate of synthesis of human milk using computerized breast measurement. *Exp Physiol.* 1992;77:79-87.
51. Daly S, Kent J, Owens R, Hartmann P. Frequency and degree of milk removal and the short-term control of human milk synthesis. *Exp Physiol.* 1996;81:861-875.
52. Daly SE, Kent JC, Huynh DQ, et al. The determination of short-term breast volume changes and the rate of synthesis of human milk using computerized breast measurement. *Exp Physiol.* 1992;77:79-87.
53. Walker M. *Breastfeeding Management for the Clinician: Using the Evidence.* 4th ed. Burlington, MA: Jones & Bartlett Learning; 2017.
54. Arthur P, Smith M, Hartmann P. Milk lactose, citrate, and glucose as markers of lactogenesis in normal and diabetic women. *J Pediatr Gastroenterol Nutr.*1989;9:488-496.
55. Arthur P, Jones T, Spruce J, Hartmann P. Measuring short-term rates of milk synthesis in breast-feeding mothers. *Q J Exp Physiol.* 1989;74:419-428.
56. Febo M, Numan M, Ferris C. Functional magnetic resonance imaging shows oxytocin activates brain regions associated with mother-pup bonding during suckling. *J Neurosci.* 2005;25:11637-11644.
57. Jonas W, Wiklund I, Nissen E, Ransjö-Arvidson A, Uvnäs-Moberg K. Newborn skin temperature two days postpartum during breastfeeding related to different labour ward practices. *Early Hum Dev.* 2007;83:55-62.
58. Uvnäs-Moberg K, Petersson M. Oxytocin—biochemical link for human relations. Mediator of antistress, well-being, social interaction, growth, healing. *Lakartidningen.* 2004;101:2634-2639.
59. Winberg J. Mother and newborn baby: mutual regulation of physiology and behavior—a selective review. *Dev Psychobiol.* 2005;47:217-229.
60. Fewtrell M, Lucas P, Collier S, Lucas A. Randomized study comparing the efficacy of a novel manual breast pump with a mini-electric breast pump in mothers of term infants. *J Hum Lactation.* 2001;17:126-131.
61. Newton M, Newton N. The let-down reflex in human lactation. *J Pediatr.* 1948;33:698-704.
62. Cobo E. Effect of different doses of ethanol on the milk-ejecting reflex in lactating women. *Am J Obstet Gynecol.* 1973;115:817-821.
63. Jonas W, Johansson LM, Nissen E, Ejdebäck M, Ransjö-Arvidson AB, Uvnäs-Moberg K. Effects of intrapartum oxytocin administration and epidural analgesia on the concentration of plasma oxytocin and prolactin, in response to suckling during the second day postpartum. *Breastfeed Med.* 2009;4:71-82.
64. Jordan S, Emery S, Watkins A, Evans JD, Storey M, Morgan G. Associations of drugs routinely given in labor with breastfeeding at 48 hours: analysis of the Cardiff births survey. *Obstetric Anesthesia Digest.* 2011;31:18-19.

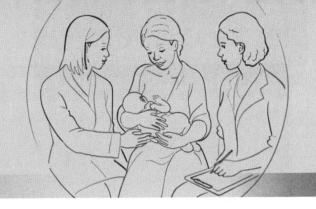

CHAPTER 7

Biochemistry of Human Milk

April Fogleman
Nicola Singletary
Jonathan C. Allen

OBJECTIVES

- Identify and describe nutritional and bioactive components of human milk.
- Characterize changes in milk composition that occur in response to infant growth requirements.
- Describe the protective function of human milk against disease.
- Compare and contrast commercial infant formula to human milk.
- Describe the nutrients in human milk and their role in infant growth and development.
- Explain how milk is a dynamic substance that changes in composition to meet the unique needs of the infant.
- Provide appropriate education regarding the importance of exclusive breastfeeding to the health of the child.

DEFINITIONS OF COMMONLY USED TERMS

alpha-lactalbumin A major whey protein in human milk. It is involved in lactose synthesis.
amino acids The building blocks of protein.
carbohydrate Macronutrient composed of one or multiple sugars.
casein A type of protein found both in solution and suspended in micelles in milk.
cholesterol A member of the group of lipids known as sterols; produced by our bodies and present in foods, including human milk.
disaccharides Pairs of single sugars linked together.
enzymes Proteins that serve as catalysts in biochemical reactions. They facilitate reactions while maintaining their structure and concentration.
fatty acid A type of lipid made of a hydrocarbon chain, with a carboxyl group on one end and a methyl group on the other end. The main component of triglycerides and phospholipids.
growth factors Proteins responsible for regulation of a variety of cellular processes, including, but not limited to, cellular growth and differentiation.

(continues)

DEFINITIONS OF COMMONLY USED TERMS *(continued)*

hormones Chemicals secreted by glands within the body that serve as messengers, acting on other organs to regulate or maintain conditions within the body.

immunoglobulin Proteins that function as antibodies. Secretory immunoglobulin A (SIgA) is an important immunoglobulin in human milk.

lactoferrin A whey protein in human milk that can modify the immune system, facilitate iron absorption, and regulate bone growth.

lipids Organic molecules that are insoluble in water. They include fatty acids, oils, waxes, sterols, phospholipids, and triglycerides.

long-chain polyunsaturated fatty acids (LCPUFAs) Fatty acids that include linoleic acid (n-6 fatty acid) (18.2 n-6, LA), alpha-linolenic acid (n-3 fatty acid) (18.3 n-3, ALA), docosahexaenoic acid (22,6 n-3, DHA), and arachidonic acid (20,4 n-4, AA).

lysozyme An enzyme found in body secretions, including human milk, saliva, tears, nasal mucus, and pancreatic juice. It is capable of breaking down the cell walls of bacteria.

macronutrients A class of nutrients that includes water and the energy-providing nutrients: proteins, lipids, and carbohydrates.

monosaccharides Single sugars.

phospholipids Similar to triglycerides, but in place of one of the fatty acids, they have a phosphorus-containing acid. They are present in cell membranes.

proteins Compounds composed of carbon, hydrogen, oxygen, and nitrogen that are arranged as strands of amino acids.

triglycerides The main form of lipid in the human diet and human body. Three fatty acids are bound to a glycerol molecule backbone, also called triacylglycerols.

whey Water-soluble fraction of milk containing proteins that include, but are not limited to, immunoglobulins, lysozyme, alpha-lactalbumin, lactoferrin, enzymes, hormones, and growth factors.

Any use of the term *mother*, *maternal*, or *breastfeeding* is not meant to exclude transgender or nonbinary parents who may be breastfeeding or providing human milk to their infant.

▶ Overview

For the first 6 months of human life, human milk is a life-sustaining food that contributes to the growth and maintenance of the rapidly growing infant. Human milk is uniquely created for the specific needs of the human infant. It provides a combination of proteins, lipids, and carbohydrates that change in proportion to meet the needs of the infant both throughout the day and over time as the child grows. In addition to these macronutrients, human milk provides vitamins and minerals as well as biologically active components that support the infant's growth and immune system.[1-4] The composition of human milk is dynamic and changes throughout the course of a feeding, throughout the day, and during the stages of lactation.[5-7] In addition to nutrients and water, human milk contains cells such as macrophages, T-cells, stem cells, and lymphocytes that protect against infection and support regeneration and repair in the body.[1,4]

Human milk is the preferred nutrition for human infants because of its distinct nutritional and health benefits. In cases where the parent's own milk or donor human milk is unavailable, appropriately prepared commercial infant formula is recommended. This chapter describes some of the components of human milk and how feeding alternatives, such as pasteurized donor human milk and commercial infant formula, compare nutritionally. The science regarding human milk is increasing exponentially. In addition, descriptions of the changes in milk composition throughout lactation, how milk meets the nutritional needs of infants, mechanisms of how milk protects against disease, and mechanisms of milk synthesis and secretion are included.

I. Macronutrients

A. Macronutrients provide energy for the infant and serve additional roles in growth and development.

B. The macronutrients in human milk are lipids, proteins, and carbohydrates.

1. Proteins provide 4 calories per gram; carbohydrates provide 4 calories per gram.

2. Lipids provide 9 calories per gram.
3. The energy provided by human milk is 60–77 kcal/100 mL (18–23 kcal/oz).[1,3,8]

II. Water

A. The majority of human milk (87.5 percent) is made of water.
B. Human milk provides all the water the infant needs for the first 6 months of life.
C. During the first 6 months of life, infants should not be given additional water, even in hot, dry climates.[4]

III. Lipids

A. Lipids are compounds composed of carbon and hydrogen atom chains.
B. Chains can vary in length and the number and location of double bonds.
C. The variations in the chains determine the function of the lipid.
D. Fatty acids are the components of lipids that are present in the greatest concentration. The majority of fatty acids are medium- and long-chain fatty acids (C:10 to C:22, where the numeral designates the number of carbons in the chain).[9]
E. Fatty acids can be cleaved from the glycerol backbone by the enzyme lipase, at which point they are known as free fatty acids.
F. Triglycerides comprise 98 percent of the total lipids in human milk; phospholipids comprise 0.8 percent, and cholesterol comprises 0.5 percent.[10] Lipids are not soluble in water, and they aid in the transport of the fat-soluble vitamins A, D, E, and K.[9]
G. Human milk lipids provide the greatest source of calories in human milk. They provide essential fat-soluble vitamins and essential fatty acids, including linoleic acid (LA; ω-6 fatty acid) and alpha-linoleic acid (ALA; ω-3 fatty acid).[11] Lipids are present in milk between 3 and 5 percent, and they exist as an emulsion, or a dispersion of tiny droplets within the aqueous (water) phase of milk.[10]
    1. Human milk contains more than 200 fatty acid structures, with oleic acid contributing 30 to 40 percent of the total fatty acids.[12]
    2. Lipids in human milk provide 40 to 50 percent of the infant's caloric requirements and are important components of neural and retinal tissues.[9]
    3. The average fat content of human milk is about 3.8 to 3.9 g/dL, but there can be a wide range of fat content among humans, ranging from 1.8 g/dL to 8.9 g/dL.[13]
    4. Breastfeeding for 6 months or longer with milk of high fat content is associated with higher developmental scores at 1 year of age. Researchers hypothesize that the supply of fat contributes energy, affects brain composition, or both.[14]
H. Alveolar cells within the mammary gland form milk fat globules, with a hydrophobic core containing triglycerides and a phospholipid membrane.[15]
    1. In milk, the fat globules are surrounded by the milk fat globule membrane (MFGM).
    2. In addition to phospholipids, the MFGM contains mucopolysaccharides, cholesterol, and enzymes.[10]
I. Lipids are the most variable portion of human milk, increasing both during a feeding and as the child gets older.[3]
J. LCPUFAs are specific for infant needs and play a role in cognitive development, vision, and nerve myelination.
    1. The amount and type of LCPUFAs can vary based on the maternal diet. In particular, the n-6 and n-3 fatty acids increase with maternal dietary intake.[16]
    2. DHA and AA are important for infant growth, immune function, vision, and brain development.[4]
K. The fat content in human milk increases from 2.0 g/dL in colostrum to 4.9 g/dL in mature milk.[9]
    1. Fat content changes during feedings and throughout the day.
        a. Fat content is about 3.0 g/dL in midday foremilk and 4.0 g/dL in midday hindmilk.
        b. Fat content is about 3.0 g/dL in early morning milk and 4.5 g/dL in evening milk.[17]

L.   Most of the fat in human milk is in the form of triglycerides, which must be broken down by enzymes called lipases before the infant can absorb them.

M.   During the third trimester, the neonate accumulates about 40 to 60 mg n-3 polyunsaturated fatty acids (PUFAs) per kilogram of body weight per day.[18] LCPUFA intake is important during lactation because an estimated 30 percent of human milk fatty acids are derived directly from the maternal diet.

1.   LCPUFAs have important effects on membrane function, photoreceptor differentiation, activation of rhodopsin, enzyme activity, ion channel function, and the levels and metabolism of neurotransmitters and eicosanoids (specific hormones).[18]

2.   Data from clinical studies in term and preterm infants comparing breastfed and formula-fed infants show enhanced development of visual function, improved retinal function, and improved visual acuity in breastfed infants due to the LCPUFAs.[17-19]

3.   Some studies have found that visual attention, problem solving, and global development are improved in infants fed LCPUFAs.[17]

N.   Nonesterified fatty acids (NEFAs, also referred to as free fatty acids) produced during the storage of human milk have been shown to have potent cytolytic effects (cell-destroying effects) on normal human blood cells and the intestinal parasites *Giardia lamblia* and *Entamoeba histolytica*, as well as gram-positive bacteria and yeast.[20]

1.   NEFAs have caused membrane disruption of enveloped viruses in cultured cells. Researchers found that lipids in fresh human milk do not inactivate viruses, but they become antiviral after storage at 4°C and 23°C, most likely when the NEFAs are released from the triglycerides.[21]

a.   Short-chain fatty acids and long-chain saturated fatty acids had little antiviral effects at the highest concentration tested; however, medium-chain saturated and long-chain unsaturated fatty acids were all antiviral at different concentrations, with polyunsaturated fatty acids having the most antiviral activity.

b.   In human milk with the most lipoprotein lipase, the antiviral activity was the highest. The fatty acids were shown to have antiviral activity by disintegrating the viral envelopes.[21]

O.   Lipid content is lower within milk that is ejected at the beginning of a feeding, before the infant feeds, and when the breast is full, compared to immediately after a feeding after the breast is softened.[22,23]

1.   More recent research investigated the change in fat and cell composition in six mothers before and after the first morning breastfeeding and at 30-minute intervals for up to 3 hours after the feeding.[24] At 30 minutes after the feeding, the fat content was eight times higher and the cell levels were 12 times higher, compared to levels before the feeding, after which point the fat and cell levels gradually decreased to the prefeeding levels.[24]

2.   Fat content of milk has been shown to change significantly throughout the day, but the concentration of lactose and protein content remains the same.[25]

IV. Proteins

A.   Proteins are composed of amino acids, which are compounds containing carbon, hydrogen, oxygen, nitrogen, and, in two cases, sulfur. Amino acids are connected into long chains and folded together to create proteins with various functions needed for survival.

B.   Human milk contains more than 400 different proteins that provide calories and bioactivity, including, but not limited to, immune factors, growth factors, hormones, and enzymes.[26]

1.   The nutritional value of protein in human milk is appreciated for many reasons, including caloric content, amino acids used for growth and development, and immunological compounds.

2.   Human milk provides all of the essential amino acids needed for infant growth and development.

C.   The total amount of protein in milk decreases from birth over the first 4 to 6 weeks of life.[1,3]

1.   The protein concentration decreases rapidly during the first month of lactation, and it decreases slowly throughout the remainder of lactation.

2.   The whey-to-casein ratio in early lactation is about 80:20, and it is about 50:50 in late lactation.[27]

3.   One study reports that the protein concentration of human milk is 14 to 16 g/L during early lactation, 8 to 10 g/L at 3 to 4 months of lactation, and 7 to 8 g/L at 6 months and later.[28]

4. However, in a longitudinal study on the changes in human milk composition, in which the researchers collected milk from the same mothers from 11 months postpartum to 17 months postpartum, the average protein concentration was 16 g/L at 11 months postpartum, and it was significantly higher at 18 g/L at 17 months postpartum.[29]

D. Human milk contains antimicrobial and immunostimulatory proteins, including SIgA, lactoperoxidase, kappa-casein, haptocorrin, casein phosphopeptides, and lactadherin, and proteins that aid in nutrient absorption, such as lactoferrin, bile-salt stimulated lipase, haptocorrin, folate-binding protein, and kappa-casein.[30]

E. Mucins, casein, and whey comprise the human milk proteins.
1. Mucins are milk fat globule membrane proteins that surround the lipid globules in milk.[31]
2. Casein is mostly found in micelles in solution in the milk.[32] The casein proteins bind calcium, which gives milk its cloudy white color and forms soft curds in the stomach.
   a. Casein concentrations are low in human milk, compared to milk of other species.[4]
   b. The casein micelle in human milk contains beta-casein, kappa-casein, and alpha$_{s1}$-casein.[28]
   c. The main subunit of human milk casein is beta-casein. Within beta-casein, there are clusters of phosphorylated serine and threonine residues close to the N-terminal end. These phosphorylated serine and threonine residues are able to complex with calcium ions, keeping calcium in a soluble state and leading to the high bioavailability of calcium in the milk.[33]
   d. As opposed to beta-casein, which is highly phosphorylated, kappa-casein is highly glycosylated[34] and may prevent the adhesion of *Helicobacter pylori* to the infant's gastric mucosa.[35]
3. Whey proteins are dissolved in the aqueous phase, and caseins are present both as casein micelles, which are suspended in solution, and dissolved monomers.[36] Micelles are casein molecules folded up into a spherical structure that is suspended in the milk. Calcium and phosphorus are found inside the micelle.
   a. Colostrum has a high protein concentration, consisting primarily of whey protein due to the low synthesis of casein during the first few days of lactation.[27]
   b. Whey proteins are water soluble and include, but are not limited to, SIgA, lysozyme, alpha-lactalbumin, lactoferrin, enzymes, hormones, and growth factors.
4. SIgA coats mucosal surfaces in the infant's gut to block pathogens, prevent inflammation, and stimulate the infant's production of SIgA.[4,26]
   a. It is generally thought that the main role of SIgA in human milk is to block the adhesion of microorganisms to the intestinal epithelium and to neutralize microbial toxins.[30]
   b. SIgA is made from proteins produced by plasma and epithelial cells of the mammary gland.
      i. Two molecules of immunoglobulin A (IgA) bind to a secretory component on the mammary gland epithelium.
      ii. The extracellular part of the secretory component, which is attached to the two molecules of IgA, is transported across the cell and secreted as SIgA.[37]
   c. The levels of SIgA vary among lactating women and the pattern of SIgA levels in milk is consistent over the course of lactation,[27] but it has been shown to increase during the second year of lactation.[29]
      i. During the first days postpartum, IgA secretion reaches 4 g/day, at which point its concentration is higher in milk than in any other bodily fluid.
      ii. IgA levels drop to about 1g/day at 10 days postpartum, and levels are detectable for the next 4 months.[30]
   d. SIgA is able to remain in the active form in the gastrointestinal tract because it is more resistant to degradation from proteases (enzymes that break down proteins) than other immunoglobulins.[27]
   e. SIgA antibodies against bacterial proteases have been found, including proteases produced by *Haemophilus influenzae*, *Streptococcus sanguis*, *Streptococcus pneumoniae*, *Proteus mirabilis*, *Escherichia coli*, *Neisseria gonorrhoeae*, and *Neisseria meningitidis*.[38]
   f. SIgA antibodies neutralize bacterial toxins and prevent binding of intestinal bacterial pathogens to epithelial cells by binding to their pili (an attachment or appendage on bacteria).[28]

g. The antibodies delivered to the infant through the milk do not harm the beneficial bacteria that is native to the gut; they have action only against pathogenic bacteria.[39]

h. As opposed to other immunoglobulins, such as immunoglobulin G (IgG) and immunoglobulin M (IgM), complexes of antigens with IgA do not activate the inflammation pathway and may help prevent inflammation by competing with IgG and IgM antibodies for antigens.[27]

5. Alpha-lactalbumin, the major whey protein in human milk, consists of 123 amino acids.[40]

  a. Alpha-lactalbumin is involved in lactose synthesis. Binding of calcium and zinc ions alters the structure in a way that increases its enzymatic activity.[4,41]

    i. Alpha-lactalbumin acts as a part of an enzyme called lactose synthase, which aids in the synthesis of lactose within the mammary gland.

    ii. Lactose synthase is composed of alpha-lactalbumin and the enzyme galactosyltransferase. Together, alpha-lactalbumin and galactosyltransferase catalyze the binding of glucose to uridine diphosphogalactose (UDPgalactose), which forms lactose.[27,42]

    iii. In addition to helping synthesize lactose, alpha-lactalbumin provides calories to the infant and is a source of the amino acids needed for protein synthesis.

  b. In addition to its role in lactose synthesis and providing nutrition, alpha-lactalbumin has been shown to inhibit the growth of cancer cells and noncancer derived cell lines.[43]

    i. Preparations of alpha-lactalbumin from human, camel, cow, and goat milk have been found to inhibit the growth of mammary epithelial cells.[44]

    ii. Antimicrobial activity has been reported when alpha-lactalbumin was folded into an active complex with oleic acid (C18:1).[45]

    iii. It was found that alpha-lactalbumin, native to human milk, did not have bactericidal activity. However, by using ion exchange chromatography in the presence of human milk casein fractions containing oleic acid, alpha-lactalbumin could be converted to an active form. The resulting complex of alpha-lactalbumin and oleic acid has activity against strains of *S. pneumoniae*, staphylococci (gram-positive), and enterococci (gram-negative).[45]

6. Lysozyme is a whey protein in human milk, representing 1 to 4 percent of whey protein nitrogen.[27]

  a. Lysozyme is an enzyme found in secretions, including human milk, saliva, tears, nasal mucus, and pancreatic juice.[27]

  b. Human milk contains about 400 µg/mL of lysozyme, which is approximately 3,000 times more than the amount of lysozyme in bovine milk.[46]

  c. Lysozyme is capable of breaking down the outer cell wall of gram-positive bacteria and some gram-negative bacteria by hydrolyzing the beta-1,4 linkages of N-acetylmuramic acid and 2-acetylamino-2-deoxy-D-glucose residues.[7,47]

  d. Lysozyme is secreted into human milk in concentrations between 2 and 6 mg/dL, which makes it the highest observed concentration among other secretions.

    i. Lysozyme concentrations stay relatively constant over the course of lactation, and levels may rise at 4 months of lactation. It is resistant to breakdown by acid and enzymes in the infant's stomach, suggesting that adequate amounts of lysozyme reach the intestinal tract.[30]

    ii. Lysozyme has been shown to kill gram-negative bacteria and inhibit the growth of gram-positive bacteria.[48]

  e. Lysozyme may work together with lactoferrin to kill gram-positive and gram-negative bacteria.[49,50] Lactoferrin binds bacterial lipopolysaccharide and removes it from the outer cell membrane of the bacteria. Lysozyme then penetrates the outer bacterial membrane and degrades the proteoglycan matrix, killing the bacteria.[50,51]

7. Lactoferrin serves as an antimicrobial, a modulator of immune function, and a facilitator of nutrient utilization.[51]

  a. Lactoferrin has a high affinity for iron and is able to suppress *E. coli* in the intestine.[52]

  b. Lactoferrin may modify immune function through a lactoferrin receptor in the intestine. After lactoferrin is bound to the receptor, it is internalized by the cell and binds to the nucleus, and then to sites on DNA, where it can regulate the expression of genes, including genes for cytokines.[51,53]

  c. Lactoferrin has been shown to facilitate iron absorption, specifically by transporting the iron across the surface of the cell membrane,[51] and to stimulate intestinal epithelial cell growth and differentiation.[54]

d. Lactoferrin is an important regulator of bone growth and has protective effects on osteoblasts (cells that synthesize bone) and inhibitory effects on osteoclasts (cells that break down bone).[55]

e. Because of its high affinity for iron, lactoferrin helps prevent pathogens from utilizing iron for growth and survival.[51]

f. Other microorganisms that are sensitive to lactoferrin include *Streptococcus mutans, S. pneumoniae, Vibrio cholerae, Pseudomonas aeruginosa, Candida albicans*, and several strains of oral streptococci.[56]

8. Human milk contains many other immunoglobulins.
   a. Research demonstrates that antibodies transfer from the breastfeeding parent to the infant through the milk.[57]
      i. Immunoglobulins provide protection to the infant's immature immune system.
      ii. Immunoglobulins, or antibodies, that are present in human milk include immunoglobulins A, G, M, D, and E, with SIgA being the most abundant.[39]
   b. Proteases, endogenous to human milk, are enzymes that break down protein.
      i. Proteases contribute to the high digestibility of milk for the infant, particularly during the neonatal period when the infant is adjusting to oral feedings rather than nutrition supplied by the placenta.[58]
      ii. Studies have indicated minimal protein digestion in the infant's stomach due to a low pepsin output[59-61] and high postprandial gastric pH.[62,63]
      iii. The pH of the infant's gastrointestinal tract is higher than that of adults (approximately 5 versus 2); therefore, proteins are not denatured (or digested) as easily within the infant's stomach due to the higher pH. As a result, the proteases in human milk aid in the digestion of protein for the infant.

V. Carbohydrates

A. Carbohydrates are a class of essential nutrients composed of carbon, hydrogen, and oxygen.
   1. Lactose, which is known as milk sugar, is the primary carbohydrate in human milk and contributes to approximately 98 percent of the carbohydrates in human milk.
      a. Lactose is made from glucose in the blood.
      b. Lactose is a disaccharide made from UDPgalactose and glucose, joined by a 1,4 beta-glycosidic bond.
      c. Lactose is synthesized by the enzyme lactose synthase in the Golgi secretory vesicle system of the lactocyte. Lactose synthase is an enzyme composed of the human milk protein alpha-lactalbumin and the enzyme beta-1,4 galactosyltransferase.
      d. The protein alpha-lactalbumin increases beta-1,4 galactosyltransferase's affinity for glucose, which facilitates the formation of lactose.[64]
      e. Human milk has one of the highest concentrations of lactose among species.
         i. Lactose averages about 7 percent in human milk and donkey milk and about 6.5 percent in milk from the red kangaroo and the horse. Lactose averages between 4 and 5 percent in milk from the cow, zebu, yak, water buffalo, goat, and sheep.[65]
         ii. Lactose digestion occurs at the brush border of the intestine by the enzyme lactase, which hydrolyzes lactose into its monosaccharide components, glucose, and galactose.
         iii. The enzymatic activity of lactose progressively decreases with age in genetically susceptible humans and most other species after weaning from lactose-containing products.[66]
   2. Human milk contains more than 200 oligosaccharides, called human milk oligosaccharides (HMOs), which are carbohydrates that are not digested by the infant. They serve as a prebiotic, providing energy to the beneficial bacteria inside the infant's intestine.
      a. Beneficial bacteria, such as *Bifidobacterium infantis*, protect the infant from disease-causing bacteria that can cause diarrhea and respiratory infections.[4,26,67] Because the beneficial bacteria are able to use HMOs for energy, they have a growth advantage over other bacteria that are unable to use HMOs because they lack the enzyme systems required for utilization.[67]

b. Most of the ingested HMOs reach the small and large intestines because they are able to resist enzymatic degradation and degradation by hydrochloric acid in the stomach. Therefore, HMOs are metabolized by intestinal bacteria or are excreted in the feces.[67-70]

c. HMOs act as decoy receptors that prevent the attachment of pathogens to the epithelial cell surface glycans (sugars) because they resemble some of the glycan structures.[67]

  i. When pathogens bind to the HMO, rather than the epithelial cell surface, the pathogens can then be excreted in the feces and leave the body without causing disease to the infant.[67]

  ii. Examples of pathogens that can bind to HMOs include norovirus, rotavirus, *Campylobacter jejuni*, and *E. coli*.[67]

d. HMOs have been shown to protect the infant by acting directly as an antimicrobial, protecting from viruses, bacteria, protozoans, and fungi, and by indirectly modifying the cellular responses of the infant's epithelial and immune cells.[67]

VI. Micronutrients

A. Micronutrient deficiencies from human milk are not common. However, some vitamins and minerals are dependent on maternal nutritional status and diet. Due to the variability of the maternal diet, taking a multivitamin during pregnancy and lactation is recommended.[1,4]

B. Minerals in human milk are bound to proteins and are more available than those in formula.[2] The nutrient needs of infants can be met by human milk for the first 6 months, after which micronutrients such as iron and zinc may become limiting.

C. Complementary foods rich in iron and zinc should begin at 6 months; in some cases oral iron drops may be needed before 6 months.[2,71,72]

D. Human milk generally contains an adequate amount of vitamins needed for infant growth, except for vitamins D and K.

1. The amount of vitamin D in human milk depends on the diet and maternal sun exposure.[8] Recommendations regarding vitamin D supplementation for breastfed infants vary.

  a. The American Academy of Pediatrics (AAP) recommends breastfed infants be given oral supplements of vitamin D (400 IU per day) to prevent vitamin D deficiency or insufficiency due to decreased sunlight exposure in modern lifestyles.[73]

  b. The World Health Organization (WHO) does not currently recommend routine vitamin D supplementation for breastfed infants, except for those who are very low birth weight.[74,75]

  c. Recent research indicates that supplementing the breastfeeding parent with high levels of vitamin D supplies the infant with adequate vitamin D via the milk.[76-78]

2. Vitamin K is low in human milk and plays a role in blood coagulation, cell cycle regulation, cell adhesion, and bone metabolism. The WHO and AAP recommend a single injection of vitamin K at birth for all infants.[1,71,74]

E. Infants of breastfeeding parents who are vegan or have had gastric bypass surgery may have an increased risk for vitamin B12 deficiency.[79]

VII. Mechanisms of Milk Secretion

A. Because milk is such a complex mixture of components there is no single physiological mechanism in the cells responsible for the secretion of all of these components.

1. Researchers have identified five main pathways responsible for the secretion of the components of milk.

2. These pathways are referred to as the Golgi and secretory vesicle pathway, a unique lipid secretion pathway, eccrine secretion of water and minerals, transcytosis, and the paracellular pathway that transports nutrients not through the epithelial cells, but between them.[64]

B. Two of the main macronutrient constituents of milk are carbohydrates (lactose and, for humans and a few other species, oligosaccharides) and protein. The secretion of these two types of macronutrients is linked with common biochemical pathways and the same subcellular organelles responsible for their movement into the milk phase.

1. Protein secretion in the mammary cells uses a pathway common to most excretory or secretory epithelial cells.
    a. The genetic information in the nucleus coding the protein sequence is transcribed from DNA to messenger RNA.
    b. Messenger RNA links to ribosomes on the rough endoplasmic reticulum membranes.
    c. The information in the messenger RNA is translated to the protein sequence in a process that inserts the newly formed protein across the membrane of the endoplasmic reticulum.
    d. Proteins mature by folding and enzymatic processing; small vesicles of the endoplasmic reticulum bud off to fuse with the Golgi apparatus.
    e. Protein processing occurs in the Golgi. Some of the enzymatically active proteins contribute to biochemical reactions, such as the synthesis of lactose.
    f. Small vesicles bud off from the Golgi and make secretory vesicles that diffuse through the cytoplasm to the apical membrane of the cell. Those secretory vesicles then fuse with the apical membrane. The contents are released into the milk space while the membrane component remains as an addition to the cell plasma membrane.[64]
2. Lactose synthesis occurs primarily in Golgi and secretory vesicles.
    a. In the Golgi, two specific proteins, called alpha-lactalbumin and galactosyltransferase, work together to make the lactose synthase enzyme complex.
    b. In the mammary cell cytosol, a molecule of glucose combines with a molecule of uridine triphosphate to make uridine diphosphoglucose (UDPglucose).
        i.   UDPglucose is isomerized to UDPgalactose.
        ii. This molecule and a molecule of glucose are transported, probably by diffusion, across the Golgi membrane to the interior of the vesicles where they are linked together by the lactose synthase complex to form lactose with the release of uridine diphosphate (UDP).
    c. Related enzymes add additional monosaccharide units to create the milk oligosaccharides.
3. Milk protein and carbohydrate coexist in the same cellular vesicles and are secreted into milk by the secretory vesicle pathway. Milk minerals that bind to proteins—such as calcium, phosphate, and zinc—also appear to enter milk primarily through this pathway.[64]

C. Milk fat is made by the movement of free fatty acids into the smooth endoplasmic reticulum, where three fatty acids are linked to a molecule of glycerol to create a triglyceride.
    1. The triglycerides diffuse out of the endoplasmic reticulum and coalesce in the cytoplasm as lipid droplets of various sizes. Very small micro lipid droplets appear to diffuse directly out of the cell into the milk, whereas larger cytoplasmic lipid droplets push against the cell membrane and enter the milk space as membrane-bound milk fat globules.
    2. The source of fatty acids for milk fat could come from the following[64]:
        a. Fatty acids stored in other adipose tissues of the body.
        b. Fatty acids absorbed directly from the diet.
        c. Fatty acids synthesized within the mammary cell from glucose or other substrates.

D. The third secretory pathway, referred to as eccrine secretion, uses transport proteins or simple diffusion through the apical cell membrane, often to create an equilibrium or steady state between the interior and exterior of the cell.
    1. Eccrine secretion is responsible for the movement of water into milk in response to an osmotic pressure gradient.
    2. Electrolytes like sodium, potassium, chloride, and other small molecules and minor milk constituents also enter the milk through this pathway.[64]
    3. As the major constituent of milk, water movement that follows lactose and electrolytes largely controls the volume of milk produced.

E. The fourth pathway, referred to as transcytosis, involves the internalization of substances that are in the extracellular fluid, bind to basolateral membrane receptors, and are taken up by an endocytotic pathway.
    1. The resulting endosomes move directly through the cytoplasm and release the contents into the milk through an exocytosis mechanism, simply reversing their mechanism of internalization.

2. The transcytosis pathway is responsible for the movement into milk of antibodies such as IgA from their site of secretion from plasma cells outside the alveolar structure.[64]

F. Milk is totally separated from blood and from the extracellular fluid and lymph space by the layers of epithelial cells.
    1. Under different conditions, the structures that hold mammary epithelial cells together to form a tight membrane are less or more permeable to molecules of different sizes.
    2. These tight junctions between cells are leaky during pregnancy, during weaning, and in cases of mastitis. Under those conditions molecules in the extracellular space, such as higher concentrations of sodium and plasma proteins, are able to move into the milk, and milk components such as lactose can leave the milk and enter the blood.[64,80]

VIII. Colostrum

A. Colostrum is the first milk produced by the breast, and its secretion begins during pregnancy.
B. It is a high-density, thick yellow milk that coats the infant's gut, blocking pathogens and promoting gut closure.
C. Colostrum is high in SIgA, white cells, growth factors, and lactoferrin.
D. Compared to mature milk, colostrum is lower in lactose, potassium, and calcium and higher in sodium, chloride, and magnesium.
E. The timing of the transition from colostrum to mature milk varies among parents, but typically begins between days 2 and 4, with complete transition to mature milk by 4 to 6 weeks after birth.[1]

IX. Pasteurized Donor Milk

A. When parental milk is not available, pasteurized human donor milk is recommended for preterm infants.
B. The heat treatment involved in pasteurization of human milk reduces bioactive components, such as SIgA and lysozyme, reducing some of the health benefits.[1,4]
C. Despite these differences, pasteurized donor milk has been shown to improve infant health outcomes, compared to formula both in the hospital and after discharge.[71] See Chapter 31, *Expression and Use of Human Milk*.

X. Infant Formula

A. Commercially prepared infant formula has a standard composition. Its production is monitored in the United States by the Food and Drug Administration (FDA) and internationally by the Codex Alimentarius of the United Nations Food and Agriculture Organization (FAO).[81,82]
    1. The standards for infant formula composition were published by the Codex Alimentarius Commission in 1981, revised based on new data in 2007, and amended through 2016 on a periodic basis.[82]
    2. The composition of infant formula is important because it is the sole source of nutrition to promote growth and development for an extended period of life.
    3. The AAP recommends that infants who are not breastfed or partially breastfed receive iron-fortified formula based on cow's milk for the first 12 months of life.[83]
B. The Codex Alimentarius standards for infant formulas provide minimum concentrations of essential nutrients and, in some cases, maximum concentrations, or guidance upper levels (GULs), if scientific evidence for adverse effects of high levels is not available.[82]
    1. The energy content of formula should be 60 to 70 kcal/100 mL, based on an intake of 750 mL per day.
    2. The protein concentration in formula should range from 1.8 to 3.0 g/100 kcal.
        a. The protein source is unspecified, but infant formula is defined as "a product based on milk of cows or other animals or a mixture thereof and/or other ingredients which have been proven to be suitable for infant feeding." [82(p2)]
        b. The Codex Alimentarius specifies minimum indispensable amino acid composition based on an average of six studies analyzing human milk protein composition published between 1979 and 1998.[82]
        c. The total protein is likely to be higher than human milk, depending on the source of the protein, although individual amino acids may be added to achieve a balanced amino acid profile.

       d.   The minimum protein concentration for soy-protein-based infant formula is 2.25 g/100 kcal, accounting for composition and bioavailability.

C.   Lipids must be present in formula at a concentration of 4.4 to 6.0 g/100 kcal.

    1.   Hydrogenated fats and oils are not allowed.

    2.   A maximum concentration level of trans fatty acids (TFAs) allows for the TFA endogenous to milk fat to be in a formula without being a violation or a hazard.

    3.   The total phospholipids should be 300 mg/100 kcal or less.

    4.   The essential fatty acids (EFAs) must be met with LA (n-6 EFA) 300 mg/100 kcal or more and ALA (n-3 EFA) 50 mg/100 kcal or more.

        a.   The LA to ALA ratio must remain between 5:1 and 15:1.

        b.   The vitamin E concentration should be increased with greater concentrations of polyunsaturated fatty acids to protect from oxidation of carbon–carbon double bonds.

    5.   Guidance values are given for the concentration of long-chain saturated fatty acids (total palmitate plus stearate is less than 20 percent of total fatty acids) and the polyunsaturated fatty acids DHA, eicosapentaenoic acid (EPA), and AA.

D.   The total carbohydrate concentration in infant formulas should be between 9 and 14 g/100 kcal, using only lactose or glucose polymers. Sucrose and fructose are prohibited because unrecognized hereditary fructose intolerance could be life threatening.

E.   The minimum and, in some cases, maximum concentrations of vitamins and essential minerals are provided in the Codex Alimentarius standards to meet infant nutritional requirements, as well as minimum concentrations of choline, myoinositol, and carnitine, nutrients that are usually synthesized adequately in adults but not necessarily in infants.[82]

F.   The Codex Alimentarius standards list generally recognized as safe (GRAS) food additives that may be included in infant formulas, such as thickeners, emulsifiers, acidulants, antioxidants, and oxygen displacers, with specified maximum concentrations or references to good manufacturing practice (GMP) levels for other foods.

G.   Commercially prepared infant formula contains proteins from nonhuman sources, commonly cow milk or soy.

    1.   They contain 60 to 70 kcal of energy per 100 mL,[4] compared to human milk energy content of 50 to 90 kcal/100 mL. The greater variation is due to fat content changing from foremilk to hindmilk.[84]

    2.   Milk-based infant formulas made from modified cow's milk have added carbohydrates, vegetable oil, vitamins, and minerals.

    3.   Formula is harder for infants to digest than human milk, in part because of the higher levels of casein found in cow's milk. Because the ratio of whey proteins and caseins in human milk is different than the ratio of whey proteins and caseins in cow's milk, most formulas are modified to increase the whey to casein ratios.

    4.   Soy-based formulas are available for infants who cannot tolerate formula made from cow's milk, whose families prefer a vegan diet for their infant, or for infants who have an allergy to cow's milk protein.

        a.   Soy formulas are more commonly made without lactose, which could benefit the rare cases of infants with galactosemia or lactose maldigestion.

        b.   Infants with milk protein allergy are likely to also have soy protein allergy, so better outcomes are associated with the use of extensively hydrolyzed protein formulas.[85]

    5.   There are several other types of formula that can be given after discussion with an infant's medical providers. These include hypoallergenic formula, lactose-free formula, and formulas that meet the need of infants with metabolic errors or special medical conditions.[4,83]

    6.   In an effort to make artificial infant formula more like human milk, manufacturers add ingredients like LCPUFAs, nucleotides, prebiotics, and probiotics. However, the evidence on the effectiveness of these additives for improving infant health and development is inconclusive.[83]

        a.   The FDA requires that any changes to the composition of an infant formula be tested in a clinical trial and shown to support adequate normal physical growth of infants.[81]

        b.   The growth standards for these clinical trials refer to the 1979 National Center for Health Statistics physical growth percentiles[86] that used a representative sample of U.S. children without regard to the breastfeeding or formula feeding history of the subjects in a 1956 to 1970 data collection sample.

▶ Key Points from This Chapter

A.   Human milk and infant formula contain macronutrients and micronutrients that provide nourishment to the human body for growth and maintenance of body tissues.

B.   Human milk contains components that are not found in formula.

C.   Each protein, carbohydrate, and lipid found in human milk provides energy to the human body. In addition to providing energy, these macronutrients have other functions that support bodily processes, including, but not limited to, immune protection and regulation of growth and metabolism.

🔍 CASE STUDY

Marytza, who is exclusively breastfeeding, calls you for help because 4-month old Andy, her baby, has confirmed gastroesophageal reflux disease (GERD). All other possible causes of GERD-like symptoms have been ruled out. The pediatrician prescribed medication to help with pain from GERD and referred Andy to a gastroenterologist. Marytza, the gastroenterologist, and the pediatrician are concerned because Andy goes through periods of weight gain when his intake is sufficient, but his weight plateaus when he is not taking in adequate volumes. Andy breastfeeds more frequently and sufficiently when the medication dose is adjusted to his weight. However, when Andy gains weight, he outgrows his dose of medicine, and he decreases his frequency of intake because of pain. Marytza reports that Andy was 1 percent for height and 0.7 percent for weight on the growth chart at the 4-month visit. Marytza tells you, "We are worried we are walking a very thin line with a feeding tube over the next month."

The gastroenterologist highly recommended infant formula based on the assumption that the formula has more calories than human milk. Marytza has ample milk production and is devastated at the thought of beginning formula. Marytza fed Andy infant formula and regularly expressed milk to maintain milk production. Andy suffered from gas and constipation from the formula, but the gastroenterologist insisted that formula was necessary for weight gain.

You ask Marytza to send milk samples to a human milk laboratory for analysis of macronutrients. The researcher asked that Marytza express five samples of milk throughout a 24-hour period, as well as two hindmilk samples. The results show that Marytza's milk is comparable to what would be expected in human milk and comparable to the caloric content of formula. The gastroenterologist found this information helpful and recommended that Marytza continue breastfeeding and cease formula feeding.

Questions

1. Why did the researcher ask Marytza to express five samples of milk throughout a 24-hour period?
2. After reviewing the caloric content measured in Marytza's milk, why did the gastroenterologist recommend that Marytza continue breastfeeding and cease formula feeding?
3. If the caloric content of the milk was not the cause of Andy's insufficient weight gain, what could have caused the insufficient weight gain?
4. Which characteristics of human milk make it easier for an infant to digest than infant formula?

References

1. Ballard O, Morrow AL. Human milk composition: nutrients and bioactive factors. *Pediatr Clin North Am.* 2013;60(1):49-74.
2. Bravi F, Wiens F, Decarli A, Dal Pont A, Agostoni C, Ferraroni M. Impact of maternal nutrition on breast-milk composition: a systematic review. *Am J Clin Nutr.* 2016;104(3):646-662.
3. Gidrewicz DA, Fenton TR. A systematic review and meta-analysis of the nutrient content of preterm and term breast milk. *BMC Pediatr.* 2014;14:216.
4. Martin CR, Ling PR, Blackburn GL. Review of infant feeding: key features of breast milk and infant formula. *Nutrients.* 2016;8(5):279.
5. Daly SE, Kent JC, Owens RA, Hartmann PE. Frequency and degree of milk removal and the short-term control of human milk synthesis. *Exp Physiol.* 1996;81(5):861-875.
6. Dewey KG, Finley DA, Lönnerdal B. Breast milk volume and composition during late lactation (7-20 months). *J Pediatr Gastroenterol Nutr.* 1984;3(5):713-720.
7. Lönnerdal B. Nutritional and physiologic significance of human milk proteins. *Am J Clin Nutr.* 2003;77(6):1537s-1543s.
8. Butte NF, King JC. Energy requirements during pregnancy and lactation. *Public Health Nutr.* 2005;8(7a):1010-1027.
9. Manson WG, Weaver LT. Fat digestion in the neonate. *Arch Dis Child Fetal Neonatal Ed.* 1997;76(3):F206-F211.
10. Jensen RG. Lipids in human milk. *Lipids.* 1999;34(12):1243-1271.
11. Koletzko B, Rodriguez-Palmero M, Demmelmair H, Fidler N, Jensen R, Sauerwald T. Physiological aspects of human milk lipids. *Early Hum Dev.* 2001;65(suppl):S3-S18.

12. Koletzko B, Mrotzek M, Bremer HJ. Fatty acid composition of mature human milk in Germany. *Am J Clin Nutr.* 1988;47(6):954-959.

13. Michaelsen KF, Skafte L, Badsberg JH, Jorgensen M. Variation in macronutrients in human bank milk: influencing factors and implications for human milk banking. *J Pediatr Gastroenterol Nutr.* 1990;11(2):229-239.

14. Agostoni C, Marangoni F, Giovannini M, Galli C, Riva E. Prolonged breast-feeding (six months or more) and milk fat content at six months are associated with higher developmental scores at one year of age within a breast-fed population. *Adv Exp Med Biol.* 2001;501:137-141.

15. Lopez C, Menard O. Human milk fat globules: polar lipid composition and in situ structural investigations revealing the heterogeneous distribution of proteins and the lateral segregation of sphingomyelin in the biological membrane. *Colloids Surf B Biointerfaces.* 2011;83(1):29-41.

16. Weseler AR, Dirix CE, Bruins MJ, Hornstra G. Dietary arachidonic acid dose-dependently increases the arachidonic acid concentration in human milk. *J Nutr.* 2008;138(11):2190-2197.

17. Jensen RG, Hagerty MM, McMahon KE. Lipids of human milk and infant formulas: a review. *Am J Clin Nutr.* 1978;31(6):990-1016.

18. Koletzko B, Lien E, Agostoni C, et al. The roles of long-chain polyunsaturated fatty acids in pregnancy, lactation and infancy: review of current knowledge and consensus recommendations. *J Perinat Med.* 2008;36(1):5-14.

19. Jensen CL, Prager TC, Fraley JK, Chen H, Anderson RE, Heird WC. Effect of dietary linoleic/alpha-linolenic acid ratio on growth and visual function of term infants. *J Pediatr.* 1997;131(2):200-209.

20. Ogundele MO. Techniques for the storage of human breast milk: implications for anti-microbial functions and safety of stored milk. *Eur J Pediatr.* 2000;159(11):793-797.

21. Thormar H, Isaacs CE, Brown HR, Barshatzky MR, Pessolano T. Inactivation of enveloped viruses and killing of cells by fatty acids and monoglycerides. *Antimicrob Agents Chemother.* 1987;31(1):27-31.

22. Mitoulas LR, Kent JC, Cox DB, Owens RA, Sherriff JL, Hartmann PE. Variation in fat, lactose and protein in human milk over 24 h and throughout the first year of lactation. *Br J Nutr.* 2002;88(1):29-37.

23. Kent JC, Mitoulas LR, Cregan MD, Ramsay DT, Doherty DA, Hartmann PE. Volume and frequency of breastfeedings and fat content of breast milk throughout the day. *Pediatrics.* 2006;117(3):e387-e395.

24. Hassiotou F, Hepworth AR, Williams TM, et al. Breastmilk cell and fat contents respond similarly to removal of breastmilk by the infant. *PLOS One.* 2013;8(11):e78232. doi:10.1371/journal.pone.0078232.

25. Khan S, Hepworth AR, Prime DK, Lai CT, Trengove NJ, Hartmann PE. Variation in fat, lactose, and protein composition in breast milk over 24 hours: associations with infant feeding patterns. *J Hum Lactation.* 2013;29(1):81-89.

26. Andreas NJ, Kampmann B, Mehring Le-Doare K. Human breast milk: a review on its composition and bioactivity. *Early Hum Dev.* 2015;91(11):629-635.

27. Atkinson SA, Lödderdal B. *Proteins and Non-protein Nitrogen in Human Milk.* Boca Raton, FL: CRC Press; 1989.

28. Newburg DS. Bioactive components of human milk: evolution, efficiency, and protection. *Adv Exp Med Biol.* 2001;501:3-10.

29. Perrin MT, Fogleman AD, Newburg DS, Allen JC. A longitudinal study of human milk composition in the second year postpartum: implications for human milk banking. *Matern Child Nutr.* 2017;13(1). [Epub ahead of print]. doi: 10.1111/mcn.12239.

30. Bernt K, Walker WA. Human milk and the response of intestinal epithelium to infection. *Advances in experimental medicine and biology.* 2001;501:11-30.

31. Patton S, Huston GE. A method for isolation of milk fat globules. *Lipids.* 1986;21(2):170-174.

32. Lönnerdal B, Woodhouse LR, Glazier C. Compartmentalization and quantitation of protein in human milk. *J Nutr.* 1987;117(8):1385-1395.

33. Sato R, Noguchi T, Naito H. Casein phosphopeptide (CPP) enhances calcium absorption from the ligated segment of rat small intestine. *J Nutr Sci Vitaminol.* 1986;32(1):67-76.

34. Brignon G, Chtourou A, Ribadeau-Dumas B. Does beta-lactoglobulin occur in human milk? *J Dairy Res.* 1985;52(2):249-254.

35. Strömqvist M, Falk P, Bergström S, et al. Human milk kappa-casein and inhibition of *Helicobacter pylori* adhesion to human gastric mucosa. *J Pediatr Gastroenterol Nutr.* 1995;21(3):288-296.

36. Jensen R. *Handbook of Milk Composition.* San Diego, CA: Academic Press Inc; 1995.

37. Lindh E. Increased risistance of immunoglobulin A dimers to proteolytic degradation after binding of secretory component. *J Immunol.* 1975;114(1 pt 2):284-286.

38. Gilbert JV, Plaut AG, Longmaid B, Lamm ME. Inhibition of microbial IgA proteases by human secretory IgA and serum. *Mol Immunol.* 1983;20(9):1039-1049.

39. Newman J. How breast milk protects newborns. *Sci Am.* 1995;273(6):76-79.

40. Phillips NI, Jenness R. Isolation and properties of human alpha-lactalbumin. *Biochim Biophys Acta.* 1971;229(2):407-410.

41. Lönnerdal B, Glazier C. Calcium binding by alpha-lactalbumin in human milk and bovine milk. *J Nutr.* 1985;115(9):1209-1216.

42. Brew K, Hill RL. Lactose biosynthesis. *Rev Physiol Biochem Pharmacol.* 1975;72:105-158.

43. Brinkmann CR, Heegaard CW, Petersen TE, Jensenius JC, Thiel S. The toxicity of bovine alpha-lactalbumin made lethal to tumor cells is highly dependent on oleic acid and induces killing in cancer cell lines and noncancer-derived primary cells. *FEBS J.* 2011;278(11):1955-1967.

44. Thompson MP, Farrell HM, Mohanam S, et al. Identification of human milk α-lactalbumin as a cell growth inhibitor. *Protoplasma.* 1992;167(3-4):134-144.

45. Hakansson A, Svensson M, Mossberg AK, et al. A folding variant of alpha-lactalbumin with bactericidal activity against *Streptococcus pneumoniae. Mol Microbiol.* 2000;35(3):589-600.

46. Florisa R, Recio I, Berkhout B, Visser S. Antibacterial and antiviral effects of milk proteins and derivatives thereof. *Curr Pharm Design.* 2003;9(16):1257-1275.

47. Chipman DM, Sharon N. Mechanism of lysozyme action. *Science.* 1969;165(3892):454-465.

48. Shah NP. Effects of milk-derived bioactives: an overview. *Br J Nutr.* 2000;84(suppl 1):S3-S10.

49. Lönnerdal B, Iyer S. Lactoferrin: molecular structure and biological function. *Ann Rev Nutr.* 1995;15:93-110.

50. Ellison RT III, Giehl TJ. Killing of gram-negative bacteria by lactoferrin and lysozyme. *J Clin Invest.* 1991;88(4):1080-1091.

51. Lönnerdal B. Bioactive proteins in human milk: health, nutrition, and implications for infant formulas. *J Pediatr.* 2016;173(suppl):S4-S9.

52. Bullen JJ. Iron-binding proteins in milk and resistance to *Escherichia coli* infection in infants. *Proc Royal Soc Med.* 1972;65(12):1086.
53. Lönnerdal B, Jiang R, Du X. Bovine lactoferrin can be taken up by the human intestinal lactoferrin receptor and exert bioactivities. *J Pediatr Gastroenterol Nutr.* 2011;53(6):606-614.
54. Liao Y, Jiang R, Lönnerdal B. Biochemical and molecular impacts of lactoferrin on small intestinal growth and development during early life. *Biochem Cell Biol.* 2012;90(3):476-484.
55. Cornish J, Callon KE, Naot D, et al. Lactoferrin is a potent regulator of bone cell activity and increases bone formation in vivo. *Endocrinology.* 2004;145(9):4366-4374.
56. Arnold RR, Brewer M, Gauthier JJ. Bactericidal activity of human lactoferrin: sensitivity of a variety of microorganisms. *Infect Immun.* 1980;28(3):893-898.
57. Silverstein AM. Paul Ehrlich: the founding of pediatric immunology. *Cell Immun.* 1996;174(1):1-6.
58. Storrs AB, Hull ME. Proteolytic enzymes in human and cow's milk. *J Dairy Sci.* 1956;39(8)1097-1103.
59. Agunod M, Yamaguchi N, Lopez R, Luhby AL, Glass GB. Correlative study of hydrochloric acid, pepsin, and intrinsic factor secretion in newborns and infants. *Am J Dig Dis.* 1969;14(6):400-414.
60. Weisselberg B, Yahav J, Reichman B, Jonas A. Basal and meal-stimulated pepsinogen secretion in preterm infants: a longitudinal study. *J Pediatr Gastroenterol Nutr.* 1992;15(1):58-62.
61. Yahav J, Carrion V, Lee PC, Lebenthal E. Meal-stimulated pepsinogen secretion in premature infants. *J Pediatr.* 1987;110(6):949-951.
62. Hamosh M, Sivasubramanian KN, Salzman-Mann C, Hamosh P. Fat digestion in the stomach of premature infants. I. Characteristics of lipase activity. *J Pediatr.* 1978;93(4):674-679.
63. Mason S. Some aspects of gastric function in the newborn. *Arch Dis Child.* 1962;37:387-391.
64. Neville MC, Allen JC, Watters CD. Mechanisms of milk secretion. In: Neville MC, ed. *Human Lactation: Physiology, Nutrition and Breast-Feeding.* Plenum, NY; 1983:49-102.
65. Jenness R. Biochemical and nutritional aspects of milk and colostrum. In: Larson BL, ed. *Lactation.* Iowa State University Press; 1985:164-197.
66. Holden C, Mace R. Phylogenetic analysis of the evolution of lactose digestion in adults. *Hum Biol.* 1997;69(5):605-628.
67. Bode L. The functional biology of human milk oligosaccharides. *Early Hum Dev.* 2015;91(11):619-622.
68. Albrecht S, Schols HA, van den Heuvel EG, Voragen AG, Gruppen H. Occurrence of oligosaccharides in feces of breast-fed babies in their first six months of life and the corresponding breast milk. *Carbohydr Res.* 2011;346(16):2540-2550.
69. Gnoth MJ, Kunz C, Kinne-Saffran E, Rudloff S. Human milk oligosaccharides are minimally digested in vitro. *J Nutr.* 2000;130(12):3014-3020.
70. Engfer MB, Stahl B, Finke B, Sawatzki G, Daniel H. Human milk oligosaccharides are resistant to enzymatic hydrolysis in the upper gastrointestinal tract. *Am J Clin Nutr.* 2000;71(6):1589-1596.
71. American Academy of Pediatrics. Breastfeeding and the use of human milk. *Pediatrics.* 2012;129(3):e827-e841.
72. WHO/UNICEF. *Global Strategy for Infant and Young Child Feeding.* Geneva, Switzerland: World Health Organization; 2003.
73. American Academy of Pediatrics. Vitamin D supplementation for infants. American Academy of Pediatrics website. https://www.aap.org/en-us/about-the-aap/aap-press-room/pages/Vitamin-D-Supplementation-for-Infants.aspx. Published March 22, 2010. Accessed September 1, 2017.
74. World Health Organization. *WHO Recommendations on Newborn Health.* Geneva, Switzerland: World Health Organization; 2017. http://www.who.int/maternal_child_adolescent/documents/newborn-health-recommendations/en/. Accessed September 1, 2017.
75. World Health Organization. Vitamin D supplementation in infants. World Health Organization website. http://www.who.int/elena/titles/vitamind_infants/en/. Accessed September 1, 2017.
76. Hollis BW, Wagner CL, Howard CR, et al. Maternal versus infant vitamin D supplementation during lactation: a randomized controlled trial. *Pediatrics.* 2015;136(4):625-634.
77. Chandy DD, Kare J, Singh SN, et al. Effect of vitamin D supplementation, directly or via breast milk for term infants, on serum 25 hydroxyvitamin D and related biochemistry, and propensity to infection: a randomised placebo-controlled trial. *Br J Nutr.* 2016;116(1):52-58.
78. Roth DE. Maternal postpartum high-dose vitamin D3 supplementation (6400 IU/day) or conventional infant vitamin D3 supplementation (400 IU/day) lead to similar vitamin D status of healthy exclusively/fully breastfeeding infants by 7 months of age. *Evidence-Based Med.* 2016;21(2):75.
79. Greer FR. Do breastfed infants need supplemental vitamins? *Pediatr Clin North Am.* 2001;48(2):415-423.
80. Allen JC. Sodium and potassium content and viability of mouse mammary gland tissue and acini. *J Dairy Sci.* 1988;71(3):633-642.
81. U.S. Food and Drug Administration. Infant formula requirements pertaining to current good manufacturing practice, quality control procedures, quality factors, records and reports, and notifications. In: Code of Federal Regulations 21CFR106. Washington, DC: US Government Publishing Office; 2017. https://www.accessdata.fda.gov/scripts/cdrh/cfdocs/cfcfr/CFRSearch.cfm?CFRPart=106&showFR=1&subpartNode=21:2.0.1.1.6.1 Accessed March 8, 2018
82. Codex Alimentarius Commission. *Standard for Infant Formula and Formulas for Special Medical Purposes Intended for Infants.* CODEX STAN 72-1981. Amendment: 1983, 1985, 1987, 2011, 2015 and 2016. Revision: 2007:17. www.fao.org/input/download/standards/288/CXS_072e_2015.pdf; Accessed March 8, 2018
83. O'Connor NR. Infant formula. *Am Fam Physician.* 2009;79(7):565-570.
84. Saarela T, Kokkonen J, Koivisto M. Macronutrient and energy contents of human milk fractions during the first six months of lactation. *Acta Paediatr.* 2005;94(9):1176-1181.
85. American Academy of Pediatrics, Committee on Nutrition. Soy protein-based formulas: recommendations for use in infant feeding. *Pediatrics.* 1998;101(1 pt 1):148-153.
86. Hamill PV, Drizd TA, Johnson CL, Reed RB, Roche AF, Moore WM. Physical growth: National Center for Health Statistics percentiles. *Am J Clin Nutr.* 1979;32(3):607-629.

Additional Resources

Formula Feeding

World Health Organization. *How to Prepare Formula for Bottle-Feeding at Home*. Geneva, Switzerland: World Health Organization; 2007. http://www.who.int/foodsafety/publications/micro/PIF_Bottle_en.pdf.

World Health Organization. *Safe Preparation, Storage and Handling of Powdered Infant Formula: Guidelines*. Geneva, Switzerland: World Health Organization; 2007. http://www.who.int/foodsafety/publications/micro/pif_guidelines.pdf.

Human Milk Bank Websites

European Milk Bank Association. http://europeanmilkbanking.com.

Human Milk Banking Association of North America. https://www.hmbana.org/.

Media Articles

Yong, E. Breast-feeding the microbiome. *The New Yorker*. July 22, 2016. http://www.newyorker.com/tech/elements/breast-feeding-the-microbiome.

Policy Documents on Infant Feeding

American Academy of Pediatrics. Policy statement: breastfeeding and the use of human milk. *Pediatrics*. 2012;129(3). http://pediatrics.aappublications.org/content/early/2012/02/22/peds.2011-3552.

World Health Organization. *WHO Recommendations on Adolescent Health*. Geneva, Switzerland: World Health Organization; 2017. http://www.who.int/maternal_child_adolescent/documents/adolescent-health-recommendations/en/.

World Health Organization. *WHO Recommendations on Child Health*. Geneva, Switzerland: World Health Organization; 2017. http://www.who.int/maternal_child_adolescent/documents/child-health-recommendations/en/.

World Health Organization. *WHO Recommendations on Maternal Health*. Geneva, Switzerland: World Health Organization; 2017. http://www.who.int/maternal_child_adolescent/documents/maternal-health-recommendations/en/.

World Health Organization. *WHO Recommendations on Newborn Health*. Geneva, Switzerland: World Health Organization; 2017. http://www.who.int/maternal_child_adolescent/documents/newborn-health-recommendations/en/.

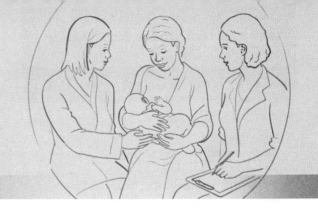

CHAPTER 8

Nutrition during Lactation

Alicia C. Simpson

DEFINITIONS OF COMMONLY USED TERMS

anorexia nervosa An eating disorder characterized by excessive calorie restriction and exercise, abnormal weight loss, and underweight.

bariatric surgery A surgical procedure performed on obese or morbidly obese individuals to assist in weight loss.

bulimia nervosa An eating disorder characterized by binge eating followed by excessive exercise, purging and vomiting food, or utilizing laxatives to quickly eliminate food from the body to maintain or lose weight.

lactogenic foods A classification of foods and herbs that are traditionally used in folk medicine to help increase the quantity of human milk produced.

(continues)

DEFINITIONS OF COMMONLY USED TERMS *(continued)*

lacto-ovo vegetarian An individual who does not eat meat but does consume dairy products and eggs.
ovo vegetarian An individual who does not eat meat or dairy products but does consume eggs.
pescatarian An individual who chooses fish as the primary source of meat in the diet and generally consumes dairy products and eggs.
tandem breastfeeding Breastfeeding more than one child at a time, typically an infant and a toddler.
vegan An individual who does not consume meat, dairy products, eggs, or animal by-products.

Any use of the term *mother, maternal,* or *breastfeeding* is not meant to exclude transgender or nonbinary parents who may be breastfeeding or providing human milk to their infant.

▶ Overview

Maternal nutrition status during lactation is directly affected by maternal nutrition status preconception and in the prenatal period. The period of lactation requires more calories from the lactating parent without requiring many more micronutrients. Lactating parents can meet their nutritional needs across a wide variety of dietary patterns. This chapter provides guidelines on proper assessment of the nutritional status of the breastfeeding parent and recommendations for macro- and micronutrient intake based on the specific health status of various world regions. Situations requiring referral to a registered dietitian or nutritionist are also discussed.

I. Initial Assessment

A. Complete a general nutrition assessment of the lactating parent.
   1. An assessment includes prenatal health and nutrition status, existing medical conditions, and birth experience.
   2. Nutrition-related disease states during pregnancy, delivery, and the immediate postpartum period can have both a positive and a negative effect on lactating parents. For example, active anorexia nervosa during pregnancy can deplete the body of essential nutrients for healthy lactation, including omega-3 fatty acids, vitamin A, vitamin C, chromium, copper, and iodine.
B. Obtain a verbal or written 24-hour food diary, including all meals, snacks, and beverages (caloric and noncaloric).
   1. In general, a lactating parent should be consuming vegetables or fruit at each meal, a grain or starchy vegetable, and a protein.
   2. If the lactating parent feels hungry between meals, there should be a small snack consisting of a combination of fruit and protein, vegetable and protein, or grains or starchy vegetable and protein.
   3. Protein foods include nuts, seeds, legumes (beans, lentils, and peas), eggs, meat, and dairy products (milk, cheese, and yogurt).
C. Ask about any supplements and medications (both prescribed and over the counter) the lactating parent took while pregnant and is presently taking. Supplements include vitamins, herbs, probiotics, tinctures, and teas.
D. Utilize the initial nutritional assessment of food intake and supplement use to determine if the lactating parent has nutritional deficits or patterns of poor nutritional intake. Severe nutritional deficits or a history of nutrition-related disease states warrant a referral to a healthcare provider or registered dietitian.

II. General Nutrition Recommendations for Lactation

A. Prepregnancy health, nutrition, and body mass index (BMI) can affect vitamin and mineral stores and maternal health while breastfeeding. When possible before conception, encourage patients to reach a healthy BMI and seek an assessment of their nutrient status (especially iron, folate, and folic acid) by a healthcare provider, nutritionist, or registered dietitian.

B.   Precautions should be taken to reduce the risk of foodborne illness. Parents should always wash their hands and all cooking surfaces before and after food preparation, thoroughly cook all meats (including eggs), and wash fresh produce in a clean source of running water.

C.   Meals should be planned with an emphasis on nonstarchy vegetables and fruits as the primary component.
1.   One fourth of a meal should consist of protein (approximately 2–4 ounces or 20–50 grams).
2.   One fourth of a meal should consist of grains or starchy vegetables (approximately one-half cup or 75 grams).

D.   The protein needs during pregnancy and lactation are nearly identical.
1.   Approximately 25 additional grams of protein per day are needed.
2.   On average, this is 71 grams of protein per day for a parent with a healthy prepregnancy BMI.
3.   However, there is significant variation based on height and prepregnancy weight (1.05 g/kg per day).[1]

E.   Carbohydrates provide the most readily available form of energy for the body and are the main fuel source that the brain utilizes.
1.   Each organ system has a nutrient that it prefers as its main fuel source. In general, the recommended intake of carbohydrates during lactation is approximately 210 grams per day, or 45 to 65 percent of daily calorie intake.[1]
2.   Refined carbohydrates should be limited in the diet. When they are eaten, they should be enriched with additional nutrients, such as iron and B vitamins, to replace the nutrients that are removed during processing. Examples of refined carbohydrates include white rice, grits, pasta, and white bread.

F.   Adipose (fat) tissue plays a vital role in the body's ability to store energy, facilitate hormone production, help protein functions, nourish vital organs, and synthesize and store vitamins, to name just a few.
1.   Essential fatty acids are fatty acids that are critical to health and must be obtained through the diet.
2.   Omega-3 fatty acids help control blood clotting and build cell membranes in the brain.[2] The omega-3 fatty acids in human milk are synthesized directly from the body's stores of omega-3 fatty acids.
3.   The adequate intake of omega-3 fatty acids has been set at 1.3 grams by the Institute of Medicine, with an acceptable macronutrient distribution range of 0.6 to 1.2 grams per day for lactating parents.
4.   Increased amounts of omega-3 fatty acids are needed during both pregnancy and lactation.
5.   Fish is an excellent source of omega-3 fatty acids.
a.   The U.S. Food and Drug Administration and the U.S. Environmental Protection Agency suggest two to three servings (4 ounces or 112 grams per serving) of fish per week for pregnant and lactating parents.
b.   Fish with the highest levels of mercury should be avoided; they include king mackerel, marlin, orange roughy, shark, swordfish, tilefish from the Gulf of Mexico, and bigeye tuna.[3]
c.   Pregnant and lactating parents who choose not to eat fish or do not have access to fish should consider supplementation with a DHA-rich omega-3 fatty acid, such as mercury-free fish oil or algae oil along with a diet rich in omega-3 fatty acids.
6.   Other foods that have high amounts of omega-3 fatty acids include walnuts, flax seed, hemp seeds, and canola oil.

G.   Water is the best primary form of hydration for lactating parents.
1.   Water should be consumed to quench thirst.
2.   Approximately 64 ounces (1,800 mL) per day of water is recommended, with variations based on climate and hydration-dependent disease states present in the parent.
3.   Increasing fluids beyond adequate intake does not increase the quality or quantity of human milk.[4]
4.   Juice and fruit juice cocktail should be limited to 2–3 ounces (60–90 mL) per day as part of a healthy diet.[5]

H.   Vegetarian and vegan diets are healthy and nutritionally adequate for lactating parents.[6]
1.   Vegetarians should ensure they are getting a wide variety of protein sources and take care to not rely on dairy-based foods for protein. They should eat a wide variety of legumes, nuts, seeds, and whole grains for protein.
2.   Vegan diets should be supplemented with vitamin B_{12}.

I.   People who follow a pescatarian diet consume fish but not meat.
1.   Organic pollutants in seafood can remain in the body for 1–5 years; therefore, it is recommended that those who rely on seafood as their primary source of protein limit its consumption.[7]
2.   Pescatarians should limit their intake of fish to 2–3 servings per week of fish with low mercury levels.

J.   When consuming a well-balanced diet, vitamin and mineral supplements are typically not needed.

1. Only a small number of vitamins and minerals have recommended daily allowances (RDAs) that are substantially greater for lactating parents than for average nonlactating parents. Only vitamin A, vitamin C, chromium, copper, and iodine are needed in quantities nearly double that of a nonlactating parent.
2. Several micronutrients in human milk are influenced by parental nutritional status and intake, including vitamins A, B_6, B_{12}, C, D, and K; thiamine; riboflavin; choline; selenium; and iodine.
3. Parental deficiencies in any of these micronutrients could result in decreased amounts in human milk, which could result in a nutritional deficiency in the infant.[8-10] However, obtaining adequate amounts of these vitamins and minerals can easily be done through diet alone. **TABLE 8-1** lists the RDA and dietary reference intake (DRI) and the sources of essential vitamins and minerals.

TABLE 8-1 Vitamins and Minerals for Lactating Parents

Nutrient Name	RDA/DRI	Tolerable Upper Limit	Benefits	Good Sources
Biotin	Ages 14+: 35 µg	n/a	Helps convert food into energy and synthesize glucose. Helps make and break down some fatty acids. Needed for healthy bones and hair.	Whole grains, organ meats, egg yolks, soybeans, fish, almonds, mushrooms, sweet potato, spinach.
Calcium	Ages 14–18: 1,300 mg Ages 19+: 1,000 mg	Ages 14–18: 3,000 mg Ages 19+: 2,500 mg	Builds and protects bones and teeth. Helps with muscle contractions and relaxation, blood clotting, and nerve impulse transmission. Good for strong bones and teeth, nerve function, muscle contraction, blood clotting.	Dairy and nondairy yogurt, cheese, dairy and nondairy milks, calcium-set tofu, sardines, salmon (with bones), beans and legumes, fortified juices, leafy green vegetables (broccoli, collards, kale).
Choline[a]	Ages 14+: 550 mg	Ages 14–18: 3.0g Ages 19+: 3.5g	Helps make and release the neurotransmitter acetylcholine, which aids in many nerve and brain activities. Plays a role in metabolizing and transporting fats.	Milk, eggs, liver, peanuts, soy milk, tofu, quinoa, broccoli.
Chromium	Ages 14–18: 44 µg Ages 19+: 45 µg	n/a	Enhances the activity of insulin, helps maintain normal blood glucose levels, and is needed to free energy from glucose. Used in the metabolism and storage of fats, proteins, and carbohydrates.	Meat, poultry, fish, some cereals, nuts, cheese, whole grains, bread, brown rice, broccoli, mushrooms, green beans, brewers' yeast, raw onions.

Nutrient Name	RDA/DRI	Tolerable Upper Limit	Benefits	Good Sources
Copper	Ages 14+: 1,300 µg	Ages 14–18: 8,000 µg Ages 19+: 10,000 µg	Plays an important role in iron metabolism. Helps make red blood cells.	Liver, shellfish, nuts, seeds, whole-grain products, beans, prunes, leafy greens (turnip greens, spinach, Swiss chard, kale, mustard greens), asparagus, summer squash.
Fluoride	Ages 14+: 3 mg	Ages 14+: 10 mg	Encourages strong bone formation. Keeps dental cavities from starting or worsening.	Water that is fluoridated, toothpaste with fluoride, marine fish, teas, dried fruit, dried beans, cocoa powder, walnuts.
Folic acid, folate	Ages 14+: 500 µg	Ages 14–18: 800 µg Ages 19+: 1,000 µg	Vital for new cell creation. Helps prevent brain and spine birth defects when taken early in pregnancy.	Fortified grains and cereals, asparagus, okra, spinach, carrots, turnip greens, broccoli, legumes (black-eyed peas, chickpeas), orange juice, tomato juice, yeast, liver, melon, apricots, pumpkin, beans, avocado.
Iodine[a]	Ages 14+: 290 µg	Ages 14–18: 900 µg Ages 19+: 1,100 µg	Part of thyroid hormone, which helps set body temperature and influences nerve and muscle function, reproduction, and growth.	Iodized salt, processed foods, seafood, cranberries, kelp, potatoes.
Iron	Ages 14–18: 10 mg Ages 19+: 9 mg	Ages 14–18: 900 µg Ages 19+: 1,100 µg	Helps hemoglobin in red blood cells and myoglobin in muscle cells ferry oxygen throughout the body. Needed for chemical reactions in the body and for making amino acids, collagen, neurotransmitters, and hormones.	Red meat, poultry, eggs, fruits, green vegetables, fortified bread and grain products, oily fish, lentils, soybeans, tofu, tempeh, lima beans, grains (quinoa, fortified cereals, brown rice, oatmeal), nuts and seeds (pumpkin, squash, pine, pistachio, sunflower, cashews).
Magnesium	Ages 14–18: 360 mg Ages 19–30: 310 mg Ages 31–50: 320 mg	Ages 14+: 350 mg	Works with calcium in muscle contraction, blood clotting, and regulation of blood pressure. Helps build bones and teeth.	Green vegetables (spinach, chard, broccoli), legumes, cashews, sunflower seeds, pumpkin seeds, almonds, black beans, halibut, whole-wheat bread, milk, nuts.
Manganese	Ages 14+: 2.6 mg	Ages 14–18: 9 mg Ages 19+: 11 mg	Helps form bones. Helps metabolize amino acids, cholesterol, and carbohydrates.	Nuts, legumes, whole grains, tea, brown rice, bran, pecans, cooked spinach.

(continues)

TABLE 8-1 Vitamins and Minerals for Lactating Parents *(continued)*

Nutrient Name	RDA/DRI	Tolerable Upper Limit	Benefits	Good Sources
Molybdenum	Ages 14+: 50 µg	Ages 14–18: 1,700 µg Ages 19+: 2,000 µg	Part of several enzymes, one of which helps ward off a form of severe neurological damage in infants that can lead to early death.	Legumes (beans, lentils, peas), nuts, grain products, milk.
Phosphorus	Ages 14–18: 1,250 mg Ages 19+: 700 mg	Ages 14+: 4g	Helps build and protect bones and teeth. Part of DNA and RNA. Helps convert food into energy.	Milk and dairy products, meat, fish, poultry, eggs, liver, green peas, broccoli, potatoes, almonds.
Potassium	Ages 14+: 5.1 g	n/a	Balances fluids in the body. Helps maintain a steady heartbeat and send nerve impulses. Needed for muscle contractions.	Meat, milk, fruits, vegetables, grains, legumes, winter squash, sweet potatoes, white beans.
Selenium[a]	Ages 14+: 70 µg	Ages 14+: 400 µg	Acts as an antioxidant, neutralizing unstable molecules that can damage cells. Helps regulate thyroid hormone activity.	Organ meats, seafood, walnuts, brazil nuts, spinach, white and shiitake mushrooms, grain products.
Sodium	Ages 14+: 1.5 g	Ages 14+: 2.3g	Balances fluids in the body. Helps send nerve impulses. Needed for muscle contractions.	Salt, soy sauce, processed foods, celery, beets.
Sulfur	n/a	n/a	Helps form bridges that shape and stabilize some protein structures. Needed for healthy hair, skin, and nails.	Protein-rich foods (meats, fish, poultry), nuts, legumes, brussels sprouts, garlic, onions, asparagus, kale, wheat germ.
Vitamin A[a]	Ages 14–18: 1,200 µg Ages 19+: 1,300 µg	Ages 14–18: 2,800 µg Ages 19+: 3,000 µg	Keeps tissues and skin healthy. Plays an important role in bone growth. Good for eyesight, growth, appetite, and taste.	Sweet potatoes, carrots, pumpkins, squash, spinach, mangoes, turnip greens, boiled carrots, raw kale, dandelion greens, dried apricots.

Nutrient Name	RDA/DRI	Tolerable Upper Limit	Benefits	Good Sources
Vitamin B$_1$ (thiamin)[a]	Ages 14+: 1.4 mg	n/a	Helps convert food into energy. Needed for healthy skin, hair, muscles, and brain. Good for nervous system, digestion, muscles, heart, alcohol-damaged nerve tissues.	Pork chops, ham, soy milk, watermelons, acorn squash, liver, yeast, egg yolk, cereal, red meat, nuts, wheat germ, black beans.
Vitamin B$_2$ (riboflavin)[a]	Ages 14+: 1.6 mg	n/a	Helps convert food into energy. Needed for healthy skin, hair, blood, and brain. Good for the breakdown of protein, fat, and carbohydrates.	Milk, yogurt, cheese, whole and enriched grains and cereals, liver, yeast, green leafy vegetables, fish, mushrooms, almonds, quinoa.
Vitamin B$_3$ (niacin)	Ages 14+: 2.0 mg	Ages 14–18: 30 mg Ages 19+: 35 mg	Helps convert food into energy. Essential for healthy skin, blood cells, brain, and nervous system.	Meat, poultry, fish, fortified and whole grains, mushrooms, potatoes, peanut butter, passion fruit, avocado.
Vitamin B$_5$ (pantothenic acid)	Ages 14+: 7 mg	n/a	Helps convert food into energy. Helps make lipids (fats), neurotransmitters, steroid hormones, and hemoglobin.	Chicken, whole grains, broccoli, mushrooms, avocados, tomato products, sunflower seeds, corn, broccoli.
Vitamin B$_6$[a]	Ages 14+: 2.0 mg	Ages 14–18: 80 mg Ages 19+: 100 mg	Helps convert tryptophan to niacin and serotonin, a neurotransmitter that plays key roles in sleep, appetite, and moods. Helps make red blood cells. Influences cognitive abilities and immune function.	Meat, fish, poultry, legumes, tofu and other soy products, potatoes, noncitrus fruits (bananas and watermelons), whole grains, dried beans.
Vitamin B$_{12}$[a]	Ages 14+: 2.8 µg	n/a	Assists in making new cells and breaking down some fatty acids and amino acids. Protects nerve cells and encourages their normal growth. Helps make red blood cells.	Meat, poultry, fish, milk, cheese, eggs, fortified cereals, fortified soy milk, shellfish, beans, mushrooms.

(continues)

TABLE 8-1 Vitamins and Minerals for Lactating Parents   (continued)

Nutrient Name	RDA/DRI	Tolerable Upper Limit	Benefits	Good Sources
Vitamin C[a]	Ages 14–18: 115 mg Ages 19+: 120 mg	Ages 14–18: 1,800 mg Ages 19+: 2,000 mg	Helps make collagen, a connective tissue that knits together wounds and supports blood vessel walls. Acts as an antioxidant, neutralizing unstable molecules that can damage cells.	Fruits and fruit juices (especially citrus), potatoes, broccoli, bell peppers, spinach, strawberries, tomatoes, brussels sprouts, berries, potatoes, green leafy vegetables, raw acerola, rosehips.
Vitamin D[a]	Ages 14+: 15 µg	Ages 14+: 100 µg	Helps maintain normal blood levels of calcium and phosphorus, which strengthen bones. Helps form teeth and bones. Supplements can reduce the number of nonspinal fractures.	Fortified milk or margarine, fortified cereals, fatty fish, sunlight, cod liver oil, sardines, herring, salmon, tuna, mushrooms, tofu.
Vitamin E	Ages 14+: 19 mg	Ages 14–18: 800 mg Ages 19+: 1,000 mg	Acts as an antioxidant, neutralizing unstable molecules that can damage cells. Protects vitamin A and certain lipids from damage.	Vegetable oils, salad dressings and margarines made with vegetable oils, wheat germ, leafy green vegetables, whole grains, nuts, soya beans, spouts, eggs.
Vitamin K[a]	Ages 14–18: 75 µg Ages 19+: 95 µg	n/a	Activates proteins and calcium; essential to blood clotting. May help prevent hip fractures.	Cabbage, liver, eggs, milk, romaine lettuce, collard greens, spinach, broccoli, sprouts, kale, brussels sprouts, scallions, prunes.
Zinc	Ages 14–18: 13 mg Ages 19+: 12 mg	Ages 14–18: 34 mg Ages 19+: 40 mg	Helps form many enzymes and proteins and creates new cells. Frees vitamin A from storage in the liver. Needed for immune system, taste, smell, and wound healing.	Nuts, cashews, seeds, beans and legumes, eggs, red meat, poultry, oysters, fortified cereals, brown rice, whole grains, dark chocolate, sesame seeds, garlic, wheat germ.

Note: RDA is recommended daily allowance; DRI is dietary reference intake.
[a]Micronutrients in human milk that are influenced by parental intake and nutritional status.

4. Maternal vitamin A deficiency reduces the amount of available vitamin A in human milk.[11] Lactating parents need 1,300 mcg (4,333 IU) of vitamin A per day, which is the equivalent of one third of a small baked sweet potato.
5. Lactating parents should get 120 mg of vitamin C per day, which is equivalent to one kiwi or a half cup of strawberries and a half cup of pineapple.
6. The requirement for chromium is 45 mcg per day. Broccoli, mushrooms, oatmeal, prunes, nuts, asparagus, whole grains, cereals, and red wine are all rich sources of chromium.

7. The requirement for copper is 1.3 mg per day. Whole grains, kale, shiitake mushrooms, sesame seeds, sunflower seeds, nuts, beans, fermented soy products (tempeh and miso), and dried fruit are good sources of copper.

8. Iodine needs for the lactating parent can be met through iodized salt, fish, kelp, or other seaweed. Because iodized salt is not available worldwide, lactation consultants should learn about local sources of iodine in their communities.

9. Prenatal vitamins are not appropriate for lactating parents.[12]

    a. The nutrient composition of prenatal vitamins is not appropriate for the nutrient needs of a lactating parent.

    b. A multivitamin or mineral supplement can be taken once per day if it does not exceed the recommended daily intake by more than 20 percent.

    c. Many foods are fortified or enriched with vitamins, in addition to supplementation.

10. In emergency or disaster situations, such as natural disasters and refugee settings, the World Health Organization (WHO) and UNICEF recommend a daily micronutrient supplement for pregnant and lactating parents. Evidence also supports the use of micronutrient supplementation, especially with iron and folic acid, for positive birth outcomes in underdeveloped and developing countries.[13]

11. Lactogenic foods and herbs, such as fenugreek and moringa, contain significant levels of micronutrients that should be considered when evaluating nutrient intake.

12. Vitamin D deficiency is a common nutrient deficiency in most industrialized countries that results from inadequate exposure to sunlight.[14,15]

    a. Very few foods contain vitamin D, and foods that do contain the vitamin do not contain sufficient levels to meet the recommended daily intake.

    b. It is recommended that lactating parents have their vitamin D levels checked. If they are deficient, they should be supplemented at a dosage of 50,000 IU once per week for 8 weeks or 6,000 IU once per day for 8 weeks.

    c. For obese parents, 10,000 IU once per day for 8 weeks is needed to correct vitamin D deficiency in lactation, followed by a maintenance dose of 3,000 to 6,000 IU daily.[16]

13. Folate is a B vitamin that plays a role in DNA synthesis.

    a. There is not a current global standardized daily intake of folate or folic acid for pregnancy or lactation.

    b. Because of this, folate and folic acid intake varies widely around the world.

14. For populations in which the prevalence of anemia in nonpregnant women of reproductive age is higher than 20 percent, it is recommended that all women of childbearing age are supplemented with 60 mg elemental iron (300 mg ferrous sulfate) once per week for 3 months, followed by 3 months of no supplementation, then repeat the cycle.[17]

III. Lactating Parent BMI

A. BMI is a measure of an individual's percentage of body fat based on sex, height, and weight.

1. BMI is a valid clinical diagnostic tool only for individuals older than 20 years. It should not be used for teenagers.

2. BMI for age or weight percentiles are a more accurate tool for assessing the weight status in children and teens.

3. Both underweight and obesity are markers for parental malnutrition.[18]

4. **TABLE 8-2** displays BMI ranges and classifications of weight status.

    a. Underweight: BMI less than 18.5.

    b. Healthy weight: BMI 18.5 to 24.99.

    c. Overweight: BMI 25 to 29.99.

    d. Obese: BMI 30 to 39.99.

    e. Morbidly obese: BMI 40 or greater.

B. Underweight parents are less likely to initiate breastfeeding than parents who have a healthy BMI. Underweight is also a predictor of lower breastfeeding initiation rates in adolescents.[19] Underweight may be indicative of a history of disordered eating patterns or poor access to food.

TABLE 8-2 International Classification of Underweight, Overweight, and Obese Adults Based on BMI

Classification	BMI (kg/m)	
	Principal Cutoff Points	**Additional Cutoff Points**
Underweight	**< 18.50**	**< 18.50**
Severe thinness	< 16.00	< 16.00
Moderate thinness	16.00–16.99	16.00–16.99
Mild thinness	17.00–18.49	17.00–18.49
Normal range	**18.50–24.99**	**18.50–22.99** **23.00–24.99**
Overweight	**≥ 25.00**	**≥ 25.00**
Preobese	25.00–29.99	25.00–27.49 27.50–29.99
Obese	**≥ 30.00**	**≥ 30.00**
Obese class I	30.00–34.99	30.00–32.49 32.50–34.99
Obese class II	35.00–39.99	35.00–37.49 37.50–39.99
Obese class III	≥ 40.00	≥ 40.00

Reproduced from World Health Organization. BMI classification. Updated 2018. Available at: http://apps.who.int/bmi/index.jsp?introPage=intro_3.html. Accessed February 23, 2018.

C. Overweight and obesity increase the risk of milk production difficulty, possibly through inhibiting the body's response to prolactin or suboptimal insulin action.[20] Starting pregnancy at a BMI greater than 25, in addition to gaining more than the recommended amount of weight during pregnancy, can delay lactogenesis II.[21] The highest prevalence of undesired weaning is reported by obese parents, followed by overweight parents.[22]

D. Obese parents in classes I, II, and III are less likely to initiate breastfeeding.[19] A prepregnancy BMI greater than 30 is significantly associated with late onset of lactogenesis II, which, in turn, leads to an increase in supplementation with formula until colostrum transitions to mature milk and an increased rate of breastfeeding discontinuation.[21,23]

1. Women who are overweight or obese at the start of their pregnancy have decreased prolactin levels in response to suckling, compared to women who have a normal BMI.[24]

2. Obesity raises the risk of birth via cesarean section, postnatal complications, and prolonged labor, all of which can have a negative impact on initiating and sustaining breastfeeding by delaying the onset of lactogenesis II.[25,26]

3. Obesity increases the risk of a macrosomic infant, which is an infant who weighs 8 pounds 13 ounces (or 4,000 g) or more at birth, irrespective of gestational age. Macrosomia, with or without the presence of gestational diabetes, decreases the initiation of breastfeeding and increases the risk of birth complications and neonatal intensive care unit (NICU) admittance.[27,28]

4. Obese parents have a higher risk of vitamin and mineral deficiencies, including vitamins B_6, B_{12}, C, D, and E; iron; zinc; phosphorus; and folic acid.[29-32] Depending on the geographic location, vitamin A can be either deficient or in excess in obese parents.[33]

IV. Energy Needs during Lactation

A. Lactating parents require approximately 500 additional calories per day.
1. Calories are supplied from a combination of increased food intake and existing fat stores.
2. Calorie needs are based on exclusive, on-demand breastfeeding.
B. One ounce of human milk contains approximately 20 calories (20 kcal per 29.5 mL).
C. Exclusively breastfed infants will consume anywhere from 19 to 30 ounces (560 to 890 mL) of human milk per day. The parental metabolic cost of breastfeeding is 380 to 600 calories per day, depending on the infant's daily consumption.

V. Importance of Exercise for Pregnant and Breastfeeding Parents

A. Exercise helps improve emotional health, reduce stress levels, improve bone density, and help with weight management.
B. For lactating parents who are exercising at a mild or moderate pace (e.g., walking, running, swimming, yoga), there is no appreciable increase in lactic acid in the milk.
C. Very strenuous exercise can increase lactic acid concentration in human milk; however, no negative side effects have been reported from the increase in lactic acid to the infant, milk production, or the quality of human milk.[34,35]

VI. Tandem Breastfeeding

A. Breastfeeding an infant and one or more older siblings most likely requires increased macro- and micronutrient needs; however, the nutrition implications of tandem breastfeeding are not well established.
B. Lactating parents who are breastfeeding both an infant and a toddler should consume at least 500 additional calories per day to meet their nutrient needs.
C. Lactating parents should be counseled to eat foods rich in omega-3 fatty acids daily because pregnancy and lactation deplete the body of this nutrient.
D. Supplementation with 500 mg per day of omega-3 fatty acid is also appropriate.

VII. Special Populations

A. The special populations outlined in this section have unique nutritional needs that can impact the volume and nutrient composition of human milk.
1. The initial assessment and interview with the parent should uncover these special dietary issues, if present.
2. All lactating parents who have special dietary conditions should be referred to a registered dietitian for a complete nutritional and diet assessment.
B. Breastfeeding adolescents should receive a nutrition consult with a registered dietitian for guidance on a healthy diet to meet both breastfeeding adolescent and infant growth and development needs. Cultural eating norms vary around the world; however, adolescent girls tend to skip meals, particularly breakfast, and consume little to no fruits and vegetables daily.[36]
1. Adolescents who are living above the poverty line in their country tend to consume more fruits, vegetables, and whole grains; however, their consumption still frequently falls below the current recommendations for daily intake.[37]
2. Teenage parents should be encouraged to breastfeed and eat a healthy, balanced diet to ensure they meet the recommended daily intake of nutrients to maintain growth through adulthood.

3. In adolescence, calcium absorption is increased when adolescents consume foods that are high in the prebiotic inulin.[38] Inulin-rich foods include bananas, plantains, garlic, leeks, onions, asparagus, and wheat.

C. Lactating parents with well-controlled Type I or Type II diabetes (hemoglobin Alc between 5.7 and 6.4) and gestational diabetes can successfully breastfeed.

1. Type 1 diabetes is caused by the pancreas not producing insulin; the parent will need to count carbohydrates and take insulin.

2. Type 2 diabetes is an inability of cell receptors for glucose to function properly. Blood glucose levels can be maintained with diet or a combination of diet and medication.

3. Gestational diabetes presents much the same way as Type 2 diabetes and responds well to dietary modifications.

4. Emerging research suggests that diabetes is a risk factor for insufficient milk production and may require additional lactation support and monitoring.[39]

5. A lack of glucose control in pregnancy results in macrosomic infants, and reactive hypoglycemia in infants, in the immediate postpartum period.

6. The milk of lactating parents with Type 2 diabetes has been shown to have two times greater insulin than that of nondiabetic parents. Higher insulin levels in human milk are associated with lower lean body mass and increased infant body weight in the first month of life.[40]

7. Altered fetal growth patterns (for both macrosomic and nonmacrosomic infants) have been observed in women with pregestational diabetes, gestational diabetes, and Type 2 diabetes in pregnancy. These altered fetal growth patterns lead to a higher rate of shoulder dystocia, which increases the risk of emergency cesarean and decreases or delays the initiation of breastfeeding.[41]

8. Gestational diabetes is an independent risk factor for delayed lactogenesis II, with or without the presence of obesity.[42]

9. Delayed lactogenesis II has been observed in Type 1 diabetes if blood glucose levels are not kept in control throughout pregnancy.[43]

10. Lactating parents with any form of diabetes should be under the supervision of an endocrinologist and dietitian throughout pregnancy and lactation to ensure good control of blood glucose levels.

D. Parents can actively attempt to lose weight while lactating through diet modification and exercise.

1. Losing weight at a rate of 1 kg per week does not negatively affect lactation.[44]

2. Losing weight by more than 1 kg per week is not recommended during lactation.

3. Exclusive breastfeeding for at least 6 months increases parental weight loss.[44-47]

4. Overall, lactating parents lose weight faster and return to their prepregnancy weights at a faster rate than their nonbreastfeeding counterparts.[45,48,49]

5. Exercise has been shown to have no negative affect on lactation, and in some cases it has been reported to improve lactation due to an increase in prolactin concentration during exercise.[44,47]

E. Bariatric surgery is becoming more common among women of childbearing age.

1. The three most common bariatric surgeries are Roux-en-Y (gastric bypass), sleeve gastrectomy, and lap band surgery.

    a. The Roux-en-Y surgery reroutes the small intestine past a large portion of absorptive area, making it more difficult for the body to utilize key nutrients including iron, zinc, magnesium, calcium, and B vitamins.

    b. Fewer nutritional deficiencies are seen postsurgery for both sleeve gastrectomy and lap band surgery.

    c. Preexisting nutritional deficiencies prior to surgery can be exacerbated postsurgery.[31]

2. Postponing pregnancy for 12 to 18 months after bariatric surgery may be suggested to avoid pregnancy during a time of rapid weight loss.[50]

3. Breastfeeding after bariatric surgery should be encouraged, but careful monitoring of both the growth and nutritional status of the infant, and the nutritional status of the lactating parent, is imperative.

4. Skin-to-skin contact with the infant immediately after birth and frequently in the neonatal period is especially important for lactating parents after bariatric surgery. Frequent feedings should be encouraged to promote the onset of lactogenesis, which can be delayed in obese or overweight lactating parents.[51]

5. Women who have had significant weight loss after bariatric surgery may have excess skin and pendulous breasts and may need assistance with positioning the infant for breastfeeding.[51]
6. Breast reduction is a common procedure after weight loss from bariatric surgery. The surgical procedure for breast reduction could impact the lactating parent's ability to produce enough milk to support normal infant growth and development of the infant.

F. Malabsorption diseases impact the nutritional status of lactating parents.
   1. Irritable bowel disease (IBD) is divided into two conditions: Crohn disease and ulcerative colitis.
   2. When the disease is active, the lactating parent will experience significant malabsorption of nutrients, including protein, essential fatty acids, calcium, vitamin D, folate, vitamin B_{12}, and zinc.

G. Anemia in the lactating parent does not negatively impact the iron levels found in human milk.[13] Because the body utilizes blood to create milk, anemia in the lactating parent can reduce the volume of milk produced while maintaining nutrient values.

H. Lactating parents with food allergies to dairy products can consume nondairy sources of calcium to meet their nutritional needs.
   1. Dairy products are quick and reliable sources of calcium.
      a. Dairy products are not the sole sources of calcium in a well-balanced diet. Breastfeeding parents who are allergic to dairy products or who are lactose intolerant can still meet their nutrient needs through nondairy calcium sources without requiring supplements.
      b. For adults, calcium needs do not increase for pregnancy and lactation. **TABLE 8-3** lists some common nondairy sources of calcium. Other nondairy foods that are high in calcium include bok choy, tofu, salmon, figs, and sardines.
      c. If calcium supplements are consumed, they should be taken 2 hours before or after any iron-containing supplements because calcium and iron compete for the same binding site in the small intestine.
         i. Calcium can decease the absorption of iron by up to 62 percent.[52]
         ii. Calcium is best absorbed in increments of 500 mg or less and in the presence of normal vitamin D levels within the body.[53]
         iii. For lactating parents who are deficient in vitamin D, taking a 500 mg calcium supplement with vitamin D helps to increase calcium absorption.

TABLE 8-3 Common Nondairy Sources of Calcium

Food Source	Serving Size	Calcium
Almond butter	2 Tbsp (43 g)	86 mg
Almonds	1/4 cup (27 g)	94 mg
Broccoli	1 cup (85 g)	94 mg
Calcium-fortified orange juice	8 oz (236 mL)	349 mg
Collard greens	1 cup (85 g)	357 mg
Edamame, cooked	1 cup (136 g)	98 mg
Kale	1 cup (85 g)	179 mg
Okra	1 cup (85 g)	136 mg
Toasted bagel	1 whole	111 mg

Data from U.S. Department of Agriculture. Nutrient Database. https://ndb.nal.usda.gov/ndb.

2. Wheat allergy, gluten allergy, and celiac disease are separate and distinct disease states.
   a. They present with an overlap in foods that must be eliminated from the diet to maintain health and proper immune function.
   b. When eliminating wheat or gluten from the diet, it is preferable to replace them with whole grains (instead of refined grains), such as brown rice, quinoa, or oats, to ensure an adequate intake of vitamins, minerals, and fiber.

I. Lactating parents of multiples have specific and unique nutrient needs and may report increased hunger or thirst.
   1. Parents who are breastfeeding multiples should drink at least 64 ounces (1,800 mL) of water daily. Drinking more than this amount has not been shown to increase the quantity of milk produced.
   2. On average, lactating parents of multiples should increase their calorie intake by 500 to 600 calories per child. Extra calories should be obtained through a well-balanced diet made up of approximately 20 percent protein, 40 percent carbohydrates, and 40 percent fat.[54]
   3. Although parents who are breastfeeding multiples have higher nutrient needs, it is not recommended that they increase micronutrient supplementation because this could lead to toxic levels of supplemental nutrients in the body. Instead, a healthy, well-balanced diet should be used to ensure adequate nutrient intake.

J. Malnutrition in the lactating parent does not generally lead to poor-quality milk.
   1. There is a decrease in the availability of certain nutrients in the milk of parents who are deficient in vitamins A, B_1, B_2, B_6, B_{12}, C, D, and K; choline; iodine; and selenium.[55]
   2. Malnutrition can be present in both obese and underweight parents. Although malnutrition in the lactating parent does not appear to negatively impact infant health in the short and long term, lactating parent starvation or severe calorie deprivation does have a negative effect on the quality and quantity of milk.
   3. There may be a link between malnutrition while breastfeeding and thyroid dysfunction in offspring that presents in adulthood.[56]

K. The many body changes that occur during pregnancy and lactation can be difficult for lactating parents who have a history of an eating disorder or body dysmorphic disease.
   1. Women who have a history of or active anorexia nervosa have a higher risk of disease relapse, postnatal depression, postnatal anxiety, and breastfeeding failure.[57]
   2. Women who have anorexia nervosa have a higher risk of giving birth to infants with low birth weight and a higher risk for birth via cesarean.[58]
   3. The data on initiating and sustaining breastfeeding in women who have anorexia nervosa is inconsistent. However, women with anorexia nervosa tend to have increased anxiety about the quality and quantity of their milk.[57]
   4. Current data shows that women with purge-type bulimia have breastfeeding initiation rates on par with the general public and similar rates of sustained exclusive breastfeeding.[58]
   5. Women with a history of an eating disorder, or an active eating disorder, should be referred to counseling professionals who specialize in these disorders to ensure appropriate care. Working with an appropriate healthcare team can help promote a positive self-image for the parent and help build healthy habits during pregnancy and lactation.[59]

▶ Key Points from This Chapter

A. Healthy lactating parents can generally meet their nutritional needs and their infant's nutritional needs by eating a well-balanced diet of protein, carbohydrates, and fats, including a variety of fruits, vegetables, grains, and starches.

B. Energy requirements for lactation are approximately 500 kcal per day over the recommended caloric intake for nonpregnant parents.

C. Several micronutrients in human milk are influenced by nutritional status and intake of the lactating parent, including vitamins A, B_6, B_{12}, C, D, and K; thiamine; riboflavin; choline; selenium; and iodine.

D.   Fish is an excellent source of omega-3 fatty acids, but it should be limited to two or three servings per week. Fish with the highest mercury levels should be avoided; they include king mackerel, marlin, orange roughy, shark, swordfish, tilefish from the Gulf of Mexico, and bigeye tuna.

E.   Fluid intake in the lactating parent plays a key role in milk production; lactating parents should drink water to quench their thirst throughout the day.

F.   Lactating parents who have chronic illnesses that result in or involve nutritional deficiencies, or those who have had a multiple birth, may benefit from vitamin and mineral supplementation and should be referred to a registered dietitian for a consultation.

🔍 CASE STUDY

Janel is 28 weeks pregnant and has recently sought prenatal care for the first time. After quite a bit of research on what foods not to eat during pregnancy, Janel finds the list to be restrictive and does not believe it fits with her current lifestyle. Janel's obstetric provider has referred her to you at an outpatient lactation clinic because she has expressed interest in breastfeeding.

Janel is a bit confused by all the conflicting information she has read about breastfeeding online. She shares with you that changing her diet in any way for pregnancy or breastfeeding is one of her biggest challenges. She wants to breastfeed but cannot imagine doing so if she must restrict her diet in any way. Janel has a BMI of 31 and considers herself to be "overweight," but does not like using the label of "obese." She does not like taking pills, even vitamins, but her obstetric provider told her she is anemic and must take iron supplements while pregnant and breastfeeding. She asks why iron status is important for breastfeeding.

Questions

1. What information can you share with Janel about food intake while breastfeeding?
2. How will you explain the benefits of normal hemoglobin values for a breastfeeding mother and what iron rich food sources will you suggest?
3. What information would you share with Janel about the immediate postpartum period and breastfeeding for a parent with a BMI greater than 30?

References

1. Procter SB, Campbell CG. Position of the Academy of Nutrition and Dietetics: nutrition and lifestyle for a healthy pregnancy outcome. *J Acad Nutr Diet.* 2014;114(7):1099-1103.
2. Innis SM. Dietary omega 3 fatty acids and the developing brain. *Brain Res.* 2008;1237:35-43.
3. U.S. Food and Drug Administration. Advice about eating fish, from the Environmental Protection Agency and Food and Drug Administration; revised fish advice; availability. Federal Register website. https://www.federalregister.gov/documents/2017/01/19/2017-01073/advice-about-eating-fish-from-the-environmental-protection-agency-and-food-and-drug-administration. Published January 19, 2017. Accessed February 8, 2018.
4. Dusdieker LB, Stumbo PJ, Booth BM, Wilmoth RN. Prolonged maternal fluid supplementation in breast-feeding. *Pediatrics.* 1990;86(5):737-740.
5. O'Neil CE, Nicklas TA, Zanovec M, Fulgoni VL. Diet quality is positively associated with 100% fruit juice consumption in children and adults in the United States: NHANES 2003-2006. *Nutr J.* 2011;10(1):17.
6. American Dietetic Association, Dietitians of Canada. Position of the American Dietetic Association and Dietitians of Canada: vegetarian diets. *J Am Diet Assoc.* 2009;109(6):1266-1282.
7. Binnington MJ, Quinn CL, McLachlan MS, Wania F. Evaluating the effectiveness of fish consumption advisories: modeling prenatal, postnatal, and childhood exposures to persistent organic pollutants. *Environ Health Perspect.* 2014;122(2):178.
8. Kominiarek MA, Rajan P. Nutrition recommendations in pregnancy and lactation. *Med Clin North Am.* 2016;100(6):1199-1215.
9. Nazeri P, Dalili H, Mehrabi Y, Hedayati M, Mirmiran P, Azizi F. Breast milk iodine concentration rather than maternal urinary iodine is a reliable indicator for monitoring iodine status of breastfed neonates. *Biol Trace Elem Res.* 2018;25:1-7.
10. Allen LH. B vitamins in breast milk: relative importance of maternal status and intake, and effects on infant status and function. *Adv Nutr.* 2012;3(3):362-369.
11. Bekele TH, Whiting SJ, Abebe H, Abuye C. Association of iron, zinc, and vitamin A maternal plasma levels with breast milk composition in rural southern Ethiopia. *European Journal of Nutrition & Food Safety.* 2015;5(5):450-451.
12. Picciano MF. Pregnancy and lactation: physiological adjustments, nutritional requirements and the role of dietary supplements. *J Nutr.* 2003;133(6):1997S-2002S.

13. Haider BA, Bhutta ZA. Multiple-micronutrient supplementation for women during pregnancy. *Cochrane Database Syst Rev.* 2015;11:CD004905. doi:10.1002/14651858.CD004905.pub4.

14. Holick MF, Chen TC. Vitamin D deficiency: a worldwide problem with health consequences. *Am J Clin Nutr.* 2008;87(4):1080S-1086S.

15. Prentice A. Vitamin D deficiency: a global perspective. *Nutr Rev.* 2008;66(10 suppl 2): S153-S164.

16. Holick MF, Binkley NC, Bischoff-Ferrari HA, et al. Evaluation, treatment, and prevention of vitamin D deficiency: an Endocrine Society clinical practice guideline. *J Clin Endocrinol Metab.* 2011;96(7):1911-1930.

17. World Health Organization. *Essential Nutrition Actions: Improving Maternal, Newborn, Infant and Young Child Health and Nutrition.* Geneva, Switzerland: World Health Organization; 2013.

18. Bose K. *Human Malnutrition: Twin Burdens of Undernutrition and Overnutrition.* Hauppauge, NY: Nova Science; 2013.

19. Thompson LA, Zhang S, Black E, et al. The association of maternal pre-pregnancy body mass index with breastfeeding initiation. *Matern Child Health J.* 2013;17(10):1842-1851.

20. Nommsen-Rivers LA. Does insulin explain the relation between maternal obesity and poor lactation outcomes? An overview of the literature. *Adv Nutr.* 2016;7(2):407-414.

21. Winkvist A, Brantsµter AL, Brandhagen M, Haugen M, Meltzer HM, Lissner L. Maternal prepregnant body mass index and gestational weight gain are associated with initiation and duration of breastfeeding among Norwegian mothers. *J Nutr.* 2015;145(6):1263-1270.

22. Stuebe AM, Willett WC, Xue F, Michels KB. Lactation and incidence of premenopausal breast cancer: a longitudinal study. *Arch Intern Med.* 2009;169(15):1364-1371.

23. Hilson JA, Rasmussen KM, Kjolhede CL. High prepregnant body mass index is associated with poor lactation outcomes among white, rural women independent of psychosocial and demographic correlates. *J Hum Lactation.* 2004;20(1):18-29.

24. Rasmussen KM, Kjolhede CL. Prepregnant overweight and obesity diminish the prolactin response to suckling in the first week postpartum. *Pediatrics.* 2004;113(5):e465-e471.

25. Zanardo V, Savona V, Cavallin F, D'Antona D, Giustardi A, Trevisanuto D. Impaired lactation performance following elective delivery at term: role of maternal levels of cortisol and prolactin. *J Matern Fetal Neonatal Med.* 2012;25(9):1595-1598.

26. Noel-Weiss J, Woodend AK, Peterson WE, Gibb W, Groll DL. An observational study of associations among maternal fluids during parturition, neonatal output, and breastfed newborn weight loss. *Int Breastfeed J.* 2011;6:9.

27. Cordero L, Oza-Frank R, Landon MB, Nankervis CA. Breastfeeding initiation among macrosomic infants born to obese nondiabetic mothers. *Breastfeed Med.* 2015;10(5):239-245.

28. Gaudet L, Wen SW, Walker M. The combined effect of maternal obesity and fetal macrosomia on pregnancy outcomes. *J Obstet Gynaecol Can.* 2014;36(9):776-784.

29. Pereira-Santos M, Costa P, Assis A, Santos D. Obesity and vitamin D deficiency: a systematic review and meta-analysis. *Obes Rev.* 2015;16(4):341-349.

30. Aigner E, Feldman A, Datz C. Obesity as an emerging risk factor for iron deficiency. *Nutrients.* 2014;6(9):3587-3600.

31. Van Rutte P, Aarts E, Smulders J, Nienhuijs S. Nutrient deficiencies before and after sleeve gastrectomy. *Obes Surg.* 2014;24(10):1639-1646.

32. Sánchez A, Rojas P, Basfi-Fer K, et al. Micronutrient deficiencies in morbidly obese women prior to bariatric surgery. *Obes Surg.* 2016;26(2):361-368.

33. Aasheim ET, Hofsø D, Hjelmesæth J, Birkeland KI, Bøhmer T. Vitamin status in morbidly obese patients: a cross-sectional study. *Am J Clin Nutr.* 2008;87(2):362-369.

34. Kam, R. Exercise and breastfeeding. Australian Breastfeeding Association website. https://www.breastfeeding.asn.au/bfinfo/exercise-and-breastfeeding. December 2012. Accessed November 1, 2017.

35. Mortensen K, Kam R. Exercise and breastfeeding. *Breastfeed Rev.* 2012;20(3):39-42.

36. Allafi A, Al-Haifi AR, Al-Fayez MA, et al. Physical activity, sedentary behaviours and dietary habits among Kuwaiti adolescents: gender differences. *Pub Health Nutr.* 2014;17(9):2045-2052.

37. Fismen A-S, Smith OR, Torsheim T, Samdal O. A school based study of time trends in food habits and their relation to socio-economic status among Norwegian adolescents, 2001–2009. *Int J Behav Nutr Phys Act.* 2014;11(1):115.

38. Abrams SA, Griffin IJ, Hawthorne KM, et al. A combination of prebiotic short- and long-chain inulin-type fructans enhances calcium absorption and bone mineralization in young adolescents. *Am J Clin Nutr.* 2005;82(2):471-476.

39. Riddle SW, Nommsen-Rivers LA. Low milk supply and the pediatrician. *Curr Opin Pediatr.* 2017;29(2):249-256.

40. Fields DA, Demerath EW. Relationship of insulin, glucose, leptin, IL-6 and TNF-α in human breast milk with infant growth and body composition. *Pediatr Obes.* 2012;7(4):304-312.

41. Hammoud NM, Visser GH, Peters SA, Graatsma E, Pistorius L, de Valk HW. Fetal growth profiles of macrosomic and non-macrosomic infants of women with pregestational or gestational diabetes. *Ultrasound Obstet Gynecol.* 2013;41(4):390-397.

42. Matias SL, Dewey KG, Quesenberry CP, Gunderson EP. Maternal prepregnancy obesity and insulin treatment during pregnancy are independently associated with delayed lactogenesis in women with recent gestational diabetes mellitus. *Am J Clin Nutr.* 2014;99(1):115-121.

43. De Bortoli J, Amir L. Is onset of lactation delayed in women with diabetes in pregnancy? A systematic review. *Diabetic Med.* 2016;33(1):17-24.

44. Dewey KG. Effects of maternal caloric restriction and exercise during lactation. *J Nutr.* 1998;128(2):386S-389S.

45. Dewey KG, Heinig MJ, Nommsen LA. Maternal weight-loss patterns during prolonged lactation. *Am J Clin Nutr.* 1993;58(2):162-166.

46. Lovelady CA, Garner KE, Moreno KL, Williams JP. The effect of weight loss in overweight, lactating women on the growth of their infants. *N Engl J Med.* 2000;342(7):449-453.

47. McCrory MA, Nommsen-Rivers LA, Molé PA, Lönnerdal B, Dewey KG. Randomized trial of the short-term effects of dieting compared with dieting plus aerobic exercise on lactation performance. *Am J Clin Nutr.* 1999;69(5):959-967.

48. Dewey KG. Impact of breastfeeding on maternal nutritional status. In: Pickering LK, Morrow AL, Ruiz-Palacios GM, Schanler R., eds. *Protecting Infants through Human Milk.* New York: Springer; 2004: 91-100.

49. Dewey KG, Cohen RJ, Brown KH, Rivera LL. Effects of exclusive breastfeeding for four versus six months on maternal nutritional status and infant motor development: results of two randomized trials in Honduras. *J Nutr.* 2001;131(2):262-267.

50. Kominiarek MA. Preparing for and managing a pregnancy after bariatric surgery. *Semin Perinatol.* 2011;35(6):356-361.

51. Lamb ML. Weight-loss surgery and breastfeeding. *Clin Lactation.* 2011;2(3):17-21.

52. Cook JD, Dassenko SA, Whittaker P. Calcium supplementation: effect on iron absorption. *Am J Clin Nutr.* 1991;53(1):106-111.

53. Heaney RP, Dowell MS, Hale CA, Bendich A. Calcium absorption varies within the reference range for serum 25-hydroxyvitamin D. *J Am Coll Nutr.* 2003;22(2):142-146.

54. Flidel-Rimon O, Shinwell ES. Breast feeding twins and high multiples. *Arch Dis Child Fetal Neonatal Ed.* 2006;91(5):F377-F380.

55. Allen L. Maternal micronutrient malnutrition: effects on breast milk and infant nutrition, and priorities for intervention. *SCN News.* 1994;11:21-24.

56. Passos M, da Fonte Ramos C, Dutra S, Mouco T, De Moura E. Long-term effects of malnutrition during lactation on the thyroid function of offspring. *Horm Metab Res.* 2002;34(01):40-43.

57. Hoffman ER, Zerwas SC, Bulik CM. Reproductive issues in anorexia nervosa. *Expert Rev Obstet Gynecol.* 2011;6(4):403-414.

58. Torgersen L, Ystrom E, Haugen M, et al. Breastfeeding practice in mothers with eating disorders. *Maternal Child Nutr.* 2010;6(3):243-252.

59. Carwell ML, Spatz DL. Eating disorders and breastfeeding. *Am J Maternal Child Nurs.* 2011;36(2):112-117.

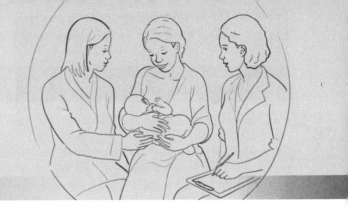

CHAPTER 9

Nutrition for the Breastfeeding Child

Alicia C. Simpson

(continues)

DEFINITIONS OF COMMONLY USED TERMS *(continued)*

exclusive breastfeeding An infant diet of exclusively human milk without the use of any artificial infant milk, infant cereal, other fluids (juices, sports drinks, herbal teas, etc.) or other solid food; however, exclusive breastfeeding does allow the infant to receive oral rehydration solution and medicinal drops and syrups (vitamins, minerals, and medicines, including sweetened pacifiers given during medical procedures).

food allergy An immune reaction when nonharmful food is consumed and causes a range of symptoms, from urticaria to gastrointestinal distress and anaphylaxis.

food sensitivity A condition in which an individual has difficulty digesting certain foods consumed in the diet, causing a variety of reactions including gastrointestinal distress, headaches, and migraines.

Any use of the term *mother, maternal,* or *breastfeeding* is not meant to exclude transgender or nonbinary parents who may be breastfeeding or providing human milk to their infant.

▶ Overview

Human milk is the optimal form of nutrition for human infants. Human milk plays an integral role in public health by decreasing the risk of mortality for children younger than age 5 years. Human milk contains the perfect amount of macro- and micronutrients to meet the unique needs of infants and plays an important role in short- and long-term disease prevention. The period of introduction of solid foods, at about 6 months of age, is a significant nutritional transition in which the breastfed infant is at the greatest risk of developing nutrient deficiency. This chapter outlines the guidelines and recommendations for infant feeding from birth through early childhood and discusses the unique requirements based on an infant's life stage and development.

I. Guidelines and Recommendations for Infant Feeding

A. The World Health Organization (WHO) Global Strategy for Infant and Young Child Feeding[1] is the guiding framework for infant nutrition.

   1. In 2003, the WHO published the Global Strategy for Infant and Young Child Feeding based on a synthesis of the global scientific evidence to date.

   2. The global public health recommendation is that infants should be exclusively breastfed for the first 6 months of life to achieve optimal growth, development, and health.

   3. To meet their evolving nutritional requirements, from the age of 6 months onward, infants should receive nutritionally adequate and safe complementary foods while breastfeeding continues for up to 2 years of age or beyond.

   4. Exclusive breastfeeding from birth is possible except for a few medical conditions. Unrestricted exclusive breastfeeding results in ample milk production.

      a. Infants should be fed on demand throughout the day and night to ensure their nutrient needs are met. Parent-led scheduled feedings have been associated with more decreased long-term cognitive and academic outcomes than in infants who were fed on demand.[2] Responsive feeding is shown to produce the best childhood outcomes across diverse cultures.[3]

      b. There is a wide variation in parental capacity to make and store milk, which can lead to a large variation in the number of times an infant breastfeeds throughout a day and the duration of each breastfeeding session.

   5. In infants, the average human milk feeding is digested in approximately 90 minutes.[4] Therefore, it is feasible for an infant with normal digestive patterns to breastfeed every 1–3 hours throughout the day and night.

B. No other fluid should be given to infants in their first 6 months of life. Juice, sports drinks, and whole cow's milk are not appropriate fluids for infants younger than 1 year. Water should be given only after the infant has accepted solid foods and is replacing a full breastfeeding session with a meal. Supplemental water is not necessary for exclusively breastfed infants younger than 6 months.[5]

C. No other foods should be mixed with human milk and fed to an infant younger than 6 months. This includes rice or other grain-based infant cereal and pureed foods.

D. Unmodified nonhuman milk should not be fed to infants younger than 12 months due to the increased risk of renal disease, diarrhea, and iron deficiency anemia.[1]

E. If human milk is not available in sufficient quantities, the infant should be fed human milk substitute that is specifically designed for infants (i.e., infant formula). Parents should receive instruction for safe preparation of human milk substitutes from healthcare workers or providers. The information given should include adequate instructions for appropriate preparation and the health hazards of inappropriate preparation and use.[1]

F. On-demand breastfeeding should continue until at least 2 years of age or as long as mutually acceptable for the lactating parent and child.[1]

G. Guidelines regarding the number of calories (kcal) an infant needs to consume each day should be calculated based on energy expenditure and energy needed for growth. A registered dietitian can assist in calculating infant nutrient needs.

CLINICAL TIP

Example calculations for calorie requirements for infants according to age and weight include the following:

a. 0 to 3 months of age = (89 + wt[kg] − 100) + 175
b. 4 to 6 months of age = (89 + wt[kg] − 100) + 56
c. 7 to 12 months of age = (89 + wt[kg] − 100) + 22
d. 13 to 35 months of age = (89 + wt[kg] − 100) + 20

H. Infants younger than 12 months should not be actively encouraged to restrict feedings to less than eight in a 24-hour period.

II. Introduction of Complementary (Solid) Foods

A. Complementary foods should be introduced at about 6 months of age. Introducing at 6 months versus 4 months decreases the incidence and severity of infectious illness in the breastfeeding infant and provides a longer duration of postpartum amenorrhea in the lactating parent.[6]

B. The transition period when complementary foods are introduced creates high nutrition risk for infants.
   1. Infants do not yet have the physiologic and developmental capabilities to eat a complete meal with all the macro- and micronutrients necessary for growth.
   2. Human milk or artificial infant milk should be the primary source of nutrients through the first year of life while the infant develops the skills necessary to replace human milk with whole foods.
   3. As stated by the WHO Global Strategy for Infant and Young Child Feeding, ensuring that nutritional needs are met requires that complementary foods have the following characteristics[1]:
      a. Timely: They are introduced when the need for energy and nutrients exceeds what can be provided through exclusive and frequent breastfeeding.
      b. Adequate: They provide sufficient energy, protein, and micronutrients to meet a growing child's nutritional needs.
      c. Safe: They are hygienically stored and prepared, and they are fed with clean hands using clean utensils, not bottles and teats.
      d. Properly fed: They are given consistent with a child's signals of appetite and satiety. Meal frequency and the feeding methods are suitable for age (actively encouraging the child, even during illness, to consume sufficient food using fingers, spoon, or self-feeding).

C. The introduction of nonpuree complementary foods between 6 and 9 months of age increases the likelihood of acceptance of a broader array of food, including fruits and vegetables, at 7 years of age.[7] Infants who are introduced to nonpuree complementary foods past 9 to 10 months of age have a higher risk of food aversions and decreased intake of vegetables in early childhood.[8]

D. When complementary foods are introduced, complete meals should be presented to the infant. A complete meal includes protein, grain or starchy vegetable, and fruit or vegetable. Offering a variety of foods ensures that nutrient needs are met.[9]

E. Complementary foods are ideally prepared from locally available fresh ingredients. Processed complementary foods are acceptable sources of nutrition if families can prepare and feed them safely. "Processed-food products for infants and young children should, when sold or otherwise distributed, meet applicable standards recommended by the Codex Alimentarius Commission and also the Codex Code of Hygienic Practice for Foods for Infants and Children."[1(p9)]

F. Frequent, on-demand breastfeeding should continue from the introduction of complementary foods until the infant is at least 2 years of age.[10]

G. Children living in poverty in both developed and developing countries are at a high risk of inappropriate infant feeding, early introduction of complementary foods, and introduction of complementary foods that are not nutritionally adequate to meet the nutrient needs of infants.

H. The early introduction of solid foods is affected by family pressure, free or discounted manufactured foods, and poverty.[11,12]

I. A new parent's principal source of child feeding education is their own mother or partner's mother, especially in low-income communities.[13] This points to a need for dietary interventions and education to be taught and supported by the entire family.

III. Breastfeeding the Toddler (1–3 Years of Age)

A. The breastfeeding toddler should be breastfed on demand while also being served three complete meals per day consisting of a grain or starchy vegetable, fruit or vegetable, and source of protein.[9] Aside from breastmilk, water should be the primary fluid consumed throughout the day to ensure adequate hydration.

B. At 12 months of age, nonhuman milk can be introduced into the toddler's diet.
   1. Although there is a correlation between increased growth rate among preschool-age children and bovine milk consumption in developing countries, there is also a strong link between the consumption and overconsumption of bovine milk to iron deficiency anemia and early dental caries.[14]
   2. Calcium and casein inhibit the absorption of nonheme iron in the small intestines, which is likely the mechanism by which bovine milk increases the risk of iron deficiency anemia.
   3. Toddlers who drink more than 16–24 ounces of bovine milk per day are at the greatest risk for severe iron deficiency anemia; therefore, bovine milk intake should be limited to less than 16 ounces per day, or two servings of bovine-milk based products like cheese or yogurt per day.[15,16]

C. Infants and toddlers who receive human milk tend to be more accepting of new foods and have a higher variation in the foods they will eat.[17] However, in Western cultures infants and toddlers consume less fruits and vegetables than the current recommendations, and they consume more sweetened beverages, candies, and desserts than other cultures, which can lead to early childhood dental caries, obesity, and malnutrition.

D. Worldwide, toddlers who are breastfed directly at the breast (not including expressed milk in bottles) have an increased risk of forming dental caries than those breastfed for less than 12 months.[18-20] However, in the United States breastfeeding duration has not been positively associated with the development of dental caries, except in low-income families.[21]
   1. Providing families with education about infant and early childhood nutrition is an effective tool to reduce the risk of dental caries.[22]
   2. Bottle feeding expressed milk at night appears to be a leading cause of dental carries in breastfeeding toddlers and therefore should be discouraged.[23]
   3. Light brushing of primary teeth starting at 9 months old with a xylitol-based toothpaste or syrup applied to teeth helps to significantly decrease the incidence of early childhood dental caries.[24]
   4. A significant relationship exists between the development of early dental caries and iron deficiency anemia.[25] Therefore, an infant's or toddler's nutrition status should be regularly examined, and infants older than 6 months should have iron-rich food incorporated into their diet.

IV. Prevention of Malnourishment

A. Infants who are underweight, growing too slowly, or failing to thrive should be supervised by a multidisciplinary team, including a lactation professional, dietitian, and pediatric healthcare provider.

    1. Childhood overweight and obesity are also markers for malnutrition.

    2. Actively screening for risk factors of malnourishment and inappropriate feeding practices is an important step to preventing malnourishment in infants and young children.

B. Slow infant growth and failure to thrive can have many different causes.

    1. Risk factors for slow infant growth and failure to thrive include prematurity, presence of an illness, inadequate nutrient intake secondary to poor feeding technique, cultural barriers, health beliefs, social and psychological problems in the family, poverty, a strict diet, severe food allergy, vomiting, diarrhea, dysphagia, infections, adenoid hypertrophy, and respiratory problems.

    2. Exclusive breastfeeding, adequate and timely introduction of complementary foods at age 6 months, along with continued breastfeeding through at least age 2 years, could save 1.5 million children younger than 5 years from death due to malnourishment.[10]

    3. Parental perception of infant body size and weight gain is a causative factor in the early introduction and inappropriate introduction of solid foods.[26]

C. Overweight and obesity are growing health concerns for infants.

    1. Many parents and healthcare providers hold the belief that the more infants weigh, the healthier they are.[13] This belief is especially prevalent in low-income communities and developing countries.

    2. New evidence has demonstrated that rapid infant weight gain, feeding practices, and high infant weight are predictors of pediatric obesity.[27,28]

        a. The combination of exclusive use of artificial infant milk and the introduction of solid foods before age 4 months has been associated with a sixfold increase in pediatric obesity.[29]

        b. Monitoring and modifying early rapid weight gain in infancy is the first step in preventing pediatric obesity, adult obesity, and obesity-related malnutrition.[27,30,31]

            i. Infant care teams must be able to understand and interpret appropriate infant weight gain and discuss these implications of too little or too much weight gain with caregivers.

            ii. Healthy growth rates for the first year of life are provided in the WHO Child Growth Standards.[32] All children younger than 5 years of age should have their height and weight measured and plotted on WHO growth charts at each primary healthcare visit as part of a comprehensive assessment of growth and nutritional status.[33,34]

            iii. An average monthly weight gain for infants in the first year of life is displayed in **TABLE 9-1**. Actual weight gain for infants in the first year of life may vary greatly from the averages presented.

    3. Infant feeding factors that affect pediatric obesity include the type of milk the infant receives (breastmilk or artificial infant milk), parental use of food to regulate infant distress, the timing of the introduction of solid foods, sweetened beverage consumption, the age of weaning from the bottle, and the introduction of solids and table foods.[30]

        a. Introducing solid foods later in infancy is associated with a lowered risk of pediatric obesity and a greater acceptance of new foods.

TABLE 9-1 Expected Weekly Weight Gain of Infants	
Age	**Grams per Week**
0–4 months	155–241
4–6 months	92–126
6–12 months	50–80

Modified from World Health Organization. *WHO Child Growth Standards: Length/Height for Age, Weight-for-Age, Weight-for-Length, Weight-for-Height and Body Mass Index-for-Age, Methods and Development.* Geneva, Switzerland: World Health Organization; 2006.

    b.   Adding infant cereal to a bottle has been shown to increase the risk of pediatric obesity.[35] The risk for early introduction of infant cereals, reported as early as day 3 of life in some studies and case reports, is significantly higher in low-income communities.[13]

    c.   The complete avoidance of sugar-sweetened beverages for infants and young children is recommended.

    d.   There is no established nutritional need for fruit juice in the diet.

        i.   Juice is not a necessary component of a healthy, well-balanced diet.

        ii.   If 100 percent fruit juices are given to an infant, they should not be given in a bottle or sippy cup, but instead an open cup, and should be limited to 4–6 ounces per day.

        iii.   Fruit juice should not take the place of milk in an infant's diet.

    4.   Early parental education on appropriate breast and bottle feeding techniques, and appropriate solid food introduction, has been shown to be an effective early intervention for the prevention of pediatric obesity.[30]

    5.   In many cultures food is associated with love and good parenting.[36]

    a.   Some families believe the more children are fed, the more they are loved and care for. This disconnect in parental feelings versus appropriate feeding practices can lead to inappropriate infant feeding.

    b.   Education about appropriate infant feeding practices should extend to as many members of the family as possible, including grandparents and other family members living in the home.

V. Macro- and Micronutrient Needs of Infants and Toddlers

    A.   Most of the macro and micronutrients in human milk are maintained despite parental nutritional status.

    1.   There are notable exceptions, including selenium, iodine, vitamin A, vitamin D, riboflavin, thiamine, vitamin B_6, vitamin B_{12}, and choline.[37]

    2.   Even though the parental diet does not influence the total amount of fat in human milk, diet does influence its fatty acid composition. For this reason, it is important for the lactating parent to consume foods abundant in omega-3 fatty acids, such as small oily fish (e.g., mackerel and sardines).

    3.   It is important to ensure that lactating parents are well nourished for their own well-being, their ability to fully care for their infant, and to optimize the quality of their milk.

    a.   In the case of vitamin B_{12}, the status during pregnancy determines the adequacy of B_{12} concentration in the milk.

    b.   Low B_{12} in the milk cannot be rescued through supplementing the lactating parent. Rather, the infant will need to be supplemented.[37]

    B.   Human milk provides all the necessary nutrients for optimal infant growth. No other foods are needed for at least the first 6 months of life to ensure healthy growth and development. Please refer to **TABLE 9-2** for a comprehensive list of the macro- and micronutrient composition of mature human milk.

    C.   Obtaining nutrients from whole foods should be a lactating parent's primary source of nutrients. However, in cases of food insecurity or scarcity a multivitamin and mineral supplement is appropriate to replete parental nutrient stores.

    D.   Approximately one third of the world's infants and children are deficient in vitamin A.[38]

    1.   The introduction of foods that are high in vitamin A should begin at age 6 months and continue throughout infancy and childhood to ensure adequate intake.

    2.   In countries where the pediatric incidence of night blindness is above 1 percent, or the prevalence of vitamin A deficiency is above 20 percent, infants and children older than 6 months should receive a daily vitamin A supplement appropriate to their nutrient needs. In these countries, for infants 6–11 months of age, a one-time supplement of 100,000 IU (30 mg RE) vitamin A is recommended.[39]

    E.   In many Western countries parental vitamin D deficiency is common.

    1.   The vitamin D status of human milk is dependent on parental status. In the first 6–8 weeks of life, infant vitamin D status is dependent predominantly on vitamin D that is acquired through placental transfer.[40]

    2.   All infants from birth to 12 months of age are recommended to receive 400 IU per day of vitamin D supplementation per day.[41]

TABLE 9-2 Macro- and Micronutrient Composition of Human Milk

Nutrients	Amount (1 fluid oz = 30.8 g)
Water	26.95 g
Energy	22 kcal
Protein	0.32 g
Total lipid (fat)	1.35 g
Carbohydrate	2.12 g
Fiber, total dietary	0 g
Sugar, total	2.12 g
Minerals	
Calcium, Ca	10 mg
Iron, Fe	0.01 mg
Magnesium, Mg	1 mg
Phosphorus, P	4 mg
Potassium, K	16 mg
Sodium, Na	5 mg
Zinc, Zn	0.05 mg
Vitamins	
Vitamin C, total ascorbic acid	1.5 mg
Thiamin	0.004 mg
Riboflavin	0.011 mg
Niacin	0.055 mg
Vitamin B_6	0.003 mg
Folate, DFE	2 mcg
Vitamin B_{12}	0.02 mcg
Vitamin A, RAE	19 mcg
Vitamin A, IU	65 IU

(continues)

TABLE 9-2 Macro- and Micronutrient Composition of Human Milk	*(continued)*
Nutrients	**Amount (1 fluid oz = 30.8 g)**
Vitamins	
Vitamin E (alpha-tocopherol)	0.02 mg
Vitamin D ($D_2 + D_3$)	Depends on maternal intake
Vitamin K (phylloquinone)	0.1 mcg
Lipids	
Fatty acids, total saturated	0.619 g
Fatty acids, total monounsaturated	0.511 g
Fatty acids, total polyunsaturated	0.153 g
Cholesterol	4 mg

3. An alternative to infant supplementation is to have the lactating parent consume at least 6,400 IU of vitamin D_3 or 4,000 IU of vitamin D_2 in supplement form daily. This is enough to transfer 400 IU per day of vitamin D to the infant via exclusive breastfeeding.[42,43]

F. Human milk is low in iron, but the form is highly bioavailable.
   1. In the first 6 months of life, the infant relies on highly bioavailable iron from the parent's milk plus iron stores accumulated in the few weeks of fetal life.
   2. By about 6 months of age, the infant requires an additional source of iron to prevent iron deficiency anemia.
      a. Risk factors for iron deficiency anemia in infancy include preterm birth, low birth weight, maternal iron deficiency in pregnancy, and early clamping of the umbilical cord.
      b. Daily iron supplementation for infants 6–23 months of age should be provided to infants who reside in countries with poor availability of iron-fortified foods and have greater than 40 percent prevalence of anemia.[10]
      c. A dietitian or healthcare provider may recommend that anemic children younger than 2 years receive 3 mg/kg iron supplement daily until hemoglobin concentrations return to normal.
      d. It is important to avoid routine iron supplementation to infants who are iron replete because multiple randomized controlled trials have reported worse outcomes in iron-supplemented infants when the infants were not anemic at baseline.[44] The reports include significantly increased incidence of gastrointestinal illnesses, less length gain, later attainment of motor milestones in infancy, and worse neurodevelopmental scores in childhood.

G. Bovine milk is a rich source of calcium and protein. However, the overconsumption of bovine milk and bovine-milk products (e.g., cheese and yogurt) can lead to iron deficiency anemia, early childhood dental caries, and pediatric obesity. Therefore, the early introduction of nondairy sources of calcium in an infant's diet is important to ensure that calcium needs are met and that bovine milk is not the sole source of calcium in a toddler's diet. Refer to **TABLE 9-3** for nonbovine sources of calcium in the diet.

H. Zinc supplementation should be recommended by a registered dietitian or healthcare provider for all children who have active diarrhea. Providing zinc supplementation in conjunction with oral rehydration salts has been shown to significantly decrease mortality for infants and children younger than 5 years.[45]

I. In countries where less than 20 percent of the population has access to iodized salt, lactating parents, infants, and children should be supplemented based on their nutrient needs.[46] There is growing concern that even in countries with access to iodized salt, the intake may not be sufficient.[47]

TABLE 9-3 Vitamin and Mineral Recommendations for Infants and Children, with Good Source Examples

Nutrient Name	RDA/DRI	Tolerable Upper Limit	Benefits	Good Sources
Biotin	Ages 0–6 months: 5 µg Ages 7–12 months: 6 µg Ages 1–3 years: 8 µg	n/a	Helps convert food into energy and synthesize glucose. Helps make and break down some fatty acids.	Whole grains, organ meats, egg yolks, soybeans, fish, almonds, mushrooms, sweet potato, spinach.
Calcium	Ages 0–6 months: 200 mg Ages 7–12 months: 260 mg Ages 1–3 years: 700 mg	Ages 0–6 months: 1,000 mg Ages 7–12 months: 1,500 mg Ages 1–3 years: 2,500 mg	Builds and protects bones and teeth. Helps with muscle contractions and relaxation, blood clotting, and nerve impulse transmission. Plays a role in hormone secretion and enzyme activation. Helps maintain healthy blood pressure.	Dairy and nondairy yogurt, cheese, dairy and nondairy milks, calcium-set tofu, sardines, salmon (with bones), beans and legumes, fortified juices, leafy green vegetables.
Choline	Ages 0–6 months: 125 mg Ages 7–12 months: 150 mg Ages 1–3 years: 200 mg	Ages 0–12 months: n/a Ages 1–3 years: 1.0 g	Helps make and release the neurotransmitter acetylcholine, which aids in many nerve and brain activities. Plays a role in metabolizing and transporting fats.	Milk, eggs, liver, peanuts, soy milk, tofu, quinoa, broccoli.
Chromium	Ages 0–6 months: 0.2 µg Ages 7–12 months: 5.5 µg Ages 1–3 years: 11 µg	n/a	Enhances the activity of insulin, helps maintain normal blood glucose levels, and is needed to free energy from glucose. Used in the metabolism and storage of fats, proteins, and carbohydrates.	Meat, poultry, fish, some cereals, nuts, cheese, whole grains, bread, brown rice, broccoli, mushrooms, green beans, brewers' yeast, raw onions.
Copper	Ages 0–6 months: 200 µg Ages 7–12 months: 220 µg Ages 1–3 years: 340 µg	Ages 0–12 months: n/a Ages 1–3 years: 1,000 µg	Plays an important role in iron metabolism. Helps make red blood cells.	Liver, shellfish, nuts, seeds, whole-grain products, beans, prunes, leafy greens (turnip greens, spinach, Swiss chard, kale, mustard greens), asparagus, summer squash.

(continues)

TABLE 9-3 Vitamin and Mineral Recommendations for Infants and Children, with Good Source Examples *(continued)*

Nutrient Name	RDA/DRI	Tolerable Upper Limit	Benefits	Good Sources
Fluoride	Ages 0–6 months: 0.01 mg 0.02 Ages 7–12 months: 0.5 mg Ages 1–3 years: 0.7 mg	Ages 0–6 months: 0.07 mg Ages 7–12 months: 0.9 mg Ages 1–3 years: 1.3 mg	Encourages strong bone formation. Keeps dental cavities from starting or worsening.	Water that is fluoridated, toothpaste with fluoride, marine fish, teas, dried fruit, dried beans, cocoa powder, walnuts.
Folic acid, folate	Ages 0–6 months: 65 µg Ages 7–12 months: 80 µg Ages 1–3 years: 150 mcg	Ages 0–12 months: n/a Ages 1–3 years: 300 µg	Vital for new cell creation.	Fortified grains and cereals, asparagus, okra, spinach, carrots, turnip greens, broccoli, legumes (black-eyed peas, chickpeas), orange juice, tomato juice, yeast, liver, melon, apricots, pumpkin, beans, avocado.
Iodine	Ages 0–6 months: 110 µg Ages 7–12 months: 130 µg Ages 1–3 years: 90 µg	Ages 0–12 months: n/a Ages 1–3 years: 200 µg	Part of thyroid hormone, which helps set body temperature and influences nerve and muscle function, reproduction, and growth. Prevents goiter and a congenital thyroid disorder.	Iodized salt, processed foods, seafood, cranberries, kelp, potatoes.
Iron	Ages 0–6 months: 0.27 mg Ages 7–12 months: 11 mg Ages 1–3 years: 7 mg	Ages 0–12 months: 40 mg Ages 1–3 years: 40 mg	Helps hemoglobin in red blood cells and myoglobin in muscle cells ferry oxygen throughout the body. Needed for chemical reactions in the body and for making amino acids, collagen, neurotransmitters, and hormones.	Red meat, poultry, eggs, fruits, green vegetables, fortified bread and grain products, oily fish, lentils, soybeans, tofu, tempeh, lima beans, grains (quinoa, fortified cereals, brown rice, oatmeal), nuts and seeds (pumpkin, squash, pine, pistachio, sunflower, cashews).
Magnesium	Ages 0–6 months: 30 mg Ages 7–12 months: 75 mg Ages 1–3 years: 80 mg	Ages 0–12 months: n/a Ages 1–3 years: 65 mg (pharmacology dose, not diet)	Needed for many chemical reactions in the body. Good for energy from food, cell repair, building strong bones, teeth, and muscles, and regulating body temperature.	Green vegetables (spinach, chard, broccoli), legumes, cashews, sunflower seeds, pumpkin seeds, almonds, black beans, halibut, whole-wheat bread, milk, nuts.

Nutrient Name	RDA/DRI	Tolerable Upper Limit	Benefits	Good Sources
Manganese	Ages 0–6 months: 0.003 mg Ages 7–12 months: 0.6 mg Ages 1–3 years: 1.2 mg	Ages 0–12 months: n/a Ages 1–3 years: 2 mg	Helps form bones. Helps metabolize amino acids, cholesterol, and carbohydrates.	Nuts, legumes, whole grains, tea, brown rice, bran, pecans, cooked spinach.
Molybdenum	Ages 0–6 months: 2 μg Ages 7–12 months: 3 μg Ages 1–3 years: 17 μg	Ages 0–12 months: n/a Ages 1–3 years: 300 μg	Part of several enzymes, one of which helps ward off a form of severe neurological damage in infants that can lead to early death.	Nuts, legumes, milk, grain products.
Phosphorus	Ages 0–6 months: 100 mg Ages 7–12 months: 275 mg Ages 1–3 years: 460 mg	Ages 0–12 months: n/a Ages 1–3 years: 3 g	Helps build and protect bones and teeth. Part of DNA and RNA. Helps convert food into energy.	Milk and dairy products, meat, fish, poultry, eggs, liver, green peas, broccoli, potatoes, almonds.
Potassium	Ages 0–6 months: 0.4 g Ages 7–12 months: 0.7 g Ages 1–3 years: 3 g	n/a	Balances fluids in the body. Helps maintain steady heartbeat and send nerve impulses. Needed for muscle contractions. A diet rich in potassium seems to lower blood pressure.	Meat, milk, fruits, vegetables, grains, legumes, winter squash, sweet potatoes, white beans.
Selenium	Ages 0–6 months: 15 μg Ages 7–12 months: 20 μg Ages 1–3 years: 20 μg	Ages 0–6 months: 45 μg Ages 7–12 months: 60 μg Ages 1–3 years: 90 μg	Acts as an antioxidant, neutralizing unstable molecules that can damage cells. Helps regulate thyroid hormone activity.	Organ meats, seafood, walnuts, brazil nuts, spinach, white and shiitake mushrooms, grain products.
Sodium	Ages 0–6 months: 0.12 g Ages 7–12 months: 0.37 g Ages 1–3 years: 1 g	Ages 0–12 months: n/a Ages 1–3 years: 1.5 g	Balances fluids in the body. Helps send nerve impulses Needed for muscle contractions. Impacts blood pressure; even modest reductions in salt consumption can lower blood pressure.	Salt, soy sauce, processed foods, celery, beets.

(continues)

TABLE 9-3 Vitamin and Mineral Recommendations for Infants and Children, with Good Source Examples   *(continued)*

Nutrient Name	RDA/DRI	Tolerable Upper Limit	Benefits	Good Sources
Sulfur	n/a	n/a	Helps form bridges that shape and stabilize some protein structures. Needed for healthy hair, skin, and nails.	Protein-rich foods (meats, fish, poultry), nuts, legumes, brussels sprouts, garlic, onions, asparagus, kale, wheat germ.
Vitamin A	Ages 0–6 months: 400 µg Ages 7–12 months: 500 µg Ages 1–3 years: 300 µg	Ages 0–12 months: 600 µg Ages 1–3 years: 600 µg	Keeps tissues and skin healthy. Plays an important role in bone growth. Good for eyesight, growth, appetite, and taste.	Sweet potatoes, carrots, pumpkins, squash, spinach, mangoes, turnip greens, boiled carrots, raw kale, dandelion greens, dried apricots.
Vitamin B_1 (thiamin)	Ages 0–6 months: 0.2 mg Ages 7–12 months: 0.3 mg Ages 1–3 years: 0.5 mg	n/a	Helps convert food into energy. Needed for healthy skin, hair, muscles, and brain. Good for nervous system, digestion, muscles, heart, alcohol-damaged nerve tissues.	Pork chops, ham, soy milk, watermelons, acorn squash, liver, yeast, egg yolk, cereal, red meat, nuts, wheat germ, black beans.
Vitamin B_2 (riboflavin)	Ages 0–6 months: 0.3 mg Ages 7–12 months: 0.4 mg Ages 1–3 years: 0.5 mg	n/a	Helps convert food into energy. Needed for healthy skin, hair, blood, and brain. Good for the breakdown of protein, fat, and carbohydrates.	Milk, yogurt, cheese, whole and enriched grains and cereals, liver, yeast, green leafy vegetables, fish, mushrooms, almonds, quinoa.
Vitamin B_3 (niacin)	Ages 0–6 months: 2 mg Ages 7–12 months: 4 mg Ages 1–3 years: 6 mg	Ages 0–12 months: n/a Ages 1–3 years: 10 mg	Helps convert food into energy. Essential for healthy skin, blood cells, brain, and nervous system.	Meat, poultry, fish, fortified and whole grains, mushrooms, potatoes, peanut butter, passion fruit, avocado.
Vitamin B_5 (pantothenic acid)	Ages 0–6 months: 1.7 mg Ages 7–12 months: 1.8 mg Ages 1–3 years: 2 mg	n/a	Helps convert food into energy. Helps make lipids (fats), neurotransmitters, steroid hormones, and hemoglobin.	Chicken, whole grains, broccoli, mushrooms, avocados, tomato products, sunflower seeds, corn, broccoli.

Nutrient Name	RDA/DRI	Tolerable Upper Limit	Benefits	Good Sources
Vitamin B$_6$	Ages 0–6 months: 0.1 mg Ages 7–12 months: 0.3 mg Ages 1–3 years: 0.5 mg	Ages 0–12 months: n/a Ages 1–3 years: 30 mg	Helps convert tryptophan to niacin and serotonin, a neurotransmitter that plays key roles in sleep, appetite, and moods. Helps make red blood cells. Influences cognitive abilities and immune function.	Meat, fish, poultry, legumes, tofu and other soy products, potatoes, noncitrus fruits (banana, watermelon), whole grains, dried beans.
Vitamin B$_{12}$	Ages 0–6 months: 0.4 μg Ages 7–12 months: 0.5 μg Ages 1–3 years: 0.9 μg	n/a	Assists in making new cells and breaking down some fatty acids and amino acids. Protects nerve cells and encourages their normal growth. Helps make red blood cells.	Meat, poultry, fish, milk, cheese, eggs, fortified cereals, fortified soy milk, shellfish, beans, mushrooms.
Vitamin C	Ages 0–6 months: 40 mg Ages 7–12 months: 50 mg Ages 1–3 years: 15 mg	Ages 0–12 months: n/a Ages 1–3 years: 300 mg	Helps make collagen. Helps make the neurotransmitters serotonin and norepinephrine. Acts as an antioxidant, neutralizing unstable molecules that can damage cells.	Fruits and fruit juices (especially citrus), potatoes, broccoli, bell peppers, spinach, strawberries, tomatoes, brussels sprouts, berries, potatoes, green leafy vegetables, raw acerola, rosehips.
Vitamin D	Ages 0–12 months: 10 μg Ages 1–13 years: 15 μg	Ages 0–6 months: 25 μg Ages 7–12 months: 38 μg Ages 1–3 years: 63 μg	Helps maintain normal blood levels of calcium and phosphorus, which strengthen bones. Helps form teeth and bones.	Fortified milk or margarine, fortified cereals, fatty fish, sunlight, cod liver oil, sardines, herring, salmon, tuna, mushrooms, tofu.
Vitamin E	Ages 0–6 months: 4 mg Ages 7–12 months: 5 mg Ages 1–3 years: 6 mg	Ages 0–12 months: n/a Ages 1–3 years: 300 mg	Acts as an antioxidant, neutralizing unstable molecules that can damage cells. Protects vitamin A and certain lipids from damage. Diets rich in vitamin E may help prevent Alzheimer disease. Supplements may protect against prostate cancer.	Vegetable oils, salad dressings and margarines made with vegetable oils, wheat germ, leafy green vegetables, whole grains, nuts, soya beans, sprouts, eggs.

(continues)

TABLE 9-3 Vitamin and Mineral Recommendations for Infants and Children, with Good Source Examples *(continued)*

Nutrient Name	RDA/DRI	Tolerable Upper Limit	Benefits	Good Sources
Vitamin K	Ages 0–6 months: 2.0 µg Ages 7–12 months: 2.5 µg Ages 1–3 years: 30 µg	n/a	Activates proteins and calcium essential to blood clotting. May help prevent hip fractures.	Cabbage, liver, eggs, milk, romaine lettuce, collard greens, spinach, broccoli, sprouts, kale, brussels sprouts, scallions, prunes.
Zinc	Ages 0–6 months: 2 mg Ages 7–12 months: 3 mg Ages 1–3 years: 3 mg	Ages 0–6 months: 4 mg Ages 7–12 months: 5 mg Ages 1–3 years: 7 mg	Helps form many enzymes and proteins and creates new cells. Frees vitamin A from storage in the liver. Needed for immune system, taste, smell, and wound healing.	Nuts, cashews, seeds, beans and legumes, eggs, red meat, poultry, oysters, fortified cereals, brown rice, whole grains, dark chocolate, sesame seeds, garlic, wheat germ.

Note: RDA is recommended daily allowance; DRI is dietary reference intake.

VI. Food Allergies and Intolerances

A. Managing food allergies in the breastfeeding dyad requires an interdisciplinary team, including a pediatric healthcare provider, a registered dietitian, and, in some cases, a pediatric gastroenterologist and a pediatric allergist.
  1. Both the lactating parent and the infant should be referred to a registered dietitian to ensure that their nutrient needs are met throughout the period of food exclusion due to allergy or intolerance.
  2. Infants should be monitored closely to ensure that proper growth and development are maintained.
B. Maternal elimination diets are often necessary when a breastfeeding infant has a food allergy or intolerance.
  1. To properly assess which foods are potential allergens or sensitivities for the infant, parents should begin by eliminating only one food item at a time rather than multiple food items at once.
  2. The process of food elimination to identify potential allergens while breastfeeding should occur under the supervision of a dietitian.
  3. Protein-based allergies are the most prevalent; therefore, elimination diets should focus on the elimination of the top eight protein-based allergens: cow's milk, soy, egg, tree nuts, peanuts, wheat, gluten, and fish.
  4. Casein, a cow's milk protein, typically takes the longest to eliminate from the body and is therefore recommended to be eliminated first.
C. Introducing foods that contain gluten (wheat, barley, and rye) in the first 3 months of life significantly increases the risk of developing celiac disease in children who have the genetic marker for the disease.[48] Individuals who carry the genetic marker for celiac disease are likely to carry the genetic marker for Type I diabetes. However, the presence of this genetic marker does not mean the infant will develop either disease.
D. A cow's milk protein allergy (CMPA) can have an adverse effect on an infant's overall health, immune function, and growth.
  1. Up to 15 percent of infants show adverse effects when exposed to casein (a protein that is present in cow's milk).
    a. The symptoms of CMPA include urticaria, angioedema, vomiting or an acute flare of atopic dermatitis, frequent regurgitation, diarrhea or constipation, blood in the stool, iron deficiency anemia, runny nose or chronic coughing (unrelated to an acute infection), wheezing, food refusal, and colic.

    b. An adverse reaction to casein, a cow's milk protein, can occur within 45 minutes of exposure. However, in more than 40 percent of cases it can take up to 24 hours to fully manifest, typically as gastrointestinal symptoms.

    c. There is no reliable test for delayed allergic manifestations of CMPA; therefore, complete elimination of cow's milk protein from the diet is the current recommendation for the identification and treatment of delayed-onset CMPA.

2. There appears to be a genetic component to CMPA. Infants with parents who have or had CMPA, or whose siblings have CMPA, are more likely to be affected.

3. Exclusive breastfeeding reduces the severity of symptoms related to CMPA. Switching a breastfed infant to a hypoallergenic formula is not recommended as the first-line treatment for CMPA. Instead, elimination of all cow's milk and casein-based products from the diet of the lactating parent is the principal treatment for CMPA in exclusively breastfed infants.[49]

4. Reactions to other foods, especially egg and soy, but also wheat, fish, peanut, and other foods, depending on the regional dietary intake, may occur in combination with CMPA. Therefore, when introducing complementary foods, these foods should be introduced in a stepwise manner, one at a time, to assess the infant's symptoms after consuming foods with potential cross reactions.[50]

5. CMPA persists in 50 percent of affected infants through their first year of life, while up to 20 percent of affected infants will have sustained CMPA throughout early childhood.[51] Therefore, the introduction of foods based on cow's milk should proceed with caution in this population. Nonmammalian milks and high-calcium plant-based foods are the most desirable options for infants and children younger than 5 years who have CMPA.

VII. Feeding in Special Populations

A. The WHO recommends that low birth weight and very low birth weight infants are fed human milk.

    1. Human milk from the infant's parent is preferred; however, if the parent's own milk is not available, donor milk is the next best option.

    2. If the parent's milk or donor milk is not available, low birth weight infants should be fed standard infant formula, and very low birth weight infants should be fed preterm infant formula (increased kcal/oz formula) if they do not gain adequate weight while consuming standard infant formula.[5]

    3. Very low birth weight infants should be given human milk fortifiers based on human milk, not bovine milk.

B. Infant colic presents as a predictable period of uncontrolled crying that can last up to 3 hours per day, at least 3 days per week, and persist in this pattern for at least 3 weeks.

    1. Infant colic appears to spontaneously dissipate at 3–4 months of life. There is some debate as to whether infant colic is truly a stand-alone diagnosis or a symptom of gastrointestinal or neurological distress (i.e., headaches or migraines) in the colicky infant.[52-54]

    2. Approximately 25 percent of infants diagnosed with colic have cow's milk dependent colic.[55] Elimination of casein-based foods from the lactating parent's diet has been shown to have a positive effect on the symptoms associated with colic.

    3. Switching the lactating parent to a low-allergen diet has been shown to improve colic symptoms in infants younger than 6 weeks.[56,57] However, food elimination diets by lactating parents should be initiated under the care of a registered dietitian, and one food at a time should be eliminated, beginning with the complete elimination of cow's milk, and products based on cow's milk, to determine which allergenic food is impacting colic symptoms in the infant.[56]

    4. *Lactobacillus reuteri* has been shown to reduce the symptoms of colic in breastfed infants younger than 3 months by increasing gastrointestinal motility and function.[55] However, the current data on *L. reuteri* is not consistent, and not all colic symptoms will resolve for all infants.[58,59]

C. Vegetarian and vegan diets are healthy and appropriate for all life cycle stages, including infancy (for infants older than 6 months) and childhood.[60,61]

    1. Children who consume vegan diets should receive guidance from healthcare providers and registered dietitians regarding necessary supplementation to meet micro- and macronutrient dietary requirements to support healthy growth and development.[62]

2. As with all diets for infants and children, special care should be taken to ensure that each meal provides a plant-based source of protein, a grain or starchy vegetable, and a fruit or vegetable, with appropriate snacks between meals.
    a. In vegetarian children, protein sources should be varied; eggs and foods based on cow's milk should not be the principal source of protein in a vegetarian infant or child's diet.
    b. The protein sources should be varied and include legumes (beans, peas, and lentils), nuts, and seeds, in addition to nonhuman milk and eggs.
3. Vegan lactating parents should regularly take vitamin B_{12} supplements and have their B_{12} status checked yearly to ensure that their milk has adequate levels of B_{12} for the breastfed infant.
    a. Vegan infants and children older than 12 months should be supplemented based on their recommended daily needs (see Table 9-3).
    b. Most vitamin B_{12} supplements are available in megadoses; therefore, daily supplementation is not recommended.
4. Due to the difference in bioavailability of heme versus nonheme iron and a higher intake of fiber in the diet, vegan and vegetarian children have a slightly higher recommendation for iron, requiring 1.8 times more iron than the current recommended daily intakes.[61] Even with their increased need for iron, vegan and vegetarian children do not have an increased risk of iron deficient anemia when compared to the general population.[63,64]
5. The calcium levels in human milk are not affected by the parental diet; therefore, a breastfeeding infant's calcium needs can be met with human milk alone.
    a. For the breastfed toddler, complementary foods that are rich in calcium should be included daily in meals.
    b. Vegan infants older than 12 months can consume a moderate amount of calcium-fortified nondairy milks throughout the day, not exceeding 16 oz (480 mL).
6. Vegan diets tend to be more deficient in omega-3 fatty acids and higher in omega-6 fatty acids.
    a. Supplementation with algae-based docosahexaenoic acid (DHA) via drops or sprays is recommended for vegan infants older than 12 months.
    b. The consumption of plant-based foods that are high in omega-3 fatty acids is also recommended; such foods include hemp seeds and oil, flax seeds and oil, chia seeds and oil, walnuts, soy products, and canola oil.
    c. It is recommended that 1 percent of the daily caloric intake come from omega-3 essential fatty acids for vegans and vegetarians.[61]

▶ Key Points from This Chapter

A. For optimal growth and health, infants should consume only human milk without the introduction of any other foods until at least 6 months of age.
B. Complementary foods should be introduced starting at 6 months of age.
C. Pediatric malnourishment can occur in both underweight and overweight infants and children.

🔍 CASE STUDY

Casey is a healthy, developmentally normal 4-month-old infant whose weight percentile has followed a steady 25th to 30th percentile range on the WHO growth charts since day 7 of life. Casey has always been tall for her age with a height percentile range of 87th to 90th since birth. Casey has been exclusively breastfed since birth without the use of bottles until she recently started daycare 4 weeks ago. Casey's daycare has noted that she is "long and thin" and the daycare providers have suggested Casey should be started on solid foods in the form of pureed fruits, carrots, and sweet potato to help Casey gain weight. Jessica, Casey's mother, has never had a reason to be concerned about Casey's weight or height as she is developmentally normal, has maintained a healthy growth rate since day 7 of life, and consistently nurses between 8 and 10 times within a 24-hour period. However, the daycare's suggestion has Jessica worried that she may be depriving her child of nutrients by not adding solid foods at 4 months of age. Jessica is anxious about which steps to take next.

🔍 CASE STUDY (continued)

Questions

1. What information can you provide to Jessica about the recommendations for introduction of solid foods to infants?
2. How will you counsel Jessica about the daycare's recommendation to add pureed fruits or root vegetables to Casey's diet to provide adequate nutrition and increase Casey's growth?
3. What resources will you provide to help ease Jessica's anxiety about Casey's weight? Which provider on Jessica's care team would be best suited to address specific concerns about infant weight gain and why?

References

1. World Health Organization, UNICEF. *Global Strategy for Infant and Young Child Feeding.* Geneva, Switzerland: World Health Organization; 2003.
2. Iacovou M, Sevilla A. Infant feeding: the effects of scheduled vs. on-demand feeding on mothers' wellbeing and children's cognitive development. *Eur J Public Health.* 2012;23(1):13-19.
3. Eshel N, Daelmans B, Mello MC, Martines J. Responsive parenting: interventions and outcomes. *Bull World Health Organ.* 2006;84(12):991-998.
4. Cavell B. Gastric emptying in infants fed human milk or infant formula. *Acta Paediatr.* 1981;70(5):639-641.
5. Williams HG. And not a drop to drink—why water is harmful for newborns. *Breastfeed Rev.* 2006;14(2):5-9.
6. World Health Organization. *The Optimal Duration of Exclusive Breastfeeding.* Geneva, Switzerland: World Health Organization; 2001.
7. Coulthard H, Harris G, Emmett P. Delayed introduction of lumpy foods to children during the complementary feeding period affects child's food acceptance and feeding at 7 years of age. *Matern Child Nutr.* 2009;5(1):75-85.
8. Northstone K, Emmett P, Nethersole F. The effect of age of introduction to lumpy solids on foods eaten and reported feeding difficulties at 6 and 15 months. *J Hum Nutr Diet.* 2001;14(1):43-54.
9. Dewey K. *Guiding Principles for Complementary Feeding of the Breastfed Child.* Washington, DC: Pan American Health Organization; 2003.
10. World Health Organization. *Essential Nutrition Actions: Improving Maternal, Newborn, Infant and Young Child Health and Nutrition.* Geneva, Switzerland: World Health Organization; 2013.
11. Alder EM, Williams FL, Anderson AS, Forsyth S, Florey CdV, Van der Velde P. What influences the timing of the introduction of solid food to infants? *Br J Nutr.* 2004;92(3):527-531.
12. Scott JA, Binns CW, Graham KI, Oddy WH. Predictors of the early introduction of solid foods in infants: results of a cohort study. *BMC Pediatr.* 2009;9(1):60.
13. Baughcum AE, Burklow KA, Deeks CM, Powers SW, Whitaker RC. Maternal feeding practices and childhood obesity: a focus group study of low-income mothers. *Arch Pediatr Adoles Med.* 1998;152(10):1010-1014.
14. Ziegler EE. Consumption of cow's milk as a cause of iron deficiency in infants and toddlers. *Nutr Rev.* 2011;69(s1):S37-S42.
15. Paoletti G, Bogen DL, Ritchey AK. Severe iron-deficiency anemia still an issue in toddlers. *Clin Pediatr.* 2014;53(14):1352-1358.
16. Elalfy MS, Hamdy AM, Abdel Maksoud SS, Abdel Megeed RI. Pattern of milk feeding and family size as risk factors for iron deficiency anemia among poor Egyptian infants 6 to 24 months old. *Nutr Res.* 2012;32(2):93-99.
17. Scott JA, Chih TY, Oddy WH. Food variety at 2 years of age is related to duration of breastfeeding. *Nutrients.* 2012;4(10):1464-1474.
18. Chaffee BW, Feldens CA, Vítolo MR. Association of long-duration breastfeeding and dental caries estimated with marginal structural models. *Ann Epidemiol.* 2014;24(6):448-454.
19. Tanaka K, Miyake Y. Association between breastfeeding and dental caries in Japanese children. *J Epidemiol.* 2012;22(1):72-77.
20. Tham R, Bowatte G, Dharmage S, et al. Breastfeeding and the risk of dental caries: a systematic review and meta-analysis. *Acta Paediatr.* 2015;104(S467):62-84.
21. Iida H, Auinger P, Billings RJ, Weitzman M. Association between infant breastfeeding and early childhood caries in the United States. *Pediatrics.* 2007;120(4):e944-e952.
22. Feldens CA, Giugliani ERJ, Duncan BB, Drachler MdL, Vítolo MR. Long-term effectiveness of a nutritional program in reducing early childhood caries: a randomized trial. *Community Dent Oral Epidemiol.* 2010;38(4):324-332.
23. Mohebbi S, Virtanen J, Vahid-Golpayegani M, Vehkalahti M. Feeding habits as determinants of early childhood caries in a population where prolonged breastfeeding is the norm. *Community Dent Oral Epidemiol.* 2008;36(4):363-369.
24. Milgrom P, Ly KA, Tut OK, et al. Xylitol pediatric topical oral syrup to prevent dental caries: a double-blind randomized clinical trial of efficacy. *Arch Pediatr Adolesc Med.* 2009;163(7):601-607.
25. Tang R-S, Huang M-C, Huang S-T. Relationship between dental caries status and anemia in children with severe early childhood caries. *Kaohsiung J Med Sci.* 2013;29(6):330-336.
26. Boyington JA, Johnson AA. Maternal perception of body size as a determinant of infant adiposity in an African-American community. *J Natl Med Assoc.* 2004;96(3):351-362.
27. Baird J, Fisher D, Lucas P, Kleijnen J, Roberts H, Law C. Being big or growing fast: systematic review of size and growth in infancy and later obesity. *BMJ.* 2005;331(7522):929.
28. Ong KK, Loos RJ. Rapid infancy weight gain and subsequent obesity: systematic reviews and hopeful suggestions. *Acta Paediatr.* 2006;95(8):904-908.
29. Huh SY, Rifas-Shiman SL, Taveras EM, Oken E, Gillman MW. Timing of solid food introduction and risk of obesity in preschool-aged children. *Pediatrics.* 2011;127(3):e544-e551.

30. Bischoff SC, Boirie Y, Cederholm T, et al. Towards a multidisciplinary approach to understand and manage obesity and related diseases. *Clin Nutr.* 2017;36(4):917-938.

31. Paul IM, Bartok CJ, Downs DS, Stifter CA, Ventura AK, Birch LL. Opportunities for the primary prevention of obesity during Infancy. *Adv Pediatr.* 2009;56(1):107-133.

32. World Health Organization. *WHO Child Growth Standards: Length/Height for Age, Weight-for-Age, Weight-for-Length, Weight-for-Height and Body Mass Index-for-Age, Methods and Development.* Geneva, Switzerland: World Health Organization; 2006.

33. World Health Organization. *Guideline: Assessing and Managing Children at Primary Health-Care Facilities to Prevent Overweight and Obesity in the Context of the Double Burden of Malnutrition.* Geneva, Switzerland: World Health Organization; 2017.

34. World Health Organization. Child growth standards: chart catalogue. WHO website. http://www.who.int/childgrowth/standards/chart_catalogue/en/. Updated 2018. Accessed February 13, 2018.

35. Shelov SP, Hannemann RE. *Caring for Your Baby and Young Child: Birth to Age 5. The Complete and Authoritative Guide.* 6th ed. New York: Bantam Books; 2014.

36. Bruss MB, Morris J, Dannison L. Prevention of childhood obesity: sociocultural and familial factors. *J Am Diet Assoc.* 2003;103(8):1042-1045.

37. Allen LH. B vitamins in breast milk: relative importance of maternal status and intake, and effects on infant status and function. *Adv Nutr.* 2012;3(3):362-369.

38. Stevens GA, Bennett JE, Hennocq Q, et al. Trends and mortality effects of vitamin A deficiency in children in 138 low-income and middle-income countries between 1991 and 2013: a pooled analysis of population-based surveys. *Lancet Glob Health.* 2015;3(9):e528-e536.

39. World Health Organization. *Guideline: Vitamin A Supplementation in Infants and Children 6-59 Months of Age.* Geneva, Switzerland: World Health Organization; 2011.

40. Mulligan ML, Felton SK, Riek AE, Bernal-Mizrachi C. Implications of vitamin D deficiency in pregnancy and lactation. *Am J Obstet Gynecol.* 2010;202(5):429.e421-429.e429.

41. Munns CF, Shaw N, Kiely M, et al. Global consensus recommendations on prevention and management of nutritional rickets. *Horm Res Paediatr.* 2016;85(2):83-106.

42. Wagner CL, Hulsey TC, Fanning D, Ebeling M, Hollis BW. High-dose vitamin D3 supplementation in a cohort of breastfeeding mothers and their infants: a 6-month follow-up pilot study. *Breastfeed Med.* 2006;1(2):59-70.

43. Hollis BW, Wagner CL, Howard CR, et al. Maternal versus infant vitamin D supplementation during lactation: a randomized controlled trial. *Pediatrics.* 2015;136(4):625-634.

44. Lönnerdal B. Excess iron intake as a factor in growth, infections, and development of infants and young children. *Am J Clin Nutr.* 2017;106(suppl):1681S-1687S.

45. World Health Organization, UNICEF. *Clinical Management of Acute Diarrhea.* Geneva, Switzerland: World Health Organization; 2004.

46. De Benoist B, Andersson M, Egli IM, El Bahi T, Allen H. *Iodine Status Worldwide: WHO Global Database on Iodine Deficiency.* Geneva, Switzerland: World Health Organization; 2004.

47. Henjum S, Lilleengen AM, Aakre I, et al. Suboptimal iodine concentration in breastmilk and inadequate iodine intake among lactating women in Norway. *Nutrients.* 2017;9(7):643.

48. Norris JM, Barriga K, Hoffenberg EJ, et al. Risk of celiac disease autoimmunity and timing of gluten introduction in the diet of infants at increased risk of disease. *JAMA.* 2005;293(19):2343-2351.

49. Vandenplas Y, Brueton M, Dupont C, et al. Guidelines for the diagnosis and management of cow's milk protein allergy in infants. *Arch Dis Child.* 2007;92(10):902-908.

50. Wood RA. The natural history of food allergy. *Pediatrics.* 2003;111(6 pt 3):1631-1637.

51. Caffarelli C, Baldi F, Bendandi B, Calzone L, Marani M, Pasquinelli P. Cow's milk protein allergy in children: a practical guide. *Ital J Pediatr.* 2010;36(1):5.

52. Gelfand AA, Thomas KC, Goadsby PJ. Before the headache: infant colic as an early life expression of migraine. *Neurology.* 2012;79(13):1392-1396.

53. Gelfand AA, Goadsby PJ, Allen IE. The relationship between migraine and infant colic: a systematic review and meta-analysis. *Cephalalgia.* 2015;35(1):63-72.

54. Shamir R, St James-Roberts I, Di Lorenzo C, et al. Infant crying, colic, and gastrointestinal discomfort in early childhood: a review of the evidence and most plausible mechanisms. *J Pediatr Gastroenterol Nutr.* 2013;57(suppl):S1-S45.

55. Savino F, Tarasco V. New treatments for infant colic. *Curr Opin Pediatr.* 2010;22(6):791-797.

56. Hill DJ, Roy N, Heine RG, et al. Effect of a low-allergen maternal diet on colic among breastfed infants: a randomized, controlled trial. *Pediatrics.* 2005;116(5):e709-e715.

57. Iacovou M, Ralston RA, Muir J, Walker KZ, Truby H. Dietary management of infantile colic: a systematic review. *Matern Child Health J.* 2012;16(6):1319-1331.

58. Sung V, Hiscock H, Tang M, et al. Probiotics to improve outcomes of colic in the community: protocol for the Baby Biotics randomised controlled trial. *BMC Pediatr.* 2012;12(1):135.

59. Sung V, Hiscock H, Tang ML, et al. Treating infant colic with the probiotic *Lactobacillus reuteri*: double blind, placebo controlled randomised trial. *BMJ.* 2014;348:g2107.

60. Position of the American Dietetic Association and Dietitians of Canada: vegetarian diets. *J Am Diet Assoc.* 2009;109(6):1266-1282.

61. Amit M. Vegetarian diets in children and adolescents. *Paediatr Child Health.* 2010;15(5):303-308.

62. Fewtrell M, Bronsky J, Campoy C, et al. Complementary feeding: a position paper by the European Society for Paediatric Gastroenterology, Hepatology, and Nutrition (ESPGHAN) Committee on Nutrition. *J Pediatr Gastroenterol Nutr.* 2017;64(1):119-132.

63. Sanders T, Manning J. The growth and development of vegan children. *J Hum Nutr Diet.* 1992;5(1):11-21.

64. Fulton JR, Hutton CW, Stitt KR. Preschool vegetarian children. Dietary and anthropometric data. *J Am Diet Assoc.* 1980;76(4):360-365.

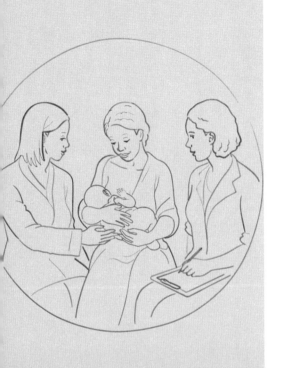

SECTION II

Management

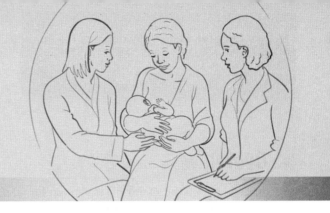

CHAPTER 10

Breastfeeding and the Transition to Parenthood

Jane Grassley

Any use of the term *mother, maternal,* or *breastfeeding* is not meant to exclude transgender or nonbinary parents who may be breastfeeding or providing human milk to their infant.

▶ Overview

Becoming a parent is a major life transition for all members of the family. This developmental transition is characterized by changes and challenges in all aspect of parents' lives. The transition to parenthood is a process that begins with an awareness of the changes that a new or additional child brings into parents' lives.[1] Parents engage in this process by seeking out information, using role models, actively preparing for the birth, and modifying their lives to accommodate the care of their new baby. Parents need support as they navigate this transition because many enter parenting with little experience of newborns, and they live away from their extended families. Because breastfeeding takes place within the social context of a family and community, lactation professionals may be a major source of support during the early stage of the transition to parenthood.

I. Transition to Parenthood

A. Becoming a parent is a major life transition for both men and women.
   1. With the birth of their first child, parents can experience changes in all aspects of their lives, such as their relationship with one another (e.g., a decrease in relational satisfaction and quality) and with their families of origin, their sexuality, and their self-esteem.[2]
   2. Becoming a parent can initially contribute to decreases in the new parents' self-esteem and sense of mastery in this new role.[3]
   3. The transition to parenthood often brings feelings of work–family conflict, which encompass how parents balance their work and household responsibilities.[2,4]
   4. Parents can experience intense emotional and physical changes during pregnancy and their child's first year of life.[2]
   5. Parents may be unprepared and ill equipped to navigate these changes in their relationships and sense of self, and they may be ill equipped to manage the practical aspects of newborn care.[5]
   6. Breastfeeding takes place in the context of this transition to parenthood.
B. The transition to parenthood occurs in stages.
   1. There are four stages identified for becoming a mother:[6]
      a. Commitment and preparation (pregnancy)
      b. Acquaintance, practice, and physical restoration (first 2 weeks)
      c. Approaching normalization (2 weeks to 4 months)
      d. Integration of maternal identity (4 months)
   2. Parental role acquisition progresses in similar stages:[7]
      a. Anticipatory: During pregnancy, parents learn about their new parental role by reading, talking with their own parents, asking questions of other family members and parents, and attending classes.
      b. Formal: After the birth, parents want to master practical childcare skills but may lack self-confidence and become easily overwhelmed and confused by conflicting information. They can develop confidence in their ability to meet their baby's basic needs when provided with concrete demonstrations and suggestions, as well as acknowledgment that they are the experts on their own baby.
      c. Informal: Parents begin interacting with their peers and others in informal interactions as they begin to relax the more rigid rules and directions used to acquire caretaking behaviors.
      d. Personal: Parents modify their practices and evolve their own unique parenting styles.
C. Social support can help parents navigate the upheaval of becoming a new parent.[5]
   1. House defined four categories of social support behaviors: informational, instrumental, emotional, and esteem.[8]
   2. Informational support behaviors include offering information, suggestions, directives, or advice.
      a. When possible, partners should be included in prenatal education that prepares parents for breastfeeding, the realities of parenthood, and changes in their relationships.[5]

      b.   Information about the importance of exclusive breastfeeding obtained during pregnancy encourages exclusive breastfeeding after birth.[9]

      c.   Parents want realistic, accurate, and sufficiently detailed information.[10]

      d.   Information support is not enough. It must be combined with instrumental or practical support.[11]

  3.   Instrumental support behaviors include practical and tangible assistance that can include offering time, modifying the environment, or helping with physical tasks.

      a.   A positive beginning to breastfeeding is essential during the postpartum period because parents' individual experiences influence the information they gather when deciding to initiate and continue breastfeeding.[10]

      b.   Postnatal parental education and environmental lactation support can promote a longer duration of exclusive breastfeeding.[9]

  4.   Emotional support behaviors convey empathy, trust, and concern.

      a.   Breastfeeding parents appreciate informational and instrumental support that is offered with empathy, trust, and concern.[11]

      b.   Adolescents need emotional, informational, and instrumental social support from nurses, their mothers, and the fathers of their babies to successfully breastfeed.[12] "The style and manner in which information, help, and support were offered was central to women's perceptions of support."[10(p53)] This approach was identified as a facilitative style, which included "realistic information, accurate and sufficiently detailed information, encouragement for breastfeeding, encouraging dialogue, and offering practical help."[10(p54)]

  5.   Esteem support behaviors encompass offering encouragement through affirmation and feedback.

      a.   Breastfeeding self-efficacy or confidence is a significant factor in the decision to initiate and continue breastfeeding, particularly for adolescents.[13]

      b.   Breastfeeding confidence is central to a parent's experiences of breastfeeding, not just when initiating or establishing breastfeeding.

      c.   Breastfeeding confidence is enhanced when expectations are congruent with actual experiences, when there is a synchronous relationship with the infant, and when at least one consistent person values the parent's decision to breastfeed.[14]

      d.   Experiences that tend to diminish confidence include the following:[14]

          i.   Feeling unprepared for the work of breastfeeding

          ii.   Difficulties initiating breastfeeding in the early postpartum period

          iii.   An infant who cries inconsolably

          iv.   Unexpected infant breastfeeding patterns

          v.   Perceived inability to produce enough milk during growth spurts or after returning to work

          vi.   Unsupportive comments from family, friends, and healthcare professionals

          vii.   Feeling overwhelmed by too many differing opinions

      e.   Hearing verbal praise from others is crucial to adolescent parents' decision to continue breastfeeding.[12]

      f.   Using a facilitative style that combines consistent information and practical help with offering encouragement through dialogue about breastfeeding is an effective way to build breastfeeding confidence.[10]

  D.   Many individuals enter parenthood with little exposure to newborns, and they experience a steep learning curve as they develop a loving, reciprocal relationship with their infant.

II. Parent–Infant Attachment

  A.   A loving relationship between parent and infant is foundational to an individual's lifetime social functioning, emotional well-being, and future intimacy.[15]

    1.   Helping parents fall in love with their infants is a major responsibility of healthcare professionals who work with new families. A healthy parent–infant attachment is essential to an individual's ability to form healthy relationships as an adult. A positive beginning to breastfeeding can be a pathway to attachment, particularly between breastfeeding parents and their babies.

2. "The infant and young child should experience a warm, intimate, and continuous relationship with his mother (or permanent mother substitute) in which both find satisfaction and enjoyment."[16(p13)]
   a. A secure attachment helps the infant develop a sense of security.
   b. The first 6 months of life are considered a sensitive period when the infant develops a trusting relationship with the caregiver.
3. There are three general patterns of infant-to-parent attachment: avoidant, ambivalent, and secure.[17]
   a. Avoidant infants show little distress during separation, treat a stranger the same way as the parent, and avoid proximity or interaction with the parent during a reunion after separation.
   b. Ambivalent infants resist contact with a stranger and might be angry or resistant to the parent upon reunion following a separation; after contact with the parent is initiated, the infant seeks to maintain it.
   c. Securely attached infants seek proximity and contact with the parent (especially during reunions) and also explore the environment.
B. Parent–infant attachment is a commitment by the parents to love and care for their infant.
   1. Parent–infant attachment is characterized by proximity, reciprocity, and commitment.[18]
   2. Because attachment is an interactional process, parents need proximity to their infant, which is defined as physical and emotional closeness to the infant.
      a. Parents become acquainted with their infants and enhance bonding and attachment by being near them and avoiding unnecessary separations.
      b. The sensitive period following birth is important in establishing attachment. Although humans are capable of adaptation and growth in this area, the concept might be of special importance to parents who are at risk of developing maladaptive parent–child relationships.[19]
      c. Attachment behaviors are enhanced by avoiding epidurals and other birth interventions and keeping the dyad together in a rooming-in environment.
      d. Skin-to-skin contact promotes proximity through the sensory experience of touching, holding, and gazing at the newborn.
      e. Proximity encompasses parents' feelings of emotional closeness to the infant.
      f. Parents' ability to differentiate their needs from their infant's needs and to respond appropriately is another aspect of proximity.
   3. Newborns have the capacity to engage in social exchange, defined as reciprocity.[15]
      a. The parent's role is one of sensitivity and responsiveness to the infant's cues.
      b. Proximity promotes the parent's ability to observe the infant and respond appropriately to the infant's cues in a timely manner.
      c. The infant is an active partner in this interaction. The infant's behavioral cues reinforce the parent's caregiving efforts; for example, parents with infants who are difficult to console or whose needs are difficult to meet might struggle with feeling competent.
      d. Parents who are sensitive and responsive to the infant's needs during the early months and who promptly meet the infant's needs foster the development of secure attachment relationships.
   4. Commitment refers to the centrality of the infant to the parents' lives and family as they assume responsibility for the well-being and safety of their new child.[18] As parents explore their new role, they begin to integrate a new identity as a parent and reorganize their lives around becoming a parent.
   5. The parent–infant attachment process begins during pregnancy.[18]
   6. Attachment with the nonbreastfeeding parent is enhanced by being actively involved in the pregnancy and birth and having extended contact with the infant during the newborn period.[20]
      a. Partners have unique ways of interacting with their infants, frequently called engrossment, in the early period.
      b. Partners often feel as though they lost a mate because the breastfeeding parent seems immersed in the care of the baby.
   7. Rigid baby training programs that prescribe scheduled feedings, limited contact, and specified sleep periods can interfere with parent–infant attachment. Babies who are left to "cry it out" might sleep through the night sooner, but the development of trust can be hampered and breastfeeding can fail.[21]
   8. The environmental context in which early parent–infant interactions take place needs to be nurturing and supportive.

III. A Nurturing and Supportive Environment

A. Uncertainty in the transition to parenthood can be eased when new parents are surrounded by a nurturing and supportive environment. Healthcare professionals and others in the parents' social network nurture the new parents so they have the energy to nurture their new baby.

B. Creating a nurturing and supportive environment in which parents and their infants can thrive while breastfeeding involves understanding the complex social domains that influence decisions to initiate and continue breastfeeding.

1. The social ecological model identifies the domains that influence parents' decisions about infant feeding (e.g., individual, interpersonal, community, organizational, and public policy).[22]

2. The return to work provides a useful example of the complex dynamics involved in breastfeeding decisions.

a. Returning to work after the birth of a child has been identified as a common barrier in a parent's ability to meet the breastfeeding goals set by the American Academy of Pediatrics and Healthy People 2020. (See Chapter 11, *Breastfeeding and Employment*.)

b. Factors that influence the decision to return to work need to be addressed to create a supportive environment in which optimal breastfeeding can occur. The factors include the following:

i. Personal or financial reasons for returning to work (individual)

ii. Partner's earnings and the availability of family or friends to provide childcare (interpersonal)

iii. The cost and quality of both childcare and breast pumps that can be purchased or rented (community)

iv. The adequacy of health insurance coverage for breast pumps, and if the employer provides time and a place to express milk (organizational)

v. The lack of sufficient paid maternity leave or a living wage in the United States (policy)[22]

C. The transition to parenthood can be eased if parents are able to develop a supportive network that includes their partner, parents, and friends, as well as their own and their infants' doctors, lactation professionals (if available), and other breastfeeding parents online or in community support groups.

1. Parents need their infants' grandmothers to value their breastfeeding decisions rather than undermine their confidence. Parents can expend an enormous amount of energy defending and protecting breastfeeding when faced with a grandmother who may lack current knowledge about the best practices for successful breastfeeding.[23]

a. Grandmothers who did not breastfeed may not understand the expected sleep and feeding patterns of infants who breastfeed. They may perceive offering to feed their newborn grandbaby formula as helpful rather than as undermining breastfeeding and self-confidence.[23]

b. Grandmothers may view breastfeeding as a barrier to their ability to bond and care for their new grandbabies.[23]

c. The sexualized breast can be a barrier to breastfeeding, particularly in extended family environments. Some grandmothers may view breastfeeding as nasty or gross.[23]

d. Grandmothers want to be helpful and need education about how to be supportive of breastfeeding. The Grandmothers Tea Project (http://www.illinoisbreastfeeding.org/21401/21464 .html) is an online resource for educating this population.[23,24]

2. Partners are an important and often unacknowledged source of breastfeeding support.[25,26]

a. Partners often feel helpless offering support when they were excluded from prenatal breastfeeding education or postpartum care.[25,26]

b. Partners want breastfeeding information that is tailored to them and guidance for providing practical support to the breastfeeding parent.[25,26]

c. Co-mothers in lesbian relationships have different needs and different roles, compared to fathers, in offering breastfeeding support.[27]

i. The partner who did not give birth needs to be acknowledged as the co-mother and included in providing breastfeeding support.[27]

ii. Lactation professionals need to develop support strategies for helping partners, regardless of gender identity and sexual orientation.

3. Breastfeeding support from physicians, midwives, or other healthcare professionals is associated with increased breastfeeding initiation and duration. The support and advice received from providers influence breastfeeding self-efficacy.[28,29]
    a. Unfortunately, "many healthcare providers won't actively promote breastfeeding for fear of creating guilt. Even when pressed by parents, some providers will offer no preference or, worse still, tell parents that breastmilk and formula are basically equivalent, so they should choose whichever one they want."[30(p346)]
    b. The American Congress of Obstetricians and Gynecologists recommends that, during pregnancy, healthcare professionals provide families with relevant, noncommercial, accurate information so they can make informed decisions about infant feeding.[31]
    c. Nurses play a vital role in parents' early experiences with breastfeeding because most early breastfeeding experiences take place in a hospital under the supervision of nurses. Whether parents and their newborns experience a positive beginning is influenced by nurses' supportive and unsupportive behaviors.[14]
4. Lactation professionals play an essential professional role in providing breastfeeding support.
5. Support groups and individual peer counselors are traditional, global, valuable resources that improve breastfeeding rates.
    a. In the United States, peer counselors who work for the federally funded Special Supplemental Nutrition Program for Women, Infants, and Children (WIC) are a primary source of ongoing breastfeeding follow-up in many communities.[32] The Canadian Prenatal Nutrition Program (CPNP) provides similar services.[33]
    b. In the United Kingdom, a targeted peer support service increases mothers' breastfeeding confidence and influences exclusive breastfeeding rates.[34]
    c. Trained and skilled community mother support groups in India significantly improved help-seeking behaviors and infant breastfeeding rates within the community's district.[35]
6. Parents increasingly turn to online resources for breastfeeding information and support.
    a. A survey of 8,144 childbearing women found that most had access to the internet, often used it for communication, and were interested in receiving health information online.[36]
    b. Online resources—such as Facebook, text messaging, online groups like Circle of Mothers, and mobile apps—increase access to breastfeeding support.[37,38]
    c. The use of mobile devices to deliver breastfeeding education modules is effective in increasing parents' knowledge of breastfeeding and improving their feelings of support.[39]

IV. Factors That Influence the Transition to Parenthood

A. Young children experience a major transition when a new sibling is born.
    1. Children respond differently, depending on their age and developmental stage.[40]
        a. Toddlers will sense, but not understand, their parents' excitement over the coming birth of a sibling.
        b. Preschoolers may have the most difficulty adjusting to the birth of a sibling. They may feel threatened by the impending family changes and experience developmental regression.
        c. School-age children are not as threatened, but they may resent the attention given to the new baby.
    2. Each child needs time and understanding to prepare for and adjust to the arrival of a new sibling. Planning time each day when the parents' total attention is devoted to the older sibling helps the adjustment.
    3. Parents will benefit from learning strategies to help ease the siblings' transition to a new baby:[40]
        a. Reading books about babies can be helpful for both toddlers and preschoolers.
        b. Preschoolers need time to adjust to major changes in the daily routine.
        c. Prepare preschoolers for their mothers' trip to the hospital.
        d. Involve siblings in preparing for the baby.
        e. Ask family members and friends to include small gifts for siblings.
        f. Accommodate younger siblings by reading books or playing simple games with them while breastfeeding the new baby.

4. Some parents tandem breastfeed their newborn and toddler.
   a. The new baby needs to take precedence over the toddler, with access to both breasts, before the toddler nurses.
   b. If an older sibling is being weaned, do so in a gradual manner by substituting activities for breastfeedings, and feed the new baby when the older child is either not present or occupied with other things.
   c. Reserving time each day for the older sibling to breastfeed can provide special time together.
   d. Children who have previously been weaned may show a temporary interest in breastfeeding when they see the new baby at the breast. They may simply be curious about the taste of the milk, so expressing some into a cup may satisfy this curiosity.

B. Parents may be unprepared for changes in their sexual relationships.
   1. Many physicians recommend waiting to resume sexual relations until after the 6-week checkup; however, not all couples will need to wait.
   2. Having a baby interferes with freedom and sexual spontaneity, and some partners may resent the attention the baby receives.
   3. Some parents might feel tired, "touched out," or too overwhelmed to concentrate on sexual needs. Breastfeeding the baby immediately before bedtime and taking advantage of moments alone during naptime can provide the parents with an opportunity for intimacy.
   4. Breastfeeding affects how a parent physically responds to sexual intimacy.
      a. Vaginal dryness caused by hormonal changes may cause some physical discomfort when first resuming sexual intercourse. An artificial lubricant can relieve the discomfort.
      b. The breasts may be either very sensitive to touch or not sensitive.
      c. Adjustments in positioning can help alleviate physical discomfort caused by a painful incision or full breasts. Kegel exercises help with general toning and facilitate entrance in intercourse.
      d. Oxytocin released during orgasm may cause the breasts to leak. Feeding the baby or expressing milk beforehand reduces leakage during lovemaking.
      e. Experiencing increased sensuality when breastfeeding is a result of oxytocin release and is a normal response for many parents.

C. Contraception methods, as they relate to lactation, are presented in the recommendations of the Academy of Breastfeeding Medicine and in other professional resources.[41-43]
   1. The lactational amenorrhea method offers pregnancy protection during the first 6 months postpartum. Only 1.5 percent of unintended pregnancies occur when all three prerequisites of the lactational amenorrhea method are present:[44-47]
      a. The menses have not yet returned (amenorrhea).
      b. The baby is breastfed around the clock and receives no other foods or pacifiers (minimum of 8 to 12 breastfeedings per 24 hours, and no more than 6 hours between feedings, even at night).
      c. The baby is younger than 6 months.
   2. The Academy of Breastfeeding Medicine makes the following recommendations regarding postpartum contraception and breastfeeding:[41]
      a. Progestin-only oral contraceptives do not appear to interfere with milk production and are therefore acceptable during lactation.
      b. A transdermal skin patch that releases progestin and estrogen should ideally be avoided during lactation.
      c. The use of an IUD should be delayed until after breastfeeding is established.
      d. The use of medroxyprogesterone should be delayed for 6 weeks until lactation is well established.
      e. Generally, oral contraceptives that contain both estrogen and progesterone should be avoided while breastfeeding.

D. Women are particularly vulnerable to intimate partner violence during the perinatal period (e.g., 1 year before conception), with an estimated global prevalence between 4 and 9 percent.[48]
   1. Abused women often exhibit health-related behaviors such as missing prenatal appointments, delaying prenatal care until the third trimester, experiencing poor nutrition or insufficient weight gain, smoking, or using drugs. These behaviors are all associated with adverse infant birth outcomes like low birth weight, preterm birth, and small for gestational age.[49,50]

2. Recent research has identified that stress experienced during pregnancy may alter a woman's hypothalamic–pituitary–adrenal axis, resulting in higher levels of corticotrophin-releasing hormone, which could initiate labor leading to preterm birth, restrict utero-placental perfusion (low birth weight and small for gestational age), and delay lactogenesis II (insufficient milk production).[48,49]

3. Healthcare professionals should assess patients for intimate partner violence throughout the perinatal period because it can occur throughout the perinatal period.[48]

4. Past childhood sexual abuse can also affect women's health during pregnancy and in the postpartum period.[50]

    a. Research demonstrates that women who are survivors of childhood sexual abuse initiate and continue breastfeeding at rates similar to those with no history of childhood sexual abuse (after adjusting for socioeconomic factors).[50,51]

    b. Some survivors may find that putting their infant to their breast is too traumatic because it reminds them of the abuse. They may choose to pump and feed their milk through a bottle.[52]

    c. Researchers estimate that 50 percent or more of adolescent mothers experienced childhood sexual abuse. Healthcare professionals need to be sensitive to their potential for distress about breastfeeding and support their infant feeding decisions with balanced information and ongoing support.[53]

    d. Childhood sexual abuse and intimate partner violence place women at increased risk for depression and PTSD.[50] (See Chapter 18, *Maternal Mental Health and Breastfeeding*.)

E. Maternal age, both younger and older, influences the transition to parenting and the need for support.

    1. Being a parent as an adolescent is a major risk factor for low breastfeeding rates.[54]

        a. Adolescents are particularly vulnerable to early introduction of formula supplements and decreased breastfeeding duration.[55-57]

        b. Positive breastfeeding experiences in the early postpartum period can influence adolescents' decisions about continuing to breastfeed.[57]

        c. Lactation professionals who care for adolescents and their infants can influence breastfeeding rates through social support. However, professionals cannot rely on their knowledge of adults when supporting adolescents because they have needs that are unique to their development.[11,58,59]

        d. Adolescents progress through three psychosocial developmental stages:[60]

            i. Early adolescents (ages 12–14) are egocentric, concrete thinkers who fear rejection and are self-conscious.

            ii. Middle adolescents (ages 15–17) seek independence and support from their peer group as they begin to form operational thought, struggle with a sense of identity, and feel awkward or strange about themselves and their bodies.

            iii. Late adolescents (ages 18–20) are at ease with themselves, can think abstractly, and can make decisions and plans about their lives.

        e. Providing social support that builds adolescents' breastfeeding confidence can influence their decisions to continue breastfeeding.[61]

            i. Adolescents need a synergistic combination of emotional, esteem, instrumental, informational, and network support.[11]

            ii. Adolescents appreciate and value lactation professionals who take time to talk with them about breastfeeding and help them effectively position and latch their infants.[11]

            iii. Breastfeeding support for adolescents is relational and facilitative. How healthcare providers offer support appears to be as important as the information or hands-on help they provide.[11]

            iv. Support strategies designed to build breastfeeding confidence include providing individualized, intentional, accurate breastfeeding education in all settings; using relational dialogue to communicate with adolescents; engaging their support network for breastfeeding education; and examining professional attitudes about adolescents and breastfeeding.[11]

    2. Delayed childbearing has increased in high-income countries with a parallel increase in the use of assisted reproductive technology to conceive and concerns about medical risks to children.[62,63]

        a. This population experiences a higher rate of scheduled cesarean births related to the rate of multiple gestations.[62]

b.   Even with a clear intent to breastfeed, the use of assisted reproductive technology and cesarean birth increase the likelihood of introducing infant formula before discharge from the hospital and early weaning in the first 4 months postpartum.[62]

c.   Lactation professionals play an important role in providing early and ongoing support.[62]

▶ Key Points from This Chapter

A.   New parents can experience changes in all aspects of their lives, such as their relationship with one another and with their families of origin, sexuality, and self-esteem.

B.   Parents may be unprepared and ill-equipped to navigate changes in their relationships and sense of self, and to manage the practical aspects of newborn care.

C.   Social support can help parents navigate the upheaval of becoming a new parent.

D.   Use of a facilitative style that combines consistent information, practical help, and encouragement is an effective way to build breastfeeding confidence.

E.   A loving relationship between parent and infant is foundational to an individual's lifetime social functioning, emotional well-being, and future intimacy.

F.   Healthcare professionals, peer counselors, and others in parents' social networks nurture new parents so they have the energy to nurture their new baby.

G.   Women are particularly vulnerable to intimate partner violence during the perinatal period.

H.   Breastfeeding support for adolescents is relational and facilitative.

🔍 CASE STUDY

Melanie describes her early breastfeeding experiences:

We were breastfeeding in the hospital, my baby was rooming in . . . and every day he just kept losing weight. He wasn't latching well; he would latch sometimes and not latch other times. Then he lost down to 10 percent of his birth weight. I didn't get any sleep at night because he would fuss, wanting to breatfeed. He would try to latch, and then he'd get off and try to get back on; it was constant.

When we left the hospital I was still trying and I was confused about when I was supposed to be feeding him. He was always crying, and part of the time I think he was starving. It got really confusing and upsetting and it was not a good experience for me. I went to the pediatrician with him every other day, and they would weigh him. I remember thinking, "Don't go to the restroom so you gain weight." I just really wanted them to think I was a good mother and could take care of my baby. It was becoming the focus of our lives. I would think, "He's not thriving . . . you don't have enough milk . . . it's not working . . . he's not thriving. I must not be a good mother."

I think one of the hardest parts about breastfeeding is that you don't have quantitative numbers to be able to prove that you're taking good care of your child. I never really had signs that I had an abundance of milk. I had a friend who said, "Your milk looks really blue, that must mean there is no fat, I'm a cream factory." My mother-in-law saw him and said, "Oh, he's so skinny, is he getting enough to eat? When I was breastfeeding, I was always leaking, and you don't ever leak? Your milk doesn't have enough fat. Let me give him a bottle."

I got really radical; I tried everything. I had heard that if you take fenugreek and blessed thistle that would increase your supply. I would feed him and then I would bottle supplement him and then I would pump. It was awful because it was a constant thing. I would pump until I was sore because I kept thinking, if I would do it right . . . This whole process of breastfeeding, feeding bottle, pumping . . . so it finally got to where I would pump and feed him the expressed milk first and then I would give him the formula. I labored at it for months because I wanted it to work. It became the focus of my whole life, trying to get this milk to produce. I remember thinking, "I want to be able to do this . . . I want to be able to do this . . . everyone says I'm supposed to do this."

Questions

1. What kinds of social support (e.g., House's theory) do Melanie and her family need to breastfeed effectively?
2. What kinds of support did Melanie receive, and from whom? Was it helpful?
3. Define some strategies that healthcare providers and family members could use to nurture and support Melanie's family. What do they need to breastfeed successfully?
4. How are breastfeeding challenges affecting Melanie's ability to attach with her baby?

References

1. Meleis AI, Sawyer LM, Im EO, Hilfinger Messias DK, Schumacher K. Experiencing transitions: an emerging middle-range theory. *ANS Adv Nurs Sci.* 2000;23(1):12-28.
2. Klobučar NR. The role of spirituality in transition to parenthood: qualitative research using transformative learning theory. *J Relig Health.* 2016;55(4):1345-1358.
3. Chen EY, Enright RD, Tung EY. The influence of family unions and parenthood transitions on self-development. *J Fam Psychol.* 2016;30(3):341-352.
4. Kaufman G, Bernhardt E. Gender, work and childbearing: couple analysis of work adjustments after the transition to parenthood. *Community Work Fam.* 2015;18(1):1-18.
5. Deave T, Johnson D, Ingram J. Transition to parenthood: the needs of parents in pregnancy and early parenthood. *BMC Pregnancy Childbirth.* 2008;8:30.
6. Mercer R. Becoming a mother vs maternal role attainment. *J Nurs Scholarsh.* 2004;36(3):226-232.
7. Bocar DL, Moore K. Acquiring the parental role: a theoretical perspective. In: Auerbach, K ed., *Lactation Consultant Series.* Franklin Park, IL: La Leche League International; 1987.
8. House JS. *Work, Stress and Social Support.* Reading, MA: Addison-Wesley; 1981.
9. Nnebe-Agumadu UH, Racine EF, Laditka SB, Coffman MJ. Associations between perceived value of exclusive breastfeeding among pregnant women in the United States and exclusive breastfeeding to three and six months postpartum: a prospective study. *Int Breastfeed J.* 2016;11:8.
10. Schmied V, Beake S, Sheehan A, McCourt C, Dykes F. Women's perceptions and experiences of breastfeeding support: a metasynthesis. *Birth.* 2011;38(1):49-60.
11. Grassley JS, Spencer B, Bryson C. The development and psychometric testing of the supportive needs of adolescents breastfeeding scale. *J Adv Nurs.* 2013;69(3):708-716.
12. Dykes F, Moran VH, Burt S, Edwards J. Adolescent mothers and breastfeeding: experiences and support needs—an exploratory study. *J Hum Lactation.* 2003;19(4):391-401.
13. Dennis C-L, Heaman M, Mossman M. Psychometric testing of the breastfeeding self-efficacy scale-short form among adolescents. *J Adolesc Health.* 2011;49:265-271.
14. Grassley J, Nelms TP. Understanding maternal breastfeeding confidence: a Gadamerian hermeneutic analysis of women's stories. *Health Care Women Int.* 2008;29(7):841-862.
15. Feldman R. Oxytocin and social affiliation in humans. *Horm Behav.* 2012;61(3):380-391.
16. Bowlby, J. *Attachment and Loss.* Vol 1. New York, NY: Basic Books; 1969.
17. Ainsworth MDS, Blehar MC, Waters E, Wall S. *Patterns of Attachment—Psychological Study of the Strange Situation.* Hillsdale, NJ: Lawrence Erlbaum; 1978.
18. Goulet C, Bell L, St-Cyr Tribble D, Paul E, Lang A. A concept analysis of parent–infant attachment. *J Adv Nurs.* 1998;28(5):1071-1081.
19. Klaus MH, Kennell JH. *Parent–Infant Bonding.* 2nd ed. St. Louis, MO: Mosby; 1982.
20. Sears W, Gotsch G. *Becoming a Father.* 2nd ed. Schaumburg, IL: La Leche League International; 2003.
21. Aney M. "Baby wise" linked to dehydration, failure to thrive. *AAP News.* 1998;14(4):21.
22. Dunn RL, Kalich KA, Henning MJ, Fedrizzi R. Engaging field-based professionals in a qualitative assessment of barriers and positive contributors to breastfeeding using the social ecological model. *Matern Child Health J.* 2015;19:6-16.
23. Grassley JS, Eschiti V. Grandmother breastfeeding support: what do mothers need and want? *Birth.* 2008;35(4):329-335.
24. Grassley JS, Spencer B, Law B. The grandmothers' tea: evaluating a breastfeeding support intervention. *J Perinat Educ.* 2012;21:80-89.
25. Brown A, Davies R. Fathers' experiences of supporting breastfeeding: challenges for breastfeeding promotion and education. *Matern Child Nutr.* 2014;10(4):510-526.
26. Sherriff N, Hall V. Engaging and supporting fathers to promote breastfeeding: a new role for health visitors? *Scand J Caring Sci.* 2011;25(3):467-475.
27. Spidsberg BD, Sørlie V. An expression of love—midwives' experiences in the encounter with lesbian women and their partners. *J Adv Nurs.* 2012;68(4):796-805.
28. Entwistle F, Kendall S, Mead M. Breastfeeding support—the importance of self-efficacy for low-income women. *Matern Child Nutr.* 2010;6(3):228-242.
29. Jarlenski M, McManus J, Diener-West M, Schwarz EB, Yeung E, Bennett WL. Association between support from a health professional and breastfeeding knowledge and practices among obese women: evidence from the Infant Practices Study II. *Women's Health Issues.* 2014;242(1):641-648.
30. Wolynn T. Breastfeeding—so easy even a doctor can support it. *Breastfeed Med.* 2011;6:345-347.
31. American Congress of Obstetricians and Gynecologists. ACOG clinical guidelines. American Congress of Obstetricians and Gynecologists website. https://www.acog.org/About-ACOG/ACOG-Departments/Breastfeeding/ACOG-Clinical-Guidelines. Accessed September 1, 2016.
32. Campbell LA, Wan J, Speck PM, Hartig MT. Women, infant and children (WIC) peer counselor contact with first time breastfeeding mothers. *Public Health Nurs.* 2014;31:3-9.
33. Public Health Agency of Canada (PHAC). Canada Prenatal Nutrition Program. 2013. https://www.canada.ca/en/public-health/services/health-promotion/childhood-adolescence/programs-initiatives/canada-prenatal-nutrition-program-cpnp.html. Accessed December 19, 2017.
34. Ingram J. A mixed methods evaluation of peer support in Bristol, UK: mothers', midwives' and peer supporters' views and the effects on breastfeeding. *BMC Pregnancy and Childbirth.* 2013;13:192.
35. Kushwaha KP, Sankar J, Sankar MJ, et al. Effect of peer counseling by mother support groups on infant and young child feeding practices: the Lalitpur experience. *PLOS One.* 2014;9(11):e109181.

36. Bensley RJ, Hovis A, Horton KD, Loyo JJ, Bensley KM, Phillips, D. Accessibility and preferred use of online web applications among WIC participants with Internet access. *J Nutr Educ and Behav.* 2014;46,S87-S92.
37. Asiodu IV, Waters CM, Dailey DE, Lee KA, Lyndon A. Breastfeeding and use of social media among first-time African American mothers. *J Obstet Gynecol Neonatal Nurs.* 2015;44(2):268-278.
38. Lewkowitz AK, O'Donnell BE, Nakagawa S, Vargas JE, Zlatnik MG. Social media messaging in pregnancy: comparing content of Text4baby to content of free smart phone applications of pregnancy. *J Matern Fetal Neonatal Med.* 2016;29(5):745-751.
39. Pitts A, Faucher MA, Spencer R. Incorporating breastfeeding education into prenatal care. *Breastfeed Med.* 2015;10:118-123.
40. American Academy of Pediatrics. Preparing your family for a new baby. HealthChildren.org website. https://www.healthychildren.org/English/ages-stages/prenatal/Pages/Preparing-Your-Family-for-a-New-Baby.aspx. Updated May 8, 2014. Accessed September 1, 2016.
41. Berens P, Labbok M, Academy of Breastfeeding Medicine. ABM clinical protocol #13: contraception during breastfeeding, revised 2015. *Breastfeeding Med.* 2015;10(1). http://www.bfmed.org/Media/Files/Protocols/Contraception%20During%20Breastfeeding.pdf. Published 2015. Accessed September 1, 2016.
42. Feldman-Winter L, Berens P. Contraception during breastfeeding—08/27/2015. YouTube website. https://www.youtube.com/watch?v=zad7hGt7xg0&feature=youtu.be. Published September 2, 2015. Accessed September 1, 2016.
43. Office on Women's Health. Birth control methods. Office on Women's Health website. https://www.womenshealth.gov/files/fact-sheet-birth-control-methods.pdf. Updated January 16, 2017. Accessed October 16, 2017.
44. Kennedy KI, Kotelchuck M, Visness CM, Kazi A, Ramos R. Users' understanding of the lactational amenorrhea method and the occurrence of pregnancy. *J Hum Lactation.* 1998;14:209-218.
45. Labbok MH, Hight Laukaran V, Peterson AE, Fletcher V, von Hertzen H, Van Look PF. Multicentre study of the lactational amenorrhea method (LAM). I. Efficacy, duration and implications for clinical application. *Contraception.* 1997;55:327-336.
46. Subhani A, Gill G, Islam A. Duration of lactational amenorrhoea: a hospital based survey in district Abbottabad. *J Ayub Med Coll Abbottabad.* 2008;20(1):122-124.
47. Van der Wijden C, Kleijnen J, Van den Berk T. Lactational amenorrhea for family planning. *Cochrane Database Syst Rev.* 2003;4:CD001329. doi:10.1002/14651858.CD001329.
48. Parys ASV, Verhamme A, Temmerman M, Verstraelen H. Intimate partner violence and pregnancy: a systematic review of interventions. *PLOS One.* 2016;9(1):e85084.
49. Alhusen JL, Ray E, Sharps P, Bullock L. Intimate partner violence during pregnancy: maternal and neonatal outcomes. *J Womens Health (Larchmt).* 2015;24(1):100-106.
50. Kendall-Tackett KA. Violence against women and the perinatal period: the impact of lifetime violence and abuse on pregnancy, postpartum, and breastfeeding. *Trauma Violence Abuse.* 2007;8(3):344-353.
51. Coles J, Anderson A, Loxton D. Breastfeeding duration after childhood sexual abuse: an Australian cohort study. *J Hum Lactation.* 2016;32(3):NP28-35.
52. Klingelhafer SK. Sexual abuse and breastfeeding. *J Hum Lactation.* 2007;23(2):194-197.
53. Bowman KG. When breastfeeding may be a threat to adolescent mothers. *Issues Ment Health Nurs.* 2007;28(1):89-99.
54. Feldman-Winter L, Shaikh U. Optimizing breastfeeding promotion and support in adolescent mothers. *J Hum Lactation.* 2007;23(4):362-367.
55. Grassley JS, Sauls DJ. Evaluation of the supportive needs of adolescents during childbirth intervention. *J Obstet Gynecol Neonatal Nurs.* 2012;41(1):33-44.
56. Misra R, James DCS. Breast-feeding practices among adolescent and adult mothers in the Missouri WIC population. *J Am Diet Assoc.* 2000;100(9):1071-1073.
57. Wambach KA, Aaronson L, Breedlove G, Domian EW, Rojjanasrirat W, Yeh HW. A randomized controlled trial of breastfeeding support and education for adolescent mothers. *West J Nurs Res.* 2011;33(4):486-505.
58. Wambach KA, Cohen SM. Breastfeeding experiences of urban adolescent mothers. *J Ped Nurs.* 2009;24:244-254.
59. Grassley JS. Adolescent mothers' breastfeeding social support needs. *J Obstet Gynecol Neonatal Nurs.* 2010;39(6):713-722.
60. Radzik M, Sherer S, Neinstein LS. Psychosocial development in normal adolescents. In: Neinstein LS, ed. *Adolescent Health Care: A Practical Guide.* 5th ed. Philadelphia, PA: Lippincott, Williams, & Wilkins; 2008:44-80.
61. Mossman M, Heaman M, Dennis C-L, Morris, M. The influence of adolescent mothers' breastfeeding confidence and attitudes on breastfeeding initiation and duration. *J Hum Lactation.* 2008;24:268-277.
62. Fisher J, Hammarberg K, Wynter K. Assisted conception, maternal age and breastfeeding: an Australian cohort study. *Acta Paediatr.* 2013;102:970-976.
63. Locke A, Budds K. We thought if it's going to take two years then we need to start that now: age, infertility risk and the timing of pregnancy in older first-time mothers. *Health, Risk and Soc.* 2013;15:525-542.

Suggested Reading

At-Risk Mothers

Alhusen JL, Ray E, Sharps P, Bullock L. Intimate partner violence during pregnancy: maternal and neonatal outcomes. *J Womens Health (Larchmt).* 2015;24(1):100-106.
Coles J, Anderson A, Loxton D. Breastfeeding duration after childhood sexual abuse: an Australian cohort study. *J Hum Lactation.* 2016;32(3):NP28-35.
Grassley JS. Adolescent mothers' breastfeeding social support needs. *J Obstet Gynecol Neonatal Nurs.* 2010;39(6):713-722.
Kendall-Tackett KA. Violence against women and the perinatal period: the impact of lifetime violence and abuse on pregnancy, postpartum, and breastfeeding. *Trauma Violence Abuse.* 2007;8(3):344-353.

Mossman M, Heaman M, Dennis C-L, Morris, M. The influence of adolescent mothers' breastfeeding confidence and attitudes on breastfeeding initiation and duration. *J Hum Lactation*. 2008;24:268-277.

Wambach KA, Cohen SM. Breastfeeding experiences of urban adolescent mothers. *J Ped Nurs*. 2009;24:244-254.

Breastfeeding Support

Grassley JS, Eschiti V. Grandmother breastfeeding support: what do mothers need and want? *Birth*. 2008;35(4):329-335.

Jarlenski M, McManus J, Diener-West M, Schwarz EB, Yeung E, Bennett WL. Association between support from a health professional and breastfeeding knowledge and practices among obese women: evidence from the Infant Practices Study II. *Womens Health Issues*. 2014;242(1):641-648.

Schmied V, Beake S, Sheehan A, McCourt C, Dykes F. Women's perceptions and experiences of breastfeeding support: a metasynthesis. *Birth*. 2011;38(1):49-60.

Sherriff N, Hall V. Engaging and supporting fathers to promote breastfeeding: a new role for health visitors? *Scand J Caring Sci*. 2011;25(3):467-475.

Role Transitions

Chen EY, Enright RD, Tung EY. The influence of family unions and parenthood transitions on self-development. *J Fam Psychol*. 2016;30(3):341-352.

Kaufman G, Bernhardt E. Gender, work and childbearing: couple analysis of work adjustments after the transition to parenthood. *Community Work Fam*. 2015;18(1):1-18.

Klobučar NR. The role of spirituality in transition to parenthood: qualitative research using transformative learning theory. *J Relig Health*. 2016;55(4):1345-1358.

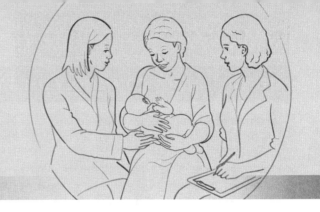

CHAPTER 11

Breastfeeding and Employment

Cathy Carothers

DEFINITIONS OF COMMONLY USED TERMS

Business Case for Breastfeeding A U.S. program designed to educate employers about the value of supporting breastfeeding employees in the workplace.
exclusive breastfeeding Receiving only human milk and no solid foods, water, or other liquids.
full-time employment Working a minimum number of hours (usually 35–45), usually with benefits not offered to part-time, temporary, or flexible workers (e.g., sick leave, health insurance, and flexible scheduling).
International Labour Organisation (ILO) A United Nations agency dealing with international labor standards, social protection, and work opportunities for all.

(continues)

DEFINITIONS OF COMMONLY USED TERMS
(continued)

lactation support program The accommodations available in the workplace that assist the new mother's transition back to work; may include physical space, resources, breaks, and breastfeeding support and may be part of employee benefits.

maternity leave A period of absence from work for an expectant or new mother, which may last from several days, weeks, or months; may be paid or unpaid depending on policies. See also paternity leave.

occupational hazards A hazard encountered in the workplace that may include chemical, biological, psychosocial, and physical hazards and is a risk accepted as a consequence of an occupation.

part-time employment Working less than what is considered full time, usually fewer than 35 hours a week and often without the benefits offered to full-time workers.

paternity leave A period of absence from work taken by a parent; length of time and monetary reimbursement dependent on location and job.

workforce Individuals in a country, area, or business who are engaged in paid employment or who are actively seeking paid employment.

working poor Individuals whose incomes fall below the poverty level.

workplace environment The place of employment, including physical geographical location as well as immediate surroundings and psychosocial feelings of safety and respect.

Any use of the term *mother*, *maternal*, or *breastfeeding* is not meant to exclude transgender or nonbinary parents who may be breastfeeding or providing human milk to their infant.

▶ Overview

Worldwide, women represent approximately 50 percent of the global labor force, including approximately 60 percent of women of childbearing age,[1] but *every* mother is a working mother. When a baby is born, the baby's care and feeding are added to an existing workload, which may already include unpaid work for the family, home, or community; income-generating employment; unpaid work in a family business; or subsistence farming. In fact, even when employed in a paid work capacity, women still carry out the larger share of unpaid household and care work, resulting in longer workdays of both paid and unpaid work.[1] Women in developing countries spend even more hours in unpaid work than women in developed countries: an average of 3 hours more per day than men.[2]

Paying jobs may be in the formal economy—working either for the government (public sector) or in business (private sector)—or in the informal economy (such as handcrafts, street vending, domestic service, small family enterprises, and many kinds of small-scale self-employment). It has been estimated that 25 percent of the world's workforce is in the informal economy, which in some nations employs more than 80 percent of workers.[3] Many of these workers who are mothers lack the safety net that is provided by labor laws and the solidarity that comes with organization by trade unions. They are among the most vulnerable and lowest-paid workers.[2] Studies also show that women are overrepresented in the lowest-paid occupations of clerical, service, and sales industries,[1] domestic work, and hourly wage jobs, which are often characterized by low pay, long hours, and lack of social protection.[2]

Much paid and unpaid work competes with breastfeeding for the employee's time and energy. Lactation consultants help clients assess these competing demands and suggest ways either to modify work demands to free up resources for breastfeeding or to modify breastfeeding to fit in with work. Lactation consultants also educate the community and advocate for policies that protect and support breastfeeding in the context of work.

Work often requires separation of a breastfeeding parent and baby, with all the challenges that separation poses. A wide range of proven strategies can help maintain the breastfeeding relationship, including (1) do the work and simultaneously care for the baby (multitasking); (2) arrange alternate childcare at or near the workplace, taking breaks from work to feed the baby; and (3) arrange alternate childcare during work, express milk at the workplace to store for later feedings, with the caregiver feeding expressed milk to the baby. Following the latter strategy with a baby who receives complementary foods or infant formula for some of the missed feedings may produce less pressure to sustain full lactation. Some babies adapt to separation by reverse cycle feeding—that is, sleeping more when the parent is away and breastfeeding more when the parent is present. Some parents, however, use artificial baby milk when they are away from their baby and breastfeed only when they are home with their baby. This can compromise milk production.

The lactation consultant assists employed mothers to reach their goals for breastfeeding through anticipatory guidance, helping them plan a course of action to support working and parenting goals. This counseling occurs during the prenatal period and continues in the early postpartum days and after resuming work. To assist parents effectively, the lactation consultant must understand the physiology of lactation to help establish and maintain adequate milk production. The lactation consultant must also be familiar with methods of milk expression, including hand expression and the use of breast pumps. Effective guidance also requires the ability to counsel on the use of alternate feeding devices, safe storage and handling of expressed human milk, and coping methods for dealing with the challenges of working and breastfeeding. The lactation consultant must be able to address employer barriers to providing work site lactation support and assist employees in navigating workplace barriers to meet their breastfeeding goals. In addition, the lactation consultant should understand the key components of job protection, nondiscrimination, lactation breaks, and paid leave.

I. Competing Demands

A. Childbearing and child rearing take place within the context of a mother's life. The amount of time and energy they can devote to these activities varies with age, socioeconomic and health status, and the multiple roles that the family and community expect them to fill, in addition to their goals as workers and parents.

B. The demands of nonparenting work can be significant, including work weeks of 80 to 100 hours for a Western physician in training as a house officer or medical resident and the 5 hours per day that a woman in an African village may spend gathering firewood and carrying water.

C. Breastfeeding lends itself to multitasking. Parents commonly combine breastfeeding with other activities, such as eating, resting, sleeping, doing household chores, using the computer and telephone, and minding older children.

D. Breastfeeding is an economic activity that provides food, health protection, and care for infants and young children. Other economic opportunities, such as a chance to work for pay, may raise the relative value of a parent's time and influence the decision to use alternative foods for the baby.[4]

E. Household tasks can be done by other people, leaving time and energy for breastfeeding. U.S. couples in which fathers routinely did a larger share of household tasks had a lower risk of early breastfeeding cessation.[5]

F. Support for breastfeeding can come from a variety of sources. A male-focused breastfeeding promotion program raised rates of breastfeeding by the partners of male employees in one U.S. corporate lactation program.[6]

G. Community support for breastfeeding varies among cultures. In many cultures, there is a traditional lying-in period, typically about 40 days of rest after birth, in which other individuals assume the new mother's normal workload.[7] The period of compulsory postpartum maternity leave in some European countries is a modern version of this practice.

H. Community programs, such as the Baby-Friendly Community Initiative in The Gambia, can build general and specific community support for mothers of young children, including a redistribution of their workload.[8]

I. Anticipatory guidance for those planning to breastfeed should include an assessment of their expected workload of family care, household tasks, and community volunteer work as well as any plans for paid employment.

II. Impact of Employment on Breastfeeding Initiation, Exclusivity, and Duration

A. Women have a higher share in the number of working poor (those whose incomes fall below the poverty level) in the world. As of 2013, nearly 50 percent of the world's working women were in vulnerable employment, often unprotected by labor legislation. The numbers are highest in east Asia (50.3 percent),

Southeast Asia and the Pacific (63.1 percent), South Asia (80.9 percent), North Africa (54.7 percent), the Middle East (33.2 percent), and sub-Saharan Africa (85.5 percent). These women are typically employed in jobs characterized by low wages, little or no job security, and fewer human rights or autonomy over their work life. These women are also more vulnerable in the face of natural disasters.[9]

B. Paid maternity leave options have a positive impact on mental health and well-being,[10] as well as breast-feeding duration rates. An international review of paid maternity leave studies found that more than half of countries around the world offer at least 14 weeks of paid maternity leave.[2] The numbers have grown, with 53 percent of 173 countries offering at least 14 weeks of maternity leave in 2015, compared to 38 percent in 1994. The numbers are higher in developed countries (90 percent), though the United States remains one of the world's nations without any paid maternity leave protection.

C. In the United States, employees return to work exceptionally soon after childbirth. For example, 33 percent are back at work within 3 months of birth, whereas only 5 percent of those in Sweden, Germany, and the United Kingdom take such a short leave.[11] Additionally, 66 percent of U.S. mothers are back on the job by 6 months after birth.[12] African Americans in the United States return to work, on average, 2 weeks earlier than those from other racial and ethnic groups.[13] An earlier return to work has been associated with a shorter duration of breastfeeding.[14]

D. Disparities contribute to issues of health equity. For example, African Americans in the United States are more likely to work in jobs with less flexible hours and social support, and they are disproportionately represented in low-income, nonmanagerial positions with high workplace stress.[15] Those with a bachelor's degree are far more likely to be employed in a job that provides paid leave—66 percent versus 19 percent of women without a high school education.[12] Those working in management and professional occupations are also more likely to initiate breastfeeding.[16]

E. A return to work affects the likelihood of breastfeeding initiation.
   1. Some studies show that intention to work can affect breastfeeding initiation. Mothers planning to work part time have been found to be more likely to initiate breastfeeding than those planning to work full time.[14,17-19]
   2. The Millennium Cohort Study conducted in Britain and Ireland found that women who returned to work within 6 weeks after delivery are less likely to initiate breastfeeding.[17] Conversely, women who have 7 or more weeks maternity leave have greater odds of initiating breastfeeding.[14] The highest breastfeeding initiation rates among working women in one study were those who delayed their maternity leave by 13 or more weeks, and the lowest rates were among those who took less than 6 weeks of leave.[14]

F. Employment also affects breastfeeding exclusivity.
   1. In a group of Italian mothers, 12 percent cited return to work as a reason to use formula.[20]
   2. Ghanaian women living near a large city considered exclusive breastfeeding to be incompatible with selling goods in a market because they had no suitable place at work to feed their babies.[21]
   3. Full-time employment is associated with lower odds of planning to exclusively breastfeed,[22] and this can, in turn, affect breastfeeding duration. A study in Yolo County, California, found that 38 percent of women working full time were almost exclusively breastfeeding at 6 months, compared to 62 percent of women working part time.[23]
   4. Expected maternity leave is associated with breastfeeding exclusivity. Those who plan to work within 6 weeks of the baby's birth had 0.60 times the odds of planning to exclusively breastfeed, compared to those who planned to delay their return to work by at least 12 weeks.[22] Paid maternity leave policies could have an additional impact on improving breastfeeding rates in African American populations.[24]

G. Employment also affects breastfeeding duration.
   1. The type of occupation affects breastfeeding duration. Mothers in occupations classified as professional, administrative, or managerial are likely to breastfeed longer than those employed in low-wage jobs or jobs requiring lower skills.[25,26] Professional, administrative, and managerial positions tend to provide more flexibility over scheduling and breaks, and they offer employees more autonomy, leading to increased access to privacy and lactation support accommodations.
   2. The number of hours worked affects duration. The more hours worked in a week, the shorter the duration of breastfeeding (see **TABLE 11-1**).[18,27]

TABLE 11-1 Breastfeeding Duration and Hours Worked				
Hours Worked per Week	Not working	20 hours	20–34 hours	35 hours
Average Duration of Breastfeeding	25.1 weeks	24.4 weeks	22.5 weeks	16.5 weeks

3. Compared with mothers who were not employed, returning to work within 12 weeks and working more than 34 hours per week were associated with a significantly shorter duration of breastfeeding.[19]

4. Positive workplace supports, such as providing physical accommodations for milk expression and implementing family-friendly policies, improves duration rates.[28] In a study of a Taiwanese manufacturing plant, having a work site lactation policy; access to a clean, dedicated space for milk expression; and support from supervisors and colleagues for needed breaks contributed to breastfeeding duration rates beyond 6 months.[27]

5. Intentional and actual breastfeeding practices can improve the duration rates of breastfeeding. Breastfeeding exclusively during the first postpartum month, with the intent to breastfeed fully or partially, is more likely to result in breastfeeding longer than 6 months after returning to work.[29]

6. Returning to work within 12 weeks postpartum is related to the greatest decrease in breastfeeding duration.[30-32] A maternity leave of 6 weeks or less is associated with fourfold higher odds of failure to establish breastfeeding and an increased probability of cessation.[30] Those who delay their return to work past 13 weeks tend to breastfeed longer.[14]

H. Other factors can affect breastfeeding outcomes.

1. High-wage and professional job settings may offer better family benefits and more flexibility of work schedules.[16] One study found that nonmanagerial jobs, inflexible job situations, and jobs with high psychosocial stress are most likely to lead to breastfeeding cessation.[30] However, even in professional work environments, such as medical residency programs, a lack of appropriate accommodations, unprotected time for milk expression, and nonsupportive colleagues can affect breastfeeding outcomes.[33]

2. The type of workplace can affect outcomes. Larger employers tend to be more likely to have designated lactation space and offer other amenities, such as access to lactation consultants, education, and resource materials.[34]

3. There is a general association between breastfeeding rates at 6 months and legislation guaranteeing breastfeeding accommodations.[35] Much progress has been made globally, though labor laws vary widely and do not always include all workers. In 2014, 71 percent (or 136) of countries guaranteed employees the right to take breastfeeding breaks during the workday to express milk.

    a. European countries are most likely to have workplace break laws for breastfeeding; countries in east Asia and the Pacific were least likely.[36]

    b. The U.S. Patient Protection and Affordable Care Act (ACA) of 2010 requires employers of nonexempt workers (those who are not exempt from overtime laws) to provide both "reasonable time for an employee to express breast milk for a nursing child for 1 year after the child's birth each time such employee has need to express the milk" and "a place, other than a bathroom, that is shielded from view and free from intrusion from coworkers and the public, which may be used by an employee to express breast milk."[37] In addition, 30 U.S. states and territories also require employers to provide basic accommodations[38]; however, the provisions vary widely in the protections, requirements, and penalties for noncompliance.

    c. Different employment sectors may have different levels of legal protection. Iranian maternity protection laws exceed International Labour Organisation (ILO) standards but apply only to government workers.[39] Malaysian workers in the public sector have 2 months of maternity leave, and those in the private sector get 3 months.[40]

4. Even when a high level of legal protection is provided, sociocultural factors, economic factors, and healthcare practices can adversely affect breastfeeding outcomes. In an Italian study, 95 percent of those who initiated breastfeeding dropped to 35 percent breastfeeding at 6 months (9 percent

exclusive) despite exemplary maternity leave and lactation break laws. Typical barriers include perceived breastmilk insufficiency, returning to work, breast problems, and other factors.[20,41]

5.   Vulnerable population groups and certain minority groups can be less likely to initiate or continue breastfeeding, implicating health equity issues.[42] For example, in the United States, breastfeeding rates tend to be lower among African American, American Indian, and Alaska Native population groups. African Americans have the lowest rates of initiation and duration across all study years, suggesting the need for more targeted support to initiate and continue breastfeeding.[43]

III. Occupational Hazards and the Breastfeeding Employee

A.   The presence of environmental contaminants has exposed human populations to elevated levels of toxins and carcinogens, some of which appear in human milk. This fact argues more for the reduction of such exposure than against breastfeeding. The long-term effects of toxic exposure via human milk are not yet known. Analyses of milk after accidental exposure to PCBs, DDE, and heptachlor have not demonstrated that infants are harmed by breastfeeding, although the level of exposure might be a mitigating factor.[44]

B.   Many employees are told to express milk or feed their baby in a restroom for needed privacy. However, public restrooms are not sanitary because they host diverse microbial communities dominated by human-associated bacteria, including those associated with skin contact such as staphylococcaceae and streptococcaceae.[45] Bacteria may be found in many surface locations, such as the toilet, toilet handle, sink, and other surfaces touched by human skin. In addition, airborne bacteria remains a concern,[46] increasing the probability of contaminating expressed milk.

C.   It is prudent during pregnancy and lactation to avoid exposure to radiation, hazardous chemicals, volatile organics, smoke, and other hazardous materials. If exposed to these substances on the job, employees should voice their concerns to the occupational health authority at the workplace, trade union, or government. Strategies to reduce exposure include the use of protective devices and clothing, reassignment to workplace tasks that avoid toxic exposures, or temporary precautionary leave without loss of pay.

D.   Protective clothing, masks, goggles, and air filters may protect employees who work around toxic materials during pregnancy and lactation. Clothing should be changed and hands washed before handling the baby.

E.   Employees face a dilemma, however, when actions taken to protect their capacity for healthy reproduction limit their choice of jobs or put them at a competitive disadvantage for promotion or better-paying jobs.

F.   Exposure to harmful substances may occur when doing unpaid family care work. For example, smoke from burning solid fuel (e.g., wood, animal dung, crop residues, and charcoal) for cooking and heating kills more than 1.6 million people every year, primarily women and children.[47]

G.   Occupational exposures typically involve trace metals, solvents, and halogenated hydrocarbons.[48]

H.   Welders, painters, artists, ceramic workers, and workers who handle weapons must beware of lead exposure.

I.   Household or agricultural herbicides and pesticides should not be directly handled or inhaled.

J.   Healthcare workers should practice universal precautions, especially given the potential for exposure to HIV and hepatitis B and C.

K.   Accidental exposure to toxins (such as hazardous chemicals or lead) or potential infections (which can include viruses, bacteria, or bodily fluids) should be reported to the employee's healthcare provider. Although milk or blood can be tested, such testing may be expensive, the process may be lengthy, and the results may not be useful in deciding what to do. In most cases, it is advised that breastfeeding continue because the risk of not breastfeeding may be greater than a potential risk of exposure to toxins. Ultimately, employees must weigh the risks and benefits of continued breastfeeding, interrupted breastfeeding, or weaning, in consultation with their physician.

L.   Other occupational hazards can include physical demands, such as long working hours, shift work (especially night shift), and job stress. One study found an association between physical work demands and low birth weight and preterm deliveries.[49]

IV. Supporting Breastfeeding Is a Win–Win–Win for Employers, Employees, and Babies

A. A positive workplace environment benefits employees, infants, and employers.[50,51] For employees, continuing to breastfeed results in the following:
1. Optimal outcomes for the baby's health, growth, and development.[52]
2. Significant reduction in numerous acute infections and chronic diseases in infants.[53]
3. Continued emotional bonding with the baby.[52]
4. Fewer missed days of work because the baby is healthier.[54]
5. Lower healthcare costs.[55]
6. Saving the energy, time, and cost to purchase, store, and prepare infant formula.
7. Benefits of oxytocin released during breastfeeding and milk expression with increased feelings of relaxation and a sense of well-being.
8. Strong sense of reconnection when the mother and child are reunited following separation at work.[56]

B. For employers, support for breastfeeding results in the following:
1. Fewer employee absences to care for a sick baby and shorter absences when employees miss work, compared to employees who do not breastfeed.[54]
2. Lower costs for employers who provide health care[54,55]; an analysis of overall healthcare costs in the United States found that suboptimal breastfeeding is associated with an excess of 3,340 premature maternal and child deaths, with $3.0 billion for total medical costs, $1.3 billion for nonmedical costs, and $14.2 billion for premature death costs.[57]
3. Reduced turnover rates and improved employee loyalty to the company.[25,51,58]
4. Higher job satisfaction.[25]
5. Community recognition as a family-friendly business.

C. For the community, workplace support for breastfeeding results in longer breastfeeding duration, with health and economic benefits.[59-61]

V. Barriers to Sustaining Lactation after Returning to Work

A. Employees experience barriers to combining breastfeeding and work.
1. Real or perceived low milk production.[62-64]
2. Lack of accommodations in the workplace to express milk.[65,66]
3. Time and scheduling issues,[65,67] with resultant diminishing milk production.[68]
4. Fatigue, stress, and exhaustion.[69-71]
5. Feeling overwhelmed with the demands of fulfilling job requirements and meeting the child's needs.[72]
6. Childcare concerns and reliance on family for help with children.[66]
7. Discomfort in discussing breastfeeding needs with a male supervisor[73] and other concerns about support from the employer and colleagues.[66,67,69]
8. Personal concerns, such as medical issues, health complications, and early breastfeeding challenges.[67]

B. Employers experience barriers for providing support to breastfeeding employees.
1. Lack of knowledge about the health benefits of breastfeeding and the differences between human milk and artificial baby milks.[73]
2. Lack of awareness about breastfeeding laws, the numbers of employees breastfeeding, or the ways breastfeeding can decrease employee absenteeism and lower healthcare costs to the company.[73-75]
3. Infrequent requests for breastfeeding accommodations.[73]
4. Belief that breastfeeding employees will be too fatigued and therefore less productive on the job.[73,75]
5. Belief that breastfeeding or milk expression in the workplace will interfere with an employee's productivity.[76]
6. Lack of space to accommodate a lactation room and lack of time for employees to express milk.[73,75]
7. Liability concerns.[73,75]
8. Belief that breastfeeding is a personal decision and not the employer's responsibility.[77]

9. Concerns that other employees will complain or resent covering for a coworker who takes time for lactation breaks.[73,75]
10. Lack of knowledge about how to set up a lactation support program.[75]
11. Prioritizing other employee benefit programs ahead of lactation support.[78]

VI. Components of a Successful Lactation Support Program[79,80]

A. Employees need space to breastfeed or express milk.
   1. A clean, private place to express milk comfortably assists with milk ejection and accommodates milk expression more effectively. The space should be accessible and easy to get to, which is especially important in companies with larger facilities or a campus[65]
   2. Options for private breastfeeding areas include the following:
      a. Converting small unused spaces, such as large closets, offices, or other small rooms.
      b. Renovating a corner of an employee lounge to create a lactation room.
      c. Flexible spaces created by installing walls, partitions, or dividers in corners or areas of rooms.
      d. Creating multiuser stations within a single room divided by partitions or curtains.
      e. Outdoor options, such as portable units or pop-up tents.
      f. Shared space among businesses (e.g., more than one business within a single building could share a milk expression room, or a business with lactation space can share its space with other small businesses nearby).
   3. Requirements for the room include the following: central area that is easy to access, private (preferably with a lock), nearby access to running water, electrical outlet, comfortable chair, table or flat surface, well lit, ventilated, and heated or air conditioned.
   4. Optional features include the following: multiuser breast pump, telephone, parenting literature, soft lighting, storage space, footstool, and breastfeeding artwork.
   5. A high-quality bilateral electric breast pump can facilitate quick milk expression.[65] Options include the following:
      a. Employer provides a hospital-grade multiuser pump and attachment kits.
      b. Employer provides a hospital-grade multiuser pump, and each employee purchases a kit.
      c. Employer provides or subsidizes a portable electric breast pump for each employee.
      d. Employees provide their own equipment.
   6. A secure place to store milk is necessary.[81] Options include the following:
      a. Employer provides a small refrigerator in the milk expression room.
      b. Employee provides an insulated container with cooler packs.
      c. Refrigerators shared with nonlactating coworkers may not be a good option because of risk that someone may tamper with the milk.
B. Employees need time to express milk.[81,82]
   1. Established lunch, morning, and afternoon breaks are usually sufficient for milk expression during a standard 8-hour workday.[83]
   2. Milk expression needs vary according to the baby's age and needs.
      a. An employee with a baby younger than 4 months may need three 20-minute milk expression breaks during a standard 8-hour work period.
      b. An employee with a 6-month-old baby may need to express milk only two times per workday because the baby is likely to be starting on solid foods.
      c. An employee with a baby older than 12 months may need to express milk only once or twice during the workday.
      d. The needs of the infant may fluctuate (e.g., during growth spurts), requiring the employee to breastfeed or express milk more often.
C. Education is critical.
   1. Standard information about the company lactation program is often included as part of new employee orientation or in employee benefits materials, wellness or work–life program initiatives, company newsletters, and posters or flyers posted in the workplace.
   2. Employers should alert their employees about available supports, such as breast pumps through their insurance company and lactation consultant services.[80]

3. Often employees are not aware of existing company policies and available resources.[65,67]
4. Identify pregnant employees and provide information. Options include information packets and lunchtime prenatal classes and support groups led by a lactation consultant.
5. Back-to-work sessions with a lactation consultant can be used to tailor a milk expression schedule to fit the job situation.
6. A resource center with books, videos, and materials should provide information on ways to maintain lactation after returning to work.
7. Promote the program with supervisors and colleagues through flyers, newsletters, email communications, and staff meeting presentations.

D. Support is critical.[61,80,82]
1. Employees are more likely to continue breastfeeding in a wide variety of workplace settings when their employers provide the needed supports. The more supports that are provided, the higher the rates of exclusive breastfeeding.[80]
2. Support from the employer is highly valued among breastfeeding employees. This often begins with a policy at the workplace that addresses the needs of breastfeeding employees and can include such components as providing flexible time and a private space to breastfeed or express milk, providing for consultations with a lactation consultant, and addressing responsibilities of the employee, supervisors, and colleagues. Although not all employers believe a policy is necessary, and it could actually limit flexibility with individuals' needs, others believe a policy may ensure consistent accommodations for employees within companies.[73]
3. Access to other breastfeeding employees enhances confidence and helps parents reach their own goals for breastfeeding.

VII. Counseling Breastfeeding Employees[84,85]

A. Consider the following during the prenatal period:
1. Help employees understand reasons to breastfeed, and continue to breastfeed after returning to work.
2. Provide practical strategies, encouragement, and support for breastfeeding.
3. Help employees understand reasons to express milk while separated from the baby, including the following:
   a. Protecting the baby from illnesses and allergies.
   b. Providing comfort from overfullness for the employee.
   c. Preventing engorgement, mastitis, and leaking.
   d. Maintaining milk production.
   e. Sustaining the breastfeeding relationship.[86]
4. Offer support and solutions to help employees reach their infant feeding goals. For example, some employees choose not to express milk at work or are unable to express because of work site constraints. They need comfort strategies when they are separated from their babies, as well as assistance with appropriate feeding strategies for the infant.
5. Refer the employee to community breastfeeding classes and support groups.
6. Develop a plan for combining employment with breastfeeding. Increasing employees' knowledge about breastfeeding and planning for their return to work helps them continue breastfeeding while employed.[87] Planning should include the following:
   a. Time the return to work with the maximum leave possible. The ILO standard for paid maternity leave is 14 weeks, and 18 weeks is recommended.
   b. Explore work options that enable the employee to spend as much time as possible with the baby. These options can include job sharing,[88] part-time employment,[89] gradual phasing in from part-time to full-time hours, or telecommuting (see **TABLE 11-2**).
7. Prepare employees to speak with their supervisor about lactation break options, including time and flexibility needed, possibilities for access to the baby, and milk expression and milk storage locations.
   a. Many employees mistakenly assume they will be unable to continue breastfeeding when they return to work and therefore do not discuss their needs with their supervisors.[90]

TABLE 11-2 Flexible Work Program Benefits

Benefit	Definition	Advantages for Employees	Advantages for Employers
Earned time	Sick leave, vacation time, and personal days are grouped into one set of paid days off. Workers take these days at their own discretion.	Employees do not have to justify time off to their supervisors. Often earned time accrues over several years, giving employees substantial paid leave after childbirth.	Promotes loyalty because workers feel trusted and valued. Workers are often willing to work extra time when needed because their needs were met.
Part time	Workers work less than 35–40 hours per week. Benefits are usually prorated to the number of hours worked.	Employees have more time at home and often can take advantage of flexible scheduling.	Retains workers with valuable experience and training, which saves time and effort to recruit and train new workers.
Job sharing	Two workers work part time and share the responsibilities and benefits of one job.	Employees have more time at home while keeping the same job.	Retains workers with valuable experience and training, which saves time and effort to recruit and train new workers.
Phase in	Workers gradually increase their hours from part time to full time over several days, weeks, or months.	Employees have a longer return-to-work adjustment period. Both the mother and the baby benefit because more time can be spent with the infant while breastfeeding is being established.	Retains workers with experience, and promotes loyalty and dedication.
Flex time	Workers arrange to work hours that suit their schedule (e.g., 7 am–3 pm, or 10 am–6 pm).	Employees can coordinate their own work hours with those of their partner to reduce childcare costs. They can arrange their hours around the best times of day to be with their baby, and they can arrange faster commutes at low-traffic times.	The workplace is covered for more hours per day. Workers are better able to focus when their schedules suit their needs.
Compressed work week	Workers work more hours on fewer days (e.g., 7 am–7 pm, 3 days per week).	Employees can spend full days at home with their baby.	Workers are better able to focus when their schedules suit their needs. Retains workers with experience and training.
Telecommuting	Workers work all or part of their jobs from home.	Employees can work around their baby's schedule. Less time is spent commuting, and less money is required for work clothing and travel expenses.	Retains workers with experience and training. Saves office and parking space.
On-site or near-site child care	Child care is provided at or near the work site and is often sponsored by the company.	Employees can visit their baby for breastfeeding during the work day. The time spent commuting is with their baby.	Promotes loyalty among workers. Workers are better able to focus when their baby is accessible.

Modified with permission from Bar-Yam N. Workplace lactation support, part 1: a return to work breastfeeding assessment tool. *J Hum Lactation*. 1998;14:249-254.[59] Copyright © 1998 by SAGE Publications, Inc.

b. Interpersonal communication between employees and managers can be challenging due to age, gender, and power dynamics, especially in male-dominated work environments. Facilitating an open conversation between employees and their supervisors can improve at-work support to continue breastfeeding.[91]

c. Begin the conversation during pregnancy to give the supervisor ample time to make adequate preparations.

8. Develop realistic milk expression schedules. Employees with job constraints that do not allow lengthy milk expression sessions can be encouraged to pump for shorter durations to relieve overfullness, then they can take a longer milk expression break during a meal period or down time.

9. Discuss strategies for managing potential schedule variations, such as interruptions or unexpected overtime.

10. Explore options for direct breastfeeding and milk expression during the workday, including bringing the baby to work,[92] having the baby brought to work during breaks, going to the childcare center to feed the baby during breaks, and using breaks to express milk. Employees who breastfeed directly during the workday, with or without additional milk expression breaks, may sustain lactation the longest.[93]

11. Advise employees about the selection of breast pump equipment and milk storage. (See Chapter 31, *Expression and Use of Human Milk*.)

12. Explore childcare options with providers who support employees' decision to breastfeed. Encourage employees to seek childcare providers close to the workplace to facilitate feeding the baby, either during the work period or immediately before and after work. (See Section IX, *Childcare Providers*, later in this chapter.)

13. Offer culturally appropriate resources to help employees learn more and to share with their supervisor. The Office on Women's Health, in the U.S. Department of Health and Human Services, created an online searchable resource called *Supporting Nursing Moms at Work: Employer Solutions*.[94] It helps parents learn positive strategies for lactation support from hundreds of businesses in all major industry sectors. The New York Department of Health also created a resource called *Making It Work Toolkit*.[95]

B. Before the employee returns to work, the lactation consultant can help by sharing information (see **TABLE 11-3**).

1. Establish breastfeeding immediately after birth, during postpartum recovery, and through the early weeks.
   a. Develop an abundant milk supply. The most frequent reason for weaning is a real or perceived insufficient milk supply.[96]
   b. Frequent breastfeeding or removal of milk during lactogenesis II increases the development of prolactin receptors that affect long-term milk production.[97]

2. Address coping strategies, including dealing with fatigue and stress, eating nutritious meals, establishing sound breastfeeding patterns, and having others do household chores to spare the employee's energy.[5]

3. Provide anticipatory guidance to assist in the prevention of engorgement, mastitis, and maintaining milk production when the employee is separated from the baby.

4. Offer realistic expectations for early pumping attempts.
   a. It is normal to not express much milk at first (about 15 mL is common in the first few pumping sessions after 3 to 4 days postpartum).
   b. With practice, the employee will learn to trigger the milk ejection reflex with hand expression, massage, or pumping.
   c. Sessions of 12 to 15 minutes are generally sufficient to obtain milk for practice feeds and to begin storing milk in the freezer.
   d. Label expressed milk with the baby's name and date of expression, and freeze it for later use.

5. Help the employee determine the amount of milk the baby will need while the two are apart.
   a. The amount needed depends on many factors, including whether the employee is exclusively breastfeeding, the baby's age, and the number of hours they are separated.
   b. Typically, as babies grow, they take less milk as they begin to eat solid foods.

TABLE 11-3 Return-to-Work Breastfeeding Assessment Work Sheet

	Notes
Type of Job	
1. What is the employee's job and setting?	
2. Does the employee have a personal office work space?	
3. Does the employee keep a personal calendar or control over personal work time?	
4. Does the job involve travel out of town or away from the workplace?	
5. Are most of the employee's colleagues men or women?[a]	
Space Restrooms are not acceptable for breastfeeding or expressing milk.	
6. Is there a designated private space in the workplace for breastfeeding or milk expression?	
7. Does the space have a sink, a chair, and electrical outlets?	
8. Are electric breast pumps available there?	
9. Where is the space in relation to the work space?	
10. How long does it take to get from the work space to the lactation area?	
11. Where will the employee store expressed milk?	
12. If there is no designated space, where will the employee express milk?	
13. Can the employee use the same space every day?	
Time Milk expression should not come at the expense of the employee's meal period.	
14. How old will the baby be when the employee returns to work?	
15. How often will the employee be expressing milk or breastfeeding when first returning to work?	
16. When will the employee express milk?	
17. Will the employee express milk manually or with a breast pump? If a pump, what type of breast pump will the employee use? Is there a double electric pump available?	
18. How many parts on the breast pump must be cleaned after each use?	

	Notes
19. Can the employee take breaks at the same time every day?	
20. If there is on-site or near-site child care, can the employee go to the baby to breastfeed?	
Support	
21. Who at work knows that the employee plans to breastfeed or express milk at work?	
22. Does the supervisor need to be informed or consulted?	
23. If so, what are the supervisor's feelings about the employee's plan?	
24. Are there other employees at work (at the same workplace, or colleagues at other workplaces) who are breastfeeding or who plan to breastfeed at work?	
25. Are there employees who have breastfed or expressed milk at work in the past?	
26. What does the employee's partner or support network think about the plan to continue breastfeeding after returning to work?	
27. Do childcare providers know how to handle expressed milk?	
28. How do they feel about it?	
29. Will on-site or near-site providers call the employee to breastfeed if the employee requests it?	
Gatekeepers	
30. If there is no lactation support program, who can help the employee find time and space to express milk or breastfeed?	
31. Who is responsible for reserving private spaces such as spare offices or conference rooms?	
32. Who keeps the calendar, answers the phone, and greets visitors?	
Supervisor	
33. Must the supervisor be consulted regarding making time or space available to express milk or breastfeed?	
34. What is the relationship between the employee and the supervisor?	
35. Has the employee addressed this issue with the supervisor?	
36. If so, what was the supervisor's response?	

(continues)

TABLE 11-3 Return-to-Work Breastfeeding Assessment Work Sheet	*(continued)*
	Notes
37. If not, what are the employee's concerns about addressing the issue with the supervisor?	
Breastfeeding-Friendly Practices	
38. Are there any policies in the workplace regarding employees who are breastfeeding?	
39. Are there any return-to-work policies regarding flexibility for employees who are breastfeeding?	
40. Does the employee have access to any of the following programs? Earned time Part time Job sharing Phase in Flex time Compressed work week Telecommuting On-site or near-site child care Other flexible work options	
41. If so, has the employee thought about taking advantage of one or more of them?	
42. What is the procedure for making special work arrangements?	
43. If not, who can help the employee arrange one or more of these programs? Supervisor Human resources officer Benefits officer Employee relations officer Other (specify)	

Note: Space for answers is not displayed to scale.

[a] In some workplaces, men are more understanding and supportive than women, and sometimes the reverse is true, but it is good information to have.

Modified with permission from Bar-Yam N. Workplace lactation support, part 1: a return-to-work breastfeeding assessment tool. *J Hum Lactation*. 1998;14:249-254.[59] Copyright © 1998 by SAGE Publications, Inc.

6. An employee who has access to a freezer can begin expressing milk about 2 to 4 weeks postpartum and store it for use after returning to work. The sooner an employee returns to work, the more frequently milk will need to be expressed when away from the baby.
7. Provide strategies to facilitate milk expression. (See Chapter 31, *Expression and Use of Human Milk*.)
8. Provide general guidelines on safe storage of human milk. (Chapter 31, *Expression and Use of Human Milk*.)
9. Provide strategies for introducing expressed milk to the baby.
   a. Milk can be offered to help the baby become accustomed to being fed by the method that the childcare provider will use.
   b. Small volumes can serve as practice feeds to familiarize the baby with alternative feeding methods.

      c.   Offer expressed milk when the baby is not overly hungry; it is difficult for babies to learn new tasks when they are uncomfortable.

      d.   Supplemental feedings can often be tolerated better by someone other than the mother.

      e.   Waiting too long to introduce a bottle can contribute to bottle refusal.[17]

      f.   Many employees use a cup for feeding expressed milk to baby. Other methods, such as a dropper or a spoon, can be used for younger infants.

  10.   Discuss realistic expectations about the first days back on the job. Suggest that the employee return to work on a part-time basis or on a partial schedule to shorten the first week away from the baby and to phase back to work gradually.

  11.   Identify community resources, such as support groups, to boost the employee's confidence in the ability to combine breastfeeding and employment.

C.   After the employee returns to work, the lactation consultant can provide information about the following:

  1.   Address lactation challenges brought on by separation from the baby (such as engorgement, leaking, and concerns about milk production).

  2.   Adapt strategies for milk expression and storage to fit the unique work and childcare situation.

  3.   Help employees deal with the baby's changing feeding patterns.

      a.   Many babies sleep long hours as a way to cope with separation. This reverse-cycle feeding means the baby wants to be held and nursed a lot when reunited with the parent.

      b.   Breastfeeding times can be viewed as a way to rest and cuddle with the baby after being apart. Support from family members will help decrease competition from other family work, such as demands from an older child.

      c.   When the dyad is separated during the day, night feedings become more important, and the baby may not sleep for long periods.

      d.   Listen and validate employees' feelings about returning to work.

VIII. Assisting Employers with Providing Lactation Support

A.   Frame the topic of lactation support as a business conversation, and make a business case to engage the employer. The Maternal and Child Health Bureau, part of the Health Resources and Services Administration in the U.S. Department of Health and Human Services, published a resource called *The Business Case for Breastfeeding*.[79]

B.   The lactation consultant is a valuable resource for employers, helping them explore solutions for supporting breastfeeding employees. Most employers are not familiar with the needs of breastfeeding employees and often welcome practical solutions.

C.   Provide information and professional materials for employers that explain the business case for breastfeeding and simple steps for establishing a lactation support program. An online searchable resource produced by the Office on Women's Health, called *Supporting Nursing Moms at Work: Employer Solutions*, provides employers with hundreds of industry-specific, practical strategies for integrating lactation support into their work environment.[94]

D.   Provide information about national, regional, provincial, or state laws related to working and breastfeeding.

E.   Offer to serve on a company task force to explore strategies for supporting breastfeeding employees or to provide training for supervisors. The Office on Women's Health has a free downloadable presentation platform that is available from the website of the United States Breastfeeding Committee; it includes hundreds of slides featuring solutions for major industry sectors.[98]

F.   Provide individual technical assistance to employers who want to establish a work site lactation program. In some cases, the lactation consultant might be employed by the company to establish a corporate lactation program or to assist employees.

G.   Provide resources for breastfeeding employees at the work site, and be available for one-on-one assistance to address breastfeeding questions and concerns.

H.   Encourage programs in the community to recognize work sites that provide support to breastfeeding employees.

IX. Childcare Providers

A.   Childcare providers can include family members or friends who provide free or low-cost care for infants, informal in-home childcare programs, and formal childcare centers.

B.   A caregiver who supports breastfeeding can make the difference between sustaining breastfeeding and stopping early. Parents should seek care providers who have a positive attitude and who have prior experience with breastfed babies or are willing to learn.

C.   Clear communication between the parent and the caregiver is crucial. They must exchange information daily about the baby's feedings, output, and general comfort level.

D.   Parents should discuss their preferences for care, such as paced bottle feeding and ample body contact (holding and carrying), with the caregiver.[99]

E.   Infants in formal childcare settings have higher rates of diarrhea and upper respiratory infections; breastfeeding helps lower the rate of these illnesses.[56]

F.   Address the childcare providers' concerns about handling expressed milk.

   1.   Milk is not classified by the U.S. Occupational Safety and Health Administration as requiring universal precautions for handling.[100]

   2.   If caregivers express concerns about handling milk, mothers can prepackage milk for individual feedings using solid, labeled containers.

   3.   Empty, used bottles are put in a bag for the mother to clean so the caregiver never handles the milk, only the bottles.

   4.   When using a formal childcare center, provide information on childcare licensing regulations, legislative requirements, and other policies related to childcare and breastfeeding. For example, the Child and Adult Care Food Program, part of the Food and Nutrition Service in the U.S. Department of Agriculture, published national guidelines allowing childcare centers to receive reimbursement when a child breastfeeds onsite at the childcare center, or when expressed milk is brought from home for the provider to feed the infant.[101]

G.   Provide information about feeding devices and methods.[56] (See Chapter 24, *Breastfeeding Devices and Topical Treatments*.)

X. The Lactation Consultant as Advocate for Working Parents

A.   The lactation consultant is in a pivotal role within the community for encouraging policies and programs to support employees with breastfeeding. A lactation consultant must know the maternity protection laws of the city, state or province, and nation; which workers the laws apply to; how the laws are implemented and monitored; and how individual workers can exercise their rights under the law.

B.   Maternity protection, as defined by the ILO, includes several key concepts:

   1.   Scope: A description of who is covered by the law.

   2.   Leave: Maternity leave, paternity leave, and family and medical leave are defined in terms of who gets it, for how long, whether it is paid, when it can be taken, and whether it is optional or compulsory.

   3.   Benefits: Provisions are discussed regarding medical care for pregnancy, birth, and recovery; income replacement during leave; and who pays for benefits (insurance or social programs, the employer, both, or neither).

   4.   Health protection: Employees are protected from workplace risks during pregnancy and lactation, have the right to return to their job or an equivalent job when the risk period is over, and can take time from work for medical care during pregnancy.

   5.   Job protection and nondiscrimination: Mothers are placed in the same job or an equivalent job when returning after leave and are treated the same on the job as employees without children.

   6.   Nursing breaks: Employees have the right to one or more paid breaks, or a daily reduction of work hours, for breastfeeding or expressing milk during the workday.

   7.   Breastfeeding facilities: A clean, private place at or near the workplace should be provided where an employee can breastfeed or express milk and securely store the milk.

   8.   Day nursery: National law in many countries requires employers to provide a day nursery at or near the workplace if they have more than a certain number of female workers.

C. Laws and programs that affect breastfeeding employees may be implemented by various government agencies, such as those that cover labor, business and industry, employment, poverty alleviation, economic development, gender, or women's affairs.

D. Be aware that legal protection alone does not guarantee optimal infant feeding. For example, Italy's breastfeeding rates are modest despite excellent national maternity protection laws.[40]

E. Advocacy for better laws can be conducted at local, state or provincial, national, regional, and international levels. Be strategic in choosing where to act.

F. Meet with your legislative representatives to discuss breastfeeding policy issues in your area.

G. Join with coalitions that advocate on behalf of workers and families. Educate them about breastfeeding issues while you learn from them about broader work-related issues, such as maternity leave and family leave.

H. Offer community education by speaking at business and service organization meetings, meetings of trade unions that employ many women (such as nurses, domestic workers, hospitality and retail workers, or teachers), or at employer organizations that meet regularly. Set up displays at job fairs or health fairs in the community to provide information about the importance of combining breastfeeding and employment.

I. Provide prenatal education about breastfeeding at lunchtime seminars with pregnant workers at selected work sites. Offer to facilitate a breastfeeding employee support group that meets at work sites in the community during lunch or in the evenings.

J. Begin a coalition, or ask the existing community breastfeeding coalition, to conduct outreach with local work sites. Provide companies with information about supporting breastfeeding and available resources in the community.

K. Alert the media about advancements in breastfeeding support in community work sites. Publicity helps parents view continued breastfeeding as the social norm, provides positive public relations to employers, and encourages other work sites to follow their lead.

▶ Key Points from This Chapter

A. Women work in a variety of paid and unpaid work settings. Although women worldwide comprise about half of the workforce, they are overrepresented in the lowest-paid occupations and in more informal jobs that are characterized by low pay, long hours, and lack of legal or social protection. These disparities contribute to issues of health equity. Parents working in these occupations, those with lower education levels, and those of certain racial and ethnic groups (e.g., African Americans in the United States) are less likely to continue breastfeeding after returning to work.

B. Returning to work has a negative impact on breastfeeding initiation, exclusivity, and duration rates. Full-time employment is more likely to shorten breastfeeding outcomes, and taking a maternity leave of 13 weeks or less is also associated with shorter breastfeeding duration. Alternatively, paid maternity leave has a positive impact on breastfeeding rates. More than half of countries worldwide offer at least 14 weeks of paid maternity leave, and 48 percent of countries now offer paternity leave. The numbers are higher in more developed countries.

C. Occupational hazards can impact an employee's health, including environmental contaminants and toxic elements that might be present. Other occupational concerns relate to physically demanding work (e.g., long hours, standing throughout the work period, and high stress), which can contribute to negative health outcomes. There are additional challenges when integrating breastfeeding with employment, including real or perceived low milk supply, lack of scheduled breaks or accommodations to express milk in the workplace, childcare concerns, and emotional issues such as stress, fatigue, and exhaustion. Employers face barriers to providing support, including lack of knowledge, a belief that breastfeeding will interfere with an employee's productivity, lack of space, concerns about liability, and lack of knowledge about the needs of breastfeeding employees.

D. Successful lactation support in the workplace includes a clean, private space to express milk comfortably, access to a high-quality breast pump, time to express milk, a secure place to store expressed milk, access to support and assistance from lactation professionals, and education about company policies and resources.

E. When advocating for breastfeeding employees, lactation consultants should present the business case for breastfeeding support, offer solutions, and provide information and technical support to assist employers with implementing supportive policies and services. The lactation consultant is in a pivotal role within the community to encourage policies and programs that support breastfeeding employees. Lactation consultants should be aware of maternity protection laws, policies of local businesses, and resources that can be shared with employers and employees.

🔍 CASE STUDY

You are approached by Rachel, a pregnant employee who works at a large factory in your community. Rachel plans to breastfeed. Your country has legislation providing 6 weeks of paid maternity leave and requires businesses to allow breastfeeding employees break time to express milk. Rachel insists that weaning will be necessary after returning to work, and is not comfortable discussing a need for support with her supervisor. Because of the rigid schedule at the factory, Rachel cannot imagine how it would work to be off the line to take the required breaks. Rachel, whose income is essential to a family of five, fears being perceived as a troublemaker and being fired.

Questions
1. What further information do you need to understand Rachel's concerns?
2. What advice can you give to assist Rachel with maintaining milk production after returning to work?
3. In what ways could you best advocate for Rachel's needs to get necessary support?

References

1. International Labour Organization. *Women at Work: Trends 2016.* Geneva, Switzerland: International Labour Office; 2016. http://www.ilo.org/wcmsp5/groups/public/---dgreports/---dcomm/---publ/documents/publication/wcms_457317.pdf. Accessed June 4, 2017.
2. United Nations Department of Economic and Social Affairs. *The World's Women 2015: Trends and Statistics.* New York, NY: United Nations; 2015. https://unstats.un.org/unsd/gender/downloads/worldswomen2015_report.pdf. Accessed June 4, 2017.
3. Maternity Protection Coalition. Maternity protection campaign kit, section 9: how to support women in the informal economy to combine their productive and reproductive roles. World Alliance for Breastfeeding Action website. http://www.waba.org.my/whatwedo/womenandwork/pdf/09.pdf. Published 2008. Accessed June 4, 2017.
4. Smith JP. Lost milk? Counting the economic value of breast milk in gross domestic product. *J Hum Lactation.* 2013;29(4):537-546.
5. Sullivan ML, Leathers SJ, Kelley MA. Family characteristics associated with duration of breastfeeding during early infancy among primiparas. *J Hum Lactation.* 2004;20(2):196-205.
6. Cohen R, Lange L, Slusser W. A description of a male-focused breastfeeding promotion corporate lactation program. *J Hum Lactation.* 2002;18(1):61-65.
7. Dennis CL, Fung K, Grigoriadis S, Robinson GE, Romans S, Ross L. Traditional postpartum practices and rituals: a qualitative systematic review. *Womens Health.* 2007;3(4):487-502.
8. Semega-Janneh IJ. *The Second Abraham Horwitz lecture. Breastfeeding: From Biology to Policy.* 1998. http://www.unscn.org/files/Awards/Horwitz_Lectures/2nd_lecture_Breastfeeding_from_biology_to_policy.pdf. Accessed on October 18, 2017.
9. International Labour Organization. *Global Employment Trends, 2014.* Geneva, Switzerland: ILO; 2014. http://www.ilo.org/global/research/global-reports/global-employment-trends/2014/WCMS_233953/lang--en/index.htm. Accessed June 4, 2017.
10. Aitken Z, Garrett CC, Hewitt B, et al. The maternal health outcomes of paid maternity leave: a systematic review. *Soc Sci Med.* 2015;130:21-41.
11. Berger LM, Hill J, Waldfogel J. Maternity leave, early maternal employment and child health and development in the US. *Econ J.* 2005;115:F29-F47.
12. U.S. Census Bureau. *Maternity Leave and Employment Patterns of First-Time Mothers: 1961-2008.* Current population reports; 2011. https://www.census.gov/prod/2011pubs/p70-128.pdf. Accessed June 4, 2017.
13. Spencer BS, Grassley JS. African American women and breastfeeding: an integrative literature review. *Health Care Women Int.* 2013;34(7):607-625.
14. Ogbuanu C, Glover S, Probst J, et al. The effect of maternity leave length and time of return to work on breastfeeding. *Pediatrics.* 2011;27(6):e1414-e1427.
15. Johnson AM, Kirk R, Muzik M. Overcoming workplace barriers: a focus group study exploring African American mothers' needs for workplace breastfeeding support. *J Hum Lactation.* 2015;31(3):425-433.
16. Ogbuanu C, Glover S, Probst J, et al. Balancing work and family: effect of employment characteristics on breastfeeding. *J Hum Lactation.* 2011;27(3): 225-238.
17. Hawkins SS, Griffiths LJ, Dezateux C, et al. Millennium cohort study child health group. Maternal employment and breast-feeding initiation: findings from the millennium cohort study. *Paediatr Perinat Epid.* 2007;21(3):242-247.
18. Fein SB, Roe B. The effect of work status on initiation and duration of breastfeeding. *Am J Pub Hlth.* 1998;88:1042-1046.
19. Mandal B, Roe B, Fein S. The differential effects of full-time and part-time work status on breastfeeding. *Health Policy,* 2001;97(1):79-86.
20. Romero SQ, Bernal R, Barbiero C, Passamonte R, Cattaneo A. A rapid ethnographic study of breastfeeding in the north and south of Italy. *Int Breastfeed J.* 2006;1:1-14.

21. Otoo G, Lartey A, Perez-Escamilla R. Perceived incentives and barriers to exclusive breastfeeding among periurban Ghanian women. *J Hum Lactation.* 2009;25(1):34-41.
22. Mirkovic KR, Perrine CG, Scanlon KS, Grummer-Strawn LM. In the United States, a mother's plans for infant feeding are associated with her plans for employment. *J Hum Lactation.* 2014;30(3):292-297.
23. Dabritz HA, Hinton BG, Babb J. Evaluation of lactation support in the workplace or school environment on 6-month breastfeeding outcomes in Yolo County, California. *J Hum Lactation.* 2009;25(2):182-193.
24. McCarter-Spaulding D, Lucas J, Gore R. Employment and breastfeeding outcomes in a sample of black women in the United States. *J Natl Black Nurses Assoc.* 2011;22(2):38-45.
25. Murtagh L, Moulton A. Working mothers, breastfeeding, and the law. *Am J Pub Hlth* 2011;101(2):217-223.
26. Hanson M, Hellerstedt WL, Desvarieux M, Duval SJ. Correlates of breast-feeding in a rural population. *Am J Hlth Beh.* 2003;27:432-444.
27. Tsai SY. Impact of a breastfeeding-friendly workplace on an employed mother's intention to continue breastfeeding after returning to work. *Breastfeed Med.* 2013;8(2):210-216.
28. Hirani SA, Karmaliani R. Evidence based workplace interventions to promote breastfeeding practices among Pakistani working mothers. *Women and Birth.* 2013;26(1):10-16.
29. Piper B, Parks PL. Predicting the duration of lactation: evidence from a national survey. *Birth.* 1996;23:7-12.
30. Guendelman S., Kosa, JL, Pearl M., et.al. Judging work and breastfeeding: effects of maternity leave and occupational charateristics. *Pediatrics.* 2009:123(1)e38-e46.
31. Galtry J. The impact on breastfeeding of labour market policy and practice in Ireland, Sweden, and the USA. *Soc Sci Med.* 2003;57:167-177.
32. Taveras E, Capra A, Braveman P, Jensvold NG, Escobar GJ, Lieu TA. Clinician support and psychosocial risk factors associated with breastfeeding discontinuation. *Pediatrics,* 2003;112:108-115.
33. Dixit A, Feldman-Winter L, Szucs KA. Frustrated, depressed, and devastated pediatric trainees: US academic medical centers fail to provide adequate workplace breastfeeding support. *J Hum Lactation.* 2015;31(2):240-248.
34. Lennon T, Willis E. Workplace lactation support in Milwaukee County 5 years after the Affordable Care Act. *J Hum Lactation.* 2017;33(1):214-219.
35. Kogan MD, Singh CK, Dee DI, Belanoff C, Grummer-Strawn LM. Multivariate analysis of state variation in breastfeeding rates in the United States. *Am J Pub Hlth.* 2008;98(10):1872-1880.
36. Atabay E, Moreno G, Nandi A, et al. Facilitating working mothers' ability to breastfeed: global trends in guaranteeing breastfeeding breaks at work, 1995-2014. *J Human Lact.* 2015;31(1):81-88.
37. U.S. Department of Labor, Wage and Hour Division. Break time for nursing mothers. U.S. Department of Labor website. https://www.dol.gov/whd/nursingmothers. Accessed June 4, 2017.
38. National Conference of State Legislatures. Breastfeeding state laws. National Conference of State Legislatures website. http://www.ncsl.org/research/health/breastfeeding-state-laws.aspx. Published August 30, 2016. Accessed June 4, 2017.
39. Olang B, Farivar K, Heidarzadeh A, Strandvik B, Yngve A. Breastfeeding in Iran: prevalence, duration and current recommendations. *Inter Breastfeeding J.* 2009;4(8). http://internationalbreastfeedingjournal.biomedcentral.com/articles/10.1186/1746-4358-4-8. Published August 5, 2009. Accessed June 4, 2017.
40. Amin R, Said Z, Sutan R, Shah SA, Darus A, Shamsuddin K. Work related determinants of breastfeeding discontinuation among employed mothers in Malaysia. *Int Breastfeed J.* 2011;6(4). http://internationalbreastfeedingjournal.biomedcentral.com/articles/10.1186/1746-4358-6-4. Published February 22, 2011. Accessed June 4, 2017.
41. Chapin EM. The state of the innocenti declaration targets in Italy. *J Human Lact.* 2001;17(3):202-206.
42. Murtagh L, Moulton AD. Strategies to protect vulnerable populations. *Am J Pub Hlth.* 2011;101(2):217-223.
43. U.S. Centers for Disease Control and Prevention. Progress in increasing breastfeeding and reducing racial/ethnic differences—United States, 2000-2008 births. *MMWR Morb Mortal Wkly Rep.* 2013;62(5):77-80. https://www.cdc.gov/mmwr/preview/mmwrhtml/mm6205a1.htm?s_cid=mm6205a1_w. Published February 8, 2013. Accessed June 4, 2017.
44. Condon M. Breast is best, but it could be better: what is in breast milk that should not be? *Ped Nurs.* 2005;31(4):333-338.
45. Flores GE, Bates ST, Knights D, et al. Microbial biogeography of public restroom surfaces. *PLOS One.* http://journals.plos.org/plosone/article?id=10.1371/journal.pone.0028132. Published November 23, 2011. Accessed June 4, 2017.
46. Johnson DL, Mead KR, Lynch RA, Hirst D. Lifting the lid on toilet plume aerosol: a literature review with suggestions for future research. *Am J Infec Control.* 2013;41(3):254-258.
47. Warwick H, Doig A. *Smoke—the Killer in the Kitchen: Indoor Air Pollution in Developing Countries.* London, England: ITDG Publishing; 2004.
48. Lindberg LD. Trends in the relationship between breastfeeding and postpartum employment in the United States. *Soc Bio.*1996;43:191-202.
49. Niedhammer I, O'Mahony D, Daly S, Morrison JJ, Kelleher CC; Lifeways Cross-Generation Cohort Study Steering Group. Lifeways cross-generation cohort study steering group. Occupational predictors of pregnancy outcomes in Irish working women in the lifeways cohort. *Brit J Ob Gyn.* 2009;116:943-952.
50. Abdulwadud OA, Snow ME. Interventions in the workplace to support breastfeeding for women in employment. *Cochrane Database Syst Rev.* 2012;10:CD006177. doi: 10.1002/14651858.CD006177.pub2.
51. Ortiz J, McGilligan K, Kelly P. Duration of breast milk expression among working mothers enrolled in an employer-sponsored lactation program. *Ped Nurs.* 2004;30:111-119.
52. Dieterich CM, Felice JP, O'Sullivan EO, Rasmussen KM. Breastfeeding and health outcomes for the mother-infant dyad. *Pediatr Clin North Am.* 2013;60(1):31-48.
53. American Academy of Pediatrics. Breastfeeding and the use of human milk. *Pediatrics,* 2012;129(3):496.
54. Cohen R, Mrtek M, Mrtek RG. Comparison of maternal absenteeism and infant illness rates among breast-feeding and formula-feeding women in two corporations. *Am J Health Promot.* 1995;10:148-153.

55. Ball T, Wright A. Health care costs of formula-feeding in the first year of life. *Pediatrics.* 1999;103:871-876.

56. Roche-Paull R. *Breastfeeding in Combat Boots: A Survival Guide to Successful Breastfeeding While Serving in the Military.* Amarillo, TX: Hale Publishing; 2010.

57. Bartick M, Schwarz EB, Green BD, et al. Suboptimal breastfeeding in the United States: maternal and pediatric health outcomes and costs. *Matern Child Nutr.* 2017;13(1). http://onlinelibrary.wiley.com/doi/10.1111/mcn.12366/full. Published September 19, 2016. Accessed June 4, 2017.

58. Lyness K, Thompson C, Francesco A, Judiesch M. Work and pregnancy: individual and organizational factors influencing organizational commitment, timing of maternity leave, and return to work. *Sex Roles.* 1999;41:485-508.

59. Bar-Yam N. Workplace lactation support, part 1: a return-to-work breastfeeding assessment tool. *J Hum Lactation.* 1998;14:249-254.

60. Cohen R, Mrtek MB. The impact of two corporate lactation programs on the incidence and duration of breastfeeding by employed mothers. *Am J Health Promot.* 1994;8:436-441.

61. Whaley S, Meehan K, Lange L, Slusser W, Jenks E. Predictors of breastfeeding duration for employees of the Special Supplemental Nutrition Program for Women, Infants, and Children (WIC). *J Am Diet Assoc.* 2002;102:1290-1293.

62. Arthur C, Saenz RB, Replogle WH. The employment-related breastfeeding decisions of physician mothers. *J MS State Med Assoc.* 2003;44:383-387.

63. Lewallen LP, Dick MJ, Flowers J, et al. Breastfeeding support and early cessation. *JOGNN.* 2006;35:166-172.

64. McLeod D, Pullon S, Cookson T. Factors influencing continuation of breastfeeding in a cohort of women. *J Hum Lactation.* 2002;18:335-343.

65. Dinour LM, Pope GA, Bai YK. Breast milk pumping beliefs, supports, and barriers on a university campus. *J Hum Lactation.* 2015;31(1):156-165.

66. Corbett-Dick P, Bezek SK. Breastfeeding promotion for the employed mother. *J Pediatr Health Care.* 1997;11:12-19.

67. Froh EB, Spatz DL. Navigating return to work and breastfeeding in a hospital with a comprehensive employee lactation program: the voices of mothers. *J Hum Lactation.* 2016;32(4):689-694.

68. Arthur CR, Saenz RB, Replogle WH. The employment-related breastfeeding decisions of physician mothers. *J Miss State Med Assoc.* 2033;44(12):383-387.

69. Frank E. Breastfeeding and maternal employment: two rights don't make a wrong. *Lancet.* 1998;352:1083-1085.

70. Nichols M, Roux G. Maternal perspectives on postpartum return to the workplace. *JOGNN.* 2004;33(4):463-471.

71. Wambach K. Maternal fatigue in breastfeeding primiparae during the first nine weeks postpartum. *J Hum Lactation.* 1998;14:219-229.

72. Hochschild A, Machung A. *The Second Shift.* New York, NY: Penguin Books. 2012.

73. Chow T, Fulmer I, Olson B. Perspectives of managers toward workplace breastfeeding support in the state of Michigan. *J Hum Lactation.* 2011;27:138-146.

74. Bai YK, Gaits SI, Wunderlich SM. Workplace lactation supports by New Jersey employers following US reasonable break time for nursing mothers law. *J Hum Lactation.* 2015;31(1):76-80.

75. Brown C, Poag S, Kasprzycki C. Exploring large employers' and small employers' knowledge, attitudes, and practices on breastfeeding support in the workplace. *J Hum Lactation.* 2001;17:39-46.

76. Libbus M, Bullock L. Breastfeeding and employment: an assessment of employer attitudes. *J Hum Lactation.* 2002;18:247-251.

77. Dunn BF, Zavela KJ, Cline AD, Cost PA. Breastfeeding practices in Colorado businesses. *J Hum Lactation.* 2004;20(2):217-218.

78. Tuttle CR, Slavit WI. Establishing the business case for breastfeeding. *Breastfeed Med.* 2009;4(suppl 1):S59-S62.

79. U.S. Department of Health and Human Services, Health Resources and Services Administration, Maternal and Child Health Bureau. *The Business Case for Breastfeeding.* Rockville, MD: HHS HRSA; 2008.

80. Dinour LM, Szaro JM. Employer-based programs to support breastfeeding among working mothers: a systematic review. *Breastfeeding Med.* 2017;12(3):131-141.

81. Stewart-Glenn J. Knowledge, perceptions, and attitudes of managers, coworkers, and employed breastfeeding mothers. *JAAOHN.* 2008;56(10):423-429.

82. Wyatt S. Challenges of the working breastfeeding mother. Workplace solutions. *AAOHN.* 2002;50(2):61-66.

83. Slusser WM, Lange L, Eickson V, Hawkes C, Cohen R. Breast milk expression in the workplace: a look at frequency and time. *J Hum Lactation.* 2004;20:164-169.

84. Angeletti MA. Breastfeeding mothers returning to work: possibilities for information, anticipatory guidance and support from US health care professionals. *J Hum Lactation.* 2009;25(2):226-232.

85. Page D. Breastfeeding and returning to work: working out the details. *J Hum Lactation.* 2008;24:85.

86. Win NN, Binns CW, Zhao Y, Scott JA, Oddy WH. Breastfeeding duration in mothers who express breast milk: a cohort study. *Int Breastfeed J.* 2006;1:28.

87. Hirani SA, Karmaliani R. The experiences of urban, professional women when combining breastfeeding with paid employment in Karachi, Pakistan: a qualitative study. *Women Birth,* 2013;26(2):147-151.

88. Vanek EP, Vanek JA. Job sharing as an employment alternative in group medical practice. *Med Group Manage J.* 2011;48:20-24.

89. Hills-Bonczyk SG, Avery MD, Savik K, Potter S, Duckett LJ.. Women's experiences with combining breastfeeding and employment. *J Nurse Midwifery,* 1993;38:257-266.

90. Bettinelli ME. Breastfeeding policies and breastfeeding support programs in the mother's workplace. *J Matern Fetal Neonatal Med.* 2012;25:73-74.

91. Anderson J, Kuehl RA, Drury SA, et al. Policies aren't enough: the importance of interpersonal communication about workplace breastfeeding support. *J Hum Lactation.* 2015;31(2):260-266.

92. Moquin C. *Babies at Work: Bringing New Life to the Workplace.* Framingham, MA: Carla Moquin; 2008.

93. Fein SB, Mandal B, Roe BE. Success of strategies for combining employment and breastfeeding. *Pediatrics.* 2008;122(suppl 2):S56-S62.

94. U.S. Department of Health and Human Services, Office on Women's Health. Supporting nursing moms at work: employer solutions. Womenshealth.gov website. https://www.womenshealth.gov/breastfeeding/employer-solutions/. Updated June 23, 2014. Accessed June 4, 2017.

95. New York State Department of Health. Making it work toolkit. Breastfeedingpartners.org website. http://breastfeedingpartners.org/index.php?option=com_content&view=article&id=164&Itemid=411. Accessed September 25, 2017.

96. Bourgoin G, Lahaie N, Rheaume B, et al. Factors influencing the duration of breastfeeding in the Sudbury region. *Can J Public Health.* 1997;88:238-241.

97. Cox DB, Owens RA, Hartmann PE. Blood and milk prolactin and the rate of milk synthesis in women. *Exper Phys.* 1996;81:1007-1020.

98. United States Breastfeeding Committee. Federal resources for supporting nursing moms at work. United States Breastfeeding Committee website. http://www.usbreastfeeding.org/SNMW-platform. Accessed June 4, 2017.

99. Kassing D. Bottle-feeding as a tool to reinforce breastfeeding. *J Hum Lactation.* 2002;18(1):56-60.

100. Kearny M, Cronenwett L. Breastfeeding and employment. *JOGNN.* 1991;20:471-480.

101. U.S. Department of Agriculture, Food and Nutrition Service. *Updated Child and Adult Care Food Program Meal Patterns: Infant Meals.* Washington, DC: USDA FNS; 2016. https://www.fns.usda.gov/sites/default/files/cacfp/CACFP_InfantMealPattern_FactSheet_V2.pdf. Accessed June 4, 2017.

Suggested Reading

Dinour LM, Szaro JM. Employer-based programs to support breastfeeding among working mothers: a systematic review. *Breastfeeding Med.* 2017;12(3):131-141.

International Labour Organization. *Global employment trends for women 2009.* Geneva, Switzerland: Author; 2009. http://www.ilo.org/wcmsp5/groups/public/@dgreports/@dcomm/documents/publication/wcms_103456.pdf. Accessed on October 18, 2017.

Lauwers J, Swisher A. When breastfeeding is interrupted. In: *Counseling the Nursing Mother.* 6th ed. Burlington, MA: Jones & Bartlett Learning; 2016:587-605.

Maternity Protection Coalition. Maternity protection campaign kit, section 9: how to support women in the informal economy to combine their productive and reproductive roles. World Alliance for Breastfeeding Action website. http://www.waba.org.my/whatwedo/womenandwork/pdf/09.pdf. Published 2008.

Mohrbacher N. *Working and Breastfeeding Made Simple.* Amarillo, TX: Praeclarus Press; 2014.

Vancour ML, Griswold MK. *Breastfeeding Best Practices in Higher Education.* Plano, TX: Hale Publishing Company; 2014.

Wambach K, Rojjanasrirat W. Maternal employment and breastfeeding. In: KA Wambach & J Riordan, eds. *Breastfeeding and Human Lactation.* 5th ed. Burlington, MA: Jones & Bartlett Learning Inc. 2016:635-666.

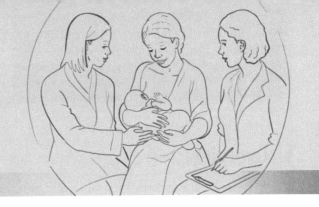

CHAPTER 12

Pregnancy, Labor, and Birth Complications

Cheryl Benn

OBJECTIVES

- Describe three conditions (hypertensive disorders, venous thromboembolism, and postpartum hemorrhage) that affect pregnancy, labor, birth, and lactation.
- Identify the signs and symptoms of each condition.
- Discuss the risks to the mother and baby of each condition.
- Outline the impact of each condition on labor and birth practices, and on lactation.
- Develop a plan of care to minimize the impact of each condition and of associated labor and birth practices on lactation.
- Promote pregnancy, labor, and birth practices that enhance lactation and breastfeeding when there are complications.

DEFINITIONS OF COMMONLY USED TERMS

atrophy The wasting away of a body organ.
cholestasis Itching of the palms of the hands and soles of the feet as bile salts build up in the body.
clonus Series of involuntary, rhythmic, muscular contractions and relaxations.
gestational Of pregnancy.
morbidity Negative and long-term health consequences following a pregnancy complicated by conditions such as hypertension.
pancytopenia Deficiency of all three cellular components of the blood (red cells, white cells, and platelets).
placenta increta Condition in which the placenta is deeply embedded into the endometrium and the uterine muscle.
placental abruption Sudden separation of the placenta.
pronurturance Combination of skin-to-skin contact and breastfeeding within 30 minutes of birth.
thrombophilia Abnormality of the blood clotting mechanisms in the body (coagulation cascade).
thromboprophylaxis Prevention of the formation of thrombi (clots).
thrombus Clot formed inside a blood vessel that obstructs the blood flow through the circulatory system.

Any use of the term *mother, maternal,* or *breastfeeding* is not meant to exclude transgender or nonbinary parents who may be breastfeeding or providing human milk to their infant.

▶ Overview

Complications during pregnancy, labor, and birth can impact the establishment and maintenance of breastfeeding and milk production. Hypertensive disorders of pregnancy complicate 10 to 15 percent of pregnancies, with 11 percent occurring in first pregnancies.[1] Although venous thromboembolism is relatively uncommon, with an incidence of 1 in 1,000–1,500 pregnancies,[2,3] it is currently the leading cause of direct maternal deaths in the United Kingdom[4] and in other developed countries.[5] Postpartum hemorrhage remains one of the major causes of death and morbidity in developing and developed countries.[6,7] Recognizing the signs and symptoms of these conditions will increase the clinician's effectiveness when working with breastfeeding families.

I. Hypertensive Disorders of Pregnancy

A. Hypertension in pregnancy is defined as systolic blood pressure greater than 140 mmHg, diastolic blood pressure greater than 90 mmHg, or both, based on at least two measurements taken 15 minutes apart using the same arm.[8]

1. Preexisting hypertension predates pregnancy or occurs before 20 weeks of pregnancy and is associated with preterm birth, abruption (sudden separation of the placenta), neonatal unit admissions, growth-restricted infants, and stillbirth.

2. Gestational hypertension occurs after 20 weeks of gestation, with preeclampsia occurring many weeks after the onset of gestational hypertension. It is characterized by gestational hypertension and new proteinuria (greater than 1+ protein in urine on dipstick), eclampsia and hemolysis, elevated liver enzymes, and low platelets (HELLP syndrome).[8]

B. Maternal and neonatal mortality and morbidity rates associated with hypertensive disorders of pregnancy remain unacceptably high in many parts of the world.[9,10]

1. The International Society for the Study of Hypertension in Pregnancy is currently undertaking two studies: Control of Hypertension in Pregnancy Study (CHIPS) and CHIPS-Child, which focuses on the long-term impact of hypertension in pregnancy on the child.

2. Globally, the hypertensive disorders of pregnancy, and preeclampsia in particular, claim some 50,000–80,000 lives annually and some 500,000 fetuses and newborns—more than 99 percent of those lives are lost in less-developed countries.

3. A key means of early detection and treatment is regular prenatal care with increasing frequency toward the end of pregnancy.[11]

4. Preterm birth, either spontaneous or medically induced, is commonly associated with hypertensive disorders in pregnancy.[12]

C. Preeclampsia or eclampsia can occur in pregnancy or present after the birth of the baby, especially in the first 24–48 hours and up to 2 weeks postpartum.

1. Preeclampsia results in multiorgan dysfunction and affects the liver, brain, kidneys, systemic blood vessels, and fetus.

2. Preeclampsia is associated with a number of predisposing factors: primigravida, first pregnancy with a particular partner, more than 10 years since the previous baby, previous history of preeclampsia, family history of preeclampsia, multiple pregnancy, and body mass index (BMI) greater than 35.

3. There is no known direct cause for preeclampsia, although it seems to be associated with abnormal development of the placenta.

4. The symptoms of preeclampsia vary dramatically among individuals. The classic presentation is high blood pressure, visual disturbances, headaches, proteinuria, epigastric pain or vomiting, liver tenderness, or signs of clonus. However, some individuals present with vague symptoms of feeling unwell; after 20 weeks of pregnancy, they should be investigated for preeclampsia.

D. Blood tests following these presentations include liver function, renal function, urea and electrolytes, and complete blood count. Raised liver enzymes—alanine aminotransferase (ALT) and aspartate aminotransferase (AST)—are classic signs of liver dysfunction in the absence of any other hepatitis conditions.

E. Magnesium sulfate (a mineral) may be administered for about 24–48 hours to prevent or treat the seizures of eclampsia if the patient is hyperreflexive, or has signs of clonus and irritability.

CLINICAL TIPS

- Consider the applicable steps from the "Ten Steps to Successful Breastfeeding" (see Chapter 29, *Initiatives to Protect, Promote, and Support Breastfeeding*):
  - Education
  - Only breastmilk unless supplements are medically indicated
  - Maintaining milk production if the mother and baby are separated
  - Rooming in
  - Support after hospital discharge
- Consider any antihypertensive drugs the mother is taking and their effects on lactation.
- Assist with expressing and storing colostrum antenatally, as well as postnatally if the mother is separated from the baby.
- Help the mother spend as much skin-to-skin time as possible with the baby to help heal the trauma of being very unwell in pregnancy and coming to terms with their anticipated pregnancy and birth and the reality of their experience.
- There will be increased and ongoing surveillance of the mother by multiple healthcare professionals through the pregnancy, labor, birth, and early postnatal period. Consider the impact on breastfeeding and how breastfeeding might help the parent focus positively on the baby.

II. Venous Thromboembolic Conditions in Pregnancy

A. The physiology of pregnancy places the mother at 5–10 times higher risk for venous thromboembolism than that of the general population.[2,13]
   1. The hormonal changes of pregnancy that affect venous stasis, the hypercoagulable state of pregnancy, and the obstruction of venous flow by the gravid uterus make pregnancy high risk.
   2. Any situation in which blood flow is slow or disrupted places the individual at risk of a thromboembolic event. Examples are long-haul flights, especially if pregnant, dehydration following severe morning sickness (hyperemesis gravidarum), or slow mobilization following surgery or a sedentary lifestyle.
   3. There are two main types of thrombus: venous (as in a deep vein thrombosis, or DVT) and arterial (as in the coronary arteries).
   4. Virchow triad is a disruption in one or more of the following[14]:
      a. Alteration of blood flow caused by injury or infection in a blood vessel
      b. Injury of the vascular endothelium
      c. Alterations to the constitution of the blood (hypercoagulability)
   5. Thrombophilia increases the risk of a thrombosis. It can be acquired (antiphospholipid syndrome) or congenital (e.g., factor V Leiden, protein C deficiency, or protein S deficiency).
   6. DVT usually occurs in one of the deep veins of the lower limb, but it can develop in pelvic and upper veins as well.

B. A clinical diagnosis is unreliable in pregnancy.
   1. Suggestive signs and symptoms include pain, especially on walking with localized tenderness, swelling of the affected area of the leg compared with the unaffected leg, and dyspnea (leg swelling and dyspnea could be related to the physiological changes of pregnancy).
   2. Objective testing to diagnose DVT or pulmonary embolus includes ultrasonography, MRI, or X-ray venography.[15,16] D-dimer is not useful in pregnancy because the levels increase progressively with advancing gestation and will be abnormal at term in an uncomplicated pregnancy.[17]

C. Individuals who smoke, are obese (BMI greater than 30 kg/m²), are sedentary, have gross varicose veins, or become dehydrated are more at risk of a DVT during childbearing.

1. A DVT may be asymptomatic and difficult to diagnose by physical examination.

2. It is important to recognize those at risk and begin thromboprophylaxis by use of compression stockings (a recent randomized controlled trial[18] did not show benefit for preventing postthrombotic syndrome) and anticoagulant therapy (use of heparin-based compounds, which alter the activity of the enzymes involved in the normal clotting process).[16]

3. Low-molecular-weight heparin (LMWH) is recommended during pregnancy and breastfeeding because it does not cross the placenta or enter breastmilk. Warfarin cannot be used in pregnancy but can be used in breastfeeding mothers in the postpartum period.[15] Thromboprophylaxis should be continued for up to 6 weeks in those who are high risk.

4. Induction of labor is performed at term for those with DVT, and LMWH should be stopped 24–48 hours before induction begins then recommended after birth or at least 4 hours after removal of the epidural catheter.[19]

5. Those at risk of DVT should not be prescribed combined oral contraceptives during the first 3 months after birth.

6. Those with a history of a thromboembolic event have an increased risk in a future pregnancy, and thromboprophylaxis should commence soon after a diagnosis of pregnancy.[19]

CLINICAL TIPS

- A consultation with a lactation consultant during pregnancy is helpful because of increased and ongoing surveillance of the mother by multiple healthcare professionals through the pregnancy, labor, birth, and early postnatal period. Consider the impact on breastfeeding.
- Support the expression and storage of colostrum prenatally.
- When taking a history from or assessing breastfeeding mothers postnatally, explore anything that might indicate the formation or presence of a thrombus and advise them to see their primary healthcare provider immediately.
- Provide parents with information about the impact on breastfeeding of CT scans, MRIs, X-ray venography, and anticoagulant drugs.
- Consider the involvement and support needs of immediate and extended family members. Consider how the lactation consultant can support them.

III. Postpartum Hemorrhage

A. Postpartum hemorrhage (PPH) is defined as blood loss of more than 500 mL, and the loss can be greater than 1,500–2,000 mL. The effect of the blood loss, whatever the volume, is suggested to be a more important measure of PPH than volume itself.[20]

1. A primary PPH occurs in the period from after birth to 24 hours postpartum.[21]

2. A secondary PPH occurs from 24 hours to 6 weeks postpartum.[21]

3. PPH is unpredictable and unexpected. Risk factors such as antepartum hemorrhage increase susceptibility to PPH. In developing countries those who have iron deficiency anemia at the end of pregnancy are more at risk of a PPH because the anemia magnifies the hemorrhage, making recovery after birth take longer.[20]

B. The causes can be related to four Ts[21]:

1. Tone: Poor tone of the uterus
2. Tissue: Retained products
3. Trauma: Lacerations of the genital tract
4. Thrombin: Disorders of coagulation (disseminated intravascular coagulation, or DIC)

C. DIC is life threatening land arises secondary to diseases and conditions that cause hypercoagulation and hemorrhage. In pregnancy, those who have a placental abruption (sudden separation of the placenta), severe preeclampsia or eclampsia, or amniotic fluid embolism are at risk for DIC in pregnancy.

    D.   Sheehan syndrome can occur after postpartum blood loss that affects blood flow to the pituitary gland.

          1.   Atrophy of the pituitary gland can affect the production of prolactin and thus the sufficiency of milk production.[22]

          2.   In rare cases pancytopenia can occur following Sheehan syndrome after a PPH.[23]

    E.   It is suggested that in most cases of PPH, the cause of insufficient milk production is related to the separation of the breastfeeding dyad and thus reduced stimulation of the breast, especially when the mother is exhausted and recovering from a significant PPH.[24]

    F.   According to a retrospective cohort study, early skin-to-skin contact and breastfeeding after birth (pro-nurturance) reduces postpartum hemorrhage for those at any level of risk of PPH, but especially for those at low risk.[25]

▶ Key Points from This Chapter

    A.   Conditions affecting pregnancy, labor, birth, and the postpartum period have the potential to affect the breastfeeding experience and present distinct challenges that should be considered when caring for these families.

    B.   Ongoing surveillance by healthcare providers and by families and friends when health challenges arise that impact on breastfeeding allows for opportunities to provide education, counseling, and care planning to meet the families' breastfeeding goals.

    C.   Alterations in the expected trajectory of pregnancy, labor, birth, and postpartum allow the lactation consultant to be included in the care team to identify potential lactation challenges and empower parents to frame their experiences in ways that support the families' breastfeeding relationships and parenting goals.

CLINICAL TIPS

- Consider the impact of ongoing surveillance of the mother by multiple different healthcare professionals, especially in the first 24 hours after birth. What might the impact be on breastfeeding?
- Consider the effect of blood loss on the mother's health, including fatigue, after birth when learning to breastfeed.
- Because any mother can experience a PPH after the birth of a baby, routinely recommend prenatal expression and storage of colostrum.
- Early and frequent skin-to-skin contact with the baby is vital, especially when the mother is in intensive care.
- Ensure assistance with latching the baby when the mother is in intensive care.
- Promote stimulating and maintaining milk production by assisting with milk expression after birth.
- Be alert for low milk production, which may be a consequence of excessive blood loss leading to Sheehan syndrome.
- Consider the best supplemental feeds for the baby, including options for human milk, and advise parents about their options to enable them to make fully informed decisions.
- Recognize that PPH may increase susceptibility to postpartum depression and posttraumatic stress disorder, which could affect breastfeeding and bonding with the baby.

🔍 CASE STUDY 1

Kate's first pregnancy was at 34 years of age. At 32 weeks of gestation, Kate started to feel unwell and showed signs of developing preeclampsia (hypertension, proteinuria, and visual disturbances, as well as some epigastric pain associated with an enlarging liver). A blood screen showed raised liver enzymes (ALT and AST), but her renal function was normal. In addition, obstetric cholestasis began (itching of the palms of the hands and soles of the feet as bile salts build up in the body). Kate was referred to the obstetric team for closer monitoring and growth scans to ensure the baby was growing well. At 36 weeks of pregnancy, a decision was made to end the pregnancy because the baby was found to be growth restricted and the preeclampsia was worsening. The baby, weighing 1880g (4lb 2oz), was born by cesarean section at 36 weeks and admitted to the neonatal unit. Kate had been encouraged to express and store colostrum so

(continues)

🔍 CASE STUDY 1 *(continued)*

the baby's first milk would be colostrum rather than formula. After birth, Kate's blood pressure increased dramatically, and labetalol and enalapril were commenced. Kate's blood pressure was monitored regularly, and the dosages of both medications were reduced until they were stopped at 6 weeks postpartum.

With both subsequent pregnancies, Kate developed preeclampsia and obstetric cholestasis. Each presentation was earlier, at 30 weeks with the second baby and 26 weeks with the third baby. In line with recommendations, Kate commenced 100 mg of low-dose aspirin between 14 and 16 weeks of gestation with each subsequent pregnancy, and the babies grew to normal size.

Questions

1. What were the challenges this parent faced with each pregnancy?
2. What implication did the prescribed drugs have for lactation?
3. What are the familiar support implications for parents in similar situations when they live in a rural area that is distant from a tertiary hospital neonatal unit?
4. How can some of these support implications be addressed?

🔍 CASE STUDY 2

Marion's third baby was born at home in a gentle water birth. The baby was immediately placed skin to skin and started breastfeeding within 1 hour. On day 7 Marion called the midwife to report extreme pain, mostly on the right side in the right-lower quadrant. On assessment there was guarding in the area, no fever, and writhing pain. Assessments were undertaken to exclude a urinary tract infection and a uterine infection. The possibility of appendicitis was considered, so a referral was made to the emergency department, where Marion was assessed by an obstetrician and a physician. Marion declined a laparoscopy to avoid being separated from the baby. A CT scan identified an ovarian vein thrombosis. This is a very rare condition that, according to published case studies, presents around day 7 postpartum and usually on the right side. Marion and the baby were admitted to the postnatal ward, where Marion was put on enoxaparin and treated with antibiotics because an associated fever is common. Marion and the baby remained together and exclusively breastfed while being treated over a 7-day period.

Questions

1. What challenges did this home-birthing parent and family face?
2. What kind of support would have been helpful?
3. What are the breastfeeding implications for the drugs and tests used in this case?
4. What advice would support their ongoing breastfeeding during treatments?

🔍 CASE STUDY 3

Louise's second baby was born at home. The third stage of labor was complicated by a retained placenta. After transfer to the hospital, it was found that Louise's placenta was deeply embedded into the endometrium and the uterine muscle (placenta increta). Surgery was required to remove the placenta because Louise had started to bleed profusely. Louise lost 2.5 to 3 liters of blood and was admitted to the intensive care unit (ICU); the baby was admitted to the neonatal unit for care. A complete hysterectomy was required to stop the bleeding. At discharge Louise felt exhausted and recalled very little of what had happened. Louise struggled with breastfeeding, worried about sufficient milk production, and felt disconnected from the baby because of the long periods of separation, even though the baby was brought to her in the ICU.

Questions

1. What are the psychosocial effects of ICU hospitalization on a new mother and family?
2. What supports are needed to facilitate skin-to-skin contact and breastfeeding while in intensive care?
3. What are the long-term implications of significant blood loss after birth?
4. How can these implications be addressed by breastfeeding and breastfeeding support?

References

1. Villar J, Say L, Shennan A, et al. Methodological and technical issues related to the diagnosis, screening, prevention and treatment of pre-eclampsia and eclampsia. *Int J Gynecol Obstet.* 2004;85(suppl 1):S28-S41.
2. McLintock, C. Venous thromboembolism and pregnancy. A search for clarity in an uncertain world. *O & G Magazine.* 2013;15(1):39-41.
3. Simcox LE, Ormesher L, Tower C, Greer IA. Pulmonary thrombo-embolism in pregnancy: diagnosis and management. Breathe. 2015;11(4):282-289.
4. Knight M, Tuffnell D, Kenyon S, Shakespeare J, Gray R, Kurinczuk JJ, eds.; MBRRACE-UK Saving Lives, Improving Mothers' Care – Surveillance of maternal deaths in the UK 2011-13 and lessons learned to inform maternity care from the UK and Ireland. Confidential Enquiries into Maternal Deaths and Morbidity 2009-13. Oxford, UK: National Perinatal Epidemiology Unit, University of Oxford; 2015.
5. Sullivan EA, Hall B, King J. Maternal deaths in Australia 2003-2005. Maternal deaths series no. 3. Sydney: AIHW National Perinatal Statistics Unit; 2008.
6. Smith JM, Gubin R, Holston MM, Fullerton J, Prata N. Misoprostol for postpartum hemorrhage prevention at home birth: an integrative review of global implementation experience to date. *BMC Pregnancy Childbirth.* 2013;13:44. doi:10.1186/1471-2393-13-44.
7. UNFPA, UNICEF, WHO, World Bank. Trends in Maternal Mortality: 1990–2010. United Nations Population Fund website. http://www.unfpa.org/public/home/publications/pid/10728. Published 2012. Accessed September 26, 2017.
8. Magee LA, Pels A, Helewa M, Rey E, von Dadelszen P; Canadian Hypertensive Disorders of Pregnancy Working Group. Diagnosis, evaluation and management of the hypertensive disorders of pregnancy: executive summary. *J Obstet Gynaecol Canada.* 2014;36(5):416-438.
9. Langenveld J, Buttinger A, van der Post J, Wolf H, Mol B, Ganzevoort W. Recurrence, risk and prediction of a delivery under 34 weeks of gestation after a history of a severe hypertensive disorder. *BJOG.* 2011;118:589-595.
10. Yucesoy G, Ozkan S, Bodur H, et al. Maternal and perinatal outcome in pregnancies complicated with hypertensive disorder of pregnancy: a seven year experience of a tertiary care center. *Arch Gynecol Obstet.* 2005;273:43-49. doi:10.1007/s00404-005-0741-3.
11. Von Dadelszen P. Pre-eclampsia in less developed countries: how to make a difference. International Society for the Study of Hypertension in Pregnancy website. http://www.isshp.org/pre-eclampsia-in-less-developed-countries-how-to-make-a-difference/. Published January 19, 2016. Accessed September 6, 2016.
12. Hofmeyr GJ, Lawrie TA, Atallah AN, Duley L, Torloni MR. Calcium supplementation during pregnancy for preventing hypertensive disorders and related problems. *Cochrane Database Syst Rev.* 2014;6:CD001059. doi:10.1002/14651858.CD001059.pub3.
13. Heit JA, Kobbervig CE, James AH, Petterson TM, Bailey KR, Melton LJ. Trends in the incidence of venous thromboembolism during pregnancy or postpartum: a 30-year population-based study. *Ann Intern Med.* 2005;143:697-706.
14. Petchet L, Alexander B. Increased clotting factors in pregnancy. *N Engl J Med.* 1961;265:1093-1097.
15. Bates SM, Jaeschke R, Stevens SM, et al. Diagnosis of DVT: Antithrombotic Therapy and Prevention of Thrombosis, 9th ed: American College of Chest Physicians evidence-based clinical practice guidelines. *Chest.* 2012;141(suppl 2):e351S-e418S.
16. Royal College of Obstetricians and Gynaecologists. *Reducing the Risk of Venous Thromboembolism during Pregnancy and the Puerperium.* Green-top guideline No. 37a. London, England: RCOG Press; 2015. https://www.rcog.org.uk/globalassets/documents/guidelines/gtg-37a.pdf. Accessed September 26, 2017.
17. Khalafallah AA, Morse M, Al-Barzan AM, et al. D-dimer levels at different stages of pregnancy in Australian Women: a single centre study using two different immunoturbidimetric assays. *Thromb Res.* 2012;130(3):e171-e177.
18. Khan SR, Shapiro S, Wells PS, et al. Compression stockings to prevent post thrombotic syndrome: a randomised placebo-controlled trial. *Lancet.* 2014;383:880-888.
19. Greer IA. Pregnancy complicated by venous thrombosis. *N Engl J Med.* 2015;373:540-547.
20. Lilley G, Burkett-St-Laurent D, Precious E, et al. Measurement of blood loss during postpartum haemorrhage. *Int J Obstet Anesth.* 2015;24:8-14.
21. Wylie L, Bryce H. *The Midwives' Guide to Key Medical Conditions: Pregnancy and Childbirth.* Edinburgh, Scotland: Elsevier; 2016.
22. Dejager S, Gerber S, Foubert S, Turpin G. Sheehan's syndrome: differential diagnosis in the acute phase. *J Intern Med.* 1998;244(3):261-266.
23. Laway BA, Bhat JB, Mir SA, Khan RSZ, Lone MI, Zargar AH. Sheehan's syndrome with pancytopenia—complete recovery after hormone replacement. *Ann Hematol.* 2010;89(3):305-308.
24. Thompson JF, Heal LJ, Roberts CL, Ellwood D. Women's breastfeeding experiences following significant primary postpartum haemorrhage: a multicentre cohort study. *Int Breastfeeding J.* 2010;5(5):1-12.
25. Saxton A, Fahy K, Rolf M, Skinner V, Hastie C. Does skin to skin contact and breastfeeding at birth affect the rates of postpartum haemorrhage: results of a cohort study. *Midwifery.* 2015;31(11):1110-1117.

Suggested Reading

American College of Obstetricians and Gynecologists. Magnesium sulfate use in obstetrics. Committee opinion no. 652. *Obstet Gynecol.* 2016;127:e52-e53.

Broekhuijsen K, van Baaren G-J, van Pampus MG, et al. Immediate delivery versus expectant monitoring for hypertensive disorders of pregnancy between 34 and 37 weeks of gestation (HYPITAT-II): an open-label, randomised controlled trial. *Lancet.* 2015;385(9986):2492-2501. http://dx.doi.org/10.1016/S0140-6736(14)61998-X.

Cowan, J, Redman, C, Walker, I. *Understanding Pre-eclampsia. A Guide for Parents and Health Professionals.* Watford, UK: Clearsay Publishing; 2017.

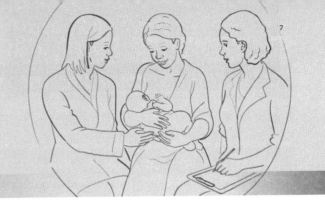

CHAPTER 13

Facilitating and Assessing Breastfeeding Initiation

Elaine Webber
Jean Benedict

OBJECTIVES

- Incorporate evidence-based strategies for the initiation of breastfeeding immediately after delivery and in the early postpartum period.
- Discuss the rationale for skin-to-skin contact between the breastfeeding dyad.
- Assess the breastfeeding dyad for adequate latch, suck, milk transfer, and infant elimination.
- Describe key positioning components of biological nurturing (laid back infant-led attachment) and mother-led attachment.
- Assess the suck cycle and differentiate between nutritive and nonnutritive sucking.
- Identify strategies for managing challenges in the initiation of breastfeeding.

DEFINITIONS OF COMMONLY USED TERMS

asymmetrical latch Infant latched onto the breast covering more of the underside of the areola, with the bottom lip covering most of the areola and the top lip covering somewhat less of the areola.

breast crawl An organized set of innate behaviors in which the infant moves toward the nipple with the intent to latch and begin breastfeeding.

chest feeding An infant feeding at the breast of a transgender man.

meconium An infant's first stool, which is black and tarry.

milk transfer The process of milk moving from the breast to the infant during a feeding session.

nipple confusion When an infant has difficulty latching effectively at the breast after being exposed to artificial nipples (teats).

nipple shield A nipple-shaped thin silicone shield that is positioned over the nipple and areola prior to nursing.

(continues)

▶ Overview

The initiation of breastfeeding in the early postpartum period is a critical time in the establishment of breastfeeding. What happens in the first few hours and days after birth, and the knowledgeable support provided by all healthcare providers, greatly influence the success of the breastfeeding dyad. What an infant needs most at the time of birth is a nurturing mother.[3] The World Health Organization (WHO) and the United Nations Children's Fund (UNICEF) recommend that all healthy infants have uninterrupted skin-to-skin care from the moment of birth until after the first feeding, prior to any medical interventions by healthcare providers.[4] Early and frequent feeds promote the development of robust milk production and prevent potential breastfeeding difficulties. This information should be communicated to families during the prenatal period, reinforced at the time of delivery, and continued throughout the postpartum period. All individuals working with breastfeeding dyads should be knowledgeable about providing breastfeeding information that is consistent with current recommended evidence-based guidelines. Providers should be skilled in the assessment of effective latch, effective suck, and indicators of adequate milk transfer. If breastfeeding difficulties are identified, a specialized interdisciplinary plan of care should be developed with lactation experts.

I. Strategies for the Initiation of Breastfeeding

   A.   Parents will benefit from anticipatory guidance prior to the birth of the baby:
      1. Encourage parents to discuss feeding plans with healthcare providers.
      2. Assist parents in identifying a support person to attend the delivery and to help with initial feeding efforts. The presence of a support person is known to enhance breastfeeding initiation and duration.[5]
      3. Assist parents in understanding the importance of initiating breastfeeding within the first hour of life.
   B.   Promote supportive breastfeeding practices after birth.
      1. Place the infant on the mother's abdomen immediately after delivery.
         a. The stable infant should be dried and placed on the mother's abdomen prior to cord clamping.[4,6,7]
         b. Infants placed skin to skin immediately after birth and left undisturbed and unmedicated will self-latch within 1 hour after delivery.[8]
         c. Extended periods of skin-to-skin time is the best initial step to encourage an infant to latch and begin feeding.[9]
         d. "Immediate, uninterrupted skin-to-skin [contact] for a minimum of one hour is among the most effective strategies . . . to promote exclusive breastfeeding."[10(p213)]
      2. Healthcare providers should be educated to delay, minimize, or eliminate neonatal and postpartum procedures that interfere with the first breastfeeding.
         a. Minimize oral suctioning.
            i. Bulb suctioning of the mouth or nares can cause physical injury or edema and stuffiness.

ii. Deep suctioning can trigger a vagal response in the infant, causing injury to the oropharynx and physiologic changes, such as increased blood pressure and changes in heart rate.[11]

iii. "Suctioning immediately following birth (including suctioning with a bulb syringe) should be reserved for babies who have obvious obstruction to spontaneous breathing or who require positive-pressure ventilation."[12(p e1402)]

iv. Aggressive suctioning can affect the infant's desire to latch as a result of pain or injury to the oropharynx; the infant may demonstrate oral defensiveness.[13]

v. "Infants who had any naso-oropharyngeal suctioning administered at birth were six times less likely to suckle effectively."[14(p1)]

vi. Wiping a healthy infant's mouth and nose has been shown to clear the airways and stimulate the initiation of respirations without the potentially adverse effects associated with bulb suctioning. This technique is especially helpful in resource-poor areas, but it should be implemented for all healthy newborns.[13,15]

b. Delay routine procedures.

i. All routine procedures, including assessments, can take place while the infant and mother are placed skin to skin, or they can be delayed until after the initial breastfeeding.[16,17]

ii. Avoid washing the mother's skin prior to initiating breastfeeding; the infant depends on olfactory cues to self-attach to the breast.[9]

iii. For a healthy newborn, weight, measurements, eye prophylaxis, and vitamin K injection can be delayed for up to 6 hours after birth to avoid interfering with the infant's self-regulatory processes.[17]

iv. Infant bathing should be delayed until well after the first feeding. Early bathing increases the risk for hypothermia, removes the mother's bacteria, and may inhibit the crawling reflex.[10]

C. Facilitate the first feeding following delivery.

1. Immediately after delivery, the infant should be dried and placed skin to skin on the mother's abdomen.[17]

2. If left undisturbed on the mother's abdomen, the healthy, unmedicated infant will latch and begin suckling within the first hour after birth.[8]

3. Encourage parents and healthcare providers to recognize and facilitate the baby's reflexes for self-attachment.

a. Organized, predictable feeding behavior develops during the first hours of life and progresses through spontaneous sucking and rooting, hand-to-mouth activity, more intense sucking, and finally sucking of the breast.[9,18-25]

b. Early optimal self-regulation occurs when the infant is given the option to progress through the nine behavioral phases (crying, relaxing, awakening, being active, crawling, resting, familiarizing, suckling, sleeping) when held skin to skin, leading to successful attachment to the breast.[9]

c. Self-attachment behaviors can be seen in the breast crawl video available at http://breastcrawl .org/video.shtml.[25]

D. See the first steps after delivery in **BOX 13-1**.

BOX 13-1 First Steps After Delivery

1. Place the infant skin to skin with the mother immediately after delivery.
2. Allow the infant to crawl to the breast and self-attach.
3. Avoid unnecessary interruptions—such as infant measurements, vitamin K injection, eye drops, or bath—until the infant has achieved the first breastfeeding.
4. Encourage frequent, unlimited feedings in a comfortable position; respond to the infant's feeding readiness.
5. Avoid the use of pacifiers or dummies.

II. Exclusive Breastfeeding in the Postpartum Period

- A. The mother and infant should remain together throughout the postpartum period, regardless of the delivery setting.
    1. Educate parents about the benefits of 24-hour rooming in (keeping babies with their mothers).
        a. Encourage extended periods of skin-to-skin contact to maximize opportunities for infant self-regulation and self-attachment.
        b. "Chest against chest, skin on skin appears to promote a searching response in the hungry, quiet alert infant . . . Eye contact and the mother's voice help the infant to remain calm, focused and in better motor control."[26(p87-88)]
        c. Evidence suggests that breastfeeding mothers get the same amount and quality of sleep when rooming in as when the baby is sent to the nursery.[17]
        d. Infants who remain with their mothers are more likely to breastfeed exclusively and for longer durations. Milk production is higher when compared to dyads who are separated.[27,28]
    2. Rooming in 24 hours per day with continuous skin-to-skin contact will lead to questions regarding co-sleeping. (See Chapter 29, *Initiatives to Protect, Promote, and Support Breastfeeding*, for a discussion of bed sharing.)
- B. Foster an environment that promotes the establishment of breastfeeding.
    1. The dyad should remain together as much as possible throughout the postpartum period.
    2. Routine infant assessments should be performed in the mother's room.
    3. Healthcare providers should be aware of the impact of interrupting an ongoing breastfeeding session. Breastfeeding should never be interrupted for nonurgent care (e.g., infant or maternal vital signs, routine exams, laboratory testing, or photographs).
    4. Provide for the mother's physical and emotional comfort.
        a. Assess the mother's comfort with visitors and family. Provide privacy to facilitate a relaxed focus on the infant to observe and respond to feeding readiness. If indicated, ask visitors to leave and return after the feeding.
        b. Eliminate distractions, such as telephone and television, to facilitate a quiet environment.
        c. If the mother is receiving pain medication, suggest that it be taken prior to feeding.
        d. Encourage adequate hydration and nutrition. (See Chapter 8, *Nutrition during Lactation*, for a discussion of nutrition during lactation).
    5. Encourage healthcare providers to cluster care to decrease intrusion into family space.

III. Management of Breastfeeding during the Early Postpartum Period

- A. Encourage the family to keep the infant skin to skin, allowing the infant to self-latch and feed as long and as often as desired.
- B. Instruct parents to observe their infant for early feeding cues. (See Chapter 4, *Normal Infant Behavior*, for a discussion of feeding cues.)
- C. Help mothers achieve effective positioning for breastfeeding.
    1. Effective positioning facilitates successful breastfeeding (see **TABLE 13-1** and **FIGURES 13-1** through **13-5**).
    2. There is no one correct position for breastfeeding.[3] Numerous variations exist and can be adapted to each couplet based on what is comfortable. Effective positioning is important to provide comfort and allow the infant to latch and feed effectively.
    3. Encourage infant-led biological nurturing utilizing a laid-back posture.
        a. Research indicates that human infants are abdominal feeders.[29,30]
        b. Placing infants in the prone position along the mother's abdomen can help trigger innate feeding behaviors; infants will often latch without assistance.[30]
        c. To initiate the laid-back position, assist mothers to lie semireclined on their back with comfortable back support. Place the infant prone on the bare abdomen or chest, resting the infant's face on or near the breast.

TABLE 13-1 Review of Basic Positions for Breastfeeding

Position	Uses	Description	Considerations
Mother Seated			
Laid-back breastfeeding or biological nurturing (**FIGURE 13-1**)	Encourages baby's natural breastfeeding instincts. Works well for first latch after delivery, following cesarean sections, and for mothers who are struggling with latch.	The mother leans back and is well supported in a bed or large recliner—not flat, but comfortably leaning back. The infant is dressed in a diaper only. The infant is placed on the mother's chest with the cheek near the breast—baby's chest to mother's chest. The infant's body rests entirely on the mother, and the infant is allowed to self-attach.	Mothers worry that the infant could fall off; use this position where the baby will be secure. Mothers have concerns that the infant could suffocate at the breast when face down on the breast; movement of the head is unrestricted and the baby can achieve a position that does not restrict breathing.
Madonna or cradle hold (**FIGURE 13-2**)	Most commonly used position. Often feels the most natural to the mother.	The infant lies across the mother's forearm on the side the mother will be using for the feeding. The infant's head is either in the bend of the mother's elbow or midway down the forearm, whichever results in the best positioning. Keeping the arm level, the mother's hand holds the infant's buttocks. The infant's lower arm can be placed around the mother's back or tucked alongside the mother's body. The infant's legs can be wrapped around the mother's waist if needed to bring the infant closer to the breast. The baby's entire body should be facing the mother, chest to chest rather than chest to ceiling. The infant's mouth should be level with the nipple. Pillows may help support the infant's body in the mother's lap to help prevent downward drift and keep the infant at breast level. Pillows may help the mother's back and arms.	Offers the least amount of control over the infant's head. Difficult to achieve a good sitting position in a hospital bed; use a chair if possible. Requires sitting; episiotomy, cesarean incision or hemorrhoids make sitting a less desirable position. Mothers tend to hunch over and take the breast to the baby, rather than bringing the baby to the breast. The infant can drift downward, which may alter the latch, put additional pressure on the nipple, or pull the breast out of the baby's mouth.
Cross-cradle hold (**FIGURE 13-3**)	Principles are the same as for the cradle hold. Useful for infants who need more direction at the breast to latch.	The infant lies across the mother's forearm that is opposite from the breast being used for the feeding (e.g., the left arm for the right breast). The infant's head is held just below the ears at the nape of the neck. The breast is supported with the hand on the same side as the breast to be used for the feeding.	Be sure the infant is chest to chest rather than chest to ceiling (turned away from the mother's body).

(continues)

TABLE 13-1 Review of Basic Positions for Breastfeeding   (continued)

Position	Uses	Description	Considerations
Mother Seated			
	May be useful for mothers with long arms.	Use a pillow to position the infant at the breast level and provide support for the mother's arm. Following the latch, the mother can bring the alternate arm underneath the infant and assume the cradle position.	
Clutch or football hold (**FIGURE 13-4**)	Often preferred when a new mother is having difficulty with latch. Improves the mother's view of the nipple, areola, and baby's mouth. Helpful after cesarean birth. Helpful for mothers with especially large breasts.	Pillows are placed at breast level, along the mother's side. The infant lies next to the mother at breast level with the hips flexed and the infant's bottom against the back of the chair, sofa, or bed, or along the wall. The infant's feet can be aiming toward the ceiling. The mother's arm is under the infant's back, with the hand at the base of the infant's head. Alternatively, the infant lies on his or her side with the entire body turned toward the mother (wrapped around the mother's side). The mother's arm is along the infant's back with the hand at the base of the infant's head.	Needs proper pillow support, which may not be available in all settings. Pressure on the occipital area of the infant's head can cause back arching. An episiotomy or hemorrhoids make sitting a less desirable position.
Mother Lying Down			
Side lying (**FIGURE 13-5**)	Mothers may experience less fatigue when breastfeeding while lying down. The lying-down position takes pressure off an episiotomy or hemorrhoids.	With the mother on her side, place a pillow behind the upper back and have the mother roll toward the pillow for stability. The infant is placed on the bed, and the mother can use her arm to hold the infant in position. Alternately, the infant can be held directly on the mother's arm, turned toward the breast.	May be a suffocation hazard if the mother has received medication that causes drowsiness. May be a falling hazard if the dyad is lying on a bed and the mother is excessively drowsy due to postlabor fatigue or medications. Lying completely at a 90° angle on the bed may make it difficult for the infant to latch. The breast may be turned in such a way that the nipple and areola are inaccessible to the infant. This may be remedied by having the infant lie on the mother's forearm rather than directly on the bed.

4. Teach techniques for mother-led attachment.
    a. Regardless of how the baby is held for feeding, assist with finding a comfortable, relaxed posture that provides support for the back and arms as needed.
    b. Bring the baby to the breast, rather than the breast to the baby.

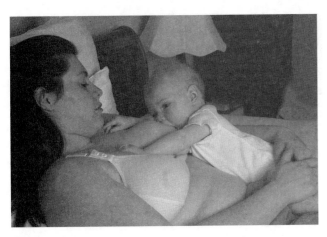

FIGURE 13-1 Laidback breastfeeding position.
Printed with permission of Nelia Box Karimi.

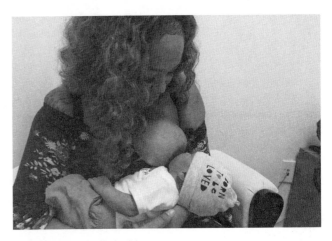

FIGURE 13-2 Cradle hold.
Photo by Regina Maria Roig-Romero. © 2016 Regina Maria Roig-Romero and Every Mother, Inc. All Rights Reserved.

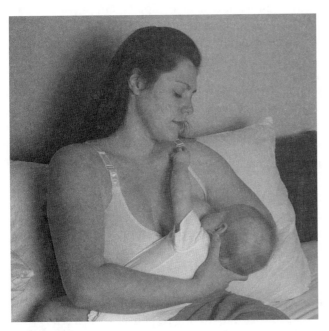

FIGURE 13-3 Cross-cradle hold.
Printed with permission of Nelia Box Karimi.

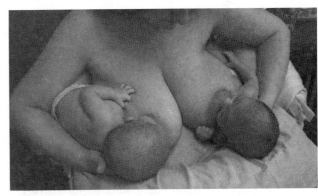

FIGURE 13-4 Clutch/football hold.
Photo by Cathy Carothers. © 2016 Cathy Carothers and Every Mother, Inc. All Rights Reserved.

   c.   Place the hand at the base of the baby's head (nape of the neck) to avoid pressure against the occiput, which can cause the baby to arch away from the breast.

   d.   Ensure the infant's body is turned toward the mother, with the ear, shoulder, and hips in alignment.

   e.   Breast support may be needed to assist with latch in the early days. The breast can be supported by cupping the hand in the shape of a "C" with four fingers below the breast and the thumb above, well behind the areola (see **FIGURE 13-6**). The fingers will generally be parallel to the infant's lips.

   f.   The scissors hold (breast grasped between the index and middle fingers) might help to support smaller breasts as long as the fingers are well away from the areola.

   g.   A rolled washcloth or towel placed under the breast may help support the weight of a larger breast.

   h.   The Dancer hold might be needed for a preterm infant or for an infant who has poor jaw support or control. Grasp the breast from below with the hand in a U shape and the baby's chin resting on the fleshy part between the thumb and index finger (see **FIGURE 13-7**). (See Chapter 14, *Breastfeeding and the Preterm Infant*, and Chapter 23, *Breastfeeding and Infant Birth Injury, Congenital Anomalies, and Illness*, for further information.)

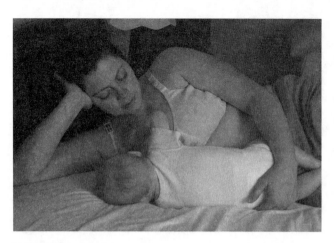

FIGURE 13-5 Side-lying position.

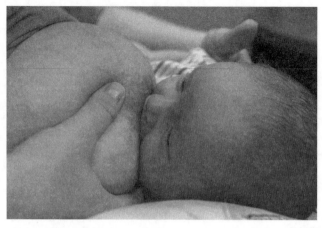

FIGURE 13-6 C-hold.

D.   Facilitate an effective latch.

1.   An effective latch can prevent many breastfeeding problems, such as nipple pain or trauma and inadequate milk transfer. See **BOX 13-2** for indicators of an effective latch.

2.   The optimal infant behavioral state for latch ranges from slightly drowsy to active alert. The quiet alert state is ideal. (See Chapter 4, *Normal Infant Behavior,* for a discussion of infant states.)

3.   Several factors may influence a successful latch.

a.   Maternal factors include:

i.   Breast anatomy including size and shape of the nipple, breast tissue elasticity, and size and shape of the breast.

ii.   Labor experience.

iii. Knowledge about breastfeeding management.

b.   Infant factors include:

i.   Oral anatomy including palate, cheeks, lip, tongue, and jaw.

ii.   Gestational age.

iii. Labor and birth experiences including medications, length of labor, and assistive labor techniques.

4.   If assistance with latch is needed, avoid forcing the infant onto the breast and offer suggestions to facilitate latch.

a.   Breastfeed any time the baby exhibits feeding cues.

b.   Brush the infant's lips lightly with the nipple to elicit the rooting response.

c.   Wait for the infant's mouth to open wide with the tongue at the floor of the mouth. A crying baby might open the mouth wide, but the tongue is often at the roof of the mouth, hindering the latch.

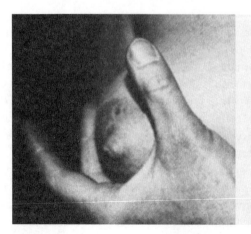
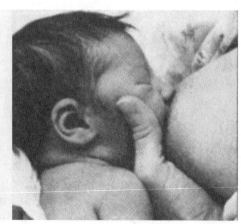

FIGURE 13-7 Dancer hold.

BOX 13-2 Indicators of Effective Latch

- The upper and lower lips are flanged outward.
- The tongue is cupped under the breast and is visible above the lower gum ridge.
- The infant is using wide gliding jaw movements.
- There is no nipple pain or trauma after feeding.

    d. As the mouth gapes open, quickly bring the baby to the breast.
       i. Aim the nipple toward the roof of the mouth.
       ii. Avoid a jerky, rapid arm movement to avoid startling the infant.
       iii. Ensure that the baby's chin touches the breast first, then bring the baby's mouth up over the areola to take in a large mouthful of breast. The chin pressing on the breast stimulates the baby to reach over the nipple and grasp a mouthful of breast to initiate the suckling response.[3] "Babies were four times more likely to suckle effectively when their chin made contact with their mother's breast as they approached the nipple."[14(p9)]
       iv. Ensure that the infant's nose is touching, or positioned close to, the breast.[31,32]
   5. Reassure parents if they have concerns about the infant's nose and the ability to breathe.
    a. If the nose is blocked, normal healthy neonates will release the breast to breathe through the mouth.
    b. Most infants have broad noses, with nares at the sides, which allows them to breathe comfortably, even when the nose is touching the breast.[33]
    c. Depressing the breast tissue to keep it away from the baby's nose is discouraged.
       i. It may alter the latch by pulling the breast out of the baby's mouth.
       ii. It may change the angle of the nipple in the baby's mouth and cause nipple trauma.
       iii. Pressure on the breast may contribute to blocked ducts.
    d. If there is concern that the infant cannot breathe, the infant can be slightly adjusted by raising the baby's buttocks or tucking the buttocks closer to the mother's body. This brings the baby's chin closer to the breast, creating more space between the infant's nose and the breast.
E. Monitor the infant's mouth position on the breast.
   1. The breast is not *placed into* the baby's mouth; the baby *draws* the breast into the mouth.
   2. "An asymmetrical, or slightly off-center latch, seems to aid in achieving a deep latch" (as opposed to a centered latch).[34(p358)]
   3. Observe the mouth for an effective latch.
    a. Lips are flanged out.
    b. Mouth is wide open.
    c. Chin is close to, or touching, the breast.
    d. Tongue is underneath the breast and over the alveolar ridge.
   4. With a proper latch, the infant maintains the latch throughout the feeding.
   5. Be alert to signs of an ineffective latch.
    a. Tight, pursed lips.
    b. Lower lip pulled in.
    c. Dimpling of the cheeks.
    d. Reports of nipple pain.
    e. Flattened or misshapen nipple following feeding.
   6. Clicking or smacking sounds during sucking may or may not indicate a problem and warrants further assessment.
   7. Observe for signs of milk transfer (swallowing).
    a. Wide jaw excursions.
    b. Audible swallow producing a *ca* sound from the throat.
    c. Deep jaw excursions with a pause preceding each swallow.[35]
    d. Adequate infant elimination based on infant age.

F.   Assess the infant's suck.
1.   In the first 24 hours after birth, term, healthy newborns exhibit less rhythmic sucking than older infants.[34]
2.   In the first 2 days of life, the infant will suck with short, rapid bursts with each swallow due to the relatively small volume of colostrum. A regular feeding rhythm begins about the 3rd to 4th day of life with the onset of lactogenesis II.[34]
3.   Teach parents how to differentiate between nutritive and nonnutritive sucking.
     a.   Nutritive sucking exhibits deep, slow sucks, about one suck per second, with a brief pause to swallow when the milk starts flowing.[36]
     b.   Nonnutritive sucking is more rapid, about two sucks per second, with little or no swallowing noted.[36]
     c.   An infant who is not displaying signs of nutritive sucking should be evaluated carefully for adequate milk intake. Nonnutritive sucking may indicate low milk volume.[1,2]
4.   Caution parents about the impact of pacifier or dummy use on breastfeeding.
     a.   Pacifiers should be used with caution during the newborn period.[17]
     b.   Earlier studies indicated that pacifier use had the potential to be detrimental to the establishment of exclusive breastfeeding.[37,38]
          i.   A 2009 systematic review of the literature did not identify a detrimental relationship between pacifier use and breastfeeding, but further study was recommended. The review did suggest that pacifier use may suppress normal infant feeding behaviors and lead to decreased feeding frequency.[39]
          ii.   A 2012 Cochrane Review found that "pacifier use in healthy term breastfeeding infants, started from birth or after lactation is established, did not significantly affect the prevalence or duration of exclusive and partial breastfeeding up to four months of age. However, evidence to assess the short-term breastfeeding difficulties . . . and long-term effect of pacifiers on infants' health is lacking."[40(p1)]
          iii. A 2013 study found that pacifier restriction resulted in increased formula supplementation.[41]
     c.   The 2016 American Academy of Pediatrics Task Force on Sudden Infant Death Syndrome continues to recommend delaying the use of a pacifier until breastfeeding is well established,[42] citing their 2012 breastfeeding policy statement.[16] The 2016 sudden infant death policy statement does not include any updated evidence regarding pacifier use and its impact on breastfeeding.[42]
     d.   The WHO continues to recommend avoiding all bottles, teats, and pacifiers to foster the establishment of exclusive breastfeeding.[43]
     e.   Further study is required to more firmly identify the impact of pacifier use on breastfeeding initiation and exclusivity in the immediate postpartum period.
G.   Monitor the frequency of feedings.
1.   Infants should be fed a minimum of eight times in 24 hours.[44,45] Watching for and responding to early feeding cues is more likely to result in an effective latch. Crying is a late indication of hunger and may make it more difficult for the infant to latch and suck effectively.
2.   Breastfed infants should be fed throughout the night.[45] WHO and UNICEF recommend that infants feed on demand and as often as the child wants, day and night.[46]
3.   Some infants may require more frequent feedings, while others may cluster feedings close together and then rest for a stretch of 4 hours or more.[45]
4.   Frequent, unrestricted feedings in the first few days of life facilitate the development of robust milk production.
5.   Skin-to-skin contact allows the opportunity to observe early feeding cues and rouse a sleepy baby.[47]
6.   Infants should be aroused for a feeding if more than 4 hours have elapsed since the beginning of the previous feed.[44]
H.   Monitor a sleepy infant.
1.   Infants may be sleepy in the first day or two of life.
2.   Evaluation and breastfeeding management may be indicated for a sleepy infant who is not feeding 8–12 times in the first 24–48 hours of life, demonstrates less than a 7 percent weight loss, and shows no signs of illness. According to the Academy of Breastfeeding Medicine, a sleepy infant may go up to 24 hours without feeding.[47]

3. Paying attention to early feeding cues and gently rousing the infant to attempt breastfeeding every 2–3 hours is more appropriate than automatic supplementation.[47]

4. Holding the infant skin to skin will trigger the infant's innate feeding reflexes and may increase feeding frequency.[9]

I. Assess for the potential need for supplementation.

1. Parents may question the adequacy of early feedings and often receive conflicting advice from friends, family, and healthcare providers.

2. Coordinated support, encouragement, and consistent information from all healthcare providers during the early days of breastfeeding are vital in promoting exclusive breastfeeding.

3. Inappropriate supplementation can undermine a parent's confidence in the ability to breastfeed.[48]
   a. A lack of confidence leads to early discontinuation of breastfeeding.[49]
   b. Psychosocial factors impact exclusive breastfeeding. In particular, self-efficacy, which includes self-confidence, is a strong predictor of long-term, exclusive breastfeeding.[50]

4. "Human milk is considered the food of choice for infants in the first 6 months of life."[51(p3)]

5. Supplementation is not immediately indicated for a sleepy infant.[47]

6. Supplementation of healthy newborns who are feeding regularly is not necessary.[43]

7. Supplementation can interfere with the normal frequency of breastfeeding[47] and impacts the infant's microbiome.[51] (See Chapter 7, *Biochemistry of Human Milk*.)

8. Concern about the adequacy of breastfeeding requires a formal evaluation of the dyad, including direct observation of a breastfeeding session, to determine the need for any supplementation.[47]
   a. Supplementation may be necessary if breastfeeding is not possible due to maternal or infant illness.
   b. A weight loss in excess of 7 percent may indicate inadequate milk transfer or milk production,[52] although a weight loss from 8 to 10 percent may be within normal limits if all else is going well and the physical exam is normal.[50,53]
   c. A 2016 systematic literature review revealed a lack of consensus on what is considered excessive weight loss in a normal breastfed infant during the first days of life.[54] A comprehensive evaluation of the breastfeeding dyad is more appropriate than using weight loss alone to determine the need for supplementation.

9. If supplementation results from parental request, educate the parents regarding the impact of supplementation on breastfeeding and document the teaching.[47]

10. If supplementation is initiated, support milk production through early, regular, and frequent milk removal. (See the discussion of milk expression in Chapter 31, *Expression and Use of Human Milk*.)

J. Understand expected infant elimination patterns.

1. In general, newborn stools go through several changes in the first few days of life. Initially infants pass black, tarry stools (meconium), followed by transitional stools that are looser and lighter in color.[51]

2. Elimination patterns that might indicate potential breastfeeding problems include the following[52]:
   a. Not passing transitional or seedy yellow stools by 4 days of age.
   b. Having fewer than six clear voids per day by 4 days of age.
   c. Appearance of urate crystals in the diaper after 3 days of age.

3. Increased stools each day during the first 5 days of life are significantly associated with decreased weight loss and an earlier return to birth weight.[55]

4. An output of fewer than four daily stools by the 4th day of life is a predictor of inadequate breastfeeding.[56]

5. A continuation of meconium stools on day 5 of life is considered a delayed stooling pattern.[47]

K. Evaluate a feeding.

1. A systematic evaluation of a feeding session should take place every 8–12 hours during the early postpartum period.[44,45]
   a. Assess for effective position and latch, and correct as needed.
   b. Maternal discomfort with continued nipple pain throughout the feeding or increased nipple trauma indicates a need to improve the latch, even when the infant is swallowing and is satisfied after feeds.
   c. Assess the infant for signs of milk transfer.
      i. Sustained, rhythmic, nutritive suck–swallow–breathe pattern with periodic pauses.
      ii. Audible swallowing, which will change based on the age of the infant.
      iii. Relaxed arms and hands.

2. Evaluate the end of the feeding.
    a. The nipple should appear rounded, with no evidence of trauma. Note any abnormal nipple shape, blister, or blanching.
    b. The mother should appear relaxed and report no shoulder, neck, or back pain.
    c. The infant should appear calm, satiated, and relaxed.
3. Complete the following tasks after the feeding:
    a. Document the encounter. (See Chapter 27, *Problem Solving and Documentation,* for information about documentation.)
    b. Consult with the healthcare team as needed for any concerns regarding milk production, adequacy of infant intake, and the overall health of the breastfeeding dyad.

IV. Managing Challenges in Initiating Breastfeeding

A. Some infants do not readily latch and effectively suck immediately after birth.
B. The reasons for failure to latch and feed are varied and complex:
    1. Drowsy mother or infant as a result of labor medications, duration of labor, or labor complications.
    2. Mechanical or physical results of labor and delivery.
    3. Separation of the dyad.
    4. Prematurity. (See Chapter 14, *Breastfeeding and the Preterm Infant.*)
    5. Infant illness or congenital anomalies, including oral anatomy. (see Chapter 23, *Breastfeeding and Infant Birth Injury, Congenital Anomalies, and Illness.*)
    6. Maternal physical or psychological health problems. (See Chapter 17, *Maternal Physical Health and Breastfeeding*, and Chapter 18, *Maternal Mental Health and Breastfeeding.*)
    7. Challenging breast anatomy. (See Chapter 20, *Breast Pathology.*)
C. When an infant has not latched effectively within the first 24 hours of life, breastfeeding may be established with the passage of time, appropriate evaluation, and timely interventions.[47]
D. If the dyad's health status allows, encourage continuous skin-to-skin contact and attempting to breastfeed whenever feeding cues are displayed. The benefits to breastfeeding of skin-to-skin contact continue beyond the immediate newborn period.[57]
    1. Dim the lights to encourage a sleepy infant to open the eyes or to help calm a fussy, overstimulated infant.[34]
    2. Avoid using a pacifier.
E. If the infant is unable to feed effectively, protect the production of milk. (See Chapter 31, *Expression and Use of Human Milk,* for information about milk expression.)
    1. Effective colostrum removal within the first hour after birth maximizes the benefits of expressing milk to protect milk production.[58]
        a. Teach hand expression of colostrum within an hour of birth. "In the early postpartum period the best way to obtain colostrum is by gentle manual expression."[59(p39)]
        b. Hand expression of colostrum onto the nipple may entice the baby to latch and feed.
        c. If the infant struggles to latch and feed, appears sleepy, does not display breast-seeking behaviors, feeds briefly, or is not satisfied after latching and feeding, the mother can express colostrum into a spoon and feed it to the baby. Often a baby will latch and feed effectively at the breast after being fed expressed colostrum.[60]
        d. If the mother is tired, ill, or otherwise unable to participate in milk expression, the nursing staff or a family member can hand express colostrum if the mother's condition is stable.
    2. Encourage continued expression eight times per 24 hours and feed the colostrum or milk to the baby until effective feeding is established.
        a. If the infant has not latched and fed effectively after 24 hours, facilitate access to an electric breast pump. Provide instruction on its use and encourage pumping 8–12 times per day. Combining pumping with hand expression maximizes milk production.[61,62]

       b.   If an electric pump is not available, teach parents how to sustain milk production through hand expression.

F.   For an infant struggling with latch, conduct a systematic evaluation of feeding attempts. Direct observation is essential when managing breastfeeding difficulties.

    1.   Teach how to soften edematous nipples with gentle pressure applied by the fingertips around the areola (reverse pressure softening).[63]

    2.   Teach how to stimulate a nonerectile nipple with hand expression to draw the nipple out and make it easier for the baby to latch.

    3.   Pain during latch or throughout a feeding requires assistance and possible correction of positioning or latch.

    4.   If pain persists beyond 24 hours, or if nipple trauma is evident and is unresolved with a change in positioning or latch, consider a referral for an evaluation of infant oral anatomy.

    5.   The use of a thin silicone nipple shield has been found to facilitate a sustained latch in some circumstances, and may reduce maternal nipple pain; however, it requires appropriate use and close monitoring.[64] (See Chapter 24, *Breastfeeding Devices and Topical Treatments,* for a discussion of nipple shield use.)

    6.   Consult with healthcare providers in other disciplines regarding complications that are outside the scope of practice for lactation consultants, such as restriction on infant tongue movement indicating possible ankyloglossia. (See Chapter 32, *Interdisciplinary Lactation Services,* for information about interdisciplinary lactation care.)

G.   Support the infant's nutritional needs while determining the cause of the breastfeeding difficulty.

    1.   In the first 24 hours of life, feed the baby hand-expressed colostrum by spoon or dropper after every breastfeeding attempt (8–12 times per 24 hours), watching for early feeding cues.

    2.   If challenges continue beyond 24–48 hours, consider supplementation at the breast utilizing a supplemental device with expressed milk, pasteurized donor milk, or artificial baby milk.

    3.   The volume of supplement to be given varies with the age of the infant; however, it should always be determined by the infant's indication of satiation.

    4.   A healthy breastfed infant's average intake of colostrum is as follows:[47]

        a.   First 24 hours: 2–10 mL.

        b.   24–48 hours: 5–15 mL.

        c.   48–72 hours: 15–30 mL.

        d.   72–96 hours: 30–60 mL.

H.   Assist when the dyad is separated or when breastfeeding is temporarily contraindicated.

    1.   Begin hand expression within the first hour after birth, and continue expressing every 2–3 hours for 8–12 sessions per 24 hours. "When oxytocin level is highest (in the first hour after delivery) colostrum is quite easy to express . . . and research supports this may be a critical window of time to maximize the benefits [of expressing]."[65(p1)]

    2.   Mothers who are separated from their sick or preterm infants should be "instructed on how to use skilled hand expression or the double set-up electric breast pump."[45(p175)]

        a.   Express at least eight times per day or approximately every 3 hours for 15 minutes (or until milk flow stops, whichever is greater).

        b.   Express around the clock and during the night.

    3.   Whenever feasible, assist the family in obtaining a quality breast pump and instruct them on using the pump within 6 hours of birth or as soon as possible after delivery. (See Chapter 31, *Expression and Use of Human Milk,* for information about milk expression.)

    4.   Combining electric pumping with hand expression increases milk production and the caloric content of the milk.[62,66]

    5.   Video instructions for a hands-on pumping technique can be found at https://med.stanford.edu/newborns/professional-education/breastfeeding/maximizing-milk-production.html.

    6.   If a breast pump is not available or feasible, continued hand expression will help to maintain milk production until the infant can begin breastfeeding.

    7.   Encourage frequent, unrestricted breastfeeding as soon as conditions permit.[45]

    8.   Offer encouragement and emotional support.

I. Complete the following tasks prior to discharge from the hospital setting:
1. Develop an appropriate plan of care.
2. Provide referral and contact information for follow up with a breastfeeding expert and other health-care providers as appropriate to the specific situation.
3. Complete any needed documentation. (See Chapter 27, *Problem Solving and Documentation,* for information about documentation.)

CLINICAL TIPS[45]

Teaching tips for the first days of life:
- Watch for *active* sucking.
- Listen for swallows.
- Monitor stool output:
  - Initial meconium (black tarry stools) (days 1–3)
  - Transition to brown-green stools (days 2–4)
- Monitor adequate urine output:
  - At least one or two wet diapers daily (days 1–3)
  - At least six wet diapers daily (by day 4)
- Pacifiers or dummies should be used with caution because they may interfere with identifying and responding to infant feeding cues.
- Request assistance for any nipple pain or trauma.

▶ Key Points from This Chapter

A. Place infant skin to skin immediately after delivery to facilitate the initiation of breastfeeding.
B. Teach parents to respond to early feeding cues; encourage rooming-in and extended periods of skin-to-skin contact, allowing for unrestricted feeding opportunities.
C. Encourage frequent breastfeeding sessions (8–12 times in 24 hours) and monitor the infant for signs of adequate milk intake.
D. Provide support and assistance with positioning and latch to the breastfeeding dyad.
E. Weight loss greater than 7 percent may indicate inadequate milk transfer or low milk production; prior to supplementation a formal evaluation of a breastfeeding session must take place.
F. If the infant is unable to initiate breastfeeding, support the infant's nutritional needs through appropriate supplementation and support the mother's milk production using evidence-based techniques for milk expression.

℗ CASE STUDY

Jasmine is a 26-year-old first time mother with a history of polycystic ovarian syndrome (PCOS). Jasmine was taking metformin to assist with conception and she continued with the medication through her 12th week of pregnancy. The pregnancy was uncomplicated, and Jasmine carried the infant, Cameron, to term. Labor was uneventful, and Cameron was delivered vaginally with no complications. Jasmine received an epidural for pain control.

Immediately after delivery, Cameron was placed skin to skin for 30 minutes. Jasmine states that Cameron latched and fed intermittently for 15 minutes, though nursing staff did not observe the feeding. Following the initial feeding session, Cameron was moved to the nursery for bathing and Jasmine was transferred to the postpartum unit. Jasmine and Cameron were separated for 3–4 hours. After they were reunited, Cameron would not latch to the breast despite hands-on assistance from the nurse. At 12 hours postpartum Jasmine was shown how to use an electric breast pump to initiate and maintain milk production. Cameron received supplemental feeds of expressed colostrum and formula, initially via syringe and eventually by bottle. When Jasmine and Cameron were discharged on day 2 postpartum,

CASE STUDY *(continued)*

Cameron was still not latching. Jasmine received instructions to continue expressing milk eight times daily with an electric breast pump and to make an appointment for routine follow-up care with Cameron's healthcare provider in 2–3 days.

Questions

1. What were some of the early actions that may have impacted Cameron's ability to latch?
2. What additional methods could have been implemented to encourage Cameron to latch and settle into a feeding?
3. What other instructions regarding milk removal would have been helpful to Jasmine in establishing and maintaining milk production?
4. What should have been included in the discharge plans to support Jasmine's breastfeeding efforts and promote breastfeeding success?

References

1. Woolridge M. The "anatomy" of infant sucking. *Midwifery*. 1986;2(4):164-171.
2. Mathew OP, Jatinder BJ. Sucking and breathing patterns during breast and bottle feeding in the term neonate. *Am J Dis Child*. 1989;143(5):588-592. doi:10.1001/archpedi.1989.02150170090030.
3. Bergman J, Bergman N. Whose choice? Advocating birthing practices according to baby's biological needs. *J Perinat Educ*. 2013;22(1):8-13. doi:10.1891/1058-1243.22.
4. World Health Organization, United Nations Children's Fund. *Baby-Friendly Hospital Initiative: Revised, Updated, and Expanded for Integrated Care*. Geneva, Switzerland: World Health Organization; 2009. https://www.unicef.org/nutrition/files/BFHI_2009_s1.pdf. Accessed September 27, 2017.
5. Kozhimannil KB, Attanasio LB, Hardeman RR, O'Brien M. Doula care supports near-universal breastfeeding initiation among diverse, low-income women. *J Midwifery Womens Health*. 2013;58(4):378-382. doi:10.1111/jmwh.12065.
6. Baby-Friendly USA. *Guidelines and Evaluation Criteria for Facilities Seeking Baby-Friendly Designation*. Albany, NY: Baby-Friendly USA; 2016. https://d14abeop4cfxkt.cloudfront.net/cms/files/386/files/original/GEC2016.pdf. Accessed September 27, 2017.
7. UNICEF UK. *The Evidence and Rationale for the UNICEF UK Baby Friendly Initiative Standards*. London, England: UNICEF UK; 2013. http://www.unicef.org.uk/Documents/Baby_Friendly/Research/baby_friendly_evidence_rationale.pdf. Accessed September 27, 2017.
8. Moore ER, Anderson GC, Berman N, Dowswell T. Early skin-to-skin contact for mothers and their healthy newborn infants. *Cochrane Database Syst Rev*. 2012;5:CD003519. doi:10.1002/14651858.CD003519.pub3.
9. Widström AM, Lilja G, Aaltomaa-Michalias P, Dahllöf M, Nissen E. Newborn behavior to locate the breast when skin-to-skin: a possible method for enabling early self-regulation. *Acta Paediatrica*. 2011;100(1):79-85.
10. Crenshaw J. Healthy birth practice #6: keep mother and baby together—it's best for mother, baby, and breastfeeding. *J Perinat Educ*. 2014;23(4):211-217. doi:10.1891/1058-1243.23.4.211.
11. Kiremitci S, Tuzun R, Yesilirmak DC, Kumral A, Duman N, Ozkan H. Is gastric aspiration needed for newborn management in delivery room? *Resuscitation*. 2011;82(1):40-44. doi:10.1016/j.resuscitation.2010.09.004.
12. Kattwinkel J, Perlman J, Aziz K, et al. Neonatal resuscitation: 2010 American Heart Association guidelines for cardiopulmonary resuscitation and emergency cardiovascular care. *Pediatrics*. 2010;126(5):e1400-e1413. doi:10.1542/peds.2010-2972E.
13. Neumann I, Mounsey A, Das N. Suctioning neonates at birth: time to change our approach. *J Fam Pract*. 2014;63(8):461-462.
14. Cantrill RM, Creedy D, Cooke M, Dykes F. Effective suckling in relation to naked maternal-infant body contact in the first hour of life: an observation study. *BMC Pregnancy Childbirth*. 2014;14:20. doi:10.1186/1471-2393-14-20.
15. Hazzani F. Is oronasopharyngeal suctioning necessary in neonatal resuscitation? *J Clin Neonatol*. 2013;2(3):118-120. doi:10.4103/2249-4847.119992.
16. American Academy of Pediatrics. Breastfeeding and the use of human milk. *Pediatrics*. 2012;129(3):e827-e841. www.pediatrics.org/cgi/doi/10.1542/peds.2011-3552. Published March 2012. Accessed September 27, 2017.
17. Holmes AV, McLeod AY, Bunik M. ABM clinical protocol #5: peripartum breastfeeding management for the healthy mother and infant at term, revision 2013. *Breastfeeding Med*. 2013;8(6):469-473. doi:10.1089/bfm.2013.9979.
18. Widström AM, Ransjo-Arvidson AB, Christensson K, Matthiesen AS, Winberg J, Ivnas-Moberg K. Gastric suction in healthy newborn infants effects on circulation and developing feeding behavior. *Acta Padiatr Scand*. 1987;76:566-572. doi:10.1111/j.1651-2227.1987.tb10522.x.
19. Righard L, Alade M. Effect of delivery room routines on success of first breastfeed. *Lancet*. 1990;336;1105-1107.
20. Varendi H, Christensson K, Winberg J, Porter RH. Soothing effect of amniotic fluid smell in newborn infants. *Early Hum Dev*. 1998;51:47-55.
21. Varendi H, Porter RH. Breast odor as the only maternal stimulus elicits crawling towards the odour source. *Acta Paediatrica*. 2001;90:372-375.
22. Widström AM, Wahlberg V, Matthiesen AS, et al. Short-term effects of early suckling and touch of the nipple on maternal behavior. *Early Hum Dev*. 1990;21(3):153-163.
23. Christensson K, Cabrera T, Christensson E, et al. Separation distress call in the human neonate in the absence of maternal body contact. *Acta Paediatrica*. 1995;84:468-473.
24. Matthiesen AS, Ransjö-Arvidson AB, Nissen E, Uvnäs-Moberg K. Postpartum maternal oxytocin release by newborns: effects of infant hand massage and sucking. *Birth*. 2001;28(1):13-19.

25. UNICEF Maharashtra. *Initiation of Breastfeeding by Breast Crawl*. Mumbai, India: UNICEF India; 2007. http://www.breastcrawl.org /pdf/breastcrawl.pdf. Accessed September 27, 2017.

26. Smillie CM. How newborns learn to latch: a neurobehavioral model for self-attachment in infancy [abstract PL9]. *Acad Breastfeeding Med News View*. 2001;7:23.

27. Bystrova K, Ivanova V, Edhborg M, et al. Early contact versus separation: effects on mother-infant interaction one year later. *Birth*. 2009;36(2):97-109. doi:10.1111/j.1523-536X.2009.00307.x.

28. Zenkner JRG, Miorim CFB, Cardoso LS, et al. Rooming in and breastfeeding: reviewing the impact on scientific production of nursing. *R Pesq Cuid Fundam Online (Revista De Pesquisa Cuidado E Fundamental Online)*. 2013;5(2):3808-3818. doi:10.9789/2175-5361.2013v5n2p3808.

29. Colson SD, Meek JH, Hawdon JM. Optimal positions for the release of primitive neonatal reflexes stimulating breastfeeding. *Early Hum Dev*. 2008;84:441-449.

30. Colson SD. Biological nurturing: the laid-back breastfeeding revolution. *Midwifery Today*. 2012;101:9-11,66.

31. Naylor AJ, Wester RA, eds. *Lactation Management Self-Study Modules: Level I*. 4th ed. Shelburne, VT: Wellstart International; 2013. http://www.wellstart.org/Self-Study-Module.pdf. Accessed September 27, 2017.

32. Wiessinger D, West D, Pitman T. *The Womanly Art of Breastfeeding*. 8th ed. New York, NY: Ballantine Books; 2010.

33. Janke J. Newborn nutrition. In Simpson KR, Creehan PA, eds. *AWHONN Perinatal Nursing*. 4th ed. Philadelphia, PA: Lippincott Williams and Wilkins; 2014:626-632.

34. Lauwers J, Swisher A. *Counseling the Nursing Mother: A Lactation Consultant's Guide*. 6th ed. Burlington, MA: Jones & Bartlett Learning; 2016.

35. Newman J, Pitman T. *The Ultimate Breastfeeding Book of Answers*. Roseville, CA: Prima Publishing, 2006.

36. Wolf LS, Glass RP. The Goldilocks problem: milk flow that is not too fast, not too slow, but *just right* (or why milk flow matters, and what to do about it). In: Genna CW, ed. *Supporting Sucking Skills in Breastfeeding Infants*. 3rd ed. Burlington, MA: Jones & Bartlett Learning; 2017:157-180.

37. Barros FC, Victora CG, Sever TC, Tonioli GS, Tomasi E, Weiderpass E. Use of pacifiers is associated with decreased breast-feeding duration. *Pediatrics*. 1995;95(4):497-499.

38. Howard CR, Howard FM, Lanphear B, et al. Randomized clinical trial of pacifier use and bottle-feeding or cupfeeding and their effect on breastfeeding. *Pediatrics*. 2003;111(3):511-518.

39. O'Connor N, Tanabe K, Siadaty M, Hauck F. Pacifiers and breastfeeding a systematic review. *Arch Pediatr Adolesc Med*. 2009;163(4):378-382.

40. Jaafer SH, Jahanfar S, Angolkar M, Ho JJ. Effect of restricted pacifier use in breastfeeding term infants for increasing duration of breastfeeding. *Cochrane Database Syst Rev*. 2012;7:CD007202. doi:10.1002/14651858.CD007202.pub3.

41. Kair LR, Kenron D, Etheredge K, Jaffer AC, Phillipi CA. Pacifier restriction and exclusive breastfeeding. *Pediatrics*. 2013:131(4):e1101-e1107. doi:10.1542/peds.2012-2203.

42. AAP Task Force on Sudden Infant Death Syndrome. SIDS and other sleep-related infant deaths: updated 2016 recommendations for a safe infant sleeping environment. *Pediatrics*. 2016;138(5):e20162938. doi:10.1542/peds.2016-2938.

43. World Health Organization. Nutrition: exclusive breastfeeding. World Health Organization website. http://www.who.int/nutrition /topics/exclusive_breastfeeding/en/. Published 2016. Retrieved September 27, 2017.

44. American Academy of Pediatrics. *Sample Hospital Breastfeeding Policy for Newborns*. Elk Grove Village, IL: American Academy of Pediatrics; 2009. https://ihcw.aap.org/Documents/POPOT/PDFs/hospital%20breastfeeding%20policy_final.pdf . Retrieved September 27, 2017.

45. Academy of Breastfeeding Medicine Protocol Committee. ABM clinical protocol #7: model breastfeeding policy: revision 2010. *Breastfeeding Med*. 2010;5(4):173-177. doi:10.1089/bfm.2010.9986.

46. World Health Organization, UNICEF. *Protecting, Promoting and Supporting Breast-Feeding: The Special Role of Maternity Services*. Geneva, Switzerland: World Health Organization; 1989. http://www.who.int/nutrition/publications/infantfeeding/9241561300/en/. Accessed September 27, 2017.

47. Academy of Breastfeeding Medicine. ABM clinical protocol #3: supplementary feedings in the healthy term breastfed neonate, revised 2017. Breastfeeding Med. 2017;1212(4): 188-198. doi:10.1089/bfm.2017.29038.ajk.

48. Blyth R, Creedy D, Dennis C, Moyle, W, Pratt, J, DeVries, SM. Effect of maternal confidence on breastfeeding duration: an application of breastfeeding self-efficacy theory. *Birth*. 2002;29(4):278-284.

49. Keister D, Kismet T, Roberts TK, Werner SL. Strategies for breastfeeding success. *Am Fam Physicians*. 2008;78(2):225-232.

50. DeJager E, Skouteris H, Broadbent J, Amir L, Mellor K. Psychosocial correlates of exclusive breastfeeding: a systematic review. *Midwifery*. 2013;29:506-518.

51. Ganduaraldi FW, Salvatori G. Effect of breast and formula feeding on gut microbiota shaping. *Newborns Front Cell Infect Microbiol*. 2012;2(94). doi:10.3389/fcimb.2012.00094.

52. Neifert M. Prevention of breastfeeding tragedies. *Pediatr Clin North Am*. 2001;48:278-297.

53. Flaherman VJ, Schaefer EW, Kuzniewicz MW, et al. Early weight loss nomograms for exclusively breastfed newborns. *Pediatrics*. 2015;135(1):e16-e23. doi:10.1542/peds.2014-1532.

54. Thulier D. Weighing the facts: a systematic review of expected patterns of weight loss in full-term, breastfed infants. *J Hum Lactation*. 2016;32(1):28-34.

55. Shrago LC, Reifsnider E, Insel K. The neonatal bowel output study: indicators of adequate breastmilk intake in neonates. *Pediatr Nurs*. 2006;32(3):195-201.

56. Nommsen-Rivers LA, Heinig MG, Cohen RJ, Dewey KG. Newborn wet and soiled diaper counts and timing of onset of lactation as indicators of breastfeeding inadequacy. *J Hum Lactation*. 2008;24(1):27-33. doi:10.1177/0890334407311538.

57. Svensson KE, Velandia MI, Matthiesen A-ST, et al. Effects of mother-infant skin-to-skin contact on severe latch-on problems in older infants: a randomized trial. *Int Breastfeeding J*. 2013;8:1. doi:10.1186/1746-4358-8-1.

58. Morton J, Hall J, Pessl M. Five steps to improve bedside breastfeeding care. *Nurs Womens Health*. 2013;17(6):478-487.

59. Ohyama M, Watabe H, Hayasaka Y. Manual expression and electric breast pumping in the first 48 hours after delivery. *Pediatr Int.* 2010;52(1):39-43. doi:10.1111/j.1442-200X.2009.02910.x.

60. Smith LJ. Why Johnny can't suck: impact of birth practices on infant suck. In: Genna CW, ed. *Supporting Sucking Skills in Breastfeeding Infants.* 3rd ed. Burlington, MA: Jones & Bartlett Learning; 2017:59-77

61. Morton J. The importance of hands. *J Hum Lactation.* 2012;28(3):276-277. doi:10.1177/0890334412444930.

62. Morton J, Hall JY, Wong RJ, et al. Combining hand techniques with electric pumping increases milk production in mothers of preterm infants. *J Perinatol.* 2009;29(11):757-764.

63. Cotterman, KJ. Reverse pressure softening: a simple tool to prepare areola for easier latching during engorgement. *J Hum Lactation.* 2004;20:227-237.

64. Chow S, Chow R, Popovic M, et al. The use of nipple shields: a review. *Frontiers Public Health.* 2015;3:236. doi:10.3389/fpubh.2015.00236.

65. Lactationmatters. Hand expression: Q & A with #ILCA 15 conference speaker Jane Morton. International Lactation Consultant Association website. https://lactationmatters.org/tag/jane-morton/. Published March 9, 2015. Accessed September 28, 2017.

66. Morton J, Wong RJ, Hall JY, et al. Combining hand techniques with electric pumping increases the caloric content of milk in mothers of preterm infants. *J. Perinatol.* 2012;28(1):11-13.

Additional Resources

Academy of Breastfeeding Medicine. www.bfmed.org.
American Academy of Family Physicians. www.aafp.org.
American Academy of Pediatrics. https://www.aap.org/en-us/Pages/Default.aspx.
American Congress of Obstetricians and Gynecologists. www.acog.org.
Baby-Friendly USA. www.babyfriendlyusa.org.
Global Health Media. Videos. https://globalhealthmedia.org/videos/breastfeeding/.
International Baby Food Action Network. www.ibfan.org.
International Lactation Consultant Association. www.ilca.org.
La Leche League International. http://www.llli.org/.
Mother and Child Health and Education Trust. Breast Crawl. http://www.breastcrawl.org/video.shtml.
Stanford Medicine. Getting Started with Breastfeeding. http://med.stanford.edu/newborns/professional-education/breastfeeding.html.
UNICEF. www.unicef.org.
Wellstart International. www.wellstart.org.
World Alliance for Breastfeeding Action. www.waba.org.my.
World Health Organization. Maternal, Newborn, Child and Adolescent Health. www.who.int/child_adolescent_health.
World Health Organization. Nutrition. www.who.int/nutrition/en.

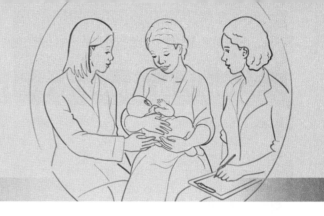

CHAPTER 14

Breastfeeding and the Preterm Infant

Kerstin Hedberg Nyqvist
Suzanne Hetzel Campbell
Laura N. Haiek

OBJECTIVES

- Understand problems associated with prematurity and their effects on the establishment of breastfeeding.
- Understand the nutritional needs of the preterm infant and the importance of human milk.
- Understand the importance of the use of pasteurized donor human milk if the mother's own milk is not available.
- List the scientific basis for breastfeeding the preterm infant.
- Describe how maturation influences suckling, swallowing, and breathing coordination and the impact on the preterm infant's ability to breastfeed.
- List the characteristics of preterm and late preterm infants that challenge successful breastfeeding.
- Understand the importance of kangaroo care (skin to skin) for mothers, infants, and establishing successful breastfeeding.
- Describe the importance of a developmentally sensitive environment in the intensive care nursery.
- Describe a discharge feeding plan for the preterm infant.

DEFINITIONS OF COMMONLY USED TERMS

birth weight The weight at which an infant is born, which comparatively may be qualified as the following:
- Extremely low birth weight: Infant weighs less than 1,000 grams at birth.
- Very low birth weight: Infant weighs less than 1,500 grams (3.3 pounds) but more than 1,000 grams (2.2 pounds) at birth.
- Low birth weight: Infant weighs less than 2,500 grams at birth.

(continues)

DEFINITIONS OF COMMONLY USED TERMS　*(continued)*

early enteral feedings　Feedings of human milk or or human milk substitutes (infant formula) via an enteral tube directly into the infant's stomach. "Early" has been defined as prior to 72 hours after birth in most cases.

family　Includes significant others and is defined by the parent (or parents) or guardian.

gastric emptying　The emptying of food from the stomach.

gastric residual　The volume of fluid remaining in a preterm infant's stomach at some point after a feeding.

gestational age　The age referred to during pregnancy to describe the time in weeks from the first day of the last menstrual cycle to the current date.

human milk feeding　Providing infants with human milk by feeding methods other than directly at the breast.

kangaroo mother care (KMC)　Early, prolonged, and continuous skin-to-skin contact between a birth parent (or substitute) and a newborn low birth weight infant, both in hospital and after early discharge, until at least about the 40th week of postmenstrual age, with ideally exclusive breastfeeding and proper follow-up.[1] May also be referred to as kangaroo care or skin-to-skin care.

lactoengineering　Tailoring breastmilk to the specific needs of a baby; may include separation of hindmilk for preterm infants for greater calorie and fat intake at a lower volume.

Luer taper　Used for making leak-free connections, it is a standardized system of small-scale fluid fittings on medical and laboratory instruments that connect a male taper fitting and its female counterpart, including hypodermic syringe tips and needles or stopcocks and needles.

neonatal intensive care unit (NICU)　A specialty unit or ward where intensive care is provided to preterm and ill newborn babies.

postmenstrual age　Corresponds to gestational age plus chronological age.

postnatal age　Corresponds to chronological age or time elapsed since birth.

preterm　Babies born alive before 37 weeks' gestation have been completed, including the following:

- Extremely preterm: Less than 28 weeks.
- Very preterm: 28 weeks to 31 weeks, 6 days.
- Moderately preterm: 32 weeks to 33 weeks, 6 days.
- Late preterm: 34 weeks to 36 weeks, 6 days.

supplementation　Feeding by other means than at the breast; can consist of human milk or human milk substitutes (infant formula).

Any use of the term *mother*, *maternal*, or *breastfeeding* is not meant to exclude transgender or nonbinary parents who may be breastfeeding or providing human milk to their infant.

▸ Overview

The overwhelming evidence of the importance of breastfeeding and human milk for the health and well-being of preterm infants is indisputable, yet establishing breastfeeding for a preterm infant can be a challenge. Globally, infants who are not fed their mother's own milk have an increased morbidity and mortality rate, and if the mother's milk is not available, pasteurized donor human milk is the next best option. Typically, the preterm infant has been treated as a medical wonder that requires oversight and direct care from specialists; therefore, it can be overwhelming for parents to envision their role in the care, protection, growth, and development of their fragile infant. Parents of preterm infants experience challenges that are unique to the preterm situation in addition to the stress that is involved in a life event that has an uncertain outcome.

Despite increasing evidence of preterm infants' early oral motor capacity, guidelines restricting initiation of breastfeeding to certain gestational age and postmenstrual ages are still common. Also erroneously, professionals may use various methods for testing infant sucking capacity and for training infants to suck before breastfeeding is introduced—interventions that only delay the initiation of breastfeeding and have been proven unnecessary.[2-4] The only criterion for initiation of breastfeeding should be infant stability, independent of gestational age, postnatal age, postmenstrual age, or weight.[5,6]

The focus of this chapter is on the strengths of preterm infants and the vitally important role of the mothers whose presence via skin-to-skin contact or kangaroo mother care, provision of human milk, and nurturing and protection are necessary for the infants' survival. Recognizing that many infants in the neonatal intensive care unit (NICU) may be critically ill and may not be able to feed at the breast or have immediate skin-to-skin care, as much as this is desired, this chapter provides encouragement and support by envisioning the possibilities and breaking down the myths surrounding feeding preterm infants and how to support dyads to successfully breastfeed. The role of the lactation consultant will also be outlined, including advocating for incorporation of the Baby-Friendly Hospital Initiative for Neonatal Wards (Neo-BFHI) policies and practices[7] that allow for the best environment, support, and resources possible for the parents of preterm infants to provide human milk for their infants and to meet their breastfeeding goals.

I. Scientific Basis for Breastfeeding the Preterm Infant

A. Breastfeeding and human milk provide numerous advantages for preterm infants.
  1. Breastfeeding (i.e., feeding at the breast) is the optimal feeding behavior for human infants, whether they are born at term or preterm.
     a. To ensure long-term healthy growth and development of infants, the World Health Organization (WHO), UNICEF, and most international organizations recommend exclusive breastfeeding for the first 6 months of life and continued for 2 years or beyond. Although this public health recommendation allows for individual practice, the recommendation for breastfeeding exclusivity and duration is the same for term and preterm infants.
     b. Expert recommendations reinforce the importance of feeding at the breast for preterm infants.[5,6]
  2. The mother's own milk, at the breast or expressed, is the optimal milk for the preterm infant.
     a. Morbidity and mortality rates increase significantly when the infant is not fed human milk.[8,9]
     b. Preterm infants who are fed human milk accrue immune system enhancement, gastrointestinal maturation, and nutrient availability.[8,10]
     c. If the mother's own milk is not available, pasteurized donor human milk is the gold standard; when it is not available, human milk substitute (preterm formula) is an option.[11,12]
  3. Human milk leads to the achievement of greater enteral feeding tolerance and more rapid advancement to full enteral feeds.
     a. Physiological amino acids and fatty acid profiles enhance the digestion and absorption of these nutrients.
     b. Human milk results in a low renal solute load.
  4. The gastric emptying time in a formula-fed preterm infant can be up to twice the time of a human milk-fed infant (51 versus 25 minutes).[13,14]
     a. A systematic review of the impact of feed protein type and degree of hydrolysis on gastric emptying confirmed that human milk has a faster gastric emptying time than formula.[15]
     b. Although some practices in the NICU may include it, another review calls into question the measurement of gastric residuals for preterm infants.[16]
  5. Human milk contains active enzymes (such as lipase, amylase, and lysozyme) that are lacking in the underdeveloped intestine or intestinal system and provide trophic factors that hasten the maturation of the preterm intestinal system.[17]
  6. Human milk provides for optimal development of visual acuity and retinal health.[8]
  7. Cognitive and neurodevelopmental outcomes are enhanced, with preterm infants who have been fed human milk showing higher intelligent quotients (IQs).[18-21] Long-chain polyunsaturated fatty acids that are present in human milk but not in many formulas are considered to be closely linked to this outcome.[19,21]
  8. Human milk provides protection from environmental pathogens.[8] This is particularly important in a special care nursery with invasive treatments and many staff members handling the infant.
B. Breastfeeding offers positive effects for children's health and development in the following areas:
  1. Respiratory benefits.[22,23]
  2. Decreased diarrheal episodes.[22-24]
  3. Decreased acute otitis media. Breastfeeding lowers the odds to contract acute otitis media (dose–response effect).[22,25-29]
  4. Decreased sudden infant death syndrome.[25,28,30-32]
  5. Decreased necrotizing enterocolitis. Human milk-fed preterm newborns have a reduced risk of necrotizing enterocolitis (dose–response effect).[25,28,33-37]
  6. Increased cognitive development (IQ). Breastfeeding is strongly associated with better intelligence test performance, even controlling for confounding variables such as maternal IQ.[22,28,29,38-41]

C. The components of preterm human milk are ideally suited to the preterm infant.
1. Preterm milk is optimally suited to the maturation of systems, immunological requirements, and growth of the preterm infant. Human milk is a medicine for both the infant and the mother—the milk for the infant, and the provision of it for the mother.[11]
2. Preterm milk is optimal for the preterm infant because of the infant's limited renal concentrating and diluting capacities, a large surface area in relation to weight, and insensible water loss.
3. When compared to full-term human milk, preterm has higher concentrations of calories, lipids, high nitrogen protein, sodium, chloride, potassium, iron, and magnesium.[17,42,43]
4. Calcium and phosphorus are the most commonly lacking macrominerals in preterm milk.[44]
5. Often extra nutrients, vitamins, and minerals are added for the very low birth weight infant, research does not yet confirm amounts or requirements.
6. The milk of mothers of preterm infants matures to the level of term milk at about 4 to 6 weeks.
7. In countries where fortification is used, research confirms that human milk with appropriate fortification for the very low birth weight infant is the standard of care.[11,12,45]

D. Preterm infants have unique needs for nutrition and optimal growth.
1. Preterm infants have special nutritional needs because they lack sufficient subcutaneous fat, brown fat, and glycogen, which contributes to an increased risk of hypothermia and hypoglycemia.
2. Optimal growth is typically based on the growth curve that would have been followed if the preterm infant had remained in utero.
    a. This target can be achieved more easily in infants who have higher gestational ages.
    b. The extremely low birth weight infant has a high energy requirement but limited volume tolerance, so the infant's intake might be restricted, which might affect their growth.
3. In some settings, early enteral feedings of human milk before the infant is actually ready to be fed by mouth are sometimes used to prime the gut.[11]
    a. Early enteral feedings are variously referred to as trickle feeds, trophic feeds, or gastrointestinal priming feeds at the following rate: 0.5 to 1.0 mL bolus of human milk via nasogastric tube every 3 or 6 hours.[46,47]
    b. Trophic feeds facilitate protective gut flora, improve bowel emptying of meconium, and decrease morbidity and mortality from necrotizing enterocolitis.[48]
    c. More mature motor patterns in the gut are seen with these small feeds.[49]
    d. If infusion pumps are used for feeding, the syringe should be tilted upward at a 25° to 45° angle so that the lipids rise to the Luer taper of the syringe and are infused first (allowing for a leak-free connection).
4. Many guidelines for the progression of preterm infant feeding exist throughout the world.
    a. Practices depend on the level and availability of technology within the country and within each individual ward or unit.
    b. Many wards or units implement kangaroo mother care (skin to skin), which is included in Step 4 of the Neo-BFHI as a key practice for initiating and maintaining breastfeeding in the preterm infant.[7]
5. Other needs of the preterm infant to facilitate normal growth and development include the following:
    a. Respiratory rate within normal range and stable.
    b. Maintain blood sugar above 2.5 mM/L (40 mg/dL) because neonatal hypoglycemia can have serious ramifications; therefore, screening and intervention are aimed at the detection and treatment of infants who are at risk.[50]
    c. Maintain body temperature within normal range.
    d. Adequate nutrition unique to each infant:
        i. The metabolized energy requirement varies according to gestational age, weight, and wellness of the preterm infant; it can vary from 109 to 140 kcal/kg per day.
        ii. Feedings for an infant at 2,000 g and more than 32 weeks' gestational age usually vary in volume and frequency from a full-term infant.
    e. Continuous or intermittent kangaroo mother care or skin-to-skin contact with mothers, whenever possible, as long and as often as the mothers are able and willing to provide this care.[7,51,52]

E. Preterm infants sometimes receive fortified human milk.
1. Human milk can be fortified with commercial fortifiers that include cow's milk–based protein, electrolytes, and a number of vitamins and minerals.[53]
2. Human milk can be fortified with specific nutrients, such as calcium and phosphorus.
3. Fortification is usually begun after feeding is established, and it is discontinued before discharge from the NICU.
4. Using the hindmilk portion of expressed milk (lactoengineering) as a concentrated source of lipids provides a high-calorie, low-volume, low-osmolar, readily absorbable supplement.[54,55]
5. Hindmilk and commercial fortifiers are used for different purposes.
    a. Commercial fortifiers are used to supplement essential nutrients.
    b. Hindmilk provides a concentrated source of lipids and calories and can be used to increase caloric intake if milk production is in excess of the infant's needs.[11]
6. Lactoengineering can further refine and tailor the milk to a specific infant's needs.[56] More research is needed on fortification in conjunction with the long-term use of hindmilk.
7. The milk can be analyzed using specialized testing techniques available in some clinical settings. The results can be used to determine the infant's fortification needs.
8. The lipid and caloric content of the milk can be estimated by creamatocrit.[57] Creamatocrit is determined by centrifuging a small milk specimen in a capillary tube, separating the lipid portion, then measuring the content as a percentage of total milk volume.[56]

F. There are numerous issues associated with fortification of human milk.
1. Significantly slower gastric emptying times and, therefore, implications for feeding intolerance.[58]
2. Neutralizing effect of some of the anti-infective (lactoferrin) properties of human milk.[59]
3. Possible increased risk of infection.
4. Higher osmolarity of fortified milk, increasing the morbidity from gastrointestinal disease.
5. Some nutrient loss can occur through enteral feeding tubes.
    a. Lipids can adhere to the lumen of a feeding tube and not reach the infant.
    b. The greatest lipid losses occur with continuous slow infusions; therefore, bolus feedings (intermittent gavage) are recommended when possible.
6. Fortification might influence short-term outcomes (such as weight gain and bone mineralization). Long-term growth and development outcomes have not been shown to be enhanced. The bone mineral content of 8- to 12-year-old children who are born preterm and are fed human milk without fortification is as high or higher than children who are born at term.[18]
7. The use of powdered fortifiers is controversial and requires surveillance and additional research.[53]
    a. Powdered fortifiers and powdered preterm formulas are not sterile.
    b. The U.S. Food and Drug Administration, European Food Safety Authority, and Centers for Disease Control and Prevention have issued guidelines stating that powdered formulas should not be used in preterm or immunocompromised infants.[60]
8. An alternative for powdered fortification is liquid fortifiers.
    a. They are often used in a 1:1 ratio with human milk, resulting in a reduction of human milk intake.
    b. They may be used when the volume of available human milk is inadequate.
9. Increasingly, hospitals are using pasteurized donor human milk when available.
    a. If the mother's own milk is not immediately available, the clinician should prioritize the use of pasteurized donor human milk, which has some of the properties of fresh human milk (e.g., immunoglobulins, growth and developmental hormones, enzymes, anti-inflammatory factors), is sterile, and reduces necrotizing enterocolitis while improving feeding tolerance.[11,12,61]
    b. When clinicians address the importance of feeding donor human milk, they demonstrate to families the value of breastfeeding.

G. There are key issues for breastfeeding related to prematurity.
1. Preterm infant characteristics:
    a. Preterm infants spend more time in a diffuse, drowsy state with frequent shifts between sleep and alertness.[62] The signs of waking are subtle (irregular respiration, gasps, grimaces, movements in lips and tongue, raised eyebrows, diffuse movements).

b. Direct light is an obstacle to eye opening, and periods of focused alertness are short. Instead, a glassy-eyed look or a surprised look with wide-open eyes is common. These responses indicate a limited ability to handle visual stimuli.

c. Voices in a normal conversational tone, activity in the visual field, and touch by stroking and tickling the skin can cause stress. This can result in irregular respiration and movements and reducing the infant's availability for activities directed at the breast. Instead, gentle, still touch and sounds of a soft voice are appropriate.

d. Habituation, the capacity to shut out common environmental stimuli, does not mature until term age. Therefore, preterm infants are easily overloaded by stimuli (touch, sounds, visual input, light), especially when they occur simultaneously. They are calm and more active with support for a position of flexed arms and legs and the hands close to the face and mouth.

2. Timing the introduction of breastfeeding:
   a. A study of infants born at a gestational age of 26 to 31 weeks concluded that breastfeeding could be safely introduced from 29 weeks postmenstrual age. In the study 12 out of 14 infants were breastfed exclusively at discharge, and two were partially breastfed. These infants' median (min–max) postmenstrual age at attainment of exclusive breastfeeding was 35 weeks (32–38 weeks).[63]
   b. The only criterion for the introduction of breastfeeding was the absence of severe apnea, bradycardia, and desaturations.

3. Suggested strategies for introducing breastfeeding to preterm infants:
   a. No tests of readiness or training for nutritive sucking at the breast are supported, and there is currently no evidence to inform clinical practice.[64]
   b. No restrictions need be applied with regard to breastfeeding frequency or duration of breast-feeding sessions.
   c. Offer parents an opportunity to be observed while breastfeeding with guidance regarding handling the infant and breastfeeding positions, strategies for assisting their baby's competence, and focused support when challenges arise or if they are identified as high risk for issues with milk production or breastfeeding difficulties.
   d. Resist hands-on support by staff, and provide guidance about preterm infants' behavioral characteristics and how to engage in a mutually responsive interaction.

4. Other strategies for successful breastfeeding:
   a. The transition from scheduled 2-hour feeds to unregulated feeding can be introduced when the infant shows signs of milk intake, such as audible swallowing.
   b. When transitioning to unregulated feeding, it is not necessary to have fixed volumes per feed or fixed intervals for supplementation.
   c. Supplementation is an area of continued debate.
      i. It can be prescribed based on an assessment of the infant's daily intake at the breast, which can be assessed by test weighing before and after breastfeeding.
      ii. If the parent does not want to weigh the infant, it may be sufficient to merely assess the infant's daily weight gain.
   d. Bottles should be avoided for supplementation or when mixed feeding (breast and bottle) is used, unless the parent explicitly states the desire to not breastfeed or to exclusively pump and bottle feed. The preferred method for oral supplementation is cup feeding.[65,66]

H. There are many common conditions associated with prematurity that may affect breastfeeding.
   1. Respiratory distress syndrome: Severe impairment of respiratory function in a preterm newborn, caused by immaturity of the lungs.
   2. Necrotizing enterocolitis: A potentially fatal inflammation with cell death in the lining of the intestines.
   3. Hyperbilirubinemia.
   4. Intracranial hemorrhage.
   5. Hypoglycemia.
   6. Bronchopulmonary dysplasia: Iatrogenic chronic lung disease that develops in preterm infants after a period of positive pressure ventilation.
   7. Patent ductus arteriosus.
   8. Sepsis.
   9. Perinatal acidosis.

10. All the preceding conditions and their treatments usually result in repeated interventions or manipulations and prolonged separation of the preterm infant and parent, resulting in a delay of establishing breastfeeding or an interruption in breastfeeding.

I. The preterm infant requires individualized developmental care.

1. Neonatal individualized developmental care can be incorporated into practice in all intensive or special care nurseries. It is based on the positive development of the five senses: sight, hearing, taste, touch, and smell.[67]

2. Some benefits of a developmentally sensitive environment include the following:
   a. Greater parental involvement and nurturing care.
   b. More time for adequate rest for the infant, which promotes brain development.
   c. Prevention of overstimulation.
   d. Reduced heart rate.
   e. Reduced need for oxygen.
   f. Earlier removal from a ventilator.
   g. Earlier initiation of breastfeeding.
   h. Better weight gain.[68,69]
   i. Reduction in rates of infection.[68]
   j. Shorter hospital stay.[68]
   k. Improved medical and neurodevelopmental outcome.[70-72]

3. The following are examples of an environmentally sensitive special care nursery[67,73,74]:
   a. Lights below 60 footcandles.[74]
   b. Blanket-covering isolette low enough to protect the infant's eyes from direct light.
   c. Day and night rhythmicity.[75]
   d. Cluster care across disciplines, allowing for longer sleep periods.
   e. Controlled noise levels:
      i. Less than 50 decibels.[76,77]
      ii. Low voice level, particularly at shift change.
      iii. Quiet trash removal.
      iv. Quiet closing of isolette doors.
      v. Quiet monitor and ventilator alarms.
      vi. Telephone rings low or silenced.

4. Examples of individualized developmental care include the following:
   a. Positioning the infant to promote feelings of security (i.e., side and foot rolls to support a position with flexed arms and legs and borders for the infant to lie or push against).
   b. Hand containment, preferably done by the parent.
   c. Gentle pressure on the infant's back or chest with an open hand to help infants organize themselves.
   d. Supporting the infant with blankets and rolls while supine or prone.
   e. Midline flexion and containment.
   f. Providing boundaries.
   g. When the infant is lying prone, wetting the fist with expressed milk and positioning it near the infant's nose and mouth.[78]
   h. Use of expressed milk for oral care to help the infant identify the parent's smell and the taste of the milk. Preterm infants have a keen sense of smell and usually respond to human milk by extending the tongue to taste milk and then opening the mouth.
      i. When the infant is comfortably positioned at the breast, the parent can express a drop of milk that remains on the tip of the nipple for the infant to smell and then taste.
      ii. Preterm infants are slow to respond to stimuli, so the parent should be patient.
   i. Recognition that breastfeeding is a developmental skill that will happen when an infant is neurobehaviorally ready.
      i. Sucking pressures are lower in preterm infants, increasing the difficulty in transferring milk.
      ii. The goal of early feedings is to allow the infant to gradually increase breastfeeding skill and stamina, which comes with time and patience.
      iii. Focusing on weight or milk transfer too early can undermine confidence and put breastfeeding at risk.

      j.   Encouraging infants to remain in skin-to-skin contact continuously, or for as long and as often every day as the parents are able and willing.[7]

      k.   Appropriate pain management.[72]

      l.   Massage therapy (for infants showing benefits from that type of touch).[67,79]

      m.   Music therapy.[80]

II. Management of the Preterm Family for Breastfeeding Success

A.   Breastfeeding is a caregiving behavior that does not have to be forfeited because of a preterm birth. Milk expression and breastfeeding can be highly significant contributions to the infant's care that represent a normalization of an abnormal event.

B.   Mothers have identified five positive outcomes or rewards from their preterm breastfeeding experience and have concluded that the rewards outweigh the efforts.[81]

    1.   The health benefits of human milk.

    2.   Knowing that they gave their infants the best possible start in life.

    3.   Enjoyment of the physical closeness and the perception that their infant preferred breastfeeding to bottle feeding.

    4.   Knowing that they made a unique contribution to the infant's care.

    5.   Belief and experience that breastfeeding was more convenient.

C.   Parents of preterm infants have special needs.

    1.   Parents may require special medical considerations resulting from a complicated pregnancy, possibly including illness, prolonged bed rest, or cesarean birth. (See Chapter 17, *Maternal Physical Health and Breastfeeding*.)

    2.   Parents may lack breastfeeding knowledge because of giving birth prior to attending prenatal courses.

    3.   Parental socioeconomic characteristics and infant gestational age, weight, and morbidity may affect successful breastfeeding.

      a.   As a result of advanced technology, the age of viability has improved so that infants of gestational age as early as 22 to 24 weeks are surviving. This situation presents a unique set of hurdles in achieving optimal short-term nutrition and long-term physical and cognitive development.

      b.   Parents of preterm infants experience challenges that are unique to the preterm situation, in addition to the stress that is involved in a life event that has an uncertain outcome.

    4.   Parents should be provided with information to make an informed decision regarding breastfeeding and providing human milk for their infants.

      a.   Withholding information in attempts to avoid making parents feel guilty if they choose not to breastfeed or provide milk denies them the right to make decisions based on factual information.[82-84]

      b.   Parents are highly influenced by the advice of professionals who care for the infant, feeling thankful for (not coerced by) their guidance and resentful if they are misinformed about human milk substitutes (e.g., formula) being equally acceptable.[82-84]

    5.   Parents will need support and education about parenting a preterm infant.

    6.   Facilitating parental infant care in the nursery will increase their confidence and self-efficacy. This approach views parents as primary caregivers and supports them to do care activities that are comfortable to them.[85,86]

    7.   Parents will need help establishing and maintaining lactation.

D.   The NICU physical environment should facilitate breastfeeding.

    1.   The unit should provide a supportive environment for breastfeeding, including adequate privacy and a quiet atmosphere at the bedside and, ideally, a separate room for breastfeeding and milk expression inside the unit.

    2.   Open, unrestricted accommodations for parents with their infants view the parents as partners and not visitors.

      a.   Parents have a need for close physical contact with their infant, such as early and frequent skin-to-skin contact. Skin-to-skin care is associated with increased amounts of milk, longer duration of breastfeeding, and breastfeeding success.[87]

   b. The NICU should be open to parents 24/7, and parents should have unrestricted access to their infants.

   c. Providing the possibility for parents to sleep in close proximity to their infants, including a family-centered environment, is ideal.

  3. Information should be consistent and correct, based on research and not personal experience or opinion. Complying with the Neo-BFHI recommendations ensures that healthcare professionals provide consistent messages based on evidence-based policies and practices; this guideline should be included in the orientation of all new NICU staff members.[7]

  4. Professionals involved in breastfeeding support need adequate preparation (knowledge, skills, and attitude) to recognize preterm infants' characteristics related to breastfeeding and to perform an observation of the breastfeeding dyad to guide parents in the interpretation of the infant's behavior at the breast.

  5. Progress is being made in enhancing a family-centered developmental care philosophy that actively involves parents in the care of their infant, yet the logistics and paradigm shift for healthcare providers continue to be an issue.[73,88]

  6. Sufficient private space needs to be provided for skin-to-skin care, breastfeeding, and milk expression.

  7. Necessary equipment includes breast pumps and comfortable chairs or beds to ensure parents' presence by their infant and for frequent skin-to-skin contact.

  8. Recognition of the value of human milk needs to be reinforced with practical ways to best acquire it.

  9. Institutions need to remove pressure for early discharge of preterm infants and provide continuity of care and follow-up once discharged.

  10. Parents require counseling regarding alternative oral feeding methods and other options to bottle feeding when the baby will be breastfed. (See Chapter 31, *Expression and Use of Human Milk.*)

  11. Feeding guidelines include strategies for transitioning from enteral feeding to breastfeeding or full oral feeding, and from scheduled feeding to demand feeding via semidemand feeding.

III. Initiatives to Support Breastfeeding the Premature Infant

 A. The Neo-BFHI is a guideline that was developed by the Nordic and Quebec working group[5-7] based on recommendations by the WHO and UNICEF in the *Baby-friendly Hospital Initiative: Revised, Updated and Expanded for Integrated Care.*[89]

  1. Hospitals may adopt the Baby-friendly Hospital Initiative (BFHI) Ten Steps to Successful Breastfeeding (Ten Steps) to integrate guidelines for preterm and sick infants.[90] The Neo-BFHI outlines the standards and criteria for each of the steps, which are expanded for neonatal care based on relevant evidence, expert opinion, and experiences implementing Baby-friendly practices in NICUs.[5-7,63] Furthermore, to take into consideration the unique needs of these infants, and to ensure that the recommended practices focus on respect for the parents, a family-centered approach, and continuity of care, the working group formulated three Guiding Principles that are meant to be basic tenets to the expanded Ten Steps.[6]

  2. More recently, the WHO and UNICEF published guidelines examining each of the recommendations in the Ten Steps to bring together recent evidence and considerations to inform practice and to include preterm, low birth weight, and sick infants, and infants admitted to NICUs.[90]

  3. Other breastfeeding-related initiatives targeting preterm and ill infants include the Humane Neonatal Care Initiative,[91] family integrated care,[92] and the U.K. Baby-Friendly Initiative.[93]

 B. Systematic reviews, meta-analyses of randomized controlled trials, and other resources describe the benefits of breastfeeding for preterm infants and the methods that best support breastfeeding in this vulnerable population. They include the following:

  1. Systematic reviews and meta-analyses of randomized controlled trials provide evidence of the scientific benefit of human milk on infant and child health.[20,29-31,38,39,41,94]

  2. A systematic review of preterm infants has demonstrated that for clinically stable infants the following have been effective in supporting breastfeeding:

   a. Kangaroo mother care (skin-to-skin contact).[95]

   b. Peer support.[96]

c. Methods of expressing milk.[96]
d. Multidisciplinary staff training and Baby-friendly accreditation.[96] Skilled support from trained hospital staff was potentially cost effective.[96]

3. Other reference materials provide methods that promote human milk feeding of preterm infants,[2] guides for parents and practitioners about what to expect when breastfeeding an infant in the NICU,[3] and a book about human milk as the best medicine in the NICU.[11]

IV. Kangaroo Mother Care

A. Kangaroo Mother Care (KMC) was developed in a NICU in Bogota, Colombia, in the 1970s to prevent overcrowding and parents' abandonment of infants.[1,97] It is also referred to as kangaroo care or skin-to-skin care.

1. A study of heat and fluid loss in infants born at a gestational age of 27 weeks or less found that intermittent kangaroo mother care may be possible for these infants during the first week after birth.[98]

2. Infants born at a gestational age of 32 weeks or greater can be cared for with continuous (24/7) skin-to-skin contact.
   a. It is essential that the infant is placed with most of the body, including the head, in direct skin-to-skin contact with the parent.
   b. Skin-to-skin contact directly after birth should be considered the norm unless there is a justifiable reason for not encouraging it.[7,68,95]

3. For infants born at a gestational age of 28 to 31 weeks, continuous skin-to-skin care directly after birth is possible, and the incubator should be used only when necessary.
   a. An individual decision should be made based on an assessment of the fluid and electrolyte balance, physiologic stability, and need for incubator temperature in every instance before the infant is taken out of the incubator.
   b. Ideally, the minimum duration of skin-to-skin care sessions should be 2 hours.
   c. From the 2nd week of life, the same guidelines apply as for infants born at 28 weeks or more gestation.[99,100]

B. Professionals should assist the parents when introducing kangaroo mother care.

1. Help with positioning the infant comfortably for effective feeding.
2. Provide appropriate clothing so that all skin surfaces are adequately covered, including the head, to ensure there is no temperature leakage. The ambient room temperature should be sufficient to support the infant's temperature, including during transfer.
3. The transfer of sensitive infants to and from the parent should be performed by staff members with adequate training. For sensitive infants, continuous temperature monitoring is essential.
4. Stable infants can be transferred by parents and placed skin-to-skin, with assistance from staff members when required.
5. Staff members should make sure the parents are comfortable when they hold their babies skin-to-skin, ask them if they need anything, offer them something to drink, and be available for assistance.
6. Privacy should be ensured as much as possible.
7. Early breastfeeding practice can be a component of kangaroo mother care, with skin-to-skin care gradually transitioning to breastfeeding.[51,97]

C. Skin-to-skin care can begin when the infant is stable and still intubated [101,102] or while receiving continuous positive airway pressure (CPAP) treatment.

1. The infant and parent should maintain skin-to-skin contact.
2. The infant is held mostly upright and snuggled between the breastfeeding parent's breasts or against the partner's bare chest.
   a. The infant's torso is bare except for a diaper.
   b. The infant's back is covered by the parent's hand, clothing, or blanket.
   c. The infant's head is covered with a cap or blanket.

D. A Cochrane Review[95] that examined kangaroo mother care and the reduction of morbidity and mortality in low birth weight infants found high-quality evidence that supported a statistically significant reduction in the risk of mortality, nosocomial infection or sepsis, and hypothermia. It found moderate-quality evidence that demonstrated an increase in weight gain, length gain, head circumference gain, and positive exclusive breastfeeding rates at discharge and at 1 to 3 months follow-up. It also found low-quality evidence showing improvement on some measures of maternal–infant attachment and the home environment.[95] Other documented benefits of kangaroo mother care for infants include the following[51,97]:

1. Stable heart rate.[95,103,104]
2. More regular breathing, with a 75 percent decrease in apneic episodes.[103,104]
3. Improved oxygen saturation levels.[105,106]
4. No cold stress and greater temperature stability.[106]
5. Longer periods of sleep.[107]
6. More rapid weight gain.[68]
7. Less caloric expenditures.[107]
8. Decreased cortisol levels.[108]
9. More rapid brain development.[109]
10. Reduction of purposeless activity (flailing of arms and legs).
11. Decreased crying.[110]
12. Longer periods of alertness.
13. More successful breastfeeding episodes.[111]
14. Increased breastfeeding duration.[111,112]
15. Reduced morbidity and mortality in low birth weight infants.[95]
16. Earlier hospital discharge.[68]

E. There are many benefits of kangaroo mother care for parents[97]:
1. Increased bonding because of increased serum oxytocin levels.[113]
2. Promotes confidence in the parents' caregiving.[114]
3. Parents feel more in control.
4. Relief of parental stress over having an infant in the intensive care nursery.[115]
5. Increased milk production.[116]
6. Earlier discharge from the hospital.
7. Significantly reduced cost, resulting from decreased length of stay.[68]

V. Professional Support for Parents of Preterm Infants

A. Skilled healthcare professionals who are knowledgeable about breastfeeding management are an important element of helping parents reach their goal to breastfeed.
1. Ideally, all parents are offered prenatal information about the importance of breastfeeding and human milk and the negative consequences of human milk substitute (e.g., formula) feeding for their infants and themselves.
2. The parent and healthcare team should establish a breastfeeding plan that is regularly reviewed to ensure that it reflects the infant's current state of development.
3. Support and appropriate management in establishing and maintaining milk production when the infant is unable to initiate breastfeeding are critical to a successful outcome.
4. Professionals should encourage the initiation of regular breastfeeding on demand as soon as possible after delivery and be observant of problems with milk production.
5. During the infant's entire hospital stay, parents should have access to lactation and breastfeeding support from staff members who have adequate knowledge and experience in breastfeeding counseling.

B. Breastfeeding the preterm infant requires a commitment of parental and family time and energy, and nurturing support and compassion from the healthcare team. Lactation support must be a team effort that is research based and comprehensive.
1. A multidisciplinary collaborative team may include lactation consultants, nurses, physicians, nutritionists, occupational therapists, physiotherapists, massage therapists, social workers, developmental specialists, and discharge planners.

    2.   Whenever possible, the interdisciplinary team supports guiding the family in initiating kangaroo mother care, or skin-to-skin contact, from birth.

        a.   A meta-analysis and systematic review on early interventions that taught skills to parents and involved them in the preterm infants' care demonstrated a positive neurobehavioral affect that enhanced child development.[94]

        b.   Although this improvement was not sustained at 36 months, it did demonstrate clinically meaningful results when parents were involved in care.[94]

C.   Each healthcare profession has an important role in supporting the parents and caring for the preterm infant.

    1.   Lactation consultants:

        a.   Provide support when the parent and the infant are ready to initiate breastfeeding and during the transition to breastfeeding and human milk feeding.

        b.   Consider the special needs of the preterm infant and incorporate a knowledge of the physiological process of breastfeeding.

    2.   Physicians:

        a.   Adhere to the breastfeeding policy.

        b.   Provide information to parents about the importance of human milk for preterm infants.

        c.   Assess and prescribe nutrition according to the infant's individual characteristics and needs while protecting the establishment of breastfeeding.

        d.   Prescribe fortification of human milk with protein and other nutrients and minerals.

        e.   Treat common breastfeeding difficulties.

        f.   Prescribe galactagogues.

        g.   Evaluate and treat ankyloglossia.

        h.   Pay attention to the compatibility between required medications and human milk.

    3.   Nurses (registered and auxiliary):

        a.   Facilitate kangaroo mother care and early initiation and continuation of lactation and breastfeeding.

        b.   Monitor milk production.

        c.   Observe breastfeeding.

        d.   Modify the physical environment to facilitate breastfeeding.

        e.   Handle human milk (when this is not done by special milk bank staff members).

    4.   Nutritionists:

        a.   Protect the use of parental milk and donor milk, when available.

        b.   Provide fortification when required.

    5.   Specialists:

        a.   Occupational therapists, depending on the models of education, may be involved in infant feeding.

        b.   Speech therapists are involved in infant feeding when infants have diagnoses associated with anatomical, neurological, or other problems with sucking and oral feeding.

VI. Establishing and Maintaining Lactation with a Preterm Infant

A.   Milk expression should ideally begin between 1 and 6 hours after birth.

    1.   A hospital-grade electric breast pump is recommended for milk expression when direct breastfeeding is not possible. (See Chapter 24, *Breastfeeding Devices and Topical Treatments*.)

    2.   Current research on pumping and hand expression found that higher milk volumes were obtained when breasts were massaged and warmed prior to pumping, when appropriate breast shield sizes were used, and when pumping was initiated within 1 hour of delivery for very low birth weight infants and the frequency was increased (four or more times per day).[2,11,117]

    3.   The recommendations are to pump eight times in 24 hours, along with hand expression during the first 3 days.[11,118] (See Chapter 31, *Expression and Use of Human Milk*.)

    4.   Pumping one breast at a time is possible, and pumping both breasts at the same time is more efficient. However, a Cochrane Review did not show any differences in results between simultaneous and sequential pumping.[117]

    5.   Ensure appropriate storage conditions of expressed milk.[119,120] (See Chapter 31, *Expression and Use of Human Milk*.)

B.   Assess when it is appropriate for the parent to start breastfeeding.
1.   The timing should be based on the infant's signs of stability, defined as absence of severe physiological instability in connection with routine care. The timing should not be based on postmenstrual or postnatal age or the infant's current weight.
2.   Breastfeeding should begin as soon as the infant shows such signs of readiness, without any unjustified delay.
a.   It is essential that healthcare providers guide parents in the interpretation of their preterm infant's behavioral characteristics.
b.   This must be done with sensitivity and focus on what parents can do to support the baby so parents do not interpret the information as meaning the baby is too fragile for suckling the breast.
c.   In some settings infants are tested for their capacity for nutritive sucking, or they receive structured training in sucking on a gloved finger before breastfeeding is introduced. However, these interventions result in unjustified delays in the introduction of breastfeeding.

C.   Help parents transition the baby to the breast.
1.   Breastfeeding facilitation includes offering a breastfeeding pillow for positioning and helping to achieve a comfortable position.
2.   In connection with the first feed at the breast, a knowledgeable healthcare professional should observe a breastfeeding, guide positioning the infant, point out signs of the baby's oral motor competence, and give suggestions about how to support the infant at the breast.
3.   The health professional describes the infant's oral motor and other activities related to breastfeeding and offers suggestions about how to support the baby to latch, stay fixed at the breast, suckle, and ingest milk.[62,63,121]
4.   The focus of this guidance is helping the infant maintain a comfortable position close to the breast with flexed arms and legs while protecting the infant from direct light in the eyes and seeing activities in the room.
a.   Preterm infants are more active at the breast when they are held with still hands; they do not appreciate stroking and tickling.
b.   Talking in a soft voice provides gentle stimulation.

D.   Help with the transition from enteral feeding to breastfeeding, and from scheduled to on-demand feeding.
1.   The transition from tube to oral feeding, and from scheduled to unregulated feeding, demands that feeding should occur with semidemand feeding as an intermediate phase.
2.   At signs of some milk intake at the breast, the transition from regular feeding to unregulated feeding (no fixed volumes, hours, or intervals) should occur while making sure the infant receives a sufficient daily milk volume.
a.   The infant is put at the breast as soon as parents notice that the infant is waking up and shows signs of interest in sucking (rooting, tongue extension, sucking movements).
b.   There are no restrictions on the frequency or intervals between breastfeeding sessions or on the duration of sessions.
c.   Complementary feeding is given with a prescription of a total daily volume of supplementation based on the infant's weight gain pattern, or based on test weighing before and after breastfeeding sessions; the last alternative is appropriate only when it is the parent's choice.

VII. Discharge Planning

A.   Parents require a detailed plan to care for their preterm infant after discharge.
B.   Ongoing care and information should include the following recommendations by the Academy of Breastfeeding Medicine (revisions are in process).[122]
1.   Watch for signs that the infant is getting enough milk by using weight checks and test weights if necessary, and count the number of wet diapers and bowel movements. (See Chapter 13, *Facilitating and Assessing Breastfeeding Initiation*.)
2.   The expected feeding patterns include at least eight feeds per 24 hours with only one prolonged sleep period of up to 5 hours and cues that indicate the infant is ready to feed.

3. Milk expression should continue until the infant is fully established at the breast, with adequate weight gain and no need for supplemental feedings.

4. Continued milk expression may be necessary after the infant has been discharged. If so, expression might be needed after each feeding or only a few times each day, depending on the number of supplemental feedings.

5. Experts recommend that, if possible, milk production should exceed what the infant needs at discharge because the increased volume helps the milk flow freely in the presence of a weaker suck.

6. Ensure that the parents understand the proper use of supplemental feeding devices, when appropriate.
    a. Cup.
    b. Feeding tube at breast.
    c. Supervision of the use of a nipple shield.
    d. Close follow-up should continue as progress is made toward full breastfeeding.

C. Parents should be counseled regarding alternative feeding methods. Cup feeding is a viable option; some studies indicate this is the preferred oral feeding alternative.[65,66] Parents should be told why bottle feeding should be avoided when the parent intends to breastfeed.[123]

1. If parents choose to bottle feed human milk during the infant's hospitalization, a lactation consultant can help transition the infant to the breast before or after discharge.

2. Indications for the use of a tube feeding device at the breast include the following:
    a. An infant who latches on to the breast but exerts low milk transfer.
    b. Lack of sucking rhythm.
    c. Parent's request to supplement at the breast with a lactation aid. Some parents want to see the amount of milk the infant takes; others prefer for the supplement to be given at the breast rather than using an alternative feeding device.
    d. When there is limited milk production. (See Chapter 22, *Low Milk Production and Infant Weight*.)
    e. Impaired milk ejection reflex.

D. The lactation consultant should conduct a postdischarge telephone follow-up.[124,125]

E. Parents should be given information about the availability of support services after discharge.
1. Primary healthcare provider.
2. International Board Certified Lactation Consultants.
3. Healthcare professional who has expertise in breastfeeding preterm infants (e.g., specially trained midwives, doulas, and peer counselors).[125]
4. Social services.
5. La Leche League or other local breastfeeding support groups.
6. Eligible national or government programs, such as Women, Infants, and Children (WIC) in the United States.

VIII. The Late Preterm Infant

A. Research shows that parents of late preterm infants also need support to successfully breastfeed.
1. Late preterm applies to infants born at gestational ages between 34 weeks and 36 weeks, 6 days.
2. These infants require particular surveillance while hospitalized and following their discharge to home until they have demonstrated that they can gain weight and grow consistently.[126]
    a. They are particularly vulnerable because they might look full term and weigh nearly the same as infants born at term, which may lead to the belief that they are as competent as full-term infants.
    b. However, they are at an increased risk for hypoglycemia, hypothermia, respiratory morbidity, apnea, severe hyperbilirubinemia, dehydration, feeding difficulties, prolonged artificial milk supplementation, weight loss, and hospital readmission.[127,128]
3. The incidence of late preterm births has been reported to be on the rise[129-134] for the following reasons:
    a. Increase in maternal age, obesity and diabetes, poor nutrition, smoking, alcohol use, and assisted reproductive technology resulting in multiple births.[135-137]
    b. Increased obstetrical surveillance that detects maternal and fetal conditions, which results in medically indicated birth (i.e., induction of labor or cesarean delivery).[135-137]

B. Special care is needed immediately after birth.
   1. Because of the wide range from 34 weeks to 36 weeks, 6 days of gestation, these infants require an individualized care plan that depends on their gestational age and capabilities.
      a. Every effort should be made for these infants to remain with the parent.
      b. The infant's gestational age and stability often determine whether the infant is cared for in a special care unit (intermediate or intensive).
      c. If the infant is cared for in a special care unit, the care often parallels that of a preterm infant.
   2. An infant who is stable should be placed skin-to-skin with the parent immediately after birth.
      a. The infant can be dried, and Apgar scoring can take place during this skin-to-skin time.
      b. A warm blanket can cover both the parent and baby, and a hat can be placed on the baby's head.
      c. Extended skin-to-skin contact keeps the infant warm, prevents crying, and allows for frequent feedings, all of which help prevent hypoglycemia and hypothermia.[138]
      d. Infants who have early skin-to-skin contact interact more with their parents, are more likely to breastfeed and to breastfeed longer, and show better cardiorespiratory stability.[139]
   3. Avoiding or delaying disruptive procedures (e.g., excessive handling, unnecessary suctioning, administration of vitamin K, eye prophylaxis, and hepatitis B vaccine) minimizes thermal and metabolic stress, improves initial feeding behavior, and enhances early parent–infant interaction immediately after birth.[140]
   4. Bathing should be delayed until after the initial parent–infant interaction.[23,140-142]
C. Parents will need help positioning the infant for breastfeeding.[127]
   1. Parents should be helped to position the infant at the breast to prevent excessive flexion of the baby's neck and trunk.
      a. The cross-cradle hold works well.
      b. When positioning the infant in the football hold, care should be taken so the weight of the breast is not on the infant's chest.
   2. The late preterm infant can have decreased muscle tone and might not be able to maintain a latch at the breast and maintain and sustain strong enough sucking to transfer milk.
      a. The use of the Dancer hold for support of the breast and chin can help the infant with jaw stability.
      b. The use of an ultrathin silicone nipple shield can be considered if the latch is difficult, cannot be sustained, or there is evidence of ineffective milk transfer.[143] However, it is best to initiate this only after other attempts at latching have been exhausted. The routine use of a nipple shield for late preterm infants is not recommended.[144,145]
   3. Because late preterm infants tend to be sleepier than full-term infants, they might need awakening every 2 to 3 hours for feeding.[146]
   4. Provisions should be made for close observation and assessment of the infant at the breast at least twice daily by two different skilled lactation professionals.[129]
      a. The determination of milk transfer is essential.
      b. The use of a breastfeeding assessment tool—such as Latch, Audible swallowing, Type of nipple, Comfort, maternal Help (LATCH) or Infant BreastFeeding Assessment Tool (IBFAT)—can be helpful.
      c. Close daily monitoring of urinary and stool patterns is important.
      d. If the amount of milk transfer and breastfeeding effectiveness are in question, the occasional use of test weights can be helpful.
   5. Milk expression should begin unless the late preterm infant is breastfeeding effectively every 2 to 3 hours (determined by skilled evaluation and documentation).
      a. Milk expression is most efficient with a combination of hand expression and electric pumping.[118]
      b. If milk expression with a breast pump does not yield sufficient colostrum, hand expression after pumping can increase milk collection.
   6. Continual skin-to-skin contact can facilitate feeding and milk production.

7. When supplementing, an alternate feeding method, such as supplementing at the breast or cup feeding, can avoid the infant becoming habituated to a bottle.[147-150] If the infant tires easily, a nasogastric tube (NGT) can be inserted.[127,151,152]

8. If supplementation is indicated, the parent's expressed milk is the first best choice, followed by pasteurized donor milk, then human milk substitute (formula), until milk production is adequate.

    a. The quantities of supplementation after breastfeeding should be small: 5 to 10 mL per feeding on day 1 and 10 to 30 mL per feeding thereafter.[122]

    b. When supplementation is necessary, small amounts should continue until the infant can transfer appropriate amounts of milk while breastfeeding and the expressed milk is sufficient for infant weight gain.

9. Milk expression should continue until the infant demonstrates the ability to sustain breastfeeding at least eight times each 24 hours and shows appropriate weight gain over time.

10. Parents of the late preterm infant should be included in their infant's care plan and can be taught to participate fully in their infant's care.

D. Discharge planning with parents should begin at birth.

1. Particularly when the late preterm infant is cared for in a special care unit, anticipatory guidance to parents and staff members should include a discussion that the late preterm infant is not a full-term baby and a discharge to home might not be within the expected 36 to 48 hours after birth.

2. Every effort should be made to keep the infant and parent together during the hospital stay.

3. Signs of discharge readiness include the following:

    a. Breastfeeding is going well, or in combination with appropriate supplementation by an alternate feeding method, and the infant demonstrates a stable or increasing weight.

    b. Evidence that milk production is becoming established.

    c. The infant can maintain normal body temperature in an open crib.

    d. Bilirubin is stable or decreasing.

4. Discharge strategies include the following:

    a. The parents demonstrate comfort with alternate feeding methods, if necessary.

    b. The parents demonstrate confidence with breastfeeding.

    c. A follow-up visit with a healthcare provider is scheduled within 24 to 48 hours of discharge, then weekly until the infant is exclusively breastfeeding.[45]

    d. A postdischarge feeding plan is developed with the family, lactation consultants, and healthcare provider.[153,154]

    e. A feeding log is provided to document the number of feedings, urinary output, and stooling pattern.

    f. The parent is given a referral for postdischarge lactation support, including a lactation consultant, peer support group, and lactation hotline number, if available.

▶ Key Points from This Chapter

A. Because of the multifaceted importance of breastfeeding and human milk feeding for preterm infants and parents, all possible and available interventions should be made for enabling them to initiate and attain successful breastfeeding according to the infant's individual situation and the parent's personal goals, without any unjustified delay.

B. There are unique challenges and opportunities to support parents of preterm, unwell, and late preterm infants. The healthcare professionals' role in advocating for infants and parents in support of their goals and needs is paramount to the present and future health and well-being of the infants and their families.

C. The healthcare system should strive to offer all parents and infants an environment that provides an organization of care and a setting that is based on accessibility, staff competence, and a physical environment that enables parents' unrestricted presence with their infants in the hospital as far as possible, and offers the provision of adequate professional and psychologically sensitive support of lactation and breastfeeding.

🔍 CASE STUDY

Greta delivered Anna at a gestational age of 30 weeks, 6 days, weighing 1,475 g. Anna required ventilator treatment during the first 3 hours of life, followed by CPAP treatment during the first 2 days. During this time Anna received expressed milk via tube feeding. At the age of 2 days (the postmenstrual age of 31 weeks, 1 day), breastfeeding was introduced. The nurse wrote in the chart, "Sucks very well, hungry." During these 2 days, Greta was a patient in the postnatal ward because of medical problems and spent most of the time in the NICU.

On day 4, Greta moved to a parent room in the NICU, and Anna was positioned at the breast whenever she showed signs of interest in sucking. On this day Anna weighed 1,445 g. The next day milk intake was noted nine times using test weighing and ranged from 1 to 25 mL. Anna required tube feeding only four times to reach the prescribed daily volume. On day 9, having reached a postmenstrual age of 32 weeks, Anna weighed 1,530 g. The next day semidemand feeding was introduced and tube feeding was required only once to attain the prescribed milk volume. On day 10, when Anna weighed 1,555 g, the incubator was exchanged for a crib with a warm water mattress, semidemand feeding was introduced, and Anna required only one tube feed to reach the prescribed daily milk volume.

The next day, at 32 weeks, 2 days (her 11th day of life), Anna attained exclusive breastfeeding with 11 recorded breastfeeding sessions and volumes ranging from 11 to 25 mL. A nurse wrote in the chart, "Spent the night in her mother's bed." Test weighing was discontinued the next day. Two days later, the warm water mattress was removed from the crib; on this day Anna weighed 1,645 g. On day 15, at the postmenstrual age of 32 weeks, 6 days, Anna's parents took her home and were supported by an early discharge program (the parents provide their baby's care at home, with access to support from the NICU). Anna was formally discharged at 33 weeks, 2 days (day 18 of life), with a weight of 1,749 g. She was scheduled for routine follow-up at the NICU, and the responsibility of her continued follow-up was transferred to the local child health center (with regular follow-up available free of charge to all infants and children up to school age). On this day, Anna weighed 1,749 g.

Questions

1. Given the early and close contact of Anna and Greta, is there any other approach you would have taken to ensure a positive environment for Anna's growth and development?
2. On day 4, as semidemand feeding is introduced, what is Anna's progress? What information is helpful in determining milk transfer? What other information would be helpful?
3. Identify the role of the lactation consultant in working with the NICU staff to support parents in meeting their infant feeding goals.

References

1. Cattaneo A, Davanzo R, Uxa F, Tamburlini G. Recommendations for the implementation of kangaroo mother care for low birthweight infants. *Acta Paediatr.* 1998;87(4):440-445.
2. Meier PP, Johnson TJ, Patel AL, Rossman B. Evidence-based methods that promote human milk feeding of preterm infants. *Clin Perinatol.* 2017;44(1):1-22.
3. Wight NE. Breastfeeding the NICU infant: what to expect. *Clin Obstet Gynecol.* 2015;58(4):840-854.
4. Greene Z, O'Donnell CPF, Walshe M. Oral stimulation for promoting oral feeding in preterm infants. *Cochrane Database Syst Rev.* 2016;9:CD009720. doi:10.1002/14651858.CD009720.pub2.
5. Nyqvist KH, Häggkvist A-P, Hansen MN, et al. Expansion of the Baby-Friendly Hospital Initiative Ten Steps to Successful Breastfeeding into Neonatal Intensive Care: expert group recommendations. *J Hum Lactation.* 2013;29(3):300-309.
6. Nyqvist KH, Häggkvist A-P, Hansen MN, et al. Expansion of the Ten Steps to Successful Breastfeeding into neonatal intensive care: expert group recommendations for three guiding principles. *J Hum Lactation.* 2012;28(3):289-296.
7. Nyqvist K, Maastrup R, Hansen MN, et al. The Neo-BFHI: the Baby-Friendly Hospital Initiative for Neonatal Wards. ILCA website. http://www.ilca.org/main/learning/resources/neo-bfhi. Published 2015. Accessed December 7, 2016.
8. Schanler RJ. Outcomes of human milk-fed premature infants. *Semin Perinatol.* 2011;35(1):29-33.
9. Schanler RJ. The use of human milk for premature infants. *Pediatr Clin North Am.* 2001;48(1):207-219.
10. Oveisi MR, Sadeghi N, Jannat B, et al. Human breast milk provides better antioxidant capacity than infant formula. *Iran J Pharm Res.* 2010;9(4):445-449.
11. Wight NE, Morton JA, Kim JH. *Best Medicine: Human Milk in the NICU.* Amarillo, TX: Hale Publishing; 2008.
12. Ziegler EE. Meeting the nutritional needs of the low-birth-weight infant. *Ann Nutr Metab.* 2011;58(suppl):8-18.
13. Van den Driessche M, Peeters K, Marien P, Ghoos Y, Devlieger H, Veereman-Wauters G. Gastric emptying in formula-fed and breast-fed infants measured with the 13C-octanoic acid breath test. *J Pediatr Gastroenterol Nutr.* 1999;29:46-51.

14. Hassan BB, Butler R, Davidson GP, et al. Patterns of antropyloric motility in fed healthy preterm infants. *Arch Dis Child Fetal Neonatal Ed.* 2002;87(2):F95-F99.

15. Meyer R, Foong R-XM, Thapar N, Kritas S, Shah N. Systematic review of the impact of feed protein type and degree of hydrolysis on gastric emptying in children. *BMC Gastroenterol.* 2015;15:137.

16. Li Y-F, Lin H-C, Torrazza RM, Parker L, Talaga E, Neu J. Gastric residual evaluation in preterm neonates: a useful monitoring technique or a hindrance? *Pediatr Neonatol.* 2014;55(5):335-340.

17. Lawrence RA, Lawrence RM. *Breastfeeding: A Guide for the Medical Profession.* 7th ed. Philadelphia, PA: Mosby-Elsevier; 2010.

18. Lucas A, Fewtrell MS, Morley R, et al. Randomized outcome trial of human milk fortification and developmental outcome in preterm infants. *Am J Clin Nutr.* 1996;64(2):142-151.

19. Lucas A, Morley R, Cole TJ, Lister G, Leeson-Payne C. Breast milk and subsequent intelligence quotient in children born preterm. *Lancet.* 1992;339(8788):261-264.

20. Vohr BR, Poindexter BB, Dusick AM, et al. Persistent beneficial effects of breast milk ingested in the neonatal intensive care unit on outcomes of extremely low birth weight infants at 30 months of age. *Pediatrics.* 2007;120(4):e953-e959.

21. Vohr BR, Poindexter BB, Dusick AM, et al. Beneficial effects of breast milk in the neonatal intensive care unit on the developmental outcome of extremely low birth weight infants at 18 months of age. *Pediatrics.* 2006;118(1):e115-e123.

22. Hörnell A, Lagström H, Lande B, Thorsdottir I. Breastfeeding, introduction of other foods and effects on health: a systematic literature review for the 5th Nordic Nutrition Recommendations. *Food Nutr Res.* 2013;57. doi:10.3402/fnr.v57i0.20823.

23. Lawn JE, Davidge R, Paul VK, et al. Born too soon: care for the preterm baby. *Reprod Health.* 2013;10(1):S5.

24. Morrow AL, Rangel JM. Human milk protection against infectious diarrhea: implications for prevention and clinical care. *Semin Pediatr Infect Dis.* 2004;15(4):221-228.

25. American Academy of Pediatrics. Breastfeeding and the use of human milk. *Pediatrics.* 2012;129(3):e827-e841.

26. Bowatte G, Tham R, Allen KJ, et al. Breastfeeding and childhood acute otitis media: a systematic review and meta-analysis. *Acta Paediatr.* 2015;104:85-95.

27. Chantry CJ, Howard CR, Auinger P. Full breastfeeding duration and associated decrease in respiratory tract infection in US children. *Pediatrics.* 2006;117(2):425-432.

28. Ip S, Chung M, Raman G, et al. *Breastfeeding and Maternal and Infant Health Outcomes in Developed Countries.* Rockville, MD: Tufts-New England Medical Center Evidence-Based Practice Center; 2007.

29. Victora CG, Bahl R, Barros AJD, et al. Breastfeeding in the 21st century: epidemiology, mechanisms, and lifelong effect. *Lancet.* 2016;387(10017):475-490.

30. Alm B, Wennergren G, Möllborg P, Lagercrantz H. Breastfeeding and dummy use have a protective effect on sudden infant death syndrome [Review]. *Acta Paediatr.* 2016;105(1):31-38.

31. Hauck FR, Thompson JMD, Tanabe KO, Moon RY, Vennemann MM. Breastfeeding and reduced risk of sudden infant death syndrome: a meta-analysis. *Pediatrics.* 2011;128(1):103-110.

32. Moon RY, Fu L. Sudden infant death syndrome: an update. *Pediatr Rev.* 2012;33(4):314-320.

33. Guthrie SO, Gordon PV, Thomas V, Thorp JA, Peabody J, Clark RH. Necrotizing enterocolitis among neonates in the United States. *J Perinatol.* 2003;23(4):278-285.

34. Henderson G, Graig F, Brocklehurst P, McGuire W. Enteral feeding regimens and necrotising enterocolitis in preterm infants: multi center case-control study. *Arch Dis Child Fetal Neonatal Ed.* 2007;94(2):F120-F123.

35. Thompson A, Bizzarro M, Yu S, Diefenbach K, Simpson BJ, Moss RL. Risk factors for necrotizing enterocolitis totalis: a case-control study. *J Perinatol.* 2011;31(11):730-738.

36. Cristofalo EA, Schanler RJ, Blanco CL, et al. Randomized trial of exclusive human milk versus preterm formula diets in extremely premature infants. *J Pediatr.* 2013;163(6):1592-1595.e1.

37. Sullivan S, Schanler RJ, Kim JH, et al. An exclusively human milk-based diet is associated with a lower rate of necrotizing enterocolitis than a diet of human milk and bovine milk-based products. *J Pediatr.* 2010;156(4):562-567.e1.

38. Horta BL, Loret de Mola C, Victora CG. Long-term consequences of breastfeeding on cholesterol, obesity, systolic blood pressure and type 2 diabetes: a systematic review and meta-analysis. *Acta Paediatr.* 2015;104:30-37.

39. Horta BL, Victoria CG. *Long-Term Effects of Breastfeeding—A Systematic Review.* Geneva, Switzerland: World Health Organization; 2013.

40. Kramer MS, Aboud F, Mironova E, et al. Breastfeeding and child cognitive development: new evidence from a large randomized trial. *Arch Gen Psychiatry.* 2008;65(5):578-584.

41. Victora CG, Horta BL, de Mola CL, et al. Association between breastfeeding and intelligence, educational attainment, and income at 30 years of age: a prospective birth cohort study from Brazil. *Lancet Glob Health.* 2015;3(4):e199-e205.

42. Gross SJ, David RJ, Bauman L, Tomarelli RM. Nutritional composition of milk from mothers delivering preterm and at term. *J Pediatr.* 1980;96(4):641-644.

43. Smilowitz JT, Gho DS, Mirmiran M, German JB, Underwood MA. Rapid measurement of human milk macronutrients in the neonatal intensive care unit: accuracy and precision of Fourier transform mid-infrared spectroscopy. *J Hum Lactation.* 2014;30(2):180-189.

44. Polberger S, Lönnerdal B. Simple and rapid macronutrient analysis of human milk for individualized fortification: basis for improved nutritional management of very-low-birth-weight infants? *J Pediatr Gastroenterol Nutr.* 1993;17(3):283-290.

45. American Academy of Pediatrics. Breastfeeding and the use of human milk. *Pediatrics.* 2005;115(2):496-506.

46. McClure RJ, Newell SJ. Randomised controlled study of clinical outcome following trophic feeding. *Arch Dis Child Fetal Neonatal Ed.* 2000;82(1):F29-F33.

47. Sallakh-Niknezhad A, Bashar-Hashemi F, Satarzadeh N, Ghojazadeh M, Sahnazarli G. Early versus late trophic feeding in very low birth weight preterm infants. *Iran J Pediatr.* 2012;22(2):171-176.

48. Li Y, Neu J, Parker L. Reply—gastric residuals, feeding intolerance, and necrotizing enterocolitis in preterm infants. *Pediatr Neonatol.* 2015;56(2):138-139.

49. Schanler RJ, Shulman RJ, Lau C, Smith EO, Heitkemper MM. Feeding strategies for premature infants: randomized trial of gastrointestinal priming and tube-feeding method. *Pediatrics.* 1999;103(2):434-439.

50. Csont GL, Groth S, Hopkins P, Guillet R. An evidence-based approach to breastfeeding neonates at risk for hypoglycemia. *J Obstet Gynecol Neonatal Nurs.* 2014;43(1):71-81.

51. Anderson GC, Chiu S-H, Dombrowski MA, Swinth JY, Albert JM, Wada N. Mother-newborn contact in a randomized trial of kangaroo (skin-to-skin) care. *J Obstet Gynecol Neonatal Nurs.* 2003;32(5):604-611.

52. Nyqvist KH. How can kangaroo mother care and high technology care be compatible? *J Hum Lactation.* 2004;20(1):72-74.

53. Schanler RJ. Human milk fortification for premature infants. *Am J Clin Nutr.* 1996;64(2):249-250.

54. Kirsten D, Bradford L. Hindmilk feedings. *Neonatal Network.* 1999;18(3):68-70.

55. Bishara R, Dunn MS, Merko SE, Darling P. Volume of foremilk, hindmilk, and total milk produced by mothers of very preterm infants born at less than 28 weeks of gestation. *J Hum Lactation.* 2009;25(3):272-279.

56. Meier PP, Engstrom JL, Fleming BA, Streeter PL, Lawrence PB. Estimating milk intake of hospitalized preterm infants who breastfeed. *J Hum Lactation.* 1996;12(1):21-26.

57. Griffin TL, Meier PP, Bradford LP, Bigger HR, Engstrom JL. Mothers' performing creamatocrit measures in the NICU: accuracy, reactions, and cost. *J Obstet Gynecol Neonatal Nurs.* 2000;29(3):249-257.

58. Ewer AK, Yu VYH. Gastric emptying in pre-term infants: the effect of breast milk fortifier. *Acta Paediatr.* 1996;85(9):1112-1115.

59. Quan R, Yang C, Rubinstein S, Lewiston NJ, Stevenson DK, Kerner JA. The effect of nutritional additives on anti-infective factors in human milk. *Clin Pediatr.* 1994;33(6):325-328.

60. American Academy of Pediatrics. CDC, FDA advise against powdered formula in NICUs. AAP News & Journals website. http://www.aappublications.org/content/20/5/219.1. Published 2002. Accessed November 4, 2017.

61. Lucas A, Cole TJ. Breast milk and neonatal necrotising enterocolitis. *Lancet.* 1990;336(8730):1519-1523.

62. Nyqvist KH, Ewald U, Sjoden P. Supporting a preterm infant's behaviour during breastfeeding: a case report. *J Hum Lactation.* 1996;12(3):221-228.

63. Nyqvist KH, Kylberg E. Application of the Baby Friendly Hospital Initiative to Neonatal Care: suggestions by Swedish mothers of very preterm infants. *J Hum Lactation.* 2008;24(3):252-262.

64. Crowe L, Chang A, Wallace K. Instruments for assessing readiness to commence suck feeds in preterm infants: effects on time to establish full oral feeding and duration of hospitalisation. *Cochrane Database Syst Rev.* 2016;8:CD005586. doi:10.1002/14651858.CD005586.pub3.

65. Flint A, New K, Davies M. Cup feeding versus other forms of supplemental enteral feeding for newborn infants unable to fully breastfeed. *Cochrane Database Syst Rev.* 2016;8:CD005092. doi:10.1002/14651858.CD005092.pub3.

66. World Health Organization. Cup-feeding for low-birth weight infants unable to fully breastfeed. WHO website. http://www.who.int/elena/titles/cupfeeding_infants/en/. Published 2017. Accessed February 1, 2018.

67. Als H, Duffy FH, McAnulty GB, et al. Early experience alters brain function and structure. *Pediatrics.* 2004;114:1738-1739.

68. Charpak N, Ruiz-Peláez JG, Figueroa de CZ, Charpak Y. A randomized, controlled trial of kangaroo mother care: results of follow-up at 1 year of corrected age. *Pediatrics.* 2001;108(5):1072-1079.

69. Ludington-Hoe SM, Swinth JY. Developmental aspects of kangaroo care. *J Obstet Gynecol Neonatal Nurs.* 1996;25(8):691-703.

70. Gupta G. NICU environment and the neonate. *J Neonatol.* 2001;15(4):7-15.

71. Tallandini MA, Scalembra C. Kangaroo mother care and mother-premature infant dyadic interaction. *Infant Ment Health J.* 2006;27(3):251-275.

72. Grunau RE. Neonatal pain in very preterm infants: long-term effects on brain, neurodevelopment and pain reactivity. *Rambam Maimonides Med J.* 2013;4(4):e0025.

73. Huppertze C, Gharavi B, Schott C, Linderkamp O. Individual development care based on Newborn Individualized Developmental Care and Assessment Program (NIDCAP). *Kinderkrankenschwester.* 2005;9:359-364.

74. White RD, Smith JA, Shepley MM. Recommended standards for newborn ICU design, eighth edition. *J Perinatol.* 2013;33(S1):S2-S16.

75. Mirmiran M, Ariagno RL. Influence of light in the NICU on the development of circadian rhythms in preterm infants. *Semin Perinatol.* 2000;24(4):247-257.

76. American Academy of Pediatrics. Noise: a hazard for the fetus and newborn. *Pediatrics.* 1997;100(4):724-727.

77. Kilpatrick SJ, Papile L, & Macones GA, eds. *Guidelines for Perinatal Care.* 8th ed. Elk Grove Village, IL: American Academy of Pediatrics & American College of Obstetricians and Gynecologists; 2017.

78. Sullivan RM, Toubas P. Clinical usefulness of maternal odor in newborns: soothing and feeding preparatory responses. *Biol Neonate.* 1998;74(6):402-408.

79. Livingston K, Beider S, Kant AJ, Gallardo CC, Joseph MH, Gold JI. Touch and massage for medically fragile infants. *Evid Based Complement Alternat Med.* 2009;6(4):473-482.

80. Bieleninik L, Gold C. Early intervention for premature infants in neonatal intensive care. *Acta Neuropsycholog.* 2014;12(2):185-203.

81. Kavanaugh K, Meier P, Zimmermann B, Mead L. The rewards outweigh the efforts: breastfeeding outcomes for mothers of preterm infants. *J Hum Lactation.* 1997;13(1):15-21.

82. Fugate K, Hernandez I, Ashmeade T, Miladinovic B, Spatz DL. Improving human milk and breastfeeding practices in the NICU. *J Obstet Gynecol Neonatal Nurs.* 2015;44(3):426-438.

83. Hoban R, Bigger H, Patel AL, Rossman B, Fogg LF, Meier P. Goals for human milk feeding in mothers of very low birth weight infants: how do goals change and are they achieved during the NICU hospitalization? *Breastfeed Med.* 2015;10(6):305-311.

84. Miracle DJ, Meier PP, Bennett PA. Mothers' decisions to change from formula to mothers' milk for very-low-birth-weight infants. *J Obstet Gynecol Neonatal Nurs.* 2004;33(6):692-703.

85. Nyqvist KH. Breastfeeding support in neonatal care: an example of the integration of international evidence and experience. *Newborn Infant Nurs Rev.* 2005;5:34-48.

86. Nyqvist KH. Breastfeeding preterm infants. In: Genna CW, ed. *Supporting Sucking Skills in Breastfeeding Infants.* 3rd ed. Burlington, MA: Jones & Bartlett Learning; 2017:181-208.

87. Furman L, Minich N, Hack M. Correlates of lactation in mothers of very low birth weight infants. *Pediatrics.* 2002;109(4):e57.

88. Schmitt J, Arnold K, Druschke D, et al. Early comprehensive care of preterm infants—effects on quality of life, childhood development, and healthcare utilization: study protocol for a cohort study linking administrative healthcare data with patient reported primary data. *BMC Pediatr.* 2016;16:104.

89. World Health Organization, UNICEF. *Baby-Friendly Hospital Initiative: Revised, Updated and Expanded for Integrated Care.* Geneva, Switzerland: World Health Organization; 2009. http://www.who.int/nutrition/publications/infantfeeding/bfhi_trainingcourse/en/. Accessed February 4, 2018.

90. World Health Organization. Protecting, promoting and supporting breastfeeding in facilities providing maternity and newborn services. WHO website. http://www.who.int/nutrition/publications/guidelines/breastfeeding-facilities-maternity-newborn/en/. Published 2017. Accessed January 19, 2018.

91. Levin A. Humane neonatal care initiative. *Acta Paediatr.* 1999;88(4):353-355.

92. Family Integrated Care. Research. FICare website. http://familyintegratedcare.com/about-ficare/research/. Accessed June 26, 2017.

93. UNICEF UK Baby-Friendly Initiative. *Guidance for Neonatal Units.* London, England: UNICEF UK Baby-Friendly Initiative; 2016. https://www.unicef.org.uk/babyfriendly/wp-content/uploads/sites/2/2015/12/Guidance-for-neonatal-units.pdf. Accessed June 26, 2017.

94. Vanderveen JA, Bassler D, Robertson CMT, Kirpalani H. Early interventions involving parents to improve neurodevelopmental outcomes of premature infants: a meta-analysis. *J Perinatol.* 2009;29(5):343-351.

95. Conde-Agudelo A, Díaz-Rossello JL. Kangaroo mother care to reduce morbidity and mortality in low birthweight infants. *Cochrane Database Syst Rev.* 2016;8:CD002771. doi:10.1002/14651858.CD002771.pub4.

96. Renfrew M, Craig D, Dyson L, et al. Breastfeeding promotion for infants in neonatal units: a systematic review and economic analysis. *Health Technol Assess.* 2009;13(40):1-146, iii-iv.

97. World Health Organization. Global strategy for infant and young child feeding. WHO website. http://www.who.int/nutrition/topics/global_strategy_iycf/en/. Published 2003. Accessed August 11, 2017.

98. Karlsson V, Heinemann A-B, Sjörs G, Nykvist KH, Agren J. Early skin-to-skin care in extremely preterm infants: thermal balance and care environment. *J Pediatr.* 2012;161(3):422-426.

99. Nyqvist KH, Sjödén P-O, Ewald U. The development of preterm infants' breastfeeding behavior. *Early Hum Dev.* 1999;55(3):247-264.

100. Hedberg K, Sjodén P-O. Advice concerning breastfeeding from mothers of infants admitted to a neonatal intensive care unit: the Roy adaptation model as a conceptual structure. *J Adv Nurs.* 1993;18(1):54-63.

101. Gale G, Franck L, Lund C. Skin-to-skin (kangaroo) holding of the intubated premature infant. *Neonatal Network.* 1993;12(6):49-57.

102. Black K. Kangaroo care and the ventilated neonate. *Infant.* 2005;1:127-132.

103. de Leeuw R, Colin EM, Dunnebier EA, Mirmiran M. Physiological effects of kangaroo care in very small preterm infants. *Biol Neonate.* 1991;59(3):149-155.

104. Ludington-Hoe SM, Swinth JV, Thompson C, Hadeed AJ. Randomized controlled trial of kangaroo care: cardiorespiratory and thermal effects on healthy preterm infants. *Neonatal Network.* 2004;23:39-48.

105. Ludington-Hoe SM, Ferreira C, Swinth J, Ceccardi JJ. Safe criteria and procedure for kangaroo care with intubated preterm infants. *J Obstet Gynecol Neonatal Nurs.* 2003;32(5):579-588.

106. Acolet D, Sleath K, Whitelaw A. Oxygenation, heart rate and temperature in very low birthweight infants during skin-to-skin contact with their mothers. *Acta Paediatr Scand.* 1989;78:189-193.

107. Ludington-Hoe SM, Kasper CE. A physiologic method of monitoring preterm infants during kangaroo care. *J Nurs Manag.* 1995;3:13-29.

108. Mooncey S, Giannakoulopoulos X, Glover V, Acolet D, Modi N. The effect of mother-infant skin-to-skin contact on plasma cortisol and β-endorphin concentrations in preterm newborns. *Infant Behav Dev.* 1997;20(4):553-557.

109. Feldman R, Eidelman AI, Sirota L, Weller A. Comparison of skin-to-skin (kangaroo) and traditional care: parenting outcomes and preterm infant development. *Pediatrics.* 2002;110(1):16-26.

110. Ludington-Hoe S, Cong X, Hashemi F. Infant crying: nature, physiologic consequences, and select interventions. *Neonatal Network.* 2002;21(2):29-36.

111. Whitlaw A, Heisterkanp G, Sleath K. Skin-to-skin contact for very low birth weight infants and their mothers. *Arch Dis Child.* 1988;63(11):1377-1381.

112. Hurst NM, Valentine CJ, Renfro L, Burns P, Ferlic L. Skin-to-skin holding in the neonatal intensive care unit influences maternal milk volume. *J Perinatol.* 1997;17(3):213-217.

113. Uvnäs-Moberg K, Eriksson M. Breastfeeding: physiological, endocrine and behavioural adaptations caused by oxytocin and local neurogenic activity in the nipple and mammary gland. *Acta Paediatr.* 1996;85(5):525-530.

114. Affonso D, Wahlberg V, Persson V. Exploration of mother's reactions to the kangaroo method of prematurity care. *Neonatal Network.* 1989;7(6):43-51.

115. Boyd S. Within these walls: moderating parental stress in the neonatal intensive care unit. *J Neonatal Nurs.* 2004;10(3):80-84.

116. Mohrbacher N, Stock J. *The Breastfeeding Answer Book.* Schaumburg, IL: La Leche League International; 2003.

117. Becker GE, Smith HA, Cooney F. Methods of milk expression for lactating women. *Cochrane Database Syst Rev.* 2016;9:CD006170. doi:10.1002/14651858.CD006170.pub5.

118. Morton J, Wong RJ, Hall JY, et al. Combining hand techniques with electric pumping increases the caloric content of milk in mothers of preterm infants. *J Perinatol.* 2012;32(10):791-796.

119. Human Milk Banking Association of North America. About HMBABA. HMBABA website. https://www.hmbana.org/about-hmbana. Published 2017. Accessed February 23, 2018.

120. Centers for Disease Control and Prevention. Proper handling and storage of human milk. CDC website. https://www.cdc.gov/breastfeeding /recommendations/handling_breastmilk.htm. Published 2017. Accessed November 4, 2017.

121. Nyqvist KH, Ewald U, Sjödén P-O. Supporting a preterm infant's behaviour during breastfeeding: a case report. *J Hum Lactation.* 1996;12(3):221-228.

122. Academy of Breastfeeding Medicine. Clinical protocol no. 12: transitioning the breastfeeding/breastmilk-fed premature infant from neonatal intensive care unit to home. ABM website. http://www.bfmed.org/protocols. Published 2004.

123. Collins CT, Gillis J, McPhee AJ, Suganuma H, Makrides M. Avoidance of bottles during the establishment of breast feeds in preterm infants. *Cochrane Database Syst Rev.* 2016;(10):CD005252. doi:10.1002/14651858.CD005252.pub4.

124. Dennis C, Kingston D. A systematic review of telephone support for women during pregnancy and the early postpartum period. *J Obstet Gynecol Neonatal Nurs.* 2008;37(3):301-314.

125. Elliott S, Reimer C. Postdischarge telephone follow-up program for breastfeeding preterm infants discharged from a special care nursery. *Neonatal Network.* 1998;17(6):41-45.

126. Meier P, Patel AL, Wright K, Engstrom JL. Management of breastfeeding during and after the maternity hospitalization for late preterm infants. *Clin Perinatol.* 2013;40(4):689-705.

127. Boies EG, Vaucher YE, Academy of Breastfeeding Medicine. ABM clinical protocol #10: breastfeeding late preterm (34-36 6/7 weeks of gestation) and early term infants (37-38 6/7 weeks gestation), 2nd revision 2016. *Breastfeed Med.* 2016;11(10):494-500.

128. Briere C-E, Lucas R, McGrath JM, Lussier M, Brownell E. Establishing breastfeeding with the late preterm infant in the NICU. *J Obstet Gynecol Neonatal Nurs.* 2015;44(1):102-113.

129. Academy of Breastfeeding Medicine. Educational objectives and skills for the physician with respect to breastfeeding. *Breastfeed Med.* 2011;6(2):99-105.

130. Engle WA. A recommendation for the definition of "late preterm" (near-term) and the birth weight-gestational age classification system. *Semin Perinatol.* 2006;30(1):2-7.

131. Raju TNK. The problem of late-preterm (near-term) births: a workshop summary. *Pediatr Res.* 2006;60(6):775-776.

132. Declercq E, Luke B, Belanoff C, et al. Perinatal outcomes associated with assisted reproductive technology: the Massachusetts Outcomes Study of Assisted Reproductive Technologies (MOSART). *Fertil Steril.* 2015;103(4):888-895.

133. Joshi N, Kissin D, Anderson JE, Session D, Macaluso M, Jamieson DJ. Trends and correlates of good perinatal outcomes in assisted reproductive technology. *Obstet Gynecol.* 2012;120(4):843-851.

134. Hallowell SG, Spatz DL. The relationship of brain development and breastfeeding in the late-preterm infant. *J Pediatr Nurs.* 2012;27(2):154-162.

135. Goldenberg RL, Culhane JF, Iams JD, Romero R. Epidemiology and causes of preterm birth. *Lancet.* 2008;371(9606):75-84.

136. Hamilton BE, Martin JA, Ventura SJ, Statitics DoV. Birth: preliminary data for 2011. *Natl Vital Stat Rep.* 2012;61(5):1-18.

137. Schieve LA, Ferre C, Peterson HB, Macaluso M, Reynolds MA, Wright VC. Perinatal outcome among singleton infants conceived through assisted reproductive technology in the United States. *Obstet Gynecol.* 2004;103:1144-1153.

138. Bergman NJ, Linley LL, Fawcus SR. Randomized controlled trial of skin-to-skin contact from birth versus conventional incubator for physiological stabilization in 1200- to 2199-gram newborns. *Acta Paediatr.* 2004;93(6):779-785.

139. Moore ER, Bergman N, Anderson GC, Medley N. Early skin-to-skin contact for mothers and their healthy newborn infants. *Cochrane Database Syst Rev.* 2016;11:CD003519. doi:10.1002/14651858.CD003519.pub4.

140. Sobel HL, Silvestre MAA, Mantaring Iii JBV, Oliveros YE, Nyunt-U S. Immediate newborn care practices delay thermoregulation and breastfeeding initiation. *Acta Paediatr.* 2011;100(8):1127-1133.

141. Black LS. Incorporating breastfeeding care into daily newborn rounds and pediatric office practice. *Pediatr Clin North Am.* 2001;48(2):299-319.

142. World Health Organization. *WHO Recommendations on Newborn Health.* Geneva, Switzerland: World Health Organization; 2017. http://www.who.int/maternal_child_adolescent/documents/newborn-health-recommendations/en/. Accessed March 24, 2018.

143. Meier PP, Brown LP, Hurst NM, et al. Nipple shields for preterm infants: effect on milk transfer and duration of breastfeeding. *J Hum Lactation.* 2000;16(2):106-114.

144. Maastrup R, Bojesen SN, Kronborg H, Hallström I. Breastfeeding support in neonatal intensive care: a national survey. *J Hum Lactation.* 2012;28(3):370-379.

145. Kronborg H, Foverskov E, Nilsson I, Maastrup R. Why do mothers use nipple shields and how does this influence duration of exclusive breastfeeding? *Matern Child Nutr.* 2017;13(1). doi:10.1111/mcn.12251.

146. California Perinatal Quality Care Collaborative. Quality improvement toolkits. CPQCC website. https://www.cpqcc.org/quality -improvement-toolkits. Accessed November 5, 2017.

147. Howard CR, de Blieck EA, ten Hoopen CB, Howard FM, Lanphear BP, Lawrence RA. Physiologic stability of newborns during cup- and bottle-feeding. *Pediatrics.* 1999;104(suppl 6):1204-1207.

148. Howard CR, Howard FM, Lanphear B, et al. Randomized clinical trial of pacifier use and bottle-feeding or cupfeeding and their effect on breastfeeding. *Pediatrics.* 2003;111(3):511-518.

149. Marinelli KA, Burke GS, Doss VL. A comparison of the safety of cup feedings and bottle feedings in premature infants whose mothers intend to breastfeed. *J Perinatol.* 2001;21(6):350-355.

150. Lanese MG. Cup feeding: a valuable tool. *J Hum Lactation.* 2011;27(1):12-13.

151. Meier P, Anderson GC. Responses of small preterm infants to bottle- and breast-feeding. *MCN Am J Matern Child Nurs.* 1987;12:97-105.

152. Meier PP, Brown LP. State of the science: breastfeeding for mothers and low birth weight infants. *Nurs Clin North Am.* 1996;31(2):351-365.

153. Walker M. Breastfeeding the late preterm infant. *J Obstet Gynecol Neonatal Nurs.* 2008;37(6):692-701.

154. Walker M. *Breastfeeding the Late Preterm Infant.* Amarillo, TX: Hale Publishing; 2009.

Additional Resources

Blencowe H, Cousens S, Chou D, et al. Born too soon: the global epidemiology of 15 million preterm births. *Reprod Health*. 2013;10(suppl):S2. doi:10.1186/1742-4755-10-S1-S2.

International Lactation Consultant Association. The Neo-BFHI: The Baby-Friendly Hospital Initiative for Neonatal Wards. ILCA website. http://www.ilca.org/main/learning/resources/neo-bfhi. Published 2018.

NCTBA.org. Feeding Challenges of the Late Preterm Infant. http://www.nctba.org/breastfeeding/feeding-challenges-of-the-late-preterm-infant. Published March 29, 2011.

World Health Organization. Cup-feeding of low-birth weight infant unable to fully breastfeed. WHO website. http://www.who.int/elena/titles/full_recommendations/feeding_lbw/en/. Published 2017.

World Health Organization. Executive summary: tracking progress for breastfeeding policies and programmes. WHO website. http://www.who.int/nutrition/publications/infantfeeding/global-bf-scorecard-2017-summary.pdf?ua=1. Published 2017.

World Health Organization. Global strategy for infant and young child feeding. WHO website. http://www.who.int/nutrition/topics/global_strategy_iycf/en/. Published 2003.

World Health Organization. Protecting, promoting and supporting breastfeeding in facilities providing maternity and newborn services. WHO website. http://www.who.int/nutrition/publications/guidelines/breastfeeding-facilities-maternity-newborn/en/. Published 2017.

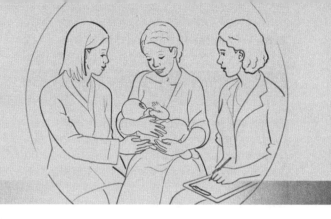

CHAPTER 15

Breastfeeding Multiples

M. Karen Kerkhoff Gromada

OBJECTIVES

- Discuss the antenatal, intrapartum, and postnatal conditions and barriers, which often affect the initiation of breastfeeding and lactation with twins and higher-order multiple births.
- Describe strategies for initiating and coordinating breastfeeding with multiple-birth neonates.
- Identify physiological and psychosocial factors that often affect the exclusivity and duration of breastfeeding or human milk feeding (HMF) with multiple-birth infants and children.

DEFINITIONS OF COMMONLY USED TERMS

artificial infant milk (AIM) Nonhuman animal or plant-derived infant milk marketed and used as a replacement for some, or all, human milk in an infant's diet. Also called infant formula.

assisted reproductive technology (ART) Techniques in which both ova and sperm are handled, including in vitro fertilization (IVF) with or without intracytoplasmic sperm injection (ICSI).

expressed human milk (EHM) Human milk obtained via milk expression by hand and breast pump.

extremely low birth weight (ELBW) Less than 1,000 grams (2.2 pounds).

dichorionic–diamniotic placentation (Di/Di or DCDA) Pregnancy in which each multiple has its own placenta with an outer chorionic and an inner amniotic sac. Multiples are usually dizygotic (DZ) but may be monozygotic (MZ).

dizygotic (DZ) Twins developing from two separate ova (eggs) that are fertilized by two separate sperm, creating two genetically unique zygotes. Also called fraternal twins.

gestational age (GA) The number of completed weeks plus days, measured beginning with the first day of the last menstrual period until the current point in pregnancy or the day of delivery. Two weeks is added to conceptual age when ART was used to achieve pregnancy.

higher-order multiples (HOM) Three or more multiples from one pregnancy, such as triplets, quadruplets, or quintuplets.

human milk fed (HMF) The feeding of expressed human milk (EHM).

in vitro fertilization (IVF) A type of MAR in which ova (eggs) are removed from a woman's ovaries and fertilized by sperm in a laboratory procedure, followed by one or more of the fertilized ova being returned to the woman's uterus.

(continues)

DEFINITIONS OF COMMONLY USED TERMS *(continued)*

intrauterine growth retardation (IUGR) A fetal weight determined by ultrasound to be below the 10th percentile for gestational age (GA).

low birth weight (LBW) Less than 2,500 grams (5.5 pounds).

medically assisted reproduction (MAR) The use of medical techniques to treat subfertility and achieve a pregnancy. Includes ovulatory induction (OI) medications, ART, or a combination of medical and surgical techniques.

monochorionic–diamniotic placentation (Mo/Di or MCDA) Shared placenta and outer chorion, but each multiple is within its own inner amniotic sac.

monochorionic–monoamniotic placentation (Mo/Mo or MCMA) Shared placenta, outer chorion, and inner amniotic sac.

monochorionic placentation (MC) MZ multiples who share a single placenta and an outer chorionic sac. The types include monochorionic–diamniotic and monochorionic–monoamniotic.

monozygotic (MZ) Twins (or HOM) developing from one ovum (egg) that is fertilized by one sperm, creating one zygote that completely divides to form two genetically identical zygotes. Also called identical twins.

mother of multiples (MOM) A woman who carries and then gives birth to two or more infants from a single pregnancy. A parent whose gestational carrier (GC) gives birth to two or more infants from a single pregnancy. A parent who adopts two or more infants born from a single pregnancy.

mother of twins (MOT) A woman who carries and then gives birth to two infants from a single pregnancy. A parent whose GC gives birth to two infants from a single pregnancy. A parent who adopts two infants born from a single pregnancy.

placentation Formation, type and structure, or arrangement, of placenta or placentas. Includes the following:

preterm (PT) Less than 37 weeks' gestation completed at birth, including the following:
- Extremely preterm (EPT): Less than 28 weeks
- Very preterm (VPT): 28 to 31 0/7 weeks
- Moderately preterm (MPT): 32 to 33 6/7 weeks
- Late preterm (LPT): 34 to 36 6/7 weeks

simultaneous feeding Feeding two infants from a set of multiples at the same time, with one at each breast. Also called tandem feeding.

small for gestational age (SGA) An infant who is smaller in size (below 10th percentile) than the normal parameters for gestational age.

term Weeks of gestation at birth. Includes the following:
- Early term (ET): 37 to 38 6/7 weeks
- Full term (FT): 39 to 40 6/7 weeks
- Late term (LT): 41 to 41 6/7 weeks
- Postterm: 42 weeks or more

twins Two infants from one pregnancy.

very low birth weight (VLBW) Less than 1,500 grams (3.3 pounds) but more than 1,000 grams (2.2 pounds).

zygosity As it pertains to twinning, the development of multiples from one or more fertilized ova (dizygotic or monozygotic).

Any use of the term *mother, maternal,* or *breastfeeding* is not meant to exclude transgender or nonbinary parents who may be breastfeeding or providing human milk to their infant.

▶ Overview

Single-infant pregnancy and birth is the norm for human mammals. Multiple pregnancy and birth strain maternal physical systems and emotional reserves, resulting in a greater risk for a number of fetal, neonatal, and maternal complications. These complications often affect breastfeeding or milk expression initiation and may have long-lasting effects on the exclusivity and duration of direct breastfeeding or human milk feeding (HMF) for one or more of the multiple-birth infants. Still, each multiple-birth infant is essentially a single infant who happened to arrive with one or more others. Each multiple-parent dyad has the same right to the breastfeeding relationship and the normal physical and psychosocial advantages that breastfeeding and lactation offer. Breastfeeding multiple infants or toddlers is affected by more than each infant's or the breastfeeding parent's ability to replicate appropriate breastfeeding mechanics or implement typical lactation management strategies with two or more infants or children. Coordinating the breastfeeding of two or more infants with varying abilities to breastfeed, or differing but normal feeding patterns and styles, may be perceived as breastfeeding problems rather than an aspect of the reality of having multiple same-aged, yet individual, infants. Also, older infant and toddler multiples often engage in interactive behaviors during breastfeeding that may affect parental coping and the perception of the breastfeeding relationship. Therefore, those who breastfeed or human milk feed multiple newborns, infants, or children are likely to need increased and specialized breastfeeding and lactation support and reinforcement.

I. Multiple-Birth Rate

A. The incidence of twin live births per year varies from approximately 7 per 1,000 to 34 per 1,000 worldwide.[1-6]

1. Higher birth rates for twins occur in industrial nations where more parents delay childbearing until an older age and where there are fewer restrictions on the number of embryos that may be transferred during in vitro fertilization.

2. The worldwide incidence for monozygotic (MZ) twins is approximately 4 per 1,000.

3. The current birth rate for triplets in certain industrialized nations is 1–2 per 1,000. In developing nations, and in industrialized nations prior to the introduction of medically assisted reproduction (MAR), the incidence is approximately 1 per 7,500–10,000 live births.

B. Medically assisted reproduction and older maternal age at conception mainly result in an increase in dizygotic (DZ) multiples. However, MAR is also associated with an increased risk for monozygotic twinning with a greater likelihood for the development of a monochorionic (MC) placenta.

C. New knowledge and improvements in medically assisted reproduction techniques have led to a steady decline in higher-order multiple births over the past 1 to 2 decades.[3,8]

II. Barriers to Breastfeeding Multiple-Birth Neonates

A. A parent intending to breastfeed multiple-birth infants deserves the best possible breastfeeding start. Yet this is challenging because twins and higher-order multiple (HOM) pregnancies have a higher risk for fetal, neonatal, and maternal complications.[9]

B. Infant-related barriers to breastfeeding initiation, duration, and exclusivity are many times more likely to affect multiple-birth neonates than single-birth infants. These include preterm (PT) birth; low birth weight (LBW); congenital anomalies; and fetal, neonatal, and infant mortality.

1. The incidence of preterm or very preterm (VPT) birth is 9–10 times higher for twins than for single-born infants, and the incidence is even greater for higher-order multiples.[10]

a. Depending on the geographic location, 50 to 60 percent of twins and more than 90 percent of higher-order multiples are born preterm.

b. Approximately 10 percent of preterm twins and 40 percent of preterm higher-order multiples are born very preterm.[5,10]

2. Twins and higher-order multiples are many times more likely than single-born neonates to be affected by low birth weight and very low birth weight (VLBW).[3,5,6] In addition to smaller size at preterm birth, one or more infants within a set of multiples may be small for gestational age (SGA) or affected by intrauterine growth restriction (IUGR). There may be central nervous system or musculoskeletal consequences[15] affecting an infant's suckling, even when multiples are born after 37 weeks of gestation.

3. Placentation is likely to affect either the timing of delivery for a set of multiples or the birth weight of one or more multiples, particularly for monozygotic twins who share a placenta.

a. The American College of Obstetricians and Gynecologists currently recommends delivery between 34 and 37 6/7 weeks of gestation for an otherwise uncomplicated monochorionic–diamniotic (Mo/Di) twin gestation, and cesarean delivery between 32 and 34 weeks for an uncomplicated monochorionic–monoamniotic (Mo/Mo) gestation.[16]

b. The findings of some recent meta-analyses suggest that, assuming close surveillance, the later gestational age parameters may be more appropriate because they decrease preterm birth-associated morbidities, including neonatal feeding difficulties, with little or no increase for fetal or neonatal mortality with each additional week of gestation.[17-19]

4. Multiples pregnancies are associated with an increased incidence of congenital anomalies, including those related to early fetal development and those associated with intrauterine crowding during the last trimester of pregnancy.[3,20-23]

   a. Chromosomal defects or malformations related to disruption during early fetal development are thought to be related to an increase in cerebral palsy and anomalies in the cardiac, gastrointestinal, genitourinary, and musculoskeletal systems.

   b. Overcrowding and malpositioning of one or more fetuses during the last trimester is more likely to result in cranial malformations, such as plagiocephaly, torticollis, and facial deviations.

   c. Whether a congenital anomaly affects one or more of multiple-birth infants, breastfeeding for both or all may be affected. (See Chapter 23, *Breastfeeding and Infant Birth Injury, Congenital Anomalies, and Illness.*)

5. The separation of the parent and one or more multiples due to a stay in a neonatal intensive care unit (NICU) or special care nursery (SCN), as well as any immaturity of physical systems affecting breastfeeding or milk expression initiation, may have short- or long-term effects on breastfeeding due to the complexity of transitioning two or more infants to the breast.[11] The exclusivity and duration of breastfeeding or human milk feeding may also be affected.[12-14]

6. Preterm birth, low birth weight, and congenital anomalies affect overall coping and attachment formation with infants, as well as time management for the breastfeeding parent.

   a. This is due, in part, to an increased need for postdischarge procedures and healthcare specialist appointments for one or more infants.

   b. The frequency or intensity of appointments and procedures may affect breastfeeding initiation, exclusivity, duration, or ongoing milk expression.

7. The rate of fetal, neonatal, and infant mortality increases with the gestation and birth of multiples.[3,24] The death of one or more multiples may affect breastfeeding, a transition to breastfeeding, or milk expression as the parent grieves or postpones grieving while forming an attachment with surviving multiples.[25,26]

C. Maternal morbidity and mortality increase during multiple pregnancy and birth.[3,16,27] Complications or conditions, and their medical treatments, may delay breastfeeding initiation or milk expression if they interfere with self-care ability. In addition, multiple pregnancy or birth is associated with increased risk for many of the complications associated with delayed lactogenesis.[28]

1. Complications that are more common with multiple pregnancy or birth include the following: hyperemesis gravidarum; hypertensive conditions, including preeclampsia and the more severe hemolysis, elevated liver enzymes, low platelets (HELLP) syndrome; gestational diabetes mellitus (GDM); antenatal and postnatal anemia; surgical delivery; postpartum hemorrhage related to uterine atony or placental anomalies, such as previa or abruption; and deep vein thrombosis (DVT).

2. Approximately 75 percent of twins[29] and almost 95 percent of higher-order multiples in the United States are now delivered via cesarean section.[30] Twin birth by cesarean section in other parts of the world ranges from 31 percent (in Iceland) to 98 percent (in Malta).[3] The differences in elective twin cesarean rates may be related to the overuse of cesarean in some wealthier countries and less access to cesarean birth in lower-income countries.[31]

3. Preconception treatment for subfertility with medically assisted reproduction is not necessarily related to insufficient milk production after delivery. However, certain maternal conditions, such as polycystic ovary syndrome (PCOS), thyroid-related conditions or obesity, which may contribute to subfertility may also result in lower milk production for some.[32]

4. Perinatal mood disorders, including depression and anxiety, are more common among mothers who have given birth to multiples, as high as 43 percent greater. Fathers also reported more symptoms of depression and anxiety.[33-35] In addition, factors associated with postnatal posttraumatic stress disorder (PTSD) symptoms are fairly common after multiple pregnancy and birth.[36]

D. Health complications and the ongoing intensity of caring for multiple infants and other children, deplete the breastfeeding parent's physical, psychological, and emotional reserves. This may affect breastfeeding or milk expression at any time during the postnatal year,[11-13,37-42] particularly if the parent lacks adequate healthcare system and social support networks and resources for breastfeeding or human milk feeding multiple infants.

III. The Right to the Breastfeeding Relationship

A. The increased incidence of pregnancy, birth, and postnatal complications for multiple-birth infants increases the importance of providing species-specific milk, particularly its immunological properties.[43-47]

B. Multiple-birth infants and their breastfeeding parent have the same right to a breastfeeding relationship, human milk, and lactation as does a single-birth infant and breastfeeding parent.[40,42,48,49]

    1. Women have breastfed or provided their milk to multiple-birth infants for periods of several hours to several years.[14,41,50-56]

    2. Parents who are expecting multiples deserve factual information so they can make informed feeding decisions.

    3. This information must take into account the increased risk of parental and neonatal complications for parents of multiples and their infants.

C. Breastfeeding and providing human milk for multiple infants requires healthcare professional, family, and social network education and support that has been adapted specifically for multiple-birth families.[12,40-42,48,49,57-60]

    1. Parents are discouraged from breastfeeding multiples by healthcare professionals for reasons based less on evidence and more on assumption, attitude, or anecdote.

    2. A healthcare professional's knowledge deficits regarding breastfeeding and lactation for multiple infants may affect a parent's confidence to initiate breastfeeding or milk expression and the ability to produce enough milk for more than one infant.

IV. Anticipatory Guidance: Prenatal Preparation for Breastfeeding Multiples

A. For parents with multiples, the intention to breastfeed or provide expressed human milk, versus breastfeeding or initiating milk expression, varies depending on the data collection method and geographic area studied.

    1. The findings of population-based research studies, including one randomized controlled trial, vary.[57,58,60-62] Geographic or cultural differences may account for significantly lower rates of breastfeeding or HMF initiation for this population when compared to single-birth infants.

    2. For studies using a convenience or self-selected sample population, parental breastfeeding intention and initiation for multiples are similar to or higher than for those with single-birth infants.[14,59]

    3. The intention to breastfeed twins was shown to be closely associated with breastfeeding them initially and at 3 months, whether the infants arrived via planned vaginal birth or cesarean birth.[63]

    4. Both exclusivity and the overall duration of breastfeeding or human milk feeding decrease over the first several weeks to months postpartum.[12,61,64] The decrease appears to occur earlier than with single-born infants. Preterm birth appears to be related to a 3- to 4-month duration for any amount of breastfeeding or human milk feeding for multiples.[14,62]

    5. Researchers found that mothers either continue to breastfeed or human milk feed all multiples or wean all of the infants at approximately the same time, indicating the duration is unrelated to individual infant need or ability.[61,65,66]

    6. Few researchers distinguish between direct breastfeeding and the feeding of expressed milk to multiples, or between exclusive breastfeeding or human milk feeding and partial direct breastfeeding or human milk feeding with partial artificial infant milk.

    7. Although the demographics for women using medically assisted reproduction to achieve pregnancy— increased maternal age, education, socioeconomic status—are associated with populations that initiate breastfeeding at higher rates, one study found that Japanese women older than 35 years were less likely to breastfeed their twins.[58]

B. Preparation for breastfeeding multiples should include an assessment of breastfeeding and lactation knowledge and any previous history of breastfeeding or milk expression.

    1. Discuss the advantages and disadvantages of breastfeeding two or more newborns for exclusive and partial breastfeeding or human milk feeding.[13,39,40,42,48,64,67]

a. The advantages that are specific to multiples may include the following:

  i. The immunological and anti-infective properties of human milk protect infants who are at greater risk of being immunocompromised at birth and who are likely to share contagious illnesses.

  ii. Parents experience an eventual time savings when simultaneously feeding two infants.

  iii. Physical contact with each infant is increased, which may enhance individual attachment formation.

  iv. Time is invested in the infants rather than in obtaining, preparing, heating, and cleaning formula for feeding of one or more infant.

  v. After the parent is past the initial learning curve, breastfeeding is easier than alternative methods.

  vi. Breastfeeding is less expensive.

  vii. Pregnancy weight may be lost more quickly due to the caloric intake required to produce milk for multiple infants.

b. Parents have reported challenges with breastfeeding multiples include the following:

  i. Initiation of breastfeeding and lactation often requires ongoing milk expression and the use of a breast pump, including related expenses.

  ii. Increased time is required for the learning curve with multiple newborns, including handling latch or suckling issues for one or more infants and dealing with any related nipple or breast trauma.

  iii. Sufficient milk production for multiple infants is a concern.

  iv. Others cannot help with feedings, including night feedings, and related sleep deprivation.

  v. Transitioning two or more preterm newborns to direct breastfeeding feels overwhelming and often burdensome due to the constant care needs for two or more infants while also continuing to express milk frequently.

  vi. Integrating breastfeeding for two or more infants is challenging when the parent returns to work.

c. When partial breastfeeding or human milk feeding is desired, a discussion of establishing and maintaining adequate milk production to achieve goals is an important aspect of preparation.

2. Assess the parent's health history for any conditions, including those related to subfertility, surgery, or injury, and examine the breasts for pregnancy-related changes or deviations that may affect breastfeeding or milk production.[67]

a. Reinforce research and case study evidence demonstrating that most parents can produce enough milk for two or more newborns through infancy and into the toddler years.[41,50,51,53]

b. Address any parental red flags that may influence adequate milk production and common neonatal issues that could affect breastfeeding initiation. (See Chapter 13, *Facilitating and Assessing Breastfeeding Initiation,* and Chapter 22, *Low Milk Production and Infant Weight.*)

C. Help parents develop realistic, individualized short- and long-term breastfeeding goals for their multiple infants.[12,39,40]

1. Identify any perceptions or concerns about caring for two or more infants, including any related to breastfeeding or human milk feeding, that may affect breastfeeding goals.[48]

2. Discuss close support systems, such as an adult partner or other adults in the household or community who influence the breastfeeding parent. Explore the level of support that may be expected from those closest to the parent.

3. Address exclusive or partial breastfeeding, and feeding of expressed milk, as it pertains to factors such as length of gestation or neonatal or parental complications.

4. Refer to literature demonstrating that many parents can, and have, breastfed twins and higher-order multiples beyond the toddler period.[40,52,54,68] There are case study reports of inducing lactation for adopted twins,[69] inducing lactation for biological twins born via a gestational carrier,[70] and exclusively breastfeeding twins on one breast after undergoing a unilateral mastectomy.[71] In addition, there are online accounts of breastfeeding twins under similar circumstances.

D. Provide anticipatory guidance, including the development of a breastfeeding plan, that may minimize the barriers commonly affecting the initiation and timing of lactogenesis II with multiple neonates.

1. Discuss the parent's pregnancy diet. Improved multiple-birth neonatal outcomes, including increased gestational age and increased birth weight, are associated with appropriate pregnancy weight gain.[72-74]

2. Provide evidence-based information about vaginal versus cesarean multiple delivery, and help the parent develop a multiples-specific birth plan that includes breastfeeding or initiating milk expression.[75]
   a. Vaginal delivery may be a safe option for an uncomplicated twin pregnancy, especially when the twin presenting first in the pelvis is in a vertex position.[76-78]
   b. Vaginal delivery could be considered for higher-order multiples when the infant presenting first is vertex.
   c. A trial of labor after cesarean may be appropriate for an expectant parent of twins who has a history of a previous low transverse surgical delivery and the twin presenting first is vertex.[16]
3. Develop strategies during pregnancy for the initiation and management of early breastfeeding or milk expression with multiple neonates, based on individual infant condition or parental complications.[42,48,49,75]
   a. Convey the importance of early (within 60–90 minutes of birth for each multiple),[79] frequent breastfeeding or milk expression to maximize milk production.[80] With an increased likelihood of late pregnancy complications or surgical birth, planning for around-the-clock help during the hospital postnatal stay can facilitate breastfeeding or milk expression. Introduce adaptations or options to accommodate healthy multiples and those who are born physically compromised.
   b. Discuss the aspects of normal breastfeeding, such as the typical frequency and duration of feedings and how they may vary among individuals within the set of multiples, and the expected breastfeeding outcomes for each baby. A good understanding of the role of milk removal to increase or maintain milk production is crucial when breastfeeding multiple infants.
   c. Explore options for obtaining donor human milk in the event that milk production is insufficient.[55]
   d. Explain the guidelines for inducing lactation, when pertinent, and the possibility of breast-feeding multiples born of a gestational carrier or surrogate, or in the case of adoptions.[69] (See Chapter 19, *Induced Lactation and Relactation*.)
4. Recommend resources, such as breastfeeding classes, community breastfeeding information and support groups, and pediatric care providers and daycare providers who are supportive of breastfeeding multiples.[75] It is particularly helpful to put parents in contact with others who are breastfeeding or have breastfed multiples.
5. Encourage extended household help during the postnatal year.[39,75,81] This may include help with an older child, household tasks, and running errands. (Postnatal doulas provide this type of assistance.) It is not realistic to care for multiple infants and still handle household duties.

V. Initiating Breastfeeding and Lactation

A. Initiating breastfeeding with each healthy multiple should mimic that for a single-born infant.[48,75] (See Chapter 13, *Facilitating and Assessing Breastfeeding Initiation*.)
B. There are elements in initiating breastfeeding that are specific to multiples.
   1. Encourage separate, rather than simultaneous, feedings at least until each infant is assessed for and demonstrates effective breastfeeding behaviors and one infant consistently latches deeply and painlessly.[37,47,75]
   2. The timing for implementing simultaneous feeding varies from the first 24 hours to several weeks or months after birth. Information, demonstration, and encouraging simultaneous breastfeeding positions help parents feel prepared when at least two of their multiples are ready.
   3. Monitor each infant for signs of effective breastfeeding and related outcomes by maintaining a simple feeding and output log for each infant until adequate weight and growth are well established.
   4. Encourage the mother to have an around-the-clock, supportive assistant (partner, relative, or friend) to help with the neonates' care and provide breastfeeding help for positioning infants, e.g., holding an infant in place if needed. This is particularly helpful after a surgical delivery. Planning for two or three assistants allows them to help in shifts so they can take breaks.
   5. Assist with effective milk removal via breastfeeding or milk expression at least eight times in 24 hours—or show a caregiver how to help—if treatment, including medications, for a complication interferes with the ability to perform these tasks independently.[82]

6. Provide appropriate discharge planning that includes the following:
   a. How to coordinate breastfeeding and infant care with two or more infants.
   b. How to monitor breastfeeding outcomes for each newborn.
   c. How to distinguish breastfeeding issues from issues related to having two or more infants.

C. Initiating breastfeeding with preterm or otherwise compromised neonates will almost always require milk expression to establish and maintain lactation until all neonates transfer milk effectively at the breast, which may take days to months.[40,83] (See Chapter 14, *Breastfeeding and the Preterm Infant.*)
   1. Help with breastfeeding any stable multiples, when appropriate. Initiate manual milk expression within 60 minutes, or at least within 6 hours, of birth.[76] Continue expressing milk bilaterally at least eight times per 24 hours to simulate the breastfeeding patterns of term neonates.
   2. Instruct the mother in the use of hands-on techniques in combination with a multiuser, double (bilateral) electric breast pump. This improves the overall volume of milk obtained, the time required to obtain it, and the fat content in the expressed milk.[80,84]
   3. Encourage frequent skin-to-skin contact, which may increase milk volume and enhance the progression to direct breastfeeding for one or more infants.[85-86] Ensuring proximity of multiples' NICU cribs or co-bedding of multiples may facilitate frequent skin-to-skin contact.
   4. Direct breastfeeding during the infants' NICU stay is associated with higher rates of continued milk expression upon discharge,[87] which may also have implications for a postdischarge transition to direct breastfeeding and a need for ongoing milk expression until all multiples breastfeed effectively.
   5. The use of a thin silicone nipple shield has been found to improve the effectiveness of milk transfer at the breast for some preterm infants.[88]
   6. Provide anticipatory guidance for NICU discharge by helping to develop a realistic feeding plan. This plan may differ from a plan for a single infant due to the complexity of ensuring adequate intake for each infant and protecting milk production while two or more infants transition to direct breastfeeding and while the parent recuperates from a more stressful or complicated pregnancy and birth.
   7. A key point in a postdischarge plan is the protection of adequate milk production for all the infants. The strategies should include the following:
      a. Postdischarge use of a high-quality multiuser (hospital-type rental) electric breast pump equipped with a double collection kit, which is associated with obtaining greater milk volumes.[89]
      b. Bilateral expression of milk at least eight times in 24 hours and the use of a simple log to monitor milk expression sessions. Although more frequent milk expression may be desired, it may not be realistic when recuperating from birth and visiting newborns in the NICU, or as each multiple is discharged to home.
      c. Milk expression more often during the daytime hours to allow for one 4–5 hour period of uninterrupted sleep at night.
      d. Manual expression and hands-on techniques during at least five of the eight or more pumping sessions per 24 hours (see the "Maximizing Milk Production with Hands-On Pumping" video).[90]
      e. Discussion of hands-free breast pumping devices and clothing, such as a camisole, bustier, or bra, that allow the parent to care for infants or accomplish another task and increase the number and duration of milk expression sessions.
      f. As-needed use of some form of power pumping for several consecutive days (in addition to the eight or more daily sessions) to boost milk production, such as alternating pumping with no pumping every 10 minutes for 1 hour,[91] or pumping for 5–10 minutes whenever possible.
   8. The infants' transition to direct breastfeeding is likely to take time and may not occur until several weeks beyond their 40-week due date. The transition time is likely to vary for each multiple because each infant is a unique individual.[28,83,92]
   9. As needed test weighing of the infants immediately before and immediately after a feeding with a digital scale that is sensitive to within 1–2 grams (0.035–0.071 ounces). Determining an infant's milk intake during a feeding may facilitate a transition to direct breastfeeding for each infant. It may also guide an infant-specific decrease in supplementation or milk expression.[93]

10. Anticipatory guidance must also consider psychosocial factors that affect NICU discharge with multiples.[40,42] Parents of multiples may face the following:
    a. Staggered infant discharge, which has the potential to affect the attachment formation process with each infant, in addition to the time available for frequent milk expression and to practice breastfeeding.
    b. Assuming the care and related concerns with the growth and development of two or more preterm or sick newborns.
    c. Coping with the individual infants' differing transitions to direct breastfeeding while maintaining adequate milk removal.
11. Ensure that the breastfeeding parent has a printed copy of community breastfeeding support resources, which should include outpatient and community-based International Board Certified Lactation Consultants (IBCLCs) and breastfeeding group leaders or meeting information.[72] Ongoing follow-up with an IBCLC should be encouraged until all multiples breastfeed effectively or until breastfeeding goals are being achieved.
12. When possible, link parents of multiples with others in the community, or in an online community, who are or have breastfed a set of same-number multiples.[47,75,83] Caution parents that lay information may not always be accurate and does not replace consulting with an appropriate expert, such as an IBCLC, if they experience a breastfeeding problem.

D. Transitioning multiple high-risk neonates to direct breastfeeding can be a challenge.[83] Milk must continue to be expressed to maintain adequate production, and alternative feeding methods must be employed to ensure adequate daily intake for each multiple while also finding time to work with each infant at the breast.[11,28,42]
1. Around-the-clock care that is required for multiple infants and the accompanying sleep deprivation while recuperating from multiple pregnancy and birth can be draining.[38]
2. Transition strategies include the following:
   a. Breastfeed, then feed expressed milk or formula, and then express milk.
   b. Block out some periods in the day strictly for breastfeeding and some periods for using alternative feeding methods plus expressing milk.[28]
3. Alternative feedings could be given by household helpers, allowing more time for milk expression and rest. One or more of the infants may be prescribed nutritional fortification for various lengths of time that last from several weeks to 1 year.
4. The use of, and the related benefits and risks of, various alternative feeding options and feeding aids or devices should be presented. If an infant feeding-bottle system is chosen, a slow-flow teat or nipple in conjunction with a cue-based or paced feeding technique will support oral feeding behavior changes that coincide with breastfeeding oral behaviors.[94-96] (See Chapter 24, *Breastfeeding Devices and Topical Treatments*.)
5. As multiple infants progress to direct breastfeeding, a frequent reassessment of each infant at the breast and a revision of interventions should occur based on each infant's changing ability.[28] Reassessments should include test weighing on an as-needed basis and observing any nipple shield use. The parent's confidence should be assessed during every encounter.
6. When one infant breastfeeds effectively but another is not yet able to do so, the parent may save time by breastfeeding the effective feeder while simultaneously pumping the other breast. This may also increase the production and improve the volume of milk obtained for the other infant.[39]
7. To protect milk production during each multiple's transition to breastfeeding, ongoing milk expression with a high-quality multiuser electric breast pump is strongly encouraged until all babies demonstrate effective breastfeeding outcomes. Some parents find that a 1–3 day breastfeeding time out, with increased milk expression and minimal breastfeeding, can help boost production.[92]
8. Because the infants are unique individuals, they will progress to direct breastfeeding at different paces. Parents, family members, and often healthcare providers tend to regard multiples as a unit, and to expect that all infants will be ready to transition to direct breastfeeding at the same time. This common early response to caring for multiple infants can interfere with the transition to breastfeeding. A lactation consultant can help parents recognize each infant's progress to effective breastfeeding.

9. With patience and persistence, each infant will usually transition to direct breastfeeding, but sometimes an infant might not. This is typically related to an ongoing health issue for the infant or simply a lack of parental time to continue working on direct breastfeeding. Some parents have reported that one or more infants finally get to the breast several months after birth.

10. Strategies for coping when one or more infants do not transition to breastfeeding include the following:
    a. Continuing to express milk with a high-quality multiuser breast pump.
    b. Pumping one breast while breastfeeding a baby on the other breast.
    c. Breastfeeding two simultaneously and pumping immediately, or waiting to pump until 30 to 60 minutes afterward for other multiples who do not go to the breast.
    d. Spending daily time skin to skin with every infant who is not breastfeeding.

VI. Biopsychosocial Issues Affecting Breastfeeding Duration with Multiples

A. The discontinuation of breastfeeding postpartum includes factors related to both the parent and the infants.[13,49,57,60,63] (See Chapter 16, *Breastfeeding and Growth: Birth through Weaning*.)

B. Postnatal mental–emotional conditions are more common after a multiple pregnancy and appear to be unrelated to the type of conception.[33,35]
    1. Caring for multiple newborn infants is associated with feelings of anxiety, being overwhelmed, and isolation.[33,38,98] Contributing to these feelings may be unrealistic parental (and family) expectations of the parents' role with multiple infants, the scope of the infants' needs and related care tasks, and a lack of physical or emotional support systems.[12,40,75]
    2. The incidence of postpartum mood disorders (PPMD) is two to three times higher in parents of multiples.[34]
    3. High-risk pregnancy and birth and a NICU experience have been associated with symptoms similar to posttraumatic stress disorder (PTSD).[99]
    4. Parents who display signs of postnatal mental–emotional conditions should be referred to their physician for depression screening and a discussion of recommended treatment.[100]
    5. IBCLCs and other healthcare providers should be aware of the increased risk of depression in the delivering parent of multiples and exercise caution in suggesting the use of galactagogues, whether medication or herbal, that have an increased risk of depressed mood or anxiety as a side effect.[101]

C. Forming an individual attachment with each infant in a set of multiples is more complex and takes longer; therefore, it is a more vulnerable process.[98] Breastfeeding may be affected positively because it may facilitate the attachment process with each infant,[40] or it may be affected negatively if it interferes with responding to an infant's feeding cues.
    1. The complexities of the process may result in short- or long-term feelings and behaviors such as the following:
        a. Forming an attachment to the multiples as a unit, rather than as individuals within the unit, which is a fairly common early response.
        b. A preferential attachment with persistent, deeper attachment for a particular baby, which presents emotional risks for all babies.
        c. A transient focus on one of the multiples for several weeks, followed by a shift to a focus on another, which may be a response to the needs of the individual infants or a normal aspect of the attachment process with multiple infants.
    2. One aspect of the attachment process is differentiation. This may include comparisons of multiples' physical and behavioral traits or the desire to treat each infant separately but also equally or fairly.[98]
    3. The process of differentiation affects breastfeeding multiples.
        a. Each infant is likely to demonstrate a unique behavioral approach or style to breastfeeding,[42] including a pattern or escalation of feeding cues, the number of feedings, and the duration of feedings.
        b. The desire to provide equal treatment, or viewing multiples as a unit, may result in ignoring individual behavioral cues that could affect weight gain and growth outcomes, as well as other physical and emotional development for one or more infant.

4. Zygosity, or type of twinning, tends to affect the infants' behavioral approaches and temperament.[102] This includes each infant's approach to breastfeeding, such as the timing, number, and duration of feedings, and infant consolability and sleep behaviors.[40] Initially, this factor may enhance or hinder the development of a daily routine.

5. The healthcare professional may enhance the attachment process and reinforce positive breastfeeding outcomes for each infant by referring to each infant by name, pointing out the infants' behavioral differences, and discussing the possible risks of failing to base breastfeeding on the individual infants' cues.

D. Concern for older children, and meeting their physical and emotional needs, can complicate the early, intense period of breastfeeding.[12,92]

VII. Maintaining Breastfeeding after All Multiples Breastfeed Effectively

A. Demonstration of effective breastfeeding by all infants is a reason for an IBCLC follow-up consult. Parents will benefit from help developing a plan for coordinating breastfeeding in a way that accommodates the individual infants' needs and feeding patterns, the parent's physical and emotional needs, and other family demands.[40,42,103]

1. Review the variations in the infants' normal breastfeeding patterns and the typical number and duration of feedings per 24 hours. Relate this information to expected breastfeeding outcome measures for each infant.

2. Reassess each infant for breastfeeding ability, effectiveness of milk transfer, and adequate breastfeeding outcomes. If two infants are feeding simultaneously, monitoring each one usually requires a higher level of alertness.

3. Until an adequate weight gain is established for each infant, encourage the use of individual 24-hour feeding logs that are clearly marked with each infant's name or color coding. Smartphone or tablet apps can track feedings, milk expression sessions, alternative feedings, and growth curves.

4. Revise the milk expression and complementary (top off) or supplementary feeding plan based on parental breastfeeding goals. If exclusive breastfeeding is the goal, the frequency and volume of pumping and alternative feedings should decrease at a pace that is sensitive to breast comfort.

5. When exclusive (or almost exclusive) direct breastfeeding is the goal, a few days of around-the-clock breastfeeding may help complete the transition, especially if one or more of the infants has just achieved effective breastfeeding behavior with appropriate milk transfer or if milk production needs a boost.

    a. Most parents find it helpful to limit this around-the-clock breastfeeding to one infant at a time.

    b. After breastfeeding decreases to a more typical number of daily feedings, it may be repeated with another infant if needed.

    c. During this intense period of feeding a household helper is needed for other tasks.[92]

B. After effective breastfeeding is assessed for each infant, any feeding rotation option can work if it is based on the individual infants' cues.[40,42,47,92]

1. The strategy of offering both breasts to each infant for each feeding is often initially used for newborns or recently transitioned infants. This strategy rarely lasts longer than a few weeks.

2. Options that include some type of alternating infants and breasts include the following:

    a. Alternating infants and breasts with every feeding, with each infant receiving only one breast per feeding.

    b. Alternating infants and breasts by assigning a particular breast to a particular infant for 24 hours, switching infants and breasts every 24 hours.

3. If all infants breastfeed effectively and both breasts produce milk adequately, the parent may consider assigning each infant a particular breast.

    a. The advantages of assigning a breast may include the following:

        i. Allows each infant to regulate a particular breast, which may be beneficial if overactive milk ejection, or reflux or gastroesophageal reflux disorder (GERD), is an issue for one or more infants.

    ii. Facilitates breastfeeding for an infant with certain positional anomalies, such as torticollis.

    iii. Minimizes cross contamination during the course of certain infective conditions, such as thrush.

  b. The disadvantages of assigning a breast may include the following:

    i. Affects milk production if attempts to monitor two feeding babies at the same time results in failing to notice ineffective breastfeeding by one infant.

    ii. Affects one infant's intake and growth if one breast produces less milk.

    iii. Contributes to infant refusal to feed on the opposite breast if one breast cannot be used for any reason or if one infant experiences a breastfeeding strike, which seems more common with multiple infants.

    iv. Results in a significant, but temporary, difference in breast sizes.

 4. Parents with triplets may rotate infants and breasts more often.

  a. Feed two infants simultaneously, then offer both breasts to the third infant. The last one to feed tends to cue sooner for a subsequent feeding.

  b. Assign a breast to two infants for a 12-hour period, and offer both breasts to the third infant.

  c. Rotate which two infants are given the 12-hour assignment and which infant is offered both breasts.

  d. Some parents maintain a rotation during the day and feed on demand during the night.

 5. Parents with quadruplets do not tend to follow a rotation, although rotation plans for twins may be adapted for an even number of multiples. Generally, the first two infants who wake are fed simultaneously. Immediately afterward, or an hour or two later, the other two infants are fed simultaneously.

 6. Parents with higher multiples often include alternative feeding in their rotation plan. For example, two infants are fed simultaneously, while the other infants receive expressed milk or formula. The infants rotate accordingly to ensure that all of them receive equal time at the breast.

 7. It is important to consider the individual infants' physical health or growth needs if supplementation is to be used. One (or more) infant may have a greater physical need for exclusive breastfeeding or human milk, or for supplementary fortification.

C. Many parents initially struggle with whether to feed twins or two higher-order multiples separately or simultaneously.[40,42,75,81,97] This decision may be affected by the infants' suckling abilities or feeding styles, and the parent's preference.

 1. The advantages of simultaneous feeding include the following:

  a. Saves time.

  b. Facilitates the development of a daytime and nighttime routine.

  c. Theoretically increases milk production (based on studies using sequential versus double breast pumping).

  d. May improve the breastfeeding behavior of one infant who is less effective at the breast by feeding with an effectively breastfeeding infant.

 2. The disadvantages of simultaneous feeding include the following:

  a. Often reinforces any ineffective latching or suckling behaviors that may reinjure nipples and potentially result in inadequate intake for one or both infants.

  b. May be difficult to manage two newborns who have little head or body control.

  c. May be difficult to facilitate latch for discreet breastfeeding during the early months, and later due to the interactions of older multiples at the breast.

  d. May be associated with feelings of aversion for some, particularly in later infancy or toddlerhood.

 3. Although some parents breastfeed only separately and some breastfeed only simultaneously, most combine simultaneous and separate feedings. Some parents also find they breastfeed mostly simultaneously at a certain period in their infants' development and breastfeed separately at another. Those periods may be quite different from one parent to another.

 4. Pillows can be helpful for support during simultaneous feedings, especially with newborns or young infants. Pillows act as extra arms. They can include household bed or sofa pillows, or larger and deeper commercial breastfeeding pillows designed specifically to support two babies at the breasts.

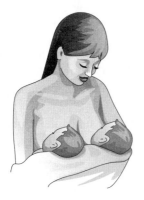

FIGURE 15-1 Combination cradle-clutch/football hold (also called a layered or parallel hold).

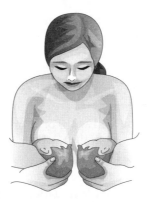

FIGURE 15-2 Double-clutch hold (also called double-football hold).

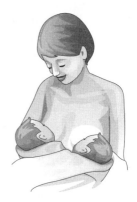

FIGURE 15-3 Cross/double cradle hold.

5.   Several positions, such as the following, can be used to hold infants for simultaneous feeding (see **FIGURE 15-1**, **FIGURE 15-2**, and **FIGURE 15-3**):
   a.   Cradle clutch combination: May also be called a layered or parallel hold.
   b.   Double clutch: May also be called a double football or double underarm hold (a variation is double perpendicular).
   c.   Double cradle: A variation is the V hold or double parallel hold, with one baby along each side of the parent in a reclined position.
   d.   Double laidback (for newborns or young infants) or double straddle (for older infants): Most often used when the parent is in a slightly reclined to semireclined position. See Figure 13-1 in Chapter 13, *Facilitating and Assessing Breastfeeding Initiation*, for an illustration of laidback breastfeeding.

D.   Breastfeeding (or milk expression) management may be easier to maintain when strategies focus on maternal recuperation and comfort.[40] Having a breastfeeding corner with snacks and beverages handy will be especially helpful to parents of multiples. (See Chapter 13, *Facilitating and Assessing Breastfeeding Initiation,* for a discussion of strategies to facilitate recuperation and comfort.)

E.   Some parents may put pressure on themselves, or experience pressure from family members, organizations for parents of multiples, and even breastfeeding and lactation support personnel, to impose a rigid feeding and infant care schedule soon after birth or upon coming home from the hospital (NICU).[40,92]
   1.   Knowledge deficits as they relate to newborn and infant emotional development, each infant's need for close contact, and the possible variations or differences for the individuals within the set should be addressed.
   2.   Some parents report that they need, or that others insist on, a strict schedule to cope with multiple infants.
      a.   A desire for some control during an intense adjustment period, with related sleep deprivation, may play a role.
      b.   Some parents may want to anticipate the infants' care and feeding needs, and this desire appears to increase with each additional infant in the set of multiples.
   3.   Many groups or professionals encourage parents of multiples to employ a nighttime infant care provider or to introduce a sleep training method. Not only may these strategies ignore the individual infants' needs, they may also interfere with effective, cue-based breastfeeding and adequate milk production, especially if no milk is removed from the breasts for a long period each night.
   4.   The pressure to develop a schedule may actually add stress rather than decrease it.

F.   Sleep deprivation is often a major issue for families throughout their multiples' infancy.[12,38,75] Significant sleep deprivation affects both the level of daytime fatigue and the infants' outcomes.[104]
   1.   Supportive strategies for breastfeeding and meeting both parental and individual infant needs include the following[40,42,48,92]:
      a.   Realistic feeding and sleep expectations for young infants and the individual infants' temperaments and behavioral patterns.

b. Risk of inadequate intake for one or more infants if an individual infant's need for more day or night feedings is ignored.

c. Possible impact on the breasts, such as increased potential for plugged ducts or mastitis and eventual decreased production, due to any sudden change in the number of hours without milk removal.

2. Developing a nighttime routine, such as the following, can be an important coping strategy[38]:

a. A consistent bedtime routine.

b. Waking a second infant to feed with, or immediately after, the first infant who feeds (and repeating for higher-order multiples), which may be adopted for all feedings, only daytime feedings, or only nighttime feedings.

3. Regular or occasional help with nighttime feedings may provide a few hours of uninterrupted sleep, which can have a positive impact on continuation of breastfeeding.[75] The risks to milk production, of plugged ducts or mastitis, and any use of infant formula should be discussed. The strategies may include the following:

a. The other parent or a helper changes the infants, brings them for breastfeeding, and afterward places them in the supine position in a nearby crib or cot.

b. Alternate feedings with all infants breastfeeding at one feeding and the helper bottle feeding them at the next feeding.

c. With higher-order multiples, breastfeed one or two infants at each feeding while the helper bottle feeds the other infants.

4. Multiple infants have an increased risk for sudden infant death syndrome (SIDS)[105] due to increased rates of preterm birth, and low birth weight or small for gestational age infants. Other factors may include bed sharing and the low incidence of exclusive breastfeeding or human milk feeding of multiples, although these variables have not been studied with multiple-birth infants.

5. Co-bedding of twins in one crib or cot, usually in the parents' room, for the first weeks to months appears to be a common sleep strategy.[103,106-107] It provides greater proximity for nighttime care-giving tasks and more synchronous sleep among the infants.[48,108] Co-bedding also saves space, may facilitate parents–infant room sharing for a longer period of time, and may enhance partner help at night.[75,109]

6. Strategies to improve the safety of co-bedding may include the following:

a. Using two (or more for higher-order multiples) smaller cribs or cots in the parents' room.

b. Attaching a standard-size crib or cot to the parents' bed to create one larger, single side-car co-sleeper.

c. Using feet-to-feet, side-by-side, or head-to-head positioning for the infants.[110] (See Chapter 13, *Facilitating and Assessing Breastfeeding Initiation,* for a discussion of safe co-bedding.)

d. Placing a bed or mattress in the infants' room to provide close proximity for breastfeeding.

VIII. Ongoing Breastfeeding Issues

A. Commonly cited difficulties associated with early cessation of breastfeeding multiples may be divided into difficulties related to the infants and those related to the parent. Limited time and energy may affect the breastfeeding parent's ability to implement what may be considered best-practice strategies for resolution.

1. Issues related to the infant include the following[12,13]:

a. Ongoing latch or suckling difficulty for one or more infant.

b. Inadequate weight gain for one or more infant.

c. Ongoing fortification of breastfeeding or human milk feeding that is prescribed for one or more infant, leading to extended triple feeding—breastfeeding, topping off, and expressing milk.

2. Issues related to the parent include the following[12,13,40,42,62,65]:

a. Milk insufficiency, whether actual or perceived.

b. Unresolved nipple or breast pain or tissue damage.

c. Recurring plugged ducts or mastitis.

d. Long-term pumping.

e. Return to work.

B. Assessments should include the following:
1. Frequency and effectiveness of milk transfer or removal via breastfeeding for each infant or during milk expression.
2. Breast history with a breast examination for lactation.
3. Physical assessment, including oral, of each infant and observation of each infant at the breast.
4. Check of equipment used for milk expression, including appropriateness of equipment for the particular situation and observation of a milk expression session.
5. Differentiation between breastfeeding or lactation difficulties and the challenges related to coping with multiple infants.
C. Contraceptive methods should be addressed. Hormonal contraceptives, including those with progestin only, may have a more deleterious impact on milk production for multiple infants than on milk production for a single infant.[108]
D. Typical interventions to resolve a difficulty may require adaptation for successful implementation. Ask if any strategy seems unrealistic or if there is uncertainty or concern about the ability to implement the intervention. If any aspect of a strategy seems unrealistic or causes concern, discuss the options for revision.

IX. Exclusive versus Partial Breastfeeding or Human Milk Feeding Options for Multiples

A. Many parents with twins, and some with triplets or quadruplets, have exclusively breastfed or human milk feeding their infants for several weeks to months until gradually introducing complementary foods. Other parents partially breastfeed one or more multiples.[40,42] (See Chapter 7, *Biochemistry of Human Milk,* for a discussion of exclusive and partial breastfeeding.)
1. Partial breastfeeding is fairly common when caring for multiple newborns or infants. It varies from occasional to regular complementary feeding, or topping off, to regular supplementary feedings that replace one or more direct breastfeedings.
2. The implementation of any exclusive or partial option may be used with one or all infants at any time during lactation, and any option may be used on a short- or long-term basis.[40-42,48]
3. The period of exclusive versus partial breastfeeding or human milk feeding can vary for one or all infants due to individual infant feeding abilities or the presence of an anomaly requiring different or additional feeding support. However, evidence indicates a tendency to use the same amount of direct breastfeeding or human milk feeding for all infants.[11,61,65]
4. Whether the rationale for feeding one or all infants the same is due to the desire for a routine, the need to treat each infant fairly and equally,[98] or for some other reason has not been studied. However, breastfeeding one infant more who is effectively breastfeeding is an option, even if another feeding method is used more often for a less effective breastfeeder.
5. To maintain adequate milk production during the first several months with partial breastfeeding, milk should be effectively removed at least 8–12 times every 24 hours. Therefore, at a minimum, each of twins would be breastfed 4–6 times, each of triplets 3–4 times, and each of quadruplets 2–3 times in 24 hours. However, depending on the particular situation, one infant may breastfeed more often than another.

X. Breastfeeding Older Infant and Toddler Multiples

A. Introducing complementary foods may be different for multiples than for singletons.
1. There is scant multiples-specific evidence to guide the introduction of complementary foods.[42] As with earlier milk feedings, parents tend to introduce complementary foods to all babies at the same time rather than to each baby based on individual signs of developmental readiness.[61]
2. Well-informed parents are more likely to introduce complementary food as an infant demonstrates developmental readiness.[111] Anticipatory guidance may promote an individualized approach.

3. Supplementary iron may be needed by one or more infants due to preterm birth, intrauterine growth restriction, or monochorionic–diamniotic placentation, which also interferes with delayed cord clamping.[19,92] Any need for supplementary iron should be based on screening, testing, and monitoring the outcomes.

4. Anticipatory guidance for the introduction of complementary food with multiple infants may include a discussion of the following:

    a. Each infant is an individual who may or may not be ready for other foods at the same time as another.

    b. The impact of gestational age at birth, including health implications of too-early solids for preterm infants.

    c. The use of thickening agents in expressed human milk or formula for reflux, gastroesophageal reflux disorder (GERD), or to help increase nighttime sleep.

    d. Signs of readiness or avoidance for each infant.

B. Breastfeeding older multiples includes an increase in interactional behaviors during breastfeeding that are associated with being multiples.[40]

    1. Increased teething-related biting during breastfeeding is common and may be related to a decreased ability to monitor infants for signs associated with the onset of biting during simultaneous feeding.

    2. Playful to more aggressive poking, pushing, and punching behaviors may occur during simultaneous feedings.

    3. When one infant requests to breastfeed, another infant may demand to breastfeed, sometimes called jealous breastfeeding.

C. Some researchers have noted more of a decrease in milk production, compared to parents with single infants between 9 and 12 months.[50] It is not clear whether the decreases were related more to physiological or situational factors.

D. Many factors may influence the cessation of breastfeeding or milk expression after the multiples' first year.[40] (See Chapter 16, *Breastfeeding and Growth: Birth through Weaning*.)

    1. An increase in breastfeeding strikes among multiples from approximately 3 months to later infancy may be related to frequent delays in bringing a cueing baby to the breast or the purposeful scheduling of breastfeeding.

    2. Cessation may result from increased use of alternative feedings for one or more infant after preterm birth, or partial breastfeeding after discharge for any reason.

E. Many multiples breastfeed for well longer than 1 year,[14,40] and some parents breastfeed one or more children from a set of multiples for 4–5 years. Continued breastfeeding generally involves all children from a set of multiples, but breastfeeding may continue longer for one (or more) child when another child (or more) stops breastfeeding.

▶ Key Points from This Chapter

A. Every multiple-birth child and parent has a right to a breastfeeding relationship and the physical and psychosocial advantages it provides.

B. Multiple-birth infants and children strain parents' physical and emotional reserves. This strain extends to breastfeeding.

C. Breastfeeding initiation and duration with multiple-birth infants are affected by more than an ability to replicate appropriate breastfeeding mechanics or typical lactation management strategies.

D. Complications for multiple-birth infants and the delivering parent often affect breastfeeding initiation and may have long-lasting effects on breastfeeding duration or the feeding pattern with one or more infant in a set of multiples.

E. Coordinating breastfeeding for two or more infants who may have varying abilities to breastfeed effectively, or who have different but normal feeding patterns and styles, may be perceived as breastfeeding problems rather than simply an aspect of having multiple infants.

F. Many older infant and toddler multiples engage in interactive behaviors during breastfeeding that can affect parents' coping and perception of breastfeeding.

G. Parents of multiples are likely to need increased and specialized breastfeeding and lactation support and reinforcement.

🔍 CASE STUDY

Marnie is a 34-year-old mother who breastfed a previous singleton for 22 months. The older child weaned completely during the fourth month of this twin pregnancy. Marnie gave birth to twins at 35 3/7 completed weeks of gestation after demonstrating signs of preeclampsia. An emergency cesarean section was performed because the presenting twin was in a breech position. Both newborns were discharged home from the NICU at 10 days of age on expressed milk. Marnie was instructed to fortify two bottles per infant per day with a powdered infant formula to increase their daily caloric intake. At discharge, the instructions were to attempt to breastfeed each infant twice a day. During a 2-week check by their pediatric care provider, Marnie was told the babies were doing well, to breastfeed as often as desired, and to feed each baby a 2-ounce (60 mL) bottle afterwards. The babies are now 4 weeks old, and Marnie feels very overwhelmed with breastfeeding, bottle feeding, pumping, and also caring for a toddler.

Marnie contacts you and reports trying to increase breastfeeding, but the babies have difficulty latching. After they latch, they often suckle for only a few minutes before drifting to sleep or slipping off the breast. Marnie repeats the process with each baby several times before supplementing with EHM or formula. A typical feeding session takes almost an hour, and by the time it is finished, it is almost time to begin again. Marnie was pumping about eight or nine times a day before trying to breastfeed each baby more often. Now the number of pumping sessions has decreased, although the number fluctuates from day to day. The amount of milk obtained during pumping is decreasing. Herbs, foods, and beverages suggested by members of a social media group do not seem to improve milk production. The toddler has been acting out more in the past 2 weeks. Marnie indicates a desire to breastfeed but may have to give up and move completely to formula feeding soon if the milk production continues to drop. You and Marnie schedule a lactation consult for the next day.

Questions

1. What information regarding Marnie's health history may be particularly pertinent in this situation? For example, was conception spontaneous or assisted? If applicable, what factors are thought to contribute to subfertility? Were there any difficulties during the previous breastfeeding experience? Is, or was, Marnie on any medication related to subfertility, preeclampsia, and so forth?

2. Prior to the changes 2 weeks ago, how was Marnie managing milk removal, both during the babies' NICU stay and after they were discharged to home? For example: Was the initiation of lactation affected by the surgical delivery or preeclampsia and any related postdelivery treatment? Does Marnie understand the relationship between the frequency and thoroughness of milk removal and the volumes obtained? What model breast pump has Marnie been using since hospital discharge? Do the breast shield or flange pieces fit properly? Did, or does, her pumping routine include hands-on pumping techniques? Has Marnie ever monitored her pumping sessions, either on paper or an app? What herbs, foods, and beverages has Marnie tried, and how did she use them?

3. What information or assessment data regarding each twin's health history is pertinent in this situation? For example: The initial call with Marnie indicates she may be regarding her newborns more as a set than as two separate individuals. Is it likely that there are no differences between each infant's ability to cue for feeding, latching, or suckling? Could her babies' current gestational age be a factor in the transition to the breast? Have any breastfeeding aids or devices been tried with either infant? Does either infant have any facial or oral deviations, whether congenital or from intrauterine position? Does Marnie breastfeed the infants separately or simultaneously?

4. What is the significance of Marnie's current support network? For example: In what ways does Marnie's partner provide emotional support and physical support for infant and toddler care, as well as household tasks? Does Marnie have family or friends nearby who help physically and emotionally? Is Marnie aware of other local resources for household help and breastfeeding support, both in general and specifically for multiples? Is Marnie aware of social media groups specifically for breastfeeding twins where she can access information and support?

References

1. Australian Bureau of Statistics. Confinements, by plurality, by state. ABS.Stat website. http://stat.data.abs.gov.au/Index.aspx?QueryId=493. Published November 8, 2016. Updated February 8, 2017. Accessed May 18, 2017.
2. Office for National Statistics. Birth characteristics in England and Wales: 2015. The small rise in the rate of women having multiple births has been driven by those aged 25 to 29. Office for National Statistics website. https://www.ons.gov.uk/peoplepopulationandcommunity/birthsdeathsandmarriages/livebirths/bulletins/birthcharacteristicsinenglandandwales/2015#the-small-rise-in-the-rate-of-women-having-multiple-births-has-been-driven-by-those-aged-25-to-29. Published October 21, 2016. Accessed May 18, 2017.
3. Zeitlin J, Mohangoo A, Delnord M, eds. *European Perinatal Health Report: Health and Care of Pregnant Women and Babies in Europe in 2010*. Paris, France: Euro-Peristat; 2013. http://www.europeristat.com/images/doc/EPHR2010_w_disclaimer.pdf. Accessed May 18, 2017.

4. Smits J, Monden C. Twinning across the developing world. *PLOS One.* 2011;6:e25239. http://journals.plos.org/plosone/article?id=10.1371/journal.pone.0025239. Published September 28, 2011. Accessed May 18, 2017.

5. Martin JA, Hamilton BE, Osterman MJK, et al. Births: final data for 2015. *Natl Vital Stat Rep.* 2017;66(1). https://www.cdc.gov/nchs/data/nvsr/nvsr66/nvsr66_01.pdf. Published January 5, 2017. Accessed May 18, 2017.

6. Statistics Canada. Table 102-4515. Live births and fetal deaths (stillbirths), by type (single or multiple), Canada, provinces and territories, annual (number). Statistics Canada website. http://www5.statcan.gc.ca/cansim/a26?lang=eng&id=1024515. Modified December 12, 2016. Accessed October 4, 2017.

7. Pison G, Monden C, Smits J. Twinning rates in developed countries: trends and explanations. *Popul Dev Rev.* 2015;41:629-649. http://onlinelibrary.wiley.com/doi/10.1111/j.1728-4457.2015.00088.x/epdf. Accessed May 18, 2017.

8. Guzoglu N, Kanmaz HG, Dilli D, Uras N, Erdeve O, Dilmen U. The impact of the new Turkish regulation, imposing single embryo transfer after assisted reproduction technology, on neonatal intensive care unit utilization: a single center experience. *Hum Reprod.* 2012;27(8):2384-2388. http://humrep.oxfordjournals.org/content/27/8/2384.long. Accessed May 18, 2017.

9. Vogel JP, Torloni MR, Seuc A, et al. Maternal and perinatal outcomes of twin pregnancy in 23 low- and middle-income countries. *PLOS One.* 2013;8:e70549. http://www.ncbi.nlm.nih.gov/pmc/articles/PMC3731264/. Accessed May18, 2017.

10. Heino A, Gissler M, Hindori-Mohangoo AD, et al. Variations in multiple birth rates and impact on perinatal outcomes in Europe. *PLOS One.* 2016;11:e0149252. http://journals.plos.org/plosone/article?id=10.1371/journal.pone.0149252. Accessed May 18, 2017.

11. Gromada KK. Breastfeeding multiples. *New Beginnings.* 2006;23:244-249. http://www.llli.org/nb/nbnovdec06p244.html/. Accessed May 18, 2017.

12. Cinar ND, Alvur TM, Kose D, Nemut T. Breastfeeding twins: a qualitative study. *J Health Popul Nutr.* 2013;31:504-509. http://www.ncbi.nlm.nih.gov/pmc/articles/PMC3905645/. Accessed May 18, 2017.

13. Damato EG, Dowling DA, Standing TS, Schuster SD. Explanation for the cessation of breastfeeding in mothers of twins. *J Hum Lactation.* 2005;21:296-304.

14. Raising Multiples. Medical birth survey data. Raising Multiples website. http://www.raisingmultiples.org/wp-content/uploads/2015/06/MBSBreastfeeding.pdf. Published June 2007. Accessed May 18, 2017.

15. Behrman RE, Butler AS. Measurement of fetal and infant maturity. In: Behrman RE, Butler AS, eds. *Preterm Birth: Causes, Consequences, and Prevention.* Washington, DC: National Academies Press; 2007:55-83. http://www.ncbi.nlm.nih.gov/books/NBK11382/. Accessed May 18, 2017.

16. American College of Obstetricians and Gynecologists. Multifetal gestations: twin, triplet, and higher-order multifetal pregnancies. *Obstet Gynecol.* 2014;123:1118-1132.

17. Shub A, Walker SP. Planned early delivery versus expectant management for monoamniotic twins. *Cochrane Database Syst Rev.* 2015;4:CD008820. doi:10.1002/14651858.CD008820.pub2.

18. Berezowsky A, Mazkereth R, Ashwal E, et al. Neonatal outcome of late preterm uncomplicated monochorionic twins: what is the optimal time for delivery? *J Matern Fetal Neonatal Med.* 2016;29:1252-1256.

19. Emery S, Bahtiyar MO, Dashe JS, et al. Network consensus statement: prenatal management of uncomplicated monochorionic gestations. *Obstet Gynecol.* 2015;125:1236-1243.

20. Boyle B, McConkey R, Garne E, et al. Trends in the prevalence, risk and pregnancy outcome of multiple births with congenital anomaly: a registry-based study in 14 European countries 1984-2007. *BJOG.* 2013;120:707-716. http://onlinelibrary.wiley.com/doi/10.1111/1471-0528.12146/full. Accessed May 18, 2017.

21. Glinianaia SV, Rankin J, Wright C. Congenital anomalies in twins: a register-based study. *Hum Reprod.* 2008;23:1306-1311. http://humrep.oxfordjournals.org/content/23/6/1306.long. Accessed May 19, 2017.

22. Tang Y, Ma C, Cui W, et al. The risk of birth defects in multiple births: a population-based study. *Matern Child Health J.* 2006;10:75-81.

23. Moh W, Graham JM, Wadhawan I, Sanchez-Lara PA. Extrinsic factors influencing fetal deformations and intrauterine growth restriction. *J Pregnancy.* 2012;750485. http://dx.doi.org/10.1155/2012/750485. Accessed May 19, 2017.

24. Mathews TJ, MacDorman MF, Thoma ME. Infant mortality statistics from the 2013 period linked birth/infant death data set. *Natl Vital Stat Rep.* 2015;64. http://www.cdc.gov/nchs/data/nvsr/nvsr64/nvsr64_09.pdf. Published August 6, 2015. Accessed May 19, 2017.

25. Pector E. How bereaved multiple-birth parents cope with hospitalization, homecoming, disposition for deceased, and attachment to survivors. *J Perinatol.* 2004;24:714-722. http://www.nature.com/jp/journal/v24/n11/full/7211170a.html. Accessed May 19, 2017.

26. Hanrahan J. Breastfeeding after the loss of a multiple. *Leaven.* 2000;36(5):102. http://www.llli.org/llleaderweb/lv/lvoctnov00p102.html. Accessed May 19, 2017.

27. Royal College of Obstetricians and Gynaecologists. *Thromboembolic Disease in Pregnancy and the Puerperium: Acute Management.* London, United Kingdom: Royal College of Obstetricians and Gynaecologists; 2015. https://www.rcog.org.uk/globalassets/documents/guidelines/gtg-37b.pdf. Accessed May 19, 2017.

28. Meier P, Patel AL, Wright K, Engstrom JL. Management of breastfeeding during and after the maternity hospitalization for late preterm infants. *Clin Perinatol.* 2013;40:689-705. http://www.ncbi.nlm.nih.gov/pmc/articles/PMC4289642/. Accessed May 19, 2017.

29. Lee HC, Gould JB, Boscardin WJ, et al. Trends in cesarean delivery for twin births in the United States: 1995-2008. *Obstet Gynecol.* 2011;118:1095-1101. https://www.ncbi.nlm.nih.gov/pmc/articles/PMC3202294/. Accessed May 19, 2017.

30. Centers for Disease Control and Prevention. Quick stats: percentage of live births by cesarean delivery, by plurality—United States, 1996, 2000, and 2006. *MMWR.* 2009;58:542. http://www.cdc.gov/mmwr/preview/mmwrhtml/mm5819a9.htm. Accessed May 17, 2017.

31. Ganchimeg T, Morisaki N, Vogel JP, et al. Mode and timing of twin delivery and perinatal outcomes in low- and middle-income countries: a secondary analysis of the WHO multicountry survey on maternal and newborn health. *BJOG.* 2014;121:89-100. http://onlinelibrary.wiley.com/doi/10.1111/1471-0528.12635/epdf. Accessed May 19, 2017.

32. West D, Marasco L. *The Breastfeeding Mother's Guide to Making More Milk.* New York, NY: McGraw-Hill; 2009.

33. Vilska S, Unkila- Kallio L, Punamäki R-L, et al. Mental health of mothers and fathers of twins conceived via assisted reproduction treatment: a 1-year prospective study. *Hum Reprod.* 2009;24:367-377. http://humrep.oxfordjournals.org/content/24/2/367.long. Accessed May 19, 2017.

34. Choi Y, Bishal D, Minkovitz CS. Multiple births are a risk factor for postpartum maternal depressive symptoms. *Pediatrics.* 2009;123:1147-1154.

35. Wenze SJ, Battle CL, Tezanos KM. Raising multiples: mental health of mothers and fathers in early parenthood. *Arch Womens Ment Health.* 2015;18:163-176. https://www.ncbi.nlm.nih.gov/pmc/articles/PMC4610720/. Accessed May 19, 2017.

36. Andersen LB, Melvaer LB, Videbach P, Lamont RF, Joergensen JS. Risk factors for developing post-traumatic stress disorder following childbirth: a systematic review. *Acta Obstetricia et Gynecologica Scandinavica.* 2012;91:1261-1272. https://www.researchgate.net/publication/225274813_Risk_factors_for_developing_post-traumatic_stress_disorder_following_childbirth_A_systematic_review. Accessed May 19, 2017.

37. McGovern T. The challenges of breastfeeding twins: a small study looks at the challenges of breastfeeding twins and what helps mothers succeed. *Nurs N Z.* 2014;20:26-27,44. http://www.thefreelibrary.com/_/print/PrintArticle.aspx?id=395846212. Accessed May 19, 2017.

38. Beck CT. Releasing the pause button: mothering twins during the first year of life. *Qual Health Res.* 2002;12:593-608.

39. Gromada K. ILCA's inside track a resource for breastfeeding mothers: twins. *J Hum Lactation.* 2010;26:331-332.

40. Gromada KK. *Mothering Multiples: Breastfeeding and Caring for Twins or More.* Rev ed. Schaumburg, IL: La Leche League International; 2007.

41. Leonard LG. Breastfeeding triplets: the at-home experience. *Public Health Nurs.* 2000;17:211-221.

42. Multiple Births Foundation. *Guidance for Health Professionals on Feeding Twins, Triplets and Higher Order Multiples.* London, United Kingdom: Multiple Births Foundation; 2011. http://www.multiplebirths.org.uk/mbf_professionals_final.pdf. Accessed May 19, 2017.

43. American Academy of Pediatrics. Breastfeeding and the use of human milk. *Pediatrics.* 2012;129:e827-e841. http://pediatrics.aappublications.org/content/pediatrics/129/3/e827.full.pdf. Accessed May 19, 2017.

44. Anatolitou F. Human milk benefits and breastfeeding. *J Pediatr Neonat Individual Med.* 2012;1:11-18. http://www.jpnim.com/index.php/jpnim/article/view/010113/18. Accessed May 19, 2017.

45. McNeil ME, Labbok MH, Abrahams SW. What are the risks associated with formula feeding? A re-analysis and review. *Birth.* 2010;37:50-58.

46. Bartick MC, Schwarz EB, Green BD, et al. Suboptimal breastfeeding in the United States: maternal and pediatric health outcomes and costs. *Maternal Child Nutr.* 2017;13(1). doi:10.1111/mcn.12366.

47. Kielbratowska B, Cwiek D, Preis K, Malinowski W, Hofman A. Breastfeeding of twins. *Arch Perinatal Med.* 2010;16:201-205. http://www.ptmp.com.pl/archives/apm/16-4/APM164-4-Kielbratowska.pdf. Accessed May 19, 2017.

48. Leonard LG, Denton J. Preparation for parenting multiple birth children. *Early Hum Dev.* 2006;82:371-378.

49. Leonard LG. Breastfeeding rights of multiple birth families and guidelines for health professionals. *Twin Res.* 2003;6:34-45.

50. Saint L, Maggiore P, Hartmann P. Yield and nutrient content of milk in eight women breast-feeding twins and one woman breast-feeding triplets. *Br J Nutr.* 1986;56:49-58. http://journals.cambridge.org/download.php?file=%2FBJN%2FBJN56_01%2FS0007114586000855a.pdf&code=63ef2cd593155e36be3d4e84592ebdd3. Accessed May 19, 2017.

51. Berlin C. "Exclusive" breastfeeding of quadruplets. *Breastfeed Med.* 2007;2:125-126.

52. Auer C, Gromada K. A case report of breastfeeding quadruplets: factors perceived as affecting breastfeeding. *J Hum Lactation.* 1998;14:135-141.

53. Mead L, Chuffo R, Lawlor-Klean P, Meier P. Breastfeeding success with preterm quadruplets. *J Obstet Gynecol Neonatal Nurs.* 1992;21:221-227.

54. Szucs KA, Axline SE, Rosenman MB. The quintuplets receiving human milk: an update. *J Hum Lactation.* 2009;25:269.

55. Szucs KA, Axline SE, Rosenman MB. Quintuplets and a mother's determination to provide human milk: it takes a village to raise a baby—how about five? *J Hum Lactation.* 2009;25:79-84.

56. Babybumper. Persistent pumping ensures milk supply. Belly Bump website. https://bellybumper.wordpress.com/2011/05/16/persistent-pumping-ensures-milk-supply/. Published May 16, 2011. Accessed May 19, 2017.

57. Östlund A, Nordström M, Dykes F, Flacking R. Breastfeeding in preterm and term twins—maternal factors associated with early cessation: a population-based study. *J Hum Lactation.* 2010;26:327-329.

58. Ooki S. Breast-feeding rates and related maternal and infants' obstetric factors in Japanese twins. *Environ Health Prev Med.* 2008;13:187-197. https://www.ncbi.nlm.nih.gov/pmc/articles/PMC2698232/. Accessed May 19, 2017.

59. Damato EG, Dowling DA, Madigan EA, Thanattherakul C. Duration of breastfeeding for mothers of twins. *J Obstet Gynecol Neonatal Nurs.* 2005;34:201-209.

60. Yokoyama Y, Wada S, Sugimoto M, Katayama M, Saito M, Sono J. Breastfeeding rates among singletons, twins and triplets in Japan: a population-based study. *Twin Res Hum Genet.* 2006;9:298-302.

61. McAndrew F, Thompson J, Fellows L, Large A, Speed M, Renfrew MJ. *Infant Feeding Survey 2010.* London, United Kingdom: Health and Social Care Information Centre; 2012. http://content.digital.nhs.uk/catalogue/PUB08694/Infant-Feeding-Survey-2010-Consolidated-Report.pdf. Accessed May 19, 2017.

62. Geraghty SR, Pinney SM, Sethurman G, Roy-Chaudhury A, Kalkwarf HJ. Breast milk feeding rates of mothers of multiples compared to mothers of singletons. *Ambul Pediatr.* 2004;4:226-231.

63. Hutton EK, Hannah ME, Ross S, et al. Maternal outcomes at 3 months after planned cesarean section versus planned vaginal birth for twin pregnancies in the twin birth study: a randomised controlled trial. *BJOG.* 2015;122:1653-1662.

64. Cinar N, Kose D, Alvur M, Dogu O. Mothers' attitudes toward feeding twin babies in the first six months of life: a sample from Sakarya, Turkey. *Iran J Pediatr.* 2016;26:e5413. doi:10.5812/ijp.5413.

65. Geraghty SR, Khoury JC, Kalkwarf HJ. Human milk pumping rates of mothers of singletons and mothers of multiples. *J Hum Lactation.* 2005;21:413-420.

66. Geraghty SR, Khoury JC, Kalkwarf HJ. Comparison of feeding among multiple birth infants. *Twin Res.* 2004;7:542-547.

67. Academy of Breastfeeding Medicine Protocol Committee. Clinical protocol number #19: breastfeeding promotion in the prenatal setting. *Breastfeeding Med.* 2009;4:43-45. http://www.bfmed.org/Media/Files/Protocols/Protocol%2019%20-%20Breastfeeding%20 Promotion%20in%20the%20Prenatal%20Setting.pdf. Accessed May 19, 2017.

68. Poulson M. Breastfeeding toddler twins. *New Beginnings.* 2009;30:14-15. http://www.lalecheleague.org/nb/nbiss56-09p14.html. Accessed May 19, 2017.

69. Szucs KA, Axline SE, Rosenman MB. Induced lactation and exclusive breast milk feeding of adopted premature twins. *J Hum Lactation.* 2010;26:309-313.

70. Farhadi R, Philip RK. Induction of lactation in the biological mother after gestational surrogacy of twins: a novel approach and review of the literature. *Breastfeed Med.* 2017;12:373-376.

71. Michaels AM, Wanner H. Breastfeeding twins after mastectomy. *J Hum Lactation.* 2013;29:20-22.

72. Fox NS, Rebarber A, Roman AS, Klauser CK, Peress D, Saltzman DH. Weight gain in twin pregnancies and adverse outcomes: examining the 2009 Institute of Medicine guidelines. *Obstet Gynecol.* 2010;116:100-106. http://journals.lww.com/greenjournal/Fulltext/2010/07000 /Weight_Gain_in_Twin_Pregnancies_and_Adverse.17.aspx#. Accessed May 19, 2017.

73. Institute of Medicine, National Research Council. *Weight Gain During Pregnancy: Reexamining the Guidelines.* Washington, DC: National Academies Press; 2009. http://www.nap.edu/catalog.php?record_id=12584. Accessed May 19, 2017.

74. Luke B. Nutrition for multiples. *Clin Obstet Gynecol.* 2015;58:585-610.

75. Gromada KK. Breastfeeding support groups for mothers of multiple-birth infants and children. In: Thorley V, Vickers MC, eds. *The 10th Step and Beyond: Mother Support for Breastfeeding.* Amarillo, TX: Praeclarus Press; 2012:171-182.

76. Seelbach-Goebel B. Twin birth considering the current results of the "twin birth study." *Geburtshilfe Frauenheilkd.* 2014;74:838-844. http://www.ncbi.nlm.nih.gov/pmc/articles/PMC4175125/. Accessed May 19, 2017.

77. de Castro H, Haas J, Schiff E, Sivan E, Yinon Y, Barzilay E. Trial of labour in twin pregnancies: a retrospective cohort study. *BJOG.* 2016;123:940-945.

78. Christopher D, Robinson BK, Peaceman AM. An evidence-based approach to determining route of delivery for twin gestations. *Rev Obstet Gynecol.* 2011;4:109-116. http://www.ncbi.nlm.nih.gov/pmc/articles/PMC3252881/. Accessed May 19, 2017.

79. Parker LA, Sullivan S, Krueger C, Kelechi T, Mueller M. Effect of early breast milk expression on milk volume and timing of lactogenesis stage II among mothers of very low birth weight infants: a pilot study. *J Perinatol.* 2012;32:205-209. http://pqcnc.org/documents /milkncccIIdoc/PQCNCBreastMilkExpressionMilkVolumeTimingPilotStudy.pdf. Accessed May 19, 2017.

80. Morton J, Hall JY, Wong RJ, Thairu L, Benitz WE, Rhine WD. Combining hand techniques with electric pumping increases milk production in mothers of preterm infants. *J Perinatol.* 2009;29:757-764. http://www.lactamed.com/increases-milk-production/. Accessed May 19, 2017.

81. La Leche League International. *Tips for Breastfeeding Twins.* Schaumburg, IL: La Leche League International; 2009. http://www.llli.org /docs/Tear-Off%20Sheets/english/10237_tips_for_breastfeeding_twins.pdf. Accessed May 19, 2017.

82. Gromada KK, Spangler A. Breastfeeding twins and higher-order multiples. *J Obstet Gynecol Neonatal Nurs.* 1998;27:441-449.

83. McGee K. What mattered most: from NICU pump dependency to exclusive breastfeeding. *Neonatal Intensive Care.* 2016;29:41-43. http://safebabybmt.paragondsi.com/wp-content/uploads/2016/08/What-Mattered-Most-From-NICU-Pump-Dependency-to-Exclusive -Breastfeeding.pdf. Accessed May 19, 2017.

84. Morton J, Wong RJ, Hall JY, et al. Combining hand techniques with electric pumping increases the caloric content of milk in mothers of preterm infants. *J Perinatol.* 2012;32:791-796.

85. Abouelfettoh A, Ludington-Hoe S. Preterm twins cardio-respiratory, thermal and maternal breast temperature responses to shared kangaroo care. *Int J Nurs Midwifery.* 2012;4:76-83. http://www.academicjournals.org/journal/IJNM/article-full-text-pdf/522AE781059. Accessed May 19, 2017.

86. Hurst NM, Valentine CJ, Renfro L, Burns P, Ferlic L. Skin-to-skin holding in the neonatal intensive care unit influences maternal milk volume. *J Perinatol.* 1997;17:213-217.

87. Pineda E. Direct breast-feeding in the neonatal intensive care unit: is it important? *J Perinatol.* 2011;31(8):540-545. http://www.pqcnc .org/documents/milkwelldoc/PQCNCDirectBreastfeedingNICU.pdf. Accessed May 19, 2017.

88. Chow S, Chow R, Popovic M, et al. The use of nipple shields: a review. *Front Public Health.* 2015;3:236. http://www.ncbi.nlm.nih.gov /pmc/articles/PMC4607874/. Accessed May 19, 2017.

89. Sisk P, Quandt S, Parson N, Tucker J. Breast milk expression and maintenance in mothers of very low birth weight infants: supports and barriers. *J Hum Lactation.* 2010;26:368-375.

90. Morton J. Maximizing milk production with hands-on pumping. Stanford Medicine website. http://med.stanford.edu/newborns /professional-education/breastfeeding/maximizing-milk-production.html. Accessed May 19, 2017.

91. Walker M. Breastfeeding the late preterm infant. *J Obstet Gynecol Neonatal Nurs.* 2008;37:692-701. http://www.allattamentoalseno.it /lavori/Breastfeeding_the_Late.pdf. Accessed May 19, 2017.

92. Gromada KK. Breastfeeding multiples: learning the dance of breastfeeding and lactation with two, three or more newborn partners. Presented at: GOLD Perinatal Online Conference; October 26 and 27, 2015.

93. Funkquizt EL, Tuvemo T, Jonsson B, Serenius F, Nyqvist KH. Influence of test weighing before/after nursing on breastfeeding in preterm infants. *Adv Neonatal Care.* 2010;10:33-39.

94. Peterson A, Harmer M. *Balancing Breast and Bottle: Reaching Your Breastfeeding Goal.* Amarillo, TX: Hale Publishing; 2009.

95. Shaker CS. Cue-based feeding in the NICU: using the infant's communication as a guide. *Neonatal Network.* 2013;32:404-408. http:// www.academyofneonatalnursing.org/NNT/FCC_CBF.pdf. Accessed May 19, 2017.

96. Kassing D. Bottle-feeding as a tool to reinforce breastfeeding. *J Hum Lactation.* 2002;18:56-60. http://www.bfar.org/bottlefeeding.pdf. Accessed May 19, 2017.

97. Fidel-Rimon O, Shinwell ES. Breast feeding twins and high multiples. *Arch Dis Child Fetal Neonatal Ed.* 2006;91:F377-F380. http:// www.ncbi.nlm.nih.gov/pmc/articles/PMC2672857/pdf/F377.pdf. Accessed May 19, 2017.

98. Beck CT. Mothering multiples: a meta-synthesis of qualitative research. *MCN Am J Matern Child Nurs.* 2002;27:214-221.

99. Furuta M, Sandall J, Bick D. A systematic review of the relationship between severe maternal morbidity and post-traumatic stress disorder. *BMC Pregnancy Childbirth.* 2012;12:125. http://bmcpregnancychildbirth.biomedcentral.com/articles/10.1186/1471-2393-12-125. Accessed May 19, 2017.

100. New Hampshire Breastfeeding Task Force. *A Breastfeeding-Friendly Approach to Depression in New Mothers.* Concord, NH: New Hampshire Breastfeeding Task Force; 2009. http://www.nhbreastfeedingtaskforce.org/pdf/breastfeeding_depression.pdf. Accessed May 19, 2017.

101. Academy of Breastfeeding Medicine Protocol Committee. Clinical protocol number #9: use of galactogogues in initiating or augmenting the rate of maternal milk secretion. *Breastfeeding Med.* 2011;6:41-49. http://www.bfmed.org/Media/Files/Protocols/Protocol%209%20-%20English%201st%20Rev.%20Jan%202011.pdf. Accessed May 19, 2017.

102. Saudino KJ. Behavioral genetics and child temperament. *J Dev Behav Pediatr.* 2005;26:214-223. https://www.ncbi.nlm.nih.gov/pmc/articles/PMC1188235/. Accessed May 19, 2017.

103. Twins and Multiple Births Association. *Breastfeeding More Than One.* Aldershot, United Kingdom: Twins and Multiple Births Association; 2013.

104. Damato EG, Burant C. Sleep patterns and fatigue in parents of twins. *J Obstet Gynecol Neonatal Nurs.* 2008;37:738-749. http://www.academia.edu/16670989/Sleep_Patterns_and_Fatigue_in_Parents_of_Twins. Accessed May 19, 2017.

105. Getahun D, Demissie K, Lu SE, Rhoads GG. Sudden infant death syndrome among twin births: United States, 1995-1998. *J Perinatol.* 2004;24:544-551. http://www.nature.com/jp/journal/v24/n9/full/7211140a.html. Accessed May 19, 2017.

106. Hutchinson BL, Stewart AW, Mitchell EA. The prevalence of cobedding and SIDS-related child care practices in twins. *Eur J Pediatr.* 2010;169:1477-1485.

107. Ball HL. Caring for twin infants: sleeping arrangements and their implications. *Evidence Based Midwifery.* 2006;4:10-16.

108. Ball HL. Together or apart? A behavioural and psychological investigation of sleeping arrangements for twin babies. *Midwifery.* 2007;23:404-412.

109. Damato EG, Brubaker JA, Burant C. Sleeping arrangements in families with twins. *Newborn Infant Nurs Rev.* 2012;12(3):171-178.

110. Twins and Multiple Births Association. Getting your twins, or more, to sleep! Twins and Multiple Births Association website. https://www.tamba.org.uk/parenting/sleep/0-12-months. Accessed May 26, 2017.

111. Chung J, Lee J, Spinazzola R, Rosen L, Milanaik R. Parental perception of premature infant growth and feeding behaviors: use of gestation-adjusted age and assessing for developmental readiness during solid food introduction. *Clin Pediatr.* 2014;53:1271-1277.

Additional Resources

Facebook Group

Mothering Multiples (Too): Breastfeeding and Caring for Twins or More. https://www.facebook.com/groups/1562320190751320/pending/. This Facebook group provides the following files:

- 30 chapters from *Mothering Multiples: Breastfeeding and Caring for Twins or More* (2007 edition)
- List of Facebook discussion groups for parents who are birthing or breastfeeding twins or other multiples
- Fill-in-the-blank birth plan for twins or triplets

Publications

Leonard LG. *Twins, Triplets & More!* Vancouver, Canada: Multiple-Births Support Program, University of British Columbia School of Nursing. https://nursing.ubc.ca/pdfs/twinstripletsandmore.pdf.

Radio Programs

Breastfeeding twins, triplets—or more! *Born to Breastfeed.* VoiceAmerica Internet Talk Radio. November 11, 2013. http://www.voiceamerica.com/episode/73969/breastfeeding-twins-tripletsor-more.

Karen Kerkhoff Gromada author of *Mothering Multiples. CAPPA Radio.* BlogTalkRadio. March 2, 2016. http://www.blogtalkradio.com/cappa-radio/2016/03/16/karen-kerkhoff-gromada-author-of-mothering-multiples.

Websites

Best for Babes. Breastfeeding Twins. http://www.bestforbabes.org/tag/breastfeeding-twins/.
Karen Kerkhoff Gromada. Mothering Multiples. http://www.karengromada.com/links/.
Naturally Parenting Twins. http://naturallyparentingtwins.net/parenting/attachment-parenting-with-multiples/.

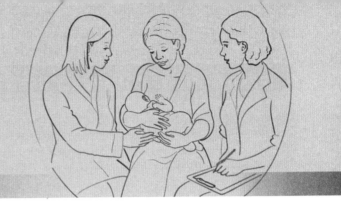

CHAPTER 16

Breastfeeding and Growth: Birth through Weaning

Debi Ferrarello
Virginia H. Carney

OBJECTIVES

- Assist parents with breastfeeding recommendations, patterns, and management challenges beyond the newborn period.
- Incorporate knowledge about the physical conditions that may affect an infant's ability to breastfeed into assessment and management techniques.
- Support later-stage breastfeeding, including toddlers, tandem breastfeeding, and breastfeeding during pregnancy.
- Interpret situations that may affect lactation or lead to early weaning (e.g., sudden refusal to breastfeed, teething, and illness).
- Individualize weaning options, strategies, and rationales.
- Incorporate cultural variations and parental decision making related to feeding and weaning into support options.

DEFINITIONS OF COMMONLY USED TERMS

comfort breastfeeding Breastfeeding used for comfort when the child is fearful, in pain, or in need of emotional support.
gastro-(o)esophageal reflux disease (GERD/GORD) Infant symptoms of reflux with symptoms of coughing, weight loss, or excessive crying where the (o)esophagus becomes irritated from stomach acid.
lactose overload Ingestion of a large volume of high-lactose, low-fat milk, causing excess gas that leads to pain.
milk stasis Stagnant milk in the breast related to milk flow issues from a variety of causes that may include poor latch, infrequent feeding, and insufficient emptying of the breast.

(continues)

▶ Overview

Breastfeeding is the physiologic norm for infants. When it is practiced naturally without interference, it provides for optimal growth. Newborns typically lose 5 to 7 percent of their birth weight in the first few days of life and regain the weight by approximately 7 to 10 days.[1] (See *Additional Resources* later in this chapter.) A weight loss of 10 percent or more requires a thorough assessment of the infant and breastfeeding.[1-3] A newborn's stomach capacity is approximately 20 mL, and it can hold 30 to 59 mL (1 to 2 oz) at a feeding by the end of the first week of life. Accounting for neonatal gastric emptying of human milk feedings, newborns are likely designed for feeding at 1-hour intervals.[4] Parents who are not prepared for this norm may wrongly conclude that their milk production is inadequate, placing breastfeeding at risk.

Breastfed infants may grow more quickly than those who are fed formula during the first weeks of life. However, breastfed infants are leaner than formula-fed infants between 3 and 4 months of age through 1 year, even after the addition of complementary foods. Most infants who are allowed to self-regulate will grow well with the recommended consumption published in dietary guidelines.[5,6] The delivery method may matter as well, with babies who are fed human milk by bottle gaining weight more quickly than those fed at the breast.[7] Growth charts provided by the World Health Organization (WHO) provide a means to track infant weight, length, and head circumference, with breastfeeding as the reference feeding method. (See *Additional Resources* later in this chapter and Chapter 13, *Facilitating and Assessing Breastfeeding Initiation*.)

This chapter will examine breastfeeding beyond the newborn period, including how breastfeeding changes as the infant matures and normal changes that can affect breastfeeding, such as the return of menstruation, another pregnancy, a sudden refusal to breastfeed, and illness. Guidance about weaning throughout the process is also discussed.

I. Breastfeeding Patterns during Infancy

A. Cultural expectations influence breastfeeding patterns. (See Chapter 13, *Facilitating and Assessing Breastfeeding Initiation*, and Chapter 22, *Low Milk Production and Infant Weight*.)

1. In some traditional cultures, babies breastfeed intensely—as often as several times each hour day and night—for 3 to 4 years.[8] In these cultures, breastfeeding parents keep their babies against their bodies as they work, and babies have ready access to the breast.

2. In many Western countries, cultural expectations are at odds with infant physiology.

   a. Breastfeeding is often regulated by the clock at intervals of no less than 2 to 3 hours.

   b. When a baby demonstrates feeding cues more frequently than every 2 to 3 hours, parents may falsely interpret the behavior as insufficient milk production.

   c. Pacifiers, dummies, and bottles are commonly used to lengthen the intervals between feedings.

   d. In many Western cultures, separation of parents and infants is considered normal and desirable, and work is usually distinct from home life, creating challenges for breastfeeding.

   e. The use of a breast pump, instead of feeding at the breast for some, most, or all feedings, is considered normal and desirable in some Western cultures.

   f. Human milk may be valued above the act of breastfeeding.

   g. Many babies are expected to self-soothe, sleep alone, and be weaned within the first year.

B. A baby's age and stomach size play a role in determining both how much milk is taken at each feeding and how many times per day a baby needs to breastfeed in order to thrive.[9] (See Chapter 13, *Facilitating and Assessing Breastfeeding Initiation.*)
   1. According to the Academy of Breastfeeding Medicine, newborns take in 2 to 10 mL per feeding on the first day of life, 5 to 15 mL per feeding on day 2, 15 to 30 mL per feeding on day 3, and 30 to 60 mL per feeding on day 4 of life.[10]
   2. Hospital feeding practices tend to exceed infants' physiologic needs, as evidenced by the large amount of artificial milk provided in 60 and 120 mL bottles. This leads to overfeeding of both breastfed and formula-fed infants.
   3. In the first day, a breastfed baby consumes an average of about 30 mL per day.[9]
   4. At about 1 week, the average intake increases to about 300 to 450 mL per day.[9]
C. Breast storage capacity affects the amount of milk a baby has access to at a feeding.[11]
   1. Breast storage capacity is the amount available to the baby during a feeding when the breast is full. Because of the multifaceted effects on milk production, the variability of breasts, and the fact that a breast is continually producing milk, it is difficult to provide exact amounts of storage capacity for individual breasts. (See the publication by Kent et al. in the *Suggested Reading* section later in this chapter.)
   2. The peak milk production rate is established by about 1 month postpartum and remains relatively stable until complementary foods are added at about 6 months of age.[11,12]
   3. By about 1 month of age, a thriving breastfed infant's intake ranges from 330 to 1,220 mL per day, with an average of about 750 to 800 mL.[13,14]
   4. Infants' energy needs change between 1 and 6 months of age.[15]
D. Individual infant feeding patterns will vary.
   1. In many cultures, babies have access to the breast throughout the day and night, and they may feed frequently.
   2. In some Western cultures, babies are encouraged to increase feeding intervals at night.
   3. It is common for babies in Western cultures to feed very often during the evening hours.
E. The length of feedings will vary.
   1. The length of feedings is highly variable, ranging from 12 to 67 minutes,[14] with no relationship between the length of the feeding and the amount of milk transferred.[15]
   2. The length of feeding time may shorten after breastfeeding is well established.
   3. When there is a fast milk flow or when the baby feeds efficiently, full feedings after the first 6 weeks may last only 5 minutes. Some parents may interpret this as breast rejection or readiness to wean.
F. Babies might return to intense breastfeeding at various times.
   1. As babies grow, they might return to intense breastfeeding to adjust milk production as needed. This is sometimes referred to as a growth spurt and often occurs at about 2 to 3 weeks, at 6 weeks, and again at 3 months.
   2. Although these high-frequency feeding days may be referred to as growth spurts, there is no evidence that babies experience a change in growth pattern that coincides with the change in feeding pattern.
G. Babies may become easily distracted while at the breast.
   1. Beginning at around 3 months, babies who were previously content and focused at the breast may become easily distracted by activities going on around them.[16]
   2. During this developmental phase, many babies breastfeed longer and drain the breast more fully at night.
   3. If a parent wants to encourage more consistent breastfeeding during the day, breastfeeding in a darkened room with fewer distractions may help keep the baby more focused and breastfeeding more effectively.
   4. If there are other children in the home, avoiding distractions during the day can be difficult.
   5. Even with distractions during breastfeeding, ready access to the breast allows a baby to consume the milk needed by feeding more often or having longer feedings at other times of day.
   6. As babies become mobile, they often become increasingly distracted during feedings.
      a. Parents may interpret this developmentally appropriate change in feeding as an interest in weaning. These parents need reassurance and education about normal changes as a baby grows.
      b. Babies may begin to take more milk at night. This may be surprising, and perhaps even disturbing, to parents who have expectations about babies sleeping through the night without feeding.

H.   Babies may clamp down on the breast during feedings for a number of reasons.
1.   The eruption of teeth may cause biting during feedings but does not signify the baby's readiness to stop breastfeeding. Clamping down on the breast can be a natural reaction to teething discomfort.
2.   Biting may be a result of holding the baby in an awkward position, causing the baby to tuck in the chin to stay attached. Shifting the baby's position for the chin to tilt back slightly, or moving the baby down in the direction of his or her own feet can reduce pressure of the top teeth on the breast.
3.   Babies cannot suck and bite at the same time. Observing when the biting occurs may lead to resolution. If biting typically occurs toward the end of a feeding, or if a change in the latch is noticed, the parent may be able to anticipate biting and remove the baby from the breast before it occurs.
4.   If a baby clamps down, first explore the cause, then proceed with possible interventions to resolve the cause and decrease the likelihood of it happening again. Possible interventions include the following:
a.   Provide the baby with a cold or frozen teething ring or age-appropriate cold food immediately prior to feeding. This soothes the gums and reduces the chance of biting.
b.   Pull the baby in close toward the breast so the baby can naturally release the breast to breathe.
c.   Try to avoid startling the baby by crying out when the baby bites. This could cause the baby to begin rejecting going to the breast.
d.   End the feeding calmly and firmly and put the baby down to signal that the feeding will not continue when the baby bites.
e.   Avoid saying the word *no* because babies may not differentiate between *no biting* and *no feeding*.
f.   Evaluate the baby's latch to prevent nipple damage caused by teething and biting.
g.   Have a finger ready to slide into the baby's mouth and break suction if the latch changes to a position indicating the baby may clamp down on the nipple.[17] It is common for the infant to clamp down at the end of a feeding when the milk flow slows. Anticipating this and removing the baby from the breast will avoid clamping down.

II. Physical Conditions That May Affect an Infant's Ability to Breastfeed

A.   Crying can adversely impact breastfeeding. (See Chapter 4, *Normal Infant Behavior*, for a discussion of infant crying.)
1.   Although some people say that a healthy infant who is fed on cue and carried frequently will seldom cry,[18] some babies who are apparently healthy do cry for many hours a day.
2.   Persistent crying is alarming to parents, may shorten the duration of breastfeeding,[19] and may put the child at risk for shaken baby syndrome.[20]
3.   Along with the infant's primary healthcare provider, the lactation consultant can assess the baby for colic, lactose overload, a gastric reflux disorder, and food intolerances.
4.   Managing feeding in these situations and helping parents to soothe their infants and develop safe coping strategies are important roles for the lactation consultant.
B.   Colic may require adjustments in breastfeeding.
1.   Colic is described as excessive crying in an otherwise healthy baby. The classic 3-3-3 definition of colic is crying for greater than 3 hours per day, for greater than 3 days per week, and for greater than 3 weeks.[21]
2.   Although there is no definite cause of colic, some theories include the following:
a.   Gastro-(o)esophageal reflex disease (GERD/GORD).
b.   Food intolerance.[22-24] (See Chapter 8, *Nutrition during Lactation*, for a discussion of infant allergies.)
c.   Lactose overload and improper feeding.[4,25]
d.   Maternal smoking.[26,27]
e.   Disruption of gastrointestinal flora.[28]
f.   Pediatric migraine headache.[21]

3. Possibly helpful interventions for colic include the following:
    a. Probiotics, in particular *Lactobacillus reuteri*, have been found to reduce symptoms.[29]
    b. Manipulation therapies, such as chiropractic treatments, have been reported as helpful in reducing symptoms; however, the evidence is not strong.[30]
    c. Changes in the maternal diet may impact the infant's symptoms.[24]
    d. Increased skin-to-skin contact and holding provide comfort to the infant.
    e. Positioning adjustments will help avoid or manage trapped gas.
4. A colicky infant may associate feeding with pain, resulting in slow weight gain or weight loss.
5. An infant in pain may frequently go to the breast for comfort, increasing milk production and resulting in overfeeding, which in turn causes more pain.
6. Continuing to breastfeed is encouraged.[31]
    a. Try positioning the infant in an upright position in the clutch hold, straddled across the parent's lap, or try a laid-back biological nurturing position. (See Chapter 13, *Facilitating and Assessing Breastfeeding Initiation*, for a discussion of positioning.)
    b. Feeding on one breast at each feeding may avoid overdistending the stomach.
    c. Feed the infant frequently.
    d. Keep the infant upright after feedings.
C. GERD/GORD is a medical condition that may be diagnosed and treated by the infant's primary healthcare provider.
    1. Reflux, including spitting up or posseting (bringing up milk during or after a feeding), is normal in infants younger than 1 year and requires no intervention.
    2. Reflux becomes GERD/GORD when symptoms such as coughing, weight loss, or excessive crying occur and the (o)esophagus becomes irritated from stomach acid.
    3. At times, feeding management alone can resolve GERD/GORD symptoms.[31]
    4. Interventions to manage GERD/GORD in infants include the following:[33]
        a. Small, frequent feedings, with the infant in an upright position.
        b. Medications such as proton pump inhibitors.
        c. Trial of removing common allergens from the maternal diet.[33]
D. Lactose overload can impact the infant's weight and cause confusion.
    1. Lactose overload occurs when a baby gets a large volume of high-lactose, low-fat milk, causing excess gas that leads to pain.[25,32]
    2. These babies often present as quite chubby after the parents interpret crying as hunger and the babies seek the breast for comfort. Frequent feedings increase milk production and thus continue the cycle of feeding, pain, crying, and more feeding.
    3. Feeding the baby from the same breast for several feedings in a row may decrease the amount of milk and lactose the baby receives per feeding and lead to more comfortable feeds. Lactation consultants can provide guidance to help minimize breast discomfort and the risk of milk stasis with this change in breastfeeding pattern.
    4. Although the symptoms are different, lactose malabsorption or lactase deficiency can be confused with an allergy to cow's milk. It can be beneficial to restrict maternal intake of cow's milk products to help relieve the infant's symptoms.
    5. The incubation of expressed milk with lactase drops may be effective if the symptoms are severe.[35]
    6. Parents often confuse lactose overload with lactose intolerance and milk allergy, and they may need help understanding the difference.
E. A sudden onset of refusal to breastfeed can occur at any time during the course of breastfeeding.
    1. Some parents experience a refusal to breastfeed as a personal rejection.
        a. It is usually temporary and is not necessarily an indication of weaning due to insufficient milk or that the baby is developmentally ready to stop breastfeeding.[36]
        b. Provide tips and reassurance, connect the parents with others who have had similar experiences, and work closely with the dyad to return to breastfeeding.
    2. The cause of a sudden refusal to breastfeed may never be discovered. Possible causes include the following:
        a. The mother's return of menses.
        b. Parental stress.

      c.   Maternal dietary changes.

      d.   Unpleasant taste in the milk.

      e.   Change in the parent's odors or aromas.

      f.   A cold restricting nasal air flow or earache in the baby.

      g.   Teething discomfort.

      h.   Episode of biting with a startle and pain reaction by the parent.

      i.   Restricted feedings because of sleep training programs.

      j.   Period of separation of the parent and baby.

      k.   The baby's increased distractibility.

      l.   Travel or changes in the home environment.

  3.   The suggested interventions for a sudden refusal to breastfeed include the following:

      a.   Breastfeed in a quiet, dark location. Make feeding special with no distractions and no other people around until regular breastfeeding resumes.

      b.   Increase the contact between the parent and the baby without actively putting the baby to the breast.

      c.   Attempt to feed when the child is sleepy or before waking from a nap.

      d.   Hold the baby skin to skin in a warm bathtub. Encourage another adult to be present for safety.

      e.   Attempt to breastfeed while walking, rocking, or dancing with the child.

      f.   Avoid startling the infant if biting occurs.

      g.   Rule out illness, oral cavity problems, or dental conditions in the infant.

      h.   Offer the breast frequently, but do not coax too much.

      i.   Breast refusal that lasts more than a day or two might require milk expression on a regular basis to protect milk production and avoid plugged ducts or mastitis.

F.   Breastfeeding should continue when the infant is ill.

  1.   An infant who is not feeling well commonly has a decreased appetite and may feed less effectively, less often, or more frequently in brief bursts.[18]

  2.   The impact the illness may have on feeding depends on its severity and duration.

  3.   Reduced feeding can impair milk production; milk expression will maintain comfort and milk volume. (See Chapter 31, *Expression and Use of Human Milk*.)

  4.   Infants with congenital, developmental, and environmental problems often undergo frequent painful procedures during treatment and care. Studies show that compared to placebo, body positioning, or no intervention, breastfeeding is best for providing pain relief.[17]

  5.   When an infant is sick, regardless of severity, breastfeeding should be encouraged and supported so lactation will continue and milk will be provided for the baby's recovery.

  6.   Discontinuing breastfeeding during an infant illness is not recommended. The baby needs the beneficial nutrients and immunities in human milk, and breastfeeding provides needed comfort for the baby during the illness.

III. Later Stages of Breastfeeding

A.   The physiological and biological human norm for weaning age is between 2.5 and 7 years.[37]

  1.   At no time is the milk of another mammal more nutritious than human milk for a human child.

  2.   Culture impacts breastfeeding practices and expectations. Some parents use code words and negotiate acceptable times and locations for breastfeeding their toddlers in cultures that do not widely accept breastfeeding beyond infancy.

  3.   Toddlers may breastfeed briefly, between other activities, and for longer periods of time when they are sleepy, ill, or need comfort.

B.   Several factors can impact breastfeeding during pregnancy.

  1.   Research indicates that 74 percent of breastfeeding women experience nipple pain while breastfeeding during subsequent pregnancies.[38]

  2.   During the second trimester, the milk production rate usually declines as the mammary gland reverts back to the secretory differentiation stage with disassembly of tight junctions between mammary

epithelial cells. This process renders the mammary gland more prone to infiltration of plasma components, including markedly increased sodium concentration, giving the milk a salty flavor.[39]

3. There is no evidence to support recommendations to wean during pregnancy or that uterine contractions during breastfeeding increase the risk of preterm labor.[39] Some healthcare professionals recommend weaning for women at high risk of repeated miscarriage.

4. Some children wean during pregnancy and resume breastfeeding after the birth of the new baby.

5. Lactation consultants can provide guidance and support for parents who choose to wean during pregnancy and for those who continue to breastfeed.

C. Tandem breastfeeding is an option for parents with an infant and an older child.

1. Continuing to breastfeed an older child after the birth of a sibling may help the child adjust to the change in the family.[1]

2. There will be sufficient milk for both children. The newborn should feed before the older child to ensure the newborn receives enough milk.

3. With the birth of the new baby, the milk will begin as colostrum and progress to mature milk. This is not harmful to older children, although their bowel movements may temporarily appear more like a newborn's and they may react to the change in the taste and consistency of the milk.

D. Consider cultural variations and perspectives regarding later-stage breastfeeding. (See Chapter 28, *Cultural Humility*.)

1. Lactation consultants should examine their own beliefs about longer-term breastfeeding.

2. Help families view breastfeeding within the context of the child's development.

3. Explain that the appropriate time to wean should be a joint decision between the parent and the child, in which they both reach a state of readiness at the same time.

4. When the baby and the parent differ in the desired time to wean, support and reassurance will help them navigate the end of breastfeeding.

E. Support parents who breastfeed an older baby.

1. In some settings, support is needed for dealing with value judgments made by others about extended breastfeeding.

2. Many who breastfeed an older child find peer support from other parents.

3. Parents may need help understanding their feelings about continuing to breastfeed and recognizing their child's needs.

IV. Weaning

A. Be alert to risk factors for early weaning.

1. Cultural pressure leads to early weaning in some settings where breastfeeding beyond infancy is not the norm.

   a. Pressure from family, friends, and even healthcare providers who are insensitive and uninformed can cause closet breastfeeding, or breastfeeding in secret at home.

   b. Cultural norms may create pressure for women to return to their prepregnancy weight.

   c. In Western cultures, parents and healthcare providers often misinterpret the recommendation of the American Academy of Pediatrics to breastfeed until the infant is at least 1 year of age, thinking of 1 year as the goal for the full duration of breastfeeding.

2. External issues relating to perceptions of sexuality, gender, or trauma can lead to early weaning and include the following:

   a. Pressure from the partner, friends, or strangers.

   b. Societal attitudes that are not in line with the feelings of parenthood and breastfeeding.

   c. Gender identity discomfort.

   d. Past trauma.

3. The return of menses can impact breastfeeding.

   a. There is a possibility of diminished milk production and tender nipples or breasts with the onset of menses each month.

   b. The baby may be reluctant to breastfeed, or may refuse the breast, right before or during the first day or two of menstruation.

4. A new pregnancy may cause any of the following:
   a. Nipple pain.
   b. Diminished milk volume.
   c. Change in the taste of the milk.[40]
5. Employment and scheduling play a significant role for many parents in the decision to wean, especially in countries without paid maternity leave.[41] Many parents believe they must wean before returning to work. To succeed, they will need the lactation consultant's support and practical information about milk expression and storage, as well as information about their employment rights. (See Chapter 11, *Breastfeeding and Employment*, and Chapter 31, *Expression and Use of Human Milk*.)
6. Cultural or religious expectations regarding weaning may affect the process.
   a. Some guidelines recommend breastfeeding until age 6 months.
   b. The Koran states that infants should be breastfed until 2 years of age.
   c. These guidelines may not consider that breastfeeding can continue alongside the introduction of solid food and for 2 years or more.
   d. Lactation consultants can support parents as they navigate their families' goals and cultural or religious time lines.

B. Optimally, weaning occurs naturally based on the needs of the child. (See Chapter 9, *Nutrition for the Breastfeeding Child*.)
   1. For some parents, weaning may refer to the process of changing from one method of feeding to another (e.g., the addition of other foods), not to the total cessation of breastfeeding.[1]
   2. The recommendation of the WHO, UNICEF, the American Academy of Pediatrics, and most major national and international maternal and child health associations is to breastfeed exclusively for 6 months.[42,43] They further recommend that breastfeeding continue for at least 1 year or beyond.
   3. Infant-initiated weaning begins with the addition of solid foods and is also referred to as *baby-led weaning*.
      a. The onset is usually between ages 5 and 9 months, with a median age of 6 months.
      b. At about age 6 months, the infant shows increased interest in exploring the environment and other foods. At times, this may be accompanied by a decreased interest in breastfeeding. These developmental behaviors facilitate infant-initiated weaning to complementary foods.
      c. Infant-initiated weaning can lead to a mutually desired transition toward complementary foods replacing breastmilk calories.
      d. Infant-initiated weaning can usually be reversed with encouragement to continue exclusive breastfeeding if the infant is younger than 6 months.[44]
   4. Breastfed infants self-regulate their total energy intake when other foods are introduced.[1]
   5. Weaning to a cup is a natural transition if the infant is at least 7 months old.
      a. Infants can learn to drink from a cup at about age 7 to 9 months.[1]
      b. Parents who desire to continue breastfeeding should provide only water during cup training. They should be made aware that the introduction of other milks or juice in a cup will severely curtail the infant's interest in breastfeeding because these other liquids contain a lot of calories. (See Chapter 9, *Nutrition for the Breastfeeding Child*.)
   6. Immunological benefits from human milk are present for the child as long as breastfeeding continues.[45-47] Human milk is an important nutritional component of the baby's diet for the first year until solid food intake gradually increases to be the primary source of calories in the second year of life.
   7. When a human milk substitute is chosen or necessary, it is important that it is prepared accurately and under sanitary conditions.
   8. Babies may start breastfeeding more frequently during the night to reconnect with a parent who has returned to work.
   9. Breastfeeding provides comfort when the child is fearful or in need of emotional support; this has been termed *comfort breastfeeding*.[1]
   10. Older babies become more distracted and may not finish feedings during the day. Therefore, they may increase nighttime feedings to make up for missed calories. The same increase in night feedings can happen if the parent is at work and away from the baby during the day.

C.   Abrupt weaning is very difficult for the child, and it carries significant health risks for the breasts.

   1.   Abrupt weaning may cause plugged ducts, mastitis, or an abscess. It may also have a negative emotional impact on the child and may not change the child's nighttime needs.

   2.   When abrupt weaning is desired or necessary, nondrug therapies may allow more comfort and prevent breast problems.

      a.   Warm showers or baths will facilitate milk release.

      b.   Hand expression or pumping can remove just enough milk for comfort and to relieve engorgement.

      c.   Wearing a supportive, comfortable bra is helpful.

      d.   Watching for plugged ducts or signs of mastitis will ensure prompt treatment.

   3.   Hold and cuddle the baby frequently to provide comfort through the transition to total weaning.

   4.   Expect this to be an emotional time for the breastfeeding parent and encourage support from others who will appreciate what is being felt.

▶ Key Points from This Chapter

A.   Breastfeeding, meaning human milk provided at the breast, provides optimal growth for infants and is the biologic norm.

B.   Breastfeeding may continue into early childhood if mutually desired by the parent and child. Breastfeeding may continue during pregnancy and after the birth of another child.

C.   When circumstances occur that threaten continued breastfeeding before the dyad is ready to wean (e.g., teething, biting, sudden refusal to breastfeed, illness, faltering growth, or social pressure), ways to preserve the relationship should be discussed to support parents in meeting their breastfeeding goals.

D.   Cultural humility and understanding are important for the lactation consultant so that traditions and cultural values are respected and trust can be established. The lactation consultant should be alert for any social and health inequities that may exist throughout the breastfeeding experience. (See Chapter 28, *Cultural Humility.*)

🔍 CASE STUDY

Maria, the birth parent of 1-month-old Thomas, who is exclusively breastfeeding, is consulting with Denae, IBCLC, because of concerns about not having enough milk. Thomas breastfeeds many times each day and never seems satisfied. He cries frequently, spits up undigested milk more than five times a day, passes gas explosively, and roots vigorously at the breast. He latches on to the breast, but often pulls off after just a few minutes and begins to cry and root again. Maria switches breasts every time Thomas pulls off. Thomas has approximately eight stools each day. Most stools are green, although some are bright yellow. Because of the frequent feedings and apparent hunger, Maria is convinced that her milk production is not sufficient, and she wants to know how to increase production.

On assessment, Denae finds that Maria's breasts are firm and full, with nipples that are graspable and intact. Thomas is in the 50th percentile for length and head circumference and is at the 80th percentile for weight. Maria reports that at the 2-week visit, Thomas was in the 50th percentile for length and 60th percentile for weight. Thomas's oral anatomy is within normal limits. His abdomen is mildly distended. He is alert and vigorous and readily makes eye contact.

Denae observes a feeding and notes that Thomas latches and breastfeeds well when the feeding begins. After 3 minutes, Thomas pulls off the breast, arches his back, cries, and passes gas. He roots for the breast, which Maria offers, and then latches and repeats the behavior. This continues for several cycles.

Denae suspects that Thomas's feeding behaviors are related to a lactose imbalance, and that his stomach quickly becomes overly full, resulting in uncomfortable gastroesophageal reflux. He is clearly gaining weight quickly, demonstrating that Maria has ample milk production. Denae suggests that Maria feed Thomas from the same breast for several feedings in a row and not change breasts sooner than 2 to 3 hours. If a breast becomes uncomfortably full,

(continues)

CASE STUDY *(continued)*

Maria should express just enough to regain comfort. Providing milk from a breast that is less full, the milk will have proportionally less lactose and more fat, which will be more comfortable for Thomas. Denae shows Maria Thomas's growth trajectory and points out his rounded cheeks and skin folds on his thighs. Denae explains that although lactose is a normal and healthy part of human milk, an excess of lactose can cause excess gas and does not promote a feeling of being satisfied. This could also explain the green stools.

Denae encourages Maria to try leaning back to breastfeed, or to feed Thomas in an upright position for the next few days to help him cope with the flow of milk. This would decrease milk production somewhat and provide a more comfortable feeding for Thomas. Denae explains that Thomas would probably feel more satisfied and be more comfortable by getting less milk overall, with more rich fat and less lactose. Denae praises Maria's response to Thomas's needs and points out Thomas's gaze fixed on her face. Maria agrees to continue the plan for 2 days and schedule a follow-up visit.

At the follow-up, Maria reports that Thomas is crying less frequently and seems more settled after feedings. His stools are consistently yellow, with only an occasional green stool. Thomas gained 60 grams in 2 days. Denae encourages Maria to continue to feed Thomas on cue and to continue offering one breast at each feeding. She praises Maria's caring behaviors and observations, such as Thomas's response to Maria's face, voice, and mannerisms. Maria receives a referral to a local parents' group led by a peer counselor so Maria can benefit from the support of other breastfeeding parents. Denae encourages further follow-up as needed.

Questions

1. Why did Denae suspect that Maria had a lactose imbalance?
2. Why did Maria assume that milk production was insufficient?
3. Why did the change in feeding pattern alter Thomas's behavior?
4. What was revealed by Denae's assessment of Maria's breasts and nipples?
5. What was the importance of Denae praising Maria?

References

1. Lawrence RA, Lawrence RM, eds. *Breastfeeding: A Guide for the Medical Profession*. 7th ed. Maryland Heights, MO: Elsevier Mosby; 2011.
2. Dewey KG, Nommsen-Rivers LA, Heinig MJ, Cohen RJ. Lactogenesis and infant weight change in the first weeks of life. *Adv Expl Med Biol*. 2002;503:159-166.
3. Flaherman VJ, Schaefer EW, Kuzniewicz MK, Li S, Walsh E, Paul IM. Newborn weight loss during birth hospitalization and breastfeeding outcomes through age 1 month. *J Hum Lactation*. 2017;33(1):225-230. doi:10.1177/0890334416680181.
4. Bergman NJ. Neonatal stomach volume and physiology suggest feeding at 1-h intervals. *Acta Paediatr*. 2013;102(8):773-777. doi:10.1111/apa.12291.
5. Dewey KG, Lonnerdal B. Infant self-regulation of breast milk intake. *Acta Paediatr Scand*. 1986;75(6):893-898.
6. Garza C, Frongillo E, Dewey KG. Implications of growth patterns of breastfed infants for growth references. *Acta Paediatr*. 1994;402(suppl):4-10.
7. Li R, Magadia J, Fein SB, Grummer-Strawn LM. Risk of bottle-feeding for rapid weight gain in the first year of life. *Arch Pediatra Adolesc Med*. 2012;166(5):431.
8. Stuart-Macadam P. Breastfeeding in prehistory. In: Stuart-Macadam P, Dettwyler K, eds. *Breastfeeding: Biocultural Perspectives*. New York, NY: Aldine de Gruyter; 1995:75-99.
9. Mohrbacher N. Breastfeeding and growth: birth through weaning. In: Mannel R, Martens PJ, Walker M, eds. *Core Curriculum for Lactation Consultant Practice*. 3rd ed. Burlington, MA: Jones & Bartlett Learning; 2012:595-596.
10. Kellams A, Harrel C, Omage S, Gregory C, Rosen-Carole C. ABM clinical protocol #3: supplementary feedings in the healthy term breastfed neonate, revised 2017. *Breastfeed Med*. 2017;12:188-198. doi:10.1089/bfm.2017.29038.ajk.
11. Kent JC. How breastfeeding works. *J Midwifery Womens Health*. 2007;52:564-570.
12. Islam MM, Peerson JM, Ahmed T, Dewey KG, Brown KH. Effects of varied energy density of complementary foods on breast-milk intakes and total energy consumption by healthy, breastfed Bangladeshi children. *Am J Clin Nutr*. 2006;83(4):851-858.
13. Kent JC, Prime DK, Garbin CP. Principles for maintaining or increasing breast milk production. *JOGNN*. 2012;41(1):114-121.
14. Kent JC, Mitoulas LR, Cregan MD, Ramsay, DT, Doherty DA, Hartmann PE. Volume and frequency of breastfeeds and fat content of breastmilk throughout the day. *Pediatrics*. 2006;117:e387-e395.
15. Ramsay DT, Kent JC, Owens RA, Hartmann PE. Ultrasound imaging of milk ejection in the breast of lactating women. *Pediatrics*. 2004;113(2):361-367.
16. Mohrbacher N. (2010). *Breastfeeding Answers Made Simple: A Guide for Helping Mothers*. Amarillo, TX: Hale Publishing; 2010.

17. La Leche League International. *Womanly Art of Breastfeeding*. New York, NY: Ballentine Books; 2004.

18. Wambach K, Riordan J. *Breastfeeding and Human Lactation*. 5th ed. Burlington, MA: Jones & Bartlett Learning; 2016.

19. Howard CR, Lanphear N, Lanphear BP, Eberly S, Lawrence RA. Parental responses to infant crying and colic: the effect on breastfeeding duration. *Breastfeed Med*. 2006;1(3):146-155.

20. Gelfand AA. Infant colic. *Semin Pediatr Neurol*. 2016;23(1):79-82. doi:10.1016/j.spen.2015.08.003.

21. Wessel MA, Cobb JC, Jackson EB, Harris GS Jr, Detwiler AC. Paroxysmal fussing in infancy, sometimes called colic. *Pediatrics*. 1954;14(5):421-435.

22. Gupta SK. Update on infantile colic and management options. *Curr Opin Investig Drugs*. 2007;8(11):921-926.

23. Estep DC, Kulczycki A Jr. Treatment of infant colic with amino acid-based infant formula: a preliminary study. *Acta Paediatr*. 2000;89(1):22-27.

24. Nocerino R, Pezzella V, Cosenza L, et al. The controversial role of food allergy in infantile colic: evidence and clinical management. *Nutrients*. 2015;7(3):2015-2025. doi:10.3390/nu7032015.

25. Woolridge MW, Fisher C. Colic, "overfeeding", and symptoms of lactose malabsorption in the breast-fed baby: a possible artifact of feed management? *Lancet*. 1988;2(8607):382-384.

26. Fleming P, Pease A, Blair P. Bed-sharing and unexpected infant deaths: what is the relationship? *Paediatra Respir Rev*. 2014;16(1):62-67. doi:10.1016/j.prrv.2014.10.008.

27. Shenassa ED, Brown MJ. Maternal smoking and infantile gastrointestinal dysregulation: the case of colic. *Pediatrics*. 2004;114(4):e497-e505. doi:10.1542/peds.2004-1036.

28. Rhoads JM, Fatheree NY, Norori J, et al. Altered fecal microflora and increased fecal calprotectin in infants with colic. *J Pediatr*. 2009;155(6):823-828. doi:10.1016/jpeds.2009.05.012.

29. Harb T, Matsuyama M, David M, Hill RJ. Infant colic—what works: a systematic review of interventions for breast-fed infants. *J Pediatr Gastroenterol Nutr*. 2016;62(5):668-686. doi:10.1097/MPG.0000000000001075.

30. Dobson D, Lucassen PL, Miller JJ, Vlieger AM, Prescott P, Lewith G. Manipulative therapies for infantile colic. *Cochrane Database Syst Rev*. 2012;12:CD004796. doi:10.1002/14651858.CD004796.pub2.

31. Boekel S. *Gastroesophageal Reflux Disease (GERD) and the Breastfeeding Baby* [independent study module]. Raleigh, NC: International Lactation Consultant Association; 2000.

32. Douglas PS. Diagnosing gastro-esophageal reflux disease or lactose intolerance in babies who cry a lot in the first few months overlooks feeding problems. *J Paediatri Child Health*. 2013;49(4):E252-E256. doi:10.1111/jpc.12153.

33. Onveador N, Paul SP, Sandhu BK. Paediatric gastroesophageal reflux clinical practice guidelines. *Arch Dis Child Educ Pract*. 2014;99(5):190-193. doi:10.1136/archdischild-2013-305253.

34. Hill DJ, Roy N, Heine RG, et al. Effect of a low-allergen maternal diet on colic among breastfed infants: a randomized, controlled trial. *Pediatrics*. 2005;116(5):e709-e715.

35. Heyman MB. Committee on nutrition: lactose intolerance in infants, children, and adolescents. *Pediatrics*. 2006:118(3):1279-1286.

36. Odom EC, Ruowei L, Kelley SS, Perrine CG, Grummer-Strawn L. Reasons for earlier than desired cessation of breastfeeding. *Pediatrics*. 2013;131(3):e726-e733.

37. Dettwyler K. A time to wean: the hominid blueprint for the natural age of weaning in modern human populations. In: Stuart-Macadam P, Dettwyler K, eds. *Breastfeeding: Biocultural Perspectives*. New York, NY: Aldine de Gruyter; 1995:39-73.

38. Mead M, Newton N. Cultural patterning of perinatal behavior. In: Richardson S, Guttmacher A, eds. *Childbearing: Its Social and Psychological Aspects*. Baltimore, MD: Williams & Wilkins; 1967:142-244.

39. Cetis I, Assandro P, Massari M, et al. Breastfeeding during pregnancy: position paper of the Italian Society of Perinatal Medicine and the Task Force on Breastfeeding, Ministry of Health, Italy. *J Hum Lactation*. 2014;30(1):20-27. doi:10.1177/0890334413514294.

40. Huggins K. *The Nursing Mother's Guide to Weaning*. Boston, MA: Harvard Common Press; 1994.

41. Hervada AR, Newman DR. Weaning: historical perspective, practical recommendations, and current controversies. *Curr Probl Pediatr*. 1992;22:223-240.

42. World Health Organization. *Joint WHO/UNICEF Meeting, Global Strategy for Infant and Young Child Feeding: Document No. A54, Information Document/4*. Geneva, Switzerland: World Health Organization; 2001.

43. American Academy of Pediatrics. Breastfeeding and the use of human milk. *Pediatrics*. 2012;129(3):e827-e841.

44. Clark SK, Harmon RJ. Infant-initiated weaning from the breast in the first year. *Early Hum Dev*. 1983;8(2):151.

45. American Academy of Pediatrics. Breastfeeding and the use of human milk. *Pediatrics*. 2012;129(3):e827-e841.

46. Perrin MT, Fogleman AD, Newburg DS, Allen JC. A longitudinal study of human milk composition in the second year postpartum: implications for human milk banking. *Matern Child Nutr*. 2016;January 18. doi:10.1111/mcn.12239.

47. Perrin MT, Fogleman AD, Allen JC. The nutritive and immunoprotective quality of human milk beyond 1 year postpartum: are lactation-duration-based donor exclusions justified? *J Hum Lactation*. 2013;29(3):341-349. doi:10.1177/0890334413487432.

Suggested Reading

Dewey KG, Cohen RJ, Rivera LL, Canahuati J, Brown KH. Do exclusively breast-fed infants require extra protein? *Pediatr Res*. 1996;39(2):303-307.

Dewey KG, Heinig MJ, Nommsen LA, Lönnerdal B. Adequacy of energy intake among breastfed infants in the DARLING study: relationships to growth velocity, morbidity, and activity levels. *J Pediatr*. 1991;119(4):538-547.

Dewey KG, Nommsen-Rivers LA, Heinig MJ, Cohen RJ. Lactogenesis and infant weight change in the first weeks of life. *Adv Exp Med Biol*. 2002;503:159-166.

Kent JC, Williams T, Sakalidis V, Hartmann PE, Lai CT. Storage capacity of the human breast. *FASEB J*. 2012;26(1):806.

Additional Resources
Professional Resources for Interpreting Growth

Centers for Disease Control and Prevention. Growth Chart Training: Using the WHO Growth Charts. http://www.cdc.gov/nccdphp/dnpao /growthcharts/who/index.htm.

Centers for Disease Control and Prevention. *Use and Interpretation of the WHO and CDC Growth Charts for Children from Birth to 20 Years in the United States.* Atlanta, GA: Centers for Disease Control and Prevention. https://www.cdc.gov/nccdphp/dnpa/growthcharts /resources/growthchart.pdf.

World Health Organization. Child Growth Standards: Weight Velocity. http://www.who.int/childgrowth/standards/w_velocity/en/.

World Health Organization. *Training Course on Child Growth Assessment.* Geneva, Switzerland: World Health Organization. http://www .who.int/childgrowth/training/module_c_interpreting_indicators.pdf.

Parent Resources

Introducing solid foods:
- Gonzalez C. *My Child Won't Eat: How to Enjoy Mealtimes without Worry.* London, United Kingdom: Pinter & Martin Ltd; 2005.
- KellyMom.com. http://kellymom.com.
- La Leche League GB. Starting Solid Food. https://www.laleche.org.uk/starting-solid-food/.

Infant food sensitivities:
- Evans M. *Could It Really Be Something They Ate? The Life Changing Impact of Addressing Food Sensitivities in Children.* Bloomington, IN: Balboa Press; 2011. http://www.dynamicchoices.ca/food-sensitivities/.
- National Institute for Health and Care Excellence. *Gastro-Oesophageal Reflux Disease in Children and Young People: Diagnosis and Management.* London, United Kingdom: National Institute for Health and Care Excellence; 2015. https://www.nice.org.uk/guidance /ng1/resources/gastrooesophageal-reflux-disease-in-children-and-young-people-diagnosis-and-management-51035086789.
- Vickerstaff Joneja J. *Dealing with Food Allergies in Babies and Children.* Boulder, CO: Bull Publishing Company; 2007.

Cultural sensitivity:
- Barber K. *The Black Woman's Guide to Breastfeeding: The Definitive Guide to Nursing for African American Mothers.* Naperville, IL: Sourcebooks; 2005.

Weaning:
- Huggins K. *The Nursing Mother's Guide to Weaning.* Boston, MA: Harvard Common Press; 1994.
- La Leche League GB. Thinking of Weaning? https://www.laleche.org.uk/thinking-of-weaning/.
- Mayo Clinic. What Role Does Breast Milk Play in an Older Baby's Diet? https://www.mayoclinic.org/healthy-lifestyle /infant-and-toddler-health/in-depth/extended-breastfeeding/art-20046962?pg=2.
- Rapley G, Murkett T. *Baby-Led Weaning: Helping Your Baby to Love Good Food.* London, United Kingdom: Vermillion; 2008.

Preparing formula:
- NHS Choices. How to Make Up Baby Formula. http://www.nhs.uk/Conditions/pregnancy-and-baby/Pages/making-up-infant -formula.aspx.
- World Health Organization. *How to Prepare Formula for Bottle-Feeding at Home.* Geneva, Switzerland: World Health Organization. http://www.who.int/foodsafety/publications/micro/PIF_Bottle_en.pdf.

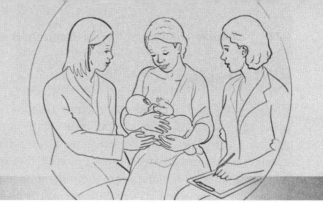

CHAPTER 17

Maternal Physical Health and Breastfeeding

Karen Wambach

OBJECTIVES

- Enumerate the effect of the birth parent's physical health on breastfeeding and lactation.
- Illustrate specific acute and chronic diseases and how they affect breastfeeding and lactation.
- Individualize management strategies to preserve breastfeeding and lactation.
- Critique the contraindications to breastfeeding and lactation.
- Describe appropriate counseling for HIV-positive families.

DEFINITIONS OF COMMONLY USED TERMS

acute illness Disease or illness that is characterized by a sudden onset and limited duration.
chronic disease Condition or illness that is characterized by long (in some cases defined as greater than 6 months) or permanent duration.
cognitive disability Condition that involves impairment in intellectual activities, such as thinking, reasoning, and remembering.
nosocomial infection An infection acquired in a hospital or other healthcare facility that is usually caused by viral, bacterial, or fungal pathogens.
physical disability Physical condition that impairs, interferes with, or limits a person's ability to engage in certain tasks or actions or to participate in typical daily activities and interactions.
physical health Refers to the conditions of the body or body systems; a continuum of health, lack of disease, or disability to states of acute or chronic illness, disability, or disease.
sensory disability Condition that involves sensory organs, such as eyes, ears, or skin (touch).

Any use of the term *mother, maternal,* or *breastfeeding* is not meant to exclude transgender or nonbinary parents who may be breastfeeding or providing human milk to their infant.

▶ Overview

Breastfeeding and lactation may occur within the context of maternal physical illness or disease states, including acute and chronic diseases or conditions, with implications for self-management and lactation consultant management. Therefore, clinical practice involves the assessment of physical, mental, and psychological states. Medical conditions may impact breastfeeding and lactation and require appropriate teaching for parents. Physical disabilities may limit the parents' handling of their infant or child. Practitioners will need to convey current recommendations on infant feeding when HIV and other chronic diseases are involved.

Most often the major concerns for the healthcare provider, and often the parent, are whether the treatment of a condition is compatible with breastfeeding. Breastfeeding is compatible with the majority of maternal diseases and illnesses, whether acute or chronic. In most cases the encouragement and support offered to any other parent can be generalized for an ill parent. (See Chapter 5, *Lactation Pharmacology*, for a discussion about the safety of medications during lactation.)

I. Acute Illnesses

A. Headaches and migraines
   1. Parents who suffer from migraine headaches, especially related to menstruation, may have a reduction of headache frequency and severity during pregnancy and lactation.[1-3]
   2. There is some evidence of lactational headaches associated with letdown and overfull breasts.[4]
   3. Common drugs for treating migraine are generally considered compatible with breastfeeding.
      a. Propranolol (lactation risk category L2) is the drug of choice.[1]
      b. Sumatriptan succinate (lactation risk category L3).
      c. Nnonsteroidal anti-inflammatory drugs (NSAIDs) such as ibuprofen (lactation risk category L1).[5]
   4. Nonpharmaceutical approaches to prevention include a healthy diet and regular meals, regular exercise, adequate rest, and plenty of sleep.[1-3]
B. Infectious diseases
   1. In most cases a common cold, an upper respiratory infection, and the flu are caused by viruses. They do not impact the ability to breastfeed.
      a. Parents are encouraged to treat the acute illness and continue breastfeeding.
      b. Rest, plenty of fluids, and symptom management are important for aiding recovery.
      c. Parents should beware of decongestants containing pseudoephedrine because it can reduce milk production, especially in parents who have poor or marginal milk production or who are in late-stage lactation.[5]
      d. If antibiotics are needed for bacterial infections, healthcare providers should use clinical guidelines for appropriate choices, dosing, and duration of treatment.
   2. Urinary tract infection is the most common problem in women who are seen by primary care providers.
      a. *Escherichia coli* is the most common pathogen in urinary tract infection and is treated with sulfamethoxazole and trimethoprim.
      b. Women may self-treat with six to eight glasses of water per day, drink cranberry juice, avoid caffeine, and urinate frequently and immediately after sexual intercourse.[6]
   3. Methicillin-resistant *Staphylococcus aureus* (MRSA) is an antibiotic-resistant staph infection that can be either hospital or community acquired.
      a. The parent, the baby, or both can be infected.[7]
      b. Individuals can also be carriers of *S. aureus*. If a breastfeeding parent becomes infected (e.g., skin lesion on the breast, mastitis, abscess, or surgical incision) breastfeeding and expressed milk should be withheld for 24 hours (pump and dump) while antibiotic therapy is initiated.
      c. The risk of MRSA and other nosocomial infections in the newborn can be decreased by exposure to nontoxic bacterial flora via skin-to-skin contact after birth.[6]

4. Group B streptococci (GBS), the leading cause of neonatal sepsis, is a common cause of neonatal morbidity and mortality.
   a. GBS is treated with antibiotics if discovered prenatally or intrapartum.
   b. GBS that is present in the vaginal or rectal area can colonize the nasopharynx of the newborn during birth.
   c. Although it is relatively rare, neonates can acquire GBS from breastmilk. The milk can be cultured, and the parent can be treated and continue breastfeeding.[8]
5. Tuberculosis is not common in developed countries, but it is very prevalent in developing countries. Individuals of childbearing age are therefore impacted by this disease.
   a. Parents who have tuberculosis at the time of birth and who are appropriately treated with isoniazid can breastfeed.
   b. In parents whose tuberculosis is discovered at the time of birth, it is necessary to separate the parent and the infant for 2 weeks. The parent must initiate therapy and express milk to protect milk production.
   c. Studies indicate that isoniazid is secreted into the milk, but the levels are considered safe.[9] Breastfeeding should be withheld for 2 hours after drug administration to avoid peak plasma concentrations.[5]
6. Zika virus, spread by two species of *Aedes* mosquitoes, can be transmitted to the fetus during pregnancy and can cause congenital Zika fever, with defects of the skull (microcephaly) being the most common result.
   a. The transmission of the Zika virus through human milk has not been confirmed, although limited research has indicated shedding of Zika viral material in the milk.[10,11]
   b. Individuals who have suspected, probable, or confirmed Zika virus infection or who live in or have traveled to areas where Zika virus is endemic can breastfeed their infants.
7. Ebola virus, first discovered in 1976 near the Ebola River in the Democratic Republic of the Congo, causes illness characterized by fever, severe headache, muscle pain, weakness, fatigue, diarrhea, vomiting, abdominal pain, and unexplained hemorrhage (bleeding or bruising).
   a. Two out of five people who contracted Ebola virus during the 2014–2016 outbreak in West Africa countries died.[12]
   b. The Ebola virus is spread by close contact. Therefore, parents who are infected should not breastfeed due to the close contact needed for breastfeeding.
   c. It is not known if the Ebola virus can be transmitted through milk, but genetic material of the virus has been detected in human milk of parents who have recovered from Ebola infection.[13]
   d. The decision about feeding the infant of a parent who is infected, or has been infected, with the Ebola virus must be weighed carefully. If there is no safe alternative to the parent's milk, the parent may have to breastfeed.[13]
8. Human immunodeficiency virus/acquired immunodeficiency syndrome (HIV/AIDS)
   a. HIV is classified as a retrovirus. A retrovirus is a group of RNA viruses that insert a DNA copy of their genome into the host cell in order to replicate. This is what occurs with HIV.
   b. When left untreated, HIV infection results in the destruction of T-cell immunity that allows recurrent, severe, and ultimately life-threatening opportunistic infections that manifest as AIDS. The progression from infection to AIDS occurs over years in adults, while in perinatally infected infants, AIDS usually presents before the first birthday.
   c. HIV infection is spread by the exchange of infected blood or by mucous membrane contact with infected blood and body fluids.
      i. In adults, intravenous drug use and sexual activity are the most common activities associated with infection.
      ii. In infants and small children, most parent-to-child transmissions of HIV infection occur either perinatally or through breastfeeding.
      iii. Since 1985, HIV-infected parents in high-resource countries have been encouraged to avoid breastfeeding.[14]
      iv. In resource-poor countries, the World Health Organization (WHO) recommends exclusive breastfeeding for 6 months and continued breastfeeding with complementary

food therafter, along with antiretroviral therapy (ART) for the mother and the baby. Breastfeeding should stop only when a nutritionally adequate and safe diet without breastmilk can be provided.[15]

d. Perinatal HIV infections have dropped dramatically in the United States and other developed countries due to routine HIV screening during pregnancy, the use of ART for the control and prevention of maternal infection, elective cesarean section in HIV-positive women, and avoidance of breastfeeding.

    i. From 1994 to 2010, interventions to prevent mother-to-child transmission accounted for approximately 22,000 prevented perinatal transmissions in the United States.[16]

    ii. Reductions in mother-to-child transmission have been accomplished in developing countries due to prevention practices. For example, in Tanzania, the rates of mother-to-child transmission dropped from 9 percent to 2.2 percent during implementation of Option B+, a WHO-recommended plan of care that uses lifelong ART for all pregnant and breastfeeding women, regardless of CD4 counts and clinical stage, and provides nevirapine or zidovudine to all HIV-exposed infants for 4 to 6 weeks, regardless of the feeding method.[17]

e. Much progress has been made in HIV detection, treatment, and parent-to-child transmission since the epidemic began in the middle 1980s. Protecting breastfeeding in underresourced countries and continued avoidance of breastfeeding in developed, high-resource countries is an important part of the fight against HIV/AIDS.

II. Chronic Illnesses

A. Asthma

    1. In the United States, the prevalence of asthma among pregnant women is 3.7 to 8.7 percent.[18]

    2. Exclusive breastfeeding offers protection for infants from families with a history of asthma.[19]

    3. Lactation should not be interrupted in asthmatic parents, and pharmacotherapy for asthma should continue.

        a. Corticosteroids administered through metered dose inhalers avoid systematic effects by delivering medication directly to the lungs.

        b. Bronchodilators (e.g., beta-agonists such as albuterol, terbutaline, and metaproterenol) are used to manage acute exacerbations.

B. Diabetes mellitus: Impaired carbohydrate metabolism is the hallmark of diabetes mellitus.

    1. Type 1 diabetes

        a. Prepregnancy diabetes can occur as Type 1, in which insulin is not produced by the beta cells of the pancreas.

        b. There are lower rates of breastfeeding among those with Type 1 diabetes.[20] Breastfeeding should be encouraged because colostrum helps to stabilize the newborn's blood glucose.[21]

        c. The parent and the infant can experience low glucose levels after birth and should be monitored closely.[22,23]

        d. Colostrum expressed prenatally can later be fed to the hypoglycemic infant of a diabetic parent.

           i. This practice is supported by evidence, and some protocols for neonatal hypoglycemia have been instituted.[24]

           ii. Recently a randomized clinical trial to examine the safety and efficacy of antenatal breast expression twice daily from 36 weeks' gestation to delivery was conducted in Victoria, Australia.[25] The outcomes indicated no differences in admission to the neonatal intensive care unit (main outcome) between experimental and control groups, and there was no difference in gestational age at birth. In addition, those in the experimental group were more likely to exclusively breastfeed in the hospital.

        e. If the infant is admitted to the neonatal intensive care unit for complications, milk expression should begin immediately.

        f. Insulin therapy is continued after giving birth. Insulin is safe during lactation due to the large size of the insulin molecule, which prevents it from crossing into the milk.[5]

g. Delayed lactogenesis (about 1 day) occurs in Type 1 diabetes.[26-28] Supportive practices, such as early and continued skin-to-skin contact, rooming in, and feeding on cue, can offset some of the factors known to delay lactogenesis.[29]

h. Diabetic parents may be at higher risk for mastitis and candidiasis, especially if they have elevated blood glucose levels.[30] (See Chapter 20, *Breast Pathology*.)

2. Type 2 diabetes

a. Prepregnancy diabetes can occur as Type 2, in which there is impaired response to insulin and beta cell dysfunction.

b. Type 2 diabetes can be part of the metabolic syndrome characterized by hypertension, obesity, dyslipidemia, and polycystic ovary syndrome (PCOS). It is much more common during pregnancy today due to higher obesity rates.[31]

c. Parents with Type 2 diabetes are less likely to breastfeed than their nondiabetic counterparts.[32]

d. Metformin is often used to treat Type 2 diabetes during and after pregnancy.[33]

e. Type 2 diabetes is associated with postpartum low milk production.[34]

f. Some research indicates that mothers with Type 2 diabetes have a shorter duration of breastfeeding than mothers with Type 1 diabetes.[35]

g. Support parents in the early postpartum period with evidence-based supportive practices similar to parents with Type 1 diabetes.

3. Gestational diabetes

a. Gestational diabetes is a glucose intolerance that occurs during pregnancy. It occurs in an estimated 9 percent of all pregnancies in the United States.[36]

b. Parents with gestational diabetes are less likely to breastfeed than their nondiabetic counterparts.[32] Breastfeeding should be encouraged because lactation improves the maternal metabolism of glucose and may prevent Type 2 diabetes.[37,38]

c. Delayed lactogenesis can occur in parents with gestational diabetes (up to one third in a recent study[39]).

d. Support is essential for parents with gestational diabetes, as noted with Type 1 and Type 2 diabetes.[29]

C. Thyroid disorders

1. Hypothyroidism

a. Optimal thyroid function is imperative to maintaining pregnancy.

b. Symptoms of hypothyroidism include thyroid swelling or nodules, cold intolerance, dry skin, thinning hair, poor appetite, extreme fatigue, and depression.

c. Untreated hypothyroidism can result in low milk production.

d. Parents who require thyroid supplementation can safely breastfeed.

e. Parents who are diagnosed postnatally will likely experience symptom relief and increased milk production.

f. Parents who took thyroid supplements during pregnancy should be reevaluated in the postpartum period because medication doses can likely be reduced to the prepregnancy level.[40]

2. Hyperthyroidism

a. Postpartum hyperthyroidism occurs in the first postpartum year in 9 percent of women.[41] Graves disease accounts for 95 percent of cases of hyperthyroidism during pregnancy[42] and only 0.2 percent of cases postnatally.[43]

b. Generally, lactation is not impacted by hyperthyroidism.

c. The treatment consists of antithyroid medications, such as methimazole or propylthiouracil, which are both considered safe during lactation. However, because of concerns that propylthiouracil is hepatotoxic, low to moderate methimazole doses are currently recommended as the first-line therapy.[43]

3. Postpartum thyroiditis

a. Postpartum thyroiditis is the most common thyroid disorder. It affects 1.1 to 16.7 percent of women in the first year after birth.[44]

b. It is believed to be an autoimmune disorder that affects those who had a normally functioning thyroid gland before pregnancy.

c. The symptoms include fatigue, depression, and anxiety.

      d.   Postpartum thyroiditis can manifest as hyperthyroidism or hypothyroidism, or it can begin as hyperthyroidism and progress to hypothyroidism.[42]

          i.   It is difficult to differentiate the hyperthyroid phase from Graves disease.

          ii.   Radioactive iodide uptake testing is required and requires temporary breastfeeding interruption.

          iii.   Due to their short half-lives, iodine 123 or technetium 99m scans may be used during lactation if milk is pumped and discarded for several days.[40]

      e.   The treatment is specific to the findings of thyroid function testing.

D.   Pituitary dysfunction

    1.   Postpartum hemorrhage and hypotension can cause the pituitary gland to cease production of gonadotropins, leading to panhypopituitarism or Sheehan syndrome.

    2.   The symptoms include lactation failure, loss of pubic and axillary hair, cold intolerance, breast and vaginal tissue atrophy, low blood pressure, secondary hypothyroidism, and adrenal failure.

    3.   In severe cases, the symptoms can occur and progress over years.

E.   Cystic fibrosis

    1.   Cystic fibrosis is a hereditary autosomal recessive genetic disorder involving the cystic fibrosis transmembrane regulator gene on chromosome 7.

    2.   Cystic fibrosis affects the apical membrane of epithelial cells lining the airways, biliary tree, intestines, vas deferens, female reproductive tract, sweat ducts, and pancreatic ducts.

    3.   The highest prevalence of cystic fibrosis is in North America, and the lowest is in Africa and Asia. About 70,000 people live with cystic fibrosis worldwide, with 30,000 in the United States.[45]

      a.   About half of people who have cystic fibrosis are older than age 18 years.

      b.   Since 1990, pregnancy rates have increased dramatically among women of childbearing age who have cystic fibrosis. In 2015, 235 women with cystic fibrosis were pregnant in the United States.[46]

    4.   Research indicates that affected individuals may or may not have increased morbidity during pregnancy and lactation. However, pregnant and lactating individuals with cystic fibrosis have increased needs for pulmonary and nutritional status monitoring and treatment (including those with diabetes).[47]

    5.   Many parents with cystic fibrosis choose to breastfeed their infants and should be supported accordingly.[48]

      a.   Human milk is not adversely affected by cystic fibrosis, although some research has indicated lower fat levels.

      b.   Additional lactation support is needed for maternal nutritional needs, pulmonary hygiene, attention to milk production (especially among those who are diabetic), infection control, and rest and sleep.

      c.   Medications that are commonly used to treat cystic fibrosis should be continued during lactation. For the most part, these medications are compatible with breastfeeding, although some medications are contraindicated (e.g., aminoglycosides, mycophenolate, and misoprostol).[49]

F.   Polycystic ovary syndrome (PCOS)

    1.   PCOS is a common endocrine disorder in women that is characterized by abnormal ovulation, clinical or laboratory indices of increased androgen levels, and polycystic ovaries.

    2.   The prevalence of the disorder is reported between 4 and 6 percent, but when the expanded Rotterdam criteria are used, the prevalence doubles.[50]

    3.   Infertility among women with PCOS is common. In women who become pregnant and give birth, lactation and breastfeeding can be challenging.[51-54]

    4.   Clinicians observe breast shape variations (tubular shape, large separation, and large nipples), little change in breast size during pregnancy, and insufficient milk production among women with PCOS.[51,52]

    5.   Insulin resistance and its compensatory hyperinsulinemia are hallmarks of PCOS, putting women with PCOS at increased risk of impaired glucose tolerance and Type 2 diabetes.

      a.   About 40 percent of women with PCOS develop impaired glucose tolerance, and 10 percent develop diabetes by age 40 years.[50]

      b.   Recent evidence speaks to the association of insulin resistance and glucose intolerance to delayed lactation and lactation insufficiency among people who are diabetic or obese.[28,34]

6. Metformin is the drug of choice for PCOS.
   a. If it is being used, it should be continued during breastfeeding.
   b. The impact of metformin on breastfeeding outcomes has not been sufficiently researched, although one trial found no difference in the duration of exclusive or partial breastfeeding in women who took metformin, compared to women who took a placebo.[55]
   c. Metformin is safe for breastfeeding infants.[5]
7. PCOS is a complex disorder with many characteristic variations. Support parents with PCOS through lactation calls and an individualized plan of care to support breastfeeding initiation, timely lactogenesis, and maintenance of milk production.

G. Autoimmune diseases
   1. Inflammatory bowel disease
      a. Two major forms of inflammatory bowel disease are ulcerative colitis and Crohn's disease. Inflammatory bowel disease most frequently presents in the childbearing years of both sexes.[56]
      b. Breastfeeding rates among individuals with inflammatory bowel disease are reported to be lower than in the general population. This is often related to concerns about the safety of prescribed medications and their transfer to the infant through the milk.[57]
         i. Research indicates that breastfeeding does not impact disease activity of either ulcerative colitis or Crohn's disease.[58,59] Breastfeeding should be encouraged.
         ii. The majority of medications used in the treatment of inflammatory bowel disease, including the biologics (e.g., anti-TNF antibodies), are considered probably compatible with breastfeeding, although methotrexate is considered teratogenic and should not be used during pregnancy or lactation.[57,60]
   2. Systemic lupus erythematous
      a. Systemic lupus erythematous is an autoimmune disorder that affects multiple body systems and occurs frequently during childbearing years.
      b. Lupus is manifested diversely and can include headache, arthritic symptoms (e.g., redness and swelling of joints), butterfly rash on the cheeks and nose, Raynaud phenomenon, fatigue, and myalgia.
      c. Miscarriage and prematurity rates are higher among women with lupus, but those who are well managed experience few flares during pregnancy. Postpartum flares can be exaggerated and call for close observation.[61]
      d. Researchers found that about half of the women in their sample of 51 pregnancies breastfed their infants. Low postpartum lupus activity, term delivery, and a plan to breastfeed early in pregnancy were significantly associated with breastfeeding in these lupus patients.[62] Breastfeeding should be encouraged.
      e. Research suggests that hydroxychloroquine, azathioprine, methotrexate, and prednisone have very limited transfer into milk and may be continued while breastfeeding.[62] However, some experts do not recommend methotrexate.[61]
      f. Considerations for a lactating parent with systemic lupus erythematous includes supportive measures for the following:
         i. Joint pain and swelling because it may impact holding the baby during feedings (e.g., positioning, pillows, laid-back breastfeeding, use of a baby sling).
         ii. Raynaud phenomenon (e.g., ensure warmth overall, apply warm compresses to the breast, avoid caffeine, and use calcium channel blockers).
   3. Multiple sclerosis
      a. Multiple sclerosis is a degenerative neurological disorder that is immune mediated; the myelin sheath covering the nerves is attacked by the immune system.
      b. There are four disease courses in multiple sclerosis[63]:
         i. Clinically isolated syndrome.
         ii. Relapsing remitting multiple sclerosis.
         iii. Secondary progressive multiple sclerosis.
         iv. Primary progressive multiple sclerosis.

    c.   The symptoms include weakness, fatigue, incoordination, paralysis, and speech and visual disturbances.

    d.   The disease is more common among women and is often diagnosed during the reproductive years (ages 20 to 40 years), thus impacting pregnancy and lactation.[64]

    e.   It is well known that the risk of relapse decreases during pregnancy, but it increases in the postpartum period—as much as 70 percent, particularly during the first 3 to 4 months—compared to before pregnancy.[64]

    f.   Although breastfeeding, and especially exclusive breastfeeding, were once thought to adversely impact disease activity, it now appears that breastfeeding reduces the risk of multiple sclerosis relapses.[65-67]

    g.   Evidence for safely using some immune-modulating therapies, also known as disease-modulating therapies, which are the mainstay of therapeutics for multiple sclerosis, during pregnancy and lactation is growing with time.

        i.   Recent evidence indicates that glatiramer acetate and interferon beta preparations are safe,[65,68] and expert opinion concurs.[69]

        ii.   For some time, interferon has been considered safe during lactation (lactation risk category L3) because of limited oral bioavailability and the large size of the molecule, meaning there is limited transfer into the milk.[5]

    h.   Individuals with multiple sclerosis should communicate closely with their healthcare providers regarding pregnancy planning and intention to breastfeed.

        i.   According to recent expert opinion, "a special challenge is the handling of women with highly active MS [multiple sclerosis], as pregnancy might not be powerful enough to suppress the risk of rebound relapses. Exclusive breastfeeding is an option for many women who want to do so, but in cases of high disease activity and those women who do not want to breastfeed, early reintroduction of MS therapies should be considered."[69(p1)]

        ii.   Lactation support, and general support for parents with multiple sclerosis, should be customized to the individual's symptomology and general health. Support should include household maintenance and childcare considerations.

    i.   Breastfeeding for 4 months or longer protects the infant against multiple sclerosis. This advantage should be discussed with parents who have multiple sclerosis and choose to breastfeed.[70] Furthermore, among women who have given birth, those with cumulative breastfeeding duration of greater than 15 months, compared to those with 0 to 4 months duration, have a reduced risk of subsequently developing multiple sclerosis.[71]

4.   Rheumatoid arthritis

    a.   Rheumatoid arthritis is a chronic inflammatory disease presumably caused by a genetically influenced autoimmune response that damages the synovial lining of the joints.

    b.   The symptoms and outcomes of the disease include pain, swelling, and stiffness of the joints; damage and deformity of the joints; fatigue; and decreased mobility. Rheumatoid arthritis can also impact the eyes, heart, lungs, or mouth; it increases morbidity and mortality from cardiovascular disease.[72]

    c.   The disease can start in early childhood and last the lifetime. It is characterized by flares and remissions in disease activity. Women are disproportionately affected by this disease, with new diagnoses of rheumatoid arthritis being two to three times higher than in men.[73]

    d.   Fertility, referenced as conceiving within 1 year, can be diminished in women with rheumatoid arthritis.[74]

        i.   For women who become pregnant, the disease activity is sometimes decreased during pregnancy, but not as much as indicated in earlier studies.[74,75]

        ii.   Like multiple sclerosis, rheumatoid arthritis flares are more common in the postpartum period, likely due to multiple hormonal and immunologic changes during pregnancy followed by the gradual return of these changes to prepregnancy values after delivery.[74]

    e.   Medication treatment for rheumatoid arthritis during lactation can differ from treatment during pregnancy.

        i.   Some antirheumatic drugs are not compatible with pregnancy or are limited in the length of time they can be used during pregnancy. For example, NSAIDs should be stopped before 32 weeks' gestation due to a risk of premature closure of ductus arteriosus in the fetus, and labor impairment in the mother. However, in general, NSAIDs are compatible with breastfeeding.[74,75]

    ii.   The nonflourinated glucocorticoids, sulfasalazine at low doses, hydroxychloroquine, and tumor necrosis factor inhibitors are compatible with pregnancy and breastfeeding.[74,75]

    iii.   Disease-modifying agents, such as methotrexate and leflunomide, are not recommended during pregnancy or lactation due to teratogen status.[74,75]

    iv.   Because of limited data on biologics such as tocilizumab, abatacept, rituximab, and anakinra, those drugs are not recommended in pregnancy or lactation.[74,75]

  f. Support for parents with rheumatoid arthritis who breastfeed should be tailored to individual needs and disease activity.

  g. Evidence-based interventions for rheumatoid arthritis are lacking.

    i.   A recent systematic review confirmed that there is a lack of evidence on pregnancy and lactation education and self-management interventions. However, it did address the major concerns of women with regard to medication safety for themselves and their children, as well as other informational needs.[76]

    ii.   Other research highlighted the complexity of decision making about childbearing in the first place and the physical and emotional issues of parenting, including breastfeeding, access to physical and emotional support services, and practical strategies for coping with daily challenges related to parenting.[76,77]

  h. Support to relieve fatigue in general, and physical bracing to support affected joints, especially in the hands and wrists, are evidence-based recommendations.

H. Other musculoskeletal and neurological injuries, disorders, and diseases

  1. Spinal cord injuries, muscular dystrophy, spinal muscular atrophy, cerebral palsy, amputation, and spina bifida can affect breastfeeding.

    a. These conditions may impact physical mobility and the ability of affected parents to hold their babies.

    b. In some cases, the injury or condition may impact the parent's ability to lactate and breastfeed (e.g., spinal cord injury above cervical vertebra 6 or at thoracic vertebrae 4 to 6).

    c. **BOX 17-1** provides baby care guidelines for breastfeeding parents who are physically disabled.

BOX 17-1 Baby Care Guidelines for Breastfeeding Parents Who Are Physically Disabled

- Parents who are confined to a wheelchair and have some upper-body strength can use a harness or a wide belt with a long strip of hook-and-loop tape to lift and retrieve a crawling baby from the floor.
- One or two special breastfeeding nests that are easily accessible and comfortable for the parent can be set up. Group together a crib or other sleeping place for the infant, diaper changing supplies, and a comfortable place to breastfeed.
- Demonstrate multiple positions for breastfeeding, and help find the best position for the parent's ability and comfort (e.g., laid-back breastfeeding or side lying).
- A small baby can be laid diagonally across the parent's knees on a pillow to breastfeed. Put other pillows under the parent's arms for support. Experiment with breastfeeding pillows to determine what works best. Elevate the parent's feet on a footrest to keep the infant secure during feeding.
- Parents who cannot elevate their feet can rest their forearm that is holding the infant on a pillow placed across their knees. This arrangement ensures that if the infant rolls, the motion will be toward the parent.
- Changing tables and cribs can be adapted so they are accessible to a parent in a wheelchair, and the room can be arranged so that moving about is minimized. A low-sided pram or baby stroller makes it easier to slide the baby onto the parent's lap without much lifting.
- A baby sling allows the parent's arms to be free and ensures that the baby is safe and supported during breastfeeding. This is also helpful when the parent has unilateral weakness or paralysis (such as from a stroke).
- A bell tied to the baby's shoes keeps track of where the mobile child is.
- When a parent is in a wheelchair, a toddler will quickly learn to climb on the parent's knee for a ride and to sit still while the chair is moving.

(continues)

BOX 17-1 Baby Care Guidelines for Breastfeeding Parents Who Are Physically Disabled *(continued)*

- The baby can be given extra cuddling, such as touching at night in bed, if there are barriers to physical contact during the day.
- A baby clothed in overalls with crossed straps can be picked up fairly easily.
- A breastfeeding bra that opens in the front and has an easy-to-fasten clip or hook-and-loop fastener that can be manipulated with one hand will facilitate breastfeeding. The usual clip for opening and closing the bra flap can be replaced with a hook-and-loop fastener. Some all-elastic bras can easily be pulled down to allow the baby to breastfeed.
- Maternity clothes can be altered to incorporate hook-and-loop openings or large-ring zippers. Antique buttonhooks are helpful to manipulate the small buttons found on many garments.
- The parent should plan rest periods during the day and should sit to work whenever possible.
- The parent can sleep with the infant or have the partner or someone else bring the baby for breastfeeding during the night.
- An intercom system or baby monitor that picks up the sound of a crying baby is helpful. If the parent is deaf, the sound can be transformed into flashing light signals.
- If it is not possible for the parent to lift the baby or themselves, consider caring for the baby on the floor, including feeding, changing, and playing. This enables the parent to roll the baby to the lap, instead of lifting, when attention is needed. A beanbag or breastfeeding pillow will support the dyad.

Modified from Morrison B, Wambach K. Women's health and breastfeeding. In: Wambach K, Riordan J, eds. *Breastfeeding and Human Lactation*. 5th ed. Burlington, MA: Jones & Bartlett Learning; 2016:553-634.[6]

---

2. Childbearing among women with disabilities appears to have increased over time.[78-80]
   a. According to a U.S. family planning survey, these women have childbearing attitudes similar to those of nondisabled women, but they have lower intentions to have a child.[81]
   b. Women with disabilities have reported that their healthcare providers were ill equipped to deal with their pregnancy and possessed negative stereotypes regarding sexuality in disabled women.[80]
   c. There is evidence that women with disabilities have many unmet needs during pregnancy and after birth. Relative to the postpartum period, these parents require breastfeeding support and accessible baby equipment, such as bassinets, cribs, changing tables, baby bath equipment, and carriers.[80]
3. Case studies provide evidence regarding breastfeeding in parents who have spinal cord injuries.
   a. Three women with injuries at the level of T4 to T6 vertebrae, which impact the milk ejection reflex, were able to successfully breastfeed with intervention (mental imagery, oxytocin spray) and to induce the milk ejection reflex for 12 to 54 weeks.[82]
   b. Another case study reported on unilateral hypogalactia experienced by a woman with C4-level quadriplegia.[83] Despite intervention to increase volume, she eventually ceased breastfeeding. It was unfortunate that lactation support for continued breastfeeding on the unaffected side was not continued.
   c. These cases demonstrate the need for lactation care for parents with spinal cord injuries and a need for additional research on these parents' breastfeeding experiences.
4. Epilepsy is the most common neurological disorder. Evidence about pregnancy and lactation among individuals with epilepsy often focuses on the safety of epilepsy medications[84,85] and preventing harm to the infant.
   a. Many epilepsy medications are safe during lactation, including carbamazepine, phenobarbital, phenytoin, primidone, and valproate. Moderately safe drugs include gabapentin, lamotrigine, levetiracetam, oxcarbazepine, pregabalin, tiagabine, topiramate, and vigabatrin.[84]
   b. With all anticonvulsants, regardless of safety category, parents should be educated on observing their infants for drowsiness, rash, breathing difficulties, feeding difficulties, weight gain, and developmental milestone achievement.[84]
   c. Due to relative infant doses greater than 10 percent, long half-life, or serious side effects observed in infants, the following anticonvulsants are contraindicated during lactation: clonazepam, diazepam, ethosuximide, and zonisamide.[84]

        d.   A recent systematic review and network meta-analysis offered evidence on outcomes of children exposed to antiepileptic drugs during pregnancy and breastfeeding.[85]

            i.   The results for cognitive developmental delay suggested that among all antiepileptic drugs, only valproate was statistically significantly associated with more children experiencing cognitive developmental delay, compared to control (nonuse of antiepileptic drugs during pregnancy and lactation).

           ii.   The results for autism suggested that oxcarbazepine, valproate, lamotrigine, and lamotrigine plus valproate were associated with significantly greater odds of developing autism, compared to control.

          iii.   The results for psychomotor developmental delay indicated that valproate, and carbamazepine plus phenobarbital and valproate, were associated with significantly greater odds of psychomotor delay, compared to control.

          iv.   These results offer evidence on longer-term outcomes for infants exposed to antiepileptic drugs during pregnancy and breastfeeding.

        e.   The other obvious issue for parents with epilepsy is the possibility of seizure during breastfeeding.

            i.   These parents may wish to breastfeed their infants in a safe location, such as a padded chair or bed. Safety precautions should be reviewed, even with parents who have not had a seizure for some time because it is possible that seizures may return or their frequency may increase due to stress, sleep deprivation, and exhaustion in the puerperium.[86]

           ii.   **BOX 17-2** outlines safety guidelines for a breastfeeding parent with epilepsy.

  I.   Vision and hearing impairment adds challenges for breastfeeding.

     1.   Blind parents may face stigma associated with their disability, especially as related to parenthood and the capacity to parent, including nurturing their infant with their own milk.[87]

     2.   These parents often have the same desires to breastfeed and deserve the same support as any other parent. Prenatal, in-hospital postpartum lactation support and postdischarge follow-up should include the following:

        a.   Prenatal education on breastfeeding benefits and anticipatory guidance in basic breastfeeding management and support needs, including the partner and family.

        b.   Seeking a pediatrician who will actively support the family in breastfeeding planning.

        c.   Prenatal breast exam to assess the breasts and nipples, as is standard for any pregnant individual.

        d.   Postpartum hospital support including the following:

            i.   Holding the newborn skin to skin immediately after birth, with continued skin-to-skin contact throughout the hospital stay so the parent can learn the infant's feeding cues.

           ii.   All other standard breastfeeding education and support, with emphasis on observation of feedings; oral instruction, support, and encouragement; and family instruction and guidance.

        e.   Postdischarge support and follow-up including the following:

            i.   Standard well-baby pediatric and breastfed infant guidelines.

           ii.   Lactation resources for postdischarge needs, including referral to other blind or partially sighted parents in the community.

        f.   Refer parents to La Leche League or other community support group for parent-to-parent support and to the National Federation of the Blind for braille and audiotape or MP3 educational resources.

BOX 17-2 Guidelines for a Breastfeeding Parent with Epilepsy

- On each level of the house, make sure there is a playpen in which to quickly place the baby when a seizure seems imminent.
- Use pillows and cushions to pad the arms of the rocker or chair where the parent usually breastfeeds.
- Place guardrails padded with pillows around the bed if the infant is taken to bed to breastfeed.
- On the baby, the stroller, and the baby carrier attach tags stating that the parent has a seizure disorder, along with other pertinent information, when away from home.

Modified from Morrison B, Wambach K. Women's health and breastfeeding. In: Wambach K, Riordan J, eds. *Breastfeeding and Human Lactation*. 5th ed. Burlington, MA: Jones & Bartlett Learning; 2016:553-634.[6]

3. Parents with hearing loss or deafness
    a. According to United States National Health and Nutrition Examination Survey, about 14.1 percent of the population in the United States is hearing impaired or deaf.[88]
    b. Childbearing individuals with hearing impairment or deafness may need breastfeeding assistance provided by an interpreter who uses sign language, a requirement in healthcare facilities in the United States under Title XI of the Civil Rights Act and the Americans with Disabilities Act.
    c. Evidence suggests that parents who are deaf desire to breastfeed their infants, are successful, and persist through difficulties.[89] Women learn about breastfeeding and gain support through their healthcare and lactation support providers and their social network.[89]
    d. Support and education for deaf parents come in many forms (e.g., videos, graphics, computer applications, written materials, and websites). They use technology such as vibration pagers, baby monitors, and telecommunications devices for the deaf (TDD) (e.g., teletypewriters [TTY] and visual displays [TDY]).

J. Accommodations may be needed for dermatological disorders.
    1. Chronic or acute dermatitis may affect any area of the body, including the breasts and nipples. It is generally caused by contact with an allergen, a virus, or a bacterium.[90]
    2. Eczema of the nipple is the most common atopic dermatitis of the breast. It presents with redness, crusting, oozing, scales, fissures, blisters, excoriations (slits), or lichenification, and it causes itching and burning.[90]
        a. The categories of dermatological disorders include the following[89]:
            i. Endogenous atopic dermatitis (predisposed to develop eczema).
            ii. Irritant contact dermatitis (direct chemical damage from detergents, soaps, bleach).
            iii. Allergic contact dermatitis (delayed hypersensitivity reaction to an allergen in a topical agent applied to the nipples, such as lanolin, topical antibiotics, chamomile, vitamin E, and fragrances); may be caused by food allergens present in residue in the baby's mouth.
        b. Management centers on cleansing (no soap), air drying after feeding, and treatment with a low- or medium-strength cortisone ointment twice per day for 2 weeks.[90]
            i. Category V or VI potency topical corticosteroid ointments are recommended.
            ii. Category I potency topical corticosteroids should be avoided.
    3. Psoriasis is a chronic immune disease identified by well-demarcated pink plaque that often appears moist and has minimal or no scale.
    4. Inframammary psoriasis may be indistinguishable clinically from seborrheic dermatitis, intertrigo (rash between folds of skin), and *Candida* infection.[90]
    5. The use of topical steroids to treat psoriasis follows the same guidelines as for eczematous processes.
        a. Calcipotriene, a topical vitamin D derivative, is considered safe to use on the nipple. Calcipotriene can be used during lactation as long as the daily body surface area coverage is less than 20 percent.[91]
        b. Systemic therapies for psoriasis include phototherapy with ultraviolet B and is considered the safest option.[91]
        c. Biologic agents, such as etanercept, adalimumab, infliximab, alefacept, and ustekinumab, are believed to be moderately safe; however, the data are very limited.[5]
    6. Bacterial infection is often caused by *S. aureus*.
        a. Parents complain of deep, dull aching breast pain during or after feedings, or both; breast tenderness, especially with deep touch; bilateral pain; and, at times, a burning quality to the pain.
        b. Parents may have failed treatment for yeast infection. Treatment is with oral antibiotics, including cephalexin, amoxicillin, or dicloxacillin for at least 2 weeks.[91]
    7. Viral infection with herpes simplex virus is fairly common and generally presents as miniature vesicles on an erythematous base.
        a. Open vesicles carry the virus, and the virus can then be transmitted to the breastfeeding infant.
        b. It is critical to rule out herpes simplex virus in infants younger than 3 months because they can develop a life-threatening infection involving the central nervous system.
            i. Herpes simplex virus should be confirmed or ruled out with a viral culture, serology, direct immunofluorescence assay, polymerase chain reaction, or Tzanck test.

ii. Parents with herpes simplex virus infection should be prescribed oral acyclovir 800 mg three times a day for 5 to 7 days.

iii. A parent should pump the breasts, instead of breastfeed, when active lesions are present.[91]

8. Raynaud phenomenon of the nipple is a vasospasm of the arterioles causing intermittent ischemia.

   a. Individuals who have experienced nipple pain for more than 4 weeks and had multiple failed rounds of antifungal or antibiotic treatment are suspected to have Raynaud phenomenon.[92]

   b. To accurately diagnose Raynaud phenomenon, sensitivity to cold, manifested as classic triphasic color change in the nipples (white, blue, and red), or biphasic color change (white and blue) should be present.[92,93]

   c. The treatment involves avoiding exposure to cold temperature, using techniques to keep the breasts and nipples warm, avoiding vasoconstrictive drugs that may precipitate symptoms, and administering nifedipine 30–60 mg/day for 2 weeks.[92]

K. Cancer and breastfeeding

1. Cancers occur in 0.05 to 0.1 percent of all pregnancies; breast, cervical, ovarian, and thyroid are the most frequently diagnosed cancers during pregnancy.[94] Pregnancy-associated breast cancer is defined as breast cancer occurring any time during gestation, during lactation, or within 1 year after delivery.[95]

2. The treatment of any cancer during lactation depends on the site, stage, and type.

3. Generally, chemotherapy and lactation are not compatible because all agents pass into the milk, albeit in low levels, and are potentially toxic to the infant.

4. Surgical treatment of cancer during lactation is possible, depending on the site, stage, and need for adjuvant therapy following surgery. Radiation of the breast may cause damage to the alveoli of the breast, although lactation with reduced volume following radiation is possible. There is no impact on the other breast.[96]

III. Assistance during Illnesses

A. Parents will need assistance when an illness leads to hospitalization or surgery. When the lactating parent needs surgery or hospitalization for another reason, it is stressful to the parent, the breastfeeding child, and the entire family.

B. Lactating parents who undergo elective surgery should plan ahead and seek lactation support at the facility. Concerns will likely center around anesthesia, postoperative analgesia, access to and handling the baby for feeding, and expressing milk. See **BOX 17-3** for guidelines to care for a breastfeeding parent who needs surgery or is hospitalized for another reason.

BOX 17-3 Guidelines to Care for Breastfeeding Parent Undergoing Surgery or Hospitalization

- Encourage the parent to plan for help at home after surgery to allow recuperation time.
- Use an outpatient surgical facility rather than an inpatient facility.
- Arrange for breastfeeding the baby immediately before the surgery.
- Assist the parent in breastfeeding as soon as awake from anesthesia.
- Make rooming in arrangements for the breastfeeding child if the parent is at an inpatient facility. Most hospitals require that another adult be present to care for the baby.
- Express and freeze a supply of milk before surgery, if needed.
- Before surgery, help the parent condition the baby to cup feedings if temporary supplementary feedings will be necessary.
- Encourage the parent to take postoperative analgesia to alleviate pain. The infant will receive only a small dose through the milk.
- If abdominal surgery is performed, show the parent how to splint the surgical area with pillows. Cover the incision area with dressings.

Modified from Morrison B, Wambach K. Women's health and breastfeeding. In: Wambach K, Riordan J, eds. *Breastfeeding and Human Lactation*. 5th ed. Burlington, MA: Jones & Bartlett Learning; 2016:553-634.[6]

    C.   Emergency surgery or hospitalization calls for more vigilant support from the family and healthcare providers to protect milk production and the breastfeeding child. Refer to Box 17-3 for guidelines that will apply in this situation.

    D.   In a critically ill parent, especially one who becomes ill during pregnancy, enhanced support from lactation specialists and the healthcare team is paramount.[97]

        1.   Evidence reveals that the needs of critically ill parents are similar to new parents in general, yet their needs are unique and traumatizing given their specific situations.

        2.   The shock of being in critical care, being a parent in critical care (e.g., loss of the birth experience, separation from the infant, and establishment of breastfeeding), being transferred out of critical care, and being discharged home require exquisite support and patience.

▶ Key Points from This Chapter

    A.   In the majority of acute and chronic diseases and illnesses, breastfeeding is not contraindicated.

    B.   The major concerns for the healthcare provider, and often the parent, are whether treatment for the condition is compatible with breastfeeding.

    C.   Individualized lactation support is key to supporting the parents and breastfeeding child.

References

1. MacGregor EA. Migraine in pregnancy and lactation. *Neurol Sci.* 2014;35(1):61-64.
2. Tepper D. Pregnancy and lactation—migraine management. Headache. *J Head Face Pain.* 2015;55(4):607-608.
3. Wells RE, Turner DP, Lee M, Bishop L, Strauss L. Managing migraine during pregnancy and lactation. *Curr Neurol Neurosci Rep.* 2016;16(4):40.
4. Thorley V. Lactational headache: a lactation consultant's diary. *J Hum Lactation.* 1997;13(1):51-53.
5. Hale TW, Rowe HE. *Medications and Mother's Milk 2014.* Plano, TX: Hale Publishing; 2014.
6. Morrison B, Wambach, K. Women's health and breastfeeding. In: Wambach K, Riordan J, eds. *Breastfeeding and Human Lactation.* 5th ed. Burlington, MA: Jones & Bartlett Learning; 2016:553-634.
7. Montalto M, Lui B. MRSA as a cause of postpartum breast abscess in infant and mother. *J Hum Lactation.* 2009;25(4):448-450.
8. Le Doare K, Kampmann B. Breast milk and group b streptococcal infection: vector of transmission or vehicle for protection? *Vaccine.* 2014;32(26):3128-3132.
9. Singh N, Golani A, Patel Z, Maitra A. Transfer of isoniazid from circulation to breast milk in lactating women on chronic therapy for tuberculosis. *Br J Clin Pharmacol.* 2008;65(3):418-422.
10. Cavalcanti MG, Cabral-Castro MJ, Gonçalves JLS, Santana LS, Pimenta ES, Peralta JM. Zika virus shedding in human milk during lactation: an unlikely source of infection? *Int J Infect Dis.* 2017;57:70-72.
11. Colt S, Garcia-Casal MN, Peña-Rosas JP, et al. Transmission of Zika virus through breast milk and other breastfeeding-related bodily-fluids: a systematic review. *PLOS Negl Trop Dis.* 2017;11(4):e0005528. https://doi.org/10.1371/journal.pntd.0005528.
12. Centers for Disease Control and Prevention. Ebola (Ebola virus disease). https://www.cdc.gov/vhf/ebola/index.html. Updated October 18, 2017. Accessed November 3, 2017.
13. Centers for Disease Control and Prevention. Recommendations for breastfeeding/infant feeding in the context of Ebola virus disease. https://www.cdc.gov/vhf/ebola/hcp/recommendations-breastfeeding-infant-feeding-ebola.html. Updated June 10, 2016. Accessed May 25, 2017.
14. Centers for Disease Control and Prevention. Recommendations for assisting in the prevention of perinatal transmission of human T-lymphotropic virus type III/lymphadenopathy-associated virus and acquired immunodeficiency syndrome. *Morbidity Mortality Weekly Rep.* 1985;34(48):721-732.
15. World Health Organization. *Consolidated Guidelines on the Use of Antiretroviral Drugs for Treating and Preventing HIV Infection.* Geneva, Switzerland: World Health Orgnization; 2016.
16. Little KM, Taylor AW, Borkowf CB, et al. Perinatal antiretroviral exposure and prevented mother-to-child HIV infections in the era of antiretroviral prophylaxis in the United States, 1994–2010. *Pediatr Infect Dis J.* 2017;36(1):66-71.
17. Gamell A, Luwanda LB, Kalinjuma AV, et al. Prevention of mother-to-child transmission of HIV Option B+ cascade in rural Tanzania: the one stop clinic model. *PLOS One.* 2017;12(7):e0181096. doi:10.1371/journal.pone.0181096.
18. Mihălțan FD, Antoniu SA, Ulmeanu R. Asthma and pregnancy: therapeutic challenges. *Arch Gynecol Obstet.* 2014;290(4):621-627.
19. Dogaru CM, Nyffenegger D, Pescatore AM, Spycher BD, Kuehni CE. Breastfeeding and childhood asthma: systematic review and meta-analysis. *Am J Epidemiol.* 2014;179(10):1153-1167.
20. Cordero L, Thung S, Landon MB, Nankervis CA. Breast-feeding initiation in women with pregestational diabetes mellitus. *Clin Pediatr.* 2014;53(1):18-25.

21. Cordero L, Ramesh S, Hillier K, Giannone PJ, Nankervis CA. Early feeding and neonatal hypoglycemia in infants of diabetic mothers. *SAGE Open Med.* 2013;1:2050312113516613.

22. Feldman AZ, Brown FM. Management of type 1 diabetes in pregnancy. *Curr Diab Rep.* 2016;16:76.

23. Yu L, Cheng M, Yang F, et al. Quantitative assessment of the effect of pre-gestational diabetes and risk of adverse maternal, perinatal and neonatal outcomes. *Oncotarget.* 2017;8(19): 61048-61056.

24. Tozier PK. Colostrum versus formula supplementation for glucose stabilization in newborns of diabetic mothers. *J Obstet Gynecol Neonatal Nurs.* 2013;42(6):619-628.

25. Forster DA, Moorhead AM, Jacobs SE, et al. Advising women with diabetes in pregnancy to express breastmilk in late pregnancy (Diabetes and Antenatal Milk Expressing [DAME]): a multicentre, unblinded, randomised controlled trial. *Lancet.* 2017;389(10085):2204-2213.

26. De Bortoli J, Amir LH. Is onset of lactation delayed in women with diabetes in pregnancy? A systematic review. *Diabetic Med.* 2016;33(1):17-24.

27. Hartmann P, Cregan M. Lactogenesis and the effects of insulin-dependent diabetes mellitus and prematurity. *J Nutr.* 2001;131(11):3016S-3020S.

28. Nommsen-Rivers LA, Chantry CJ, Peerson JM, Cohen RJ, Dewey KG. Delayed onset of lactogenesis among first-time mothers is related to maternal obesity and factors associated with ineffective breastfeeding. *Am J Clin Nutr.* 2010;92(3):574-584.

29. Fallon A, Dunne F. Breastfeeding practices that support women with diabetes to breastfeed. *Diabetes Res Clin Pract.* 2015;110(1):10-17.

30. Soltani H, Dickinson FM, Kalk J, Payne K. Breast feeding practices and views among diabetic women: a retrospective cohort study. *Midwifery.* 2008;24(4):471-479.

31. Ashwal E, Hod M. Gestational diabetes mellitus: where are we now? *Clinica Chimica Acta.* 2015;451(pt A):14-20.

32. Finkelstein SA, Keely E, Feig DS, Tu X, Yasseen AS 3rd, Walker M. Breastfeeding in women with diabetes: lower rates despite greater rewards: a population-based study. *Diabetic Med.* 2013;30(9):1094-1101.

33. Simmons D. Metformin treatment for type 2 diabetes in pregnancy? *Best Pract Res Clin Endocrinol Metab.* 2010;24(4):625-634.

34. Riddle SW, Nommsen-Rivers LA. A case control study of diabetes during pregnancy and low milk supply. *Breastfeeding Med.* 2016;11(2):80-85.

35. Herskin CW, Stage E, Barfred C, et al. Low prevalence of long-term breastfeeding among women with type 2 diabetes. *J Maternal Fetal Neonatal Med.* 2016;29(15):2513-2518.

36. DeSisto CL, Kim SY, Sharma AJ. Prevalence estimates of gestational diabetes mellitus in the United States, Pregnancy Risk Assessment Monitoring System (PRAMS), 2007–2010. *Prev Chronic Dis.* 2014;11:E104.

37. Gunderson EP, Hurston SR, Ning X, et al. Lactation and progression to type 2 diabetes mellitus after gestational diabetes mellitus: a prospective cohort study. *Ann Intern Med.* 2015;163(12):889-898.

38. Much D, Beyerlein A, Roßbauer M, Hummel S, Ziegler AG. Beneficial effects of breastfeeding in women with gestational diabetes mellitus. *Mol Metab.* 2014;3(3):284-292.

39. Matias SL, Dewey KG, Quesenberry CP Jr, Gunderson EP. Maternal prepregnancy obesity and insulin treatment during pregnancy are independently associated with delayed lactogenesis in women with recent gestational diabetes mellitus. *Am J Clin Nutr.* 2014;99(1):115-121.

40. Alexander EK, Pearce EN, Brent GA, et al. 2017 guidelines of the American Thyroid Association for the diagnosis and management of thyroid disease during pregnancy and the postpartum. *Thyroid.* 2017;27(3):315-389.

41. Goldstein AL. New-onset Graves' disease in the postpartum period. *J Midwifery Womens Health.* 2013;58(2):211-214.

42. Carney LA, Quinlan JD, West JM. Thyroid disease in pregnancy. *Am Fam Phys.* 2014;89(4):273-278.

43. Sarkar S, Bischoff LA. Management of hyperthyroidism during the preconception phase, pregnancy, and the postpartum period. *Semin Reprod Med.* 2016;34(06):317-322.

44. Yalamanchi S, Cooper DS. Thyroid disorders in pregnancy. *Curr Opinion Obstet Gynecol.* 2015;27(6):406-415.

45. Antunovic SS, Lukac M, Vujovic D. Longitudinal cystic fibrosis care. *Clin Pharmacol Ther.* 2013;93(1):86-97.

46. Cystic Fibrosis Foundation Patient Registry. Annual Data Reort 2015. Bethesda, MD. https://www.cff.org/Our-Research/CF-Patient-Registry /2015-Patient-Registry-Annual-Data-Report.pdf . Accessed June 30, 2017.

47. Schechter MS, Quittner AL, Konstan MW, et al. Long-term effects of pregnancy and motherhood on disease outcomes of women with cystic fibrosis. *Ann Am Thorac Soc.* 2013;10(3):213-219.

48. Edenborough FP, Borgo G, Knoop C, et al. Guidelines for the management of pregnancy in women with cystic fibrosis. *J Cystic Fibrosis.* 2008;7:S2-S32.

49. Panchaud A, Di Paolo ER, Koutsokera A, et al. Safety of drugs during pregnancy and breastfeeding in cystic fibrosis patients. *Respiration.* 2016;91(4):333-348.

50. Dumesic DA, Oberfield SE, Stener-Victorin E, Marshall JC, Laven JS, Legro RS. Scientific statement on the diagnostic criteria, epidemiology, pathophysiology, and molecular genetics of polycystic ovary syndrome. *Endoc Rev.* 2015;36(5):487-525.

51. Marasco L, Marmet C, Shell E. Polycystic ovary syndrome: a connection to insufficient milk supply? *J Hum Lactation.* 2000;16(2):143-148.

52. Joham AE, Nanayakkara N, Ranasinha S, et al. Obesity, polycystic ovary syndrome and breastfeeding: an observational study. *Acta Obstet Gynecol Scand.* 2016;95(4):458-466.

53. Teede H, Deeks A, Moran L. Polycystic ovary syndrome: a complex condition with psychological, reproductive and metabolic manifestations that impacts on health across the lifespan. *BMC Med.* 2010;8:41.

54. Vanky E, Isaksen H, Moen MH, Carlsen SM. Breastfeeding in polycystic ovary syndrome. *Acta Obstet Gynecol Scand.* 2008;87(5):531-535.

55. Vanky E, Nordskar JJ, Leithe H, Hjorth-Hansen AK, Martinussen M, Carlsen SM. Breast size increment during pregnancy and breastfeeding in mothers with polycystic ovary syndrome: a follow-up study of a randomised controlled trial on metformin versus placebo. *BJOG: Int J Obstet Gynaecol.* 2012;119(11):1403-1409.

56. Molodecky NA, Soon IS, Rabi DM, et al. Increasing incidence and prevalence of the inflammatory bowel diseases with time, based on systematic review. *Gastroenterology.* 2012;142(1):46-54.e42.

57. Schulze H, Esters P, Dignass A. Review article: the management of Crohn's disease and ulcerative colitis during pregnancy and lactation. *Aliment Pharmacol Ther*. 2014;40(9):991-1008.

58. Kane S, Lemieux N. The role of breastfeeding in postpartum disease activity in women with inflammatory bowel disease. *Am J Gastroenterol*. 2005;100(1):102-105.

59. Julsgaard M, Nørgaard M, Hvas CL, Grosen A, Hasseriis S, Christensen LA. Self-reported adherence to medical treatment, breastfeeding behaviour, and disease activity during the postpartum period in women with Crohn's disease. *Scand J Gastroenterol*. 2014;49(8):958-966.

60. Horst S, Kane S. The use of biologic agents in pregnancy and breastfeeding. *Gastroenterol Clin North Am*. 2014;43(3):495-508.

61. Marder W, Littlejohn EA, Somers EC. Pregnancy and autoimmune connective tissue diseases. *Best Pract Res Clin Rheumatol*. 2016;30(1):63-80.

62. Noviani M, Wasserman S, Clowse MEB. Breastfeeding in mothers with systemic lupus erythematosus. *Lupus*. 2016;25(9):973-979.

63. Lublin FD, Reingold SC, Cohen JA, et al. Defining the clinical course of multiple sclerosis: the 2013 revisions. *Neurology*. 2014;83(3):278-286.

64. Langer-Gould A, Beaber BE. Effects of pregnancy and breastfeeding on the multiple sclerosis disease course. *Clin Immunol*. 2013;149(2):244-250.

65. Hellwig K, Haghikia A, Rockhoff M, Gold R. Multiple sclerosis and pregnancy: experience from a nationwide database in Germany. *Ther Adv Neurol Disord*. 2012;5(5):247-253.

66. Hellwig K, Rockhoff M, Herbstritt S, et al. Exclusive breastfeeding and the effect on postpartum multiple sclerosis relapses. *JAMA Neurol*. 2015;72(10):1132-1138.

67. Langer-Gould A, Huang SM, Gupta R, et al. Exclusive breastfeeding and the risk of postpartum relapses in women with multiple sclerosis. *Arch Neurol*. 2009;66(8):958-963.

68. Herbstritt S, Langer-Gould A, Rockhoff M, et al. Glatiramer acetate during early pregnancy: a prospective cohort study. *Multiple Sclerosis J*. 2016;22(6):810-816.

69. Thöne J, Thiel S, Gold R, Hellwig K. Treatment of multiple sclerosis during pregnancy—safety considerations. *Expert Opin Drug Saf*. 2017;16(5):523-534.

70. Conradi S, Malzahn U, Paul F, et al. Breastfeeding is associated with lower risk for multiple sclerosis. *Multiple Sclerosis J*. 2012;19(5):553-558.

71. Langer-Gould A, Smith JB, Hellwig K, et al. Breastfeeding, ovulatory years, and risk of multiple sclerosis. *Neurology*. 2017;89(6):563-569.

72. Hollan I, Dessein PH, Ronda N, et al. Prevention of cardiovascular disease in rheumatoid arthritis. *Autoimmunity Rev*. 2015;14(10):952-969.

73. Centers for Disease Control and Prevention. Rheumatoid arthritis. https://www.cdc.gov/arthritis/basics/rheumatoid-arthritis.html. Accessed July 31, 2017.

74. de Jong PHP, Dolhain RJEM. Fertility, pregnancy, and lactation in rheumatoid arthritis. *Rheum Dis Clin North Am*. 2017;43(2):227-237.

75. Krause ML, Makol A. Management of rheumatoid arthritis during pregnancy: challenges and solutions. *Open Access Rheumatol Res Rev*. 2016;8:23-36.

76. Ackerman IN, Jordan JE, Van Doornum S, Ricardo M, Briggs AM. Understanding the information needs of women with rheumatoid arthritis concerning pregnancy, post-natal care and early parenting: a mixed-methods study. *BMC Musculoskeletal Disord*. 2015;16:194.

77. Meade T, Sharpe L, Hallab L, Aspanell D, Manolios N. Navigating motherhood choices in the context of rheumatoid arthritis: women's stories. *Musculoskeletal Care*. 2013;11(2):73-82.

78. Horner-Johnson W, Darney BG, Kulkarni-Rajasekhara S, Quigley B, Caughey AB. Pregnancy among U.S. women: differences by presence, type, and complexity of disability. *Am J Obstet Gynecol*. 2016;214(4):529.e1-529.e9.

79. Iezzoni LI, Chen Y, McLain ABJ. Current pregnancy among women with spinal cord injury: findings from the U.S. national spinal cord injury database. *Spinal Cord*. 2015;53(11):821-826.

80. Mitra M, Long-Bellil LM, Iezzoni LI, Smeltzer SC, Smith LD. Pregnancy among women with physical disabilities: unmet needs and recommendations on navigating pregnancy. *Disability Health J*. 2016;9(3):457-463.

81. Bloom TL, Mosher W, Alhusen J, Lantos H, Hughes RB. Fertility desires and intentions among U.S. women by disability status: findings from the 2011–2013 national survey of family growth. *Maternal Child Health J*. 2017;21(8):1606-1615.

82. Cowley KC. Psychogenic and pharmacologic induction of the let-down reflex can facilitate breastfeeding by tetraplegic women: a report of 3 cases. *Arch Phys Med Rehabil*. 2005;86(6):1261-1264.

83. Liu N, Krassioukov AV. Postpartum hypogalactica in a women with Brown–Séquard-plus syndrome: A case report. *Spinal Cord*. 2013;51:794-796.

84. Davanzo R, Dal Bo S, Bua J, Copertino M, Zanelli E, Matarazzo L. Antiepileptic drugs and breastfeeding. *Italian J Pediatr*. 2013;39:50.

85. Veroniki AA, Rios P, Cogo E, et al. Comparative safety of antiepileptic drugs for neurological development in children exposed during pregnancy and breast feeding: a systematic review and network meta-analysis. *BMJ Open*. 2017;7(7):e017248. doi:10.1136/bmjopen-2017-017248.

86. Crawford P. Best practice guidelines for the management of women with epilepsy. *Epilepsia*. 2005;46:117-124.

87. Frederick A. Between stigma and mother-blame: blind mothers' experiences in USA hospital postnatal care. *Sociol Health Illness*. 2015;37(8):1127-1141.

88. Hoffman HJ, Dobie, RA, Losonczy KJ, Themann CL, Flamme GA. Declining Prevalence of Hearing Loss in US Adults Aged 20 to 69 Years. *JAMA Otolaryngol Head Neck Surg*. 2017;143(3):274–285. doi:10.1001/jamaoto.2016.3527

89. Chin NP, Cuculick J, Starr M, Panko T, Widanka H, Dozier A. Deaf mothers and breastfeeding. *J Hum Lactation*. 2013;29(4):564-571.

90. Whitaker-Worth DL, Carlone V, Susser WS, Phelan N, Grant-Kels JM. Dermatologic diseases of the breast and nipple. *J Am Acad Dermatol*. 2000;43(5):733-754.

91. Barrett ME, Heller MM, Fullerton Stone H, Murase JE. Dermatoses of the breast in lactation. *Dermatol Ther*. 2013;26(4):331-336.

92. Barrett ME, Heller MM, Fullerton Stone H, Murase JE. Raynaud phenomenon of the nipple in breastfeeding mothers: an underdiagnosed cause of nipple pain. *JAMA Dermatol*. 2013;149(3):300-306.

93. Anderson JE, Held N, Wright K. Raynaud's phenomenon of the nipple: a treatable cause of painful breastfeeding. *Pediatrics*. 2004;113(4):e360-e364.

94. Albright CM, Wenstrom KD. Malignancies in pregnancy. *Best Pract Res Clin Obstet Gynaecol.* 2016;33:2-18.
95. Ruiz R, Herrero C, Strasser-Weippl K, et al. Epidemiology and pathophysiology of pregnancy-associated breast cancer: a review. *Breast.* 2017;35:136-141.
96. Leal SC, Stuart SR, Carvalho HdA. Breast irradiation and lactation: a review. *Expert Rev Anticancer Ther.* 2013;13(2):159-164.
97. Hinton L, Locock L, Knight M. Maternal critical care: what can we learn from patient experience? A qualitative study. *BMJ Open.* 2015;5(4):e006676. doi:10.1136/bmjopen-2014-006676.

Additional Resources

Center on Deafness—Inland Empire. http://codie.org/mission-and-purpose/.

DeafHealth. Provides accurate, concise, and valuable health information in American Sign Language using health information created by the Centers for Disease Control and Prevention and the National Institutes of Health. http://www.deafhealth.org.

La Leche League International. Resources. http://www.llli.org/resources.html.

National Federation of the Blind. Blind Parents. https://nfb.org/blindparents.

U.S. Department of Justice, Civil Rights Division, Disability Rights Section. ADA Business BRIEF: Communicating with People Who Are Deaf or Hard of Hearing in Hospital Settings. https://www.ada.gov/hospcombr.htm.

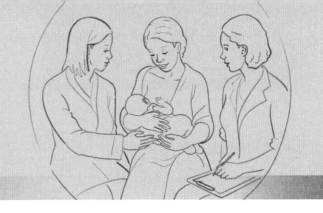

CHAPTER 18

Maternal Mental Health and Breastfeeding

Kathleen Kendall-Tackett

OBJECTIVES

- Recognize the symptoms of depression and related disorders in the early postpartum period, such as posttraumatic stress disorder (PTSD) and anxiety disorders.
- Describe the role of the inflammatory response system in the etiology of depression.
- Describe how breastfeeding protects the birth parent's mental health.
- Recognize that breastfeeding problems increase the risk of depression and need to be addressed promptly.
- Recognize that depression increases the risk for breastfeeding cessation.
- Provide information to families on treatment options for depression that are compatible with breastfeeding.

DEFINITIONS OF COMMONLY USED TERMS

anhedonia The inability to experience pleasure in normally pleasurable activities.
antenatal depression Depression during pregnancy.
anxiety disorders Excessive worry or anxiety characterized by restlessness, hypervigilance, irritability, sleep problems, and fears. Includes obsessive-compulsive disorder, phobias, and generalized anxiety disorder.
inflammatory response system A key part of the stress response. It is the underlying physiological mechanism behind depression, anxiety, PTSD, and other perinatal mood disorders.
postpartum depression (postnatal depression) Major depressive disorder during the first year after birth. Symptoms include sadness, anhedonia, agitation, social withdrawal, sleep problems, and irritability that last more than 2 weeks.
posttraumatic stress disorder (PTSD) A disorder that can occur following a traumatic event.
traumatic event According to the *Diagnostic and Statistical Manual of Mental Disorders (DSM-5)*, an event meets the exposure criteria for PTSD if it includes death or threatened death, actual or threatened physical harm, or actual or threatened sexual violation. The event can be directly experienced, or it can be witnessed; additionally, the event may have happened to a loved one.

Any use of the term *mother, maternal,* or *breastfeeding* is not meant to exclude transgender or nonbinary parents who may be breastfeeding or providing human milk to their infant.

▶ Overview

Mental health is a critical part of lactation care. Postpartum mood disorders, including depression, anxiety disorders, PTSD, and other conditions, can lead to breastfeeding cessation and have a negative impact on both parent and baby.[1,2] Providers must learn how to recognize symptoms of depression and make referrals so parents can get the help they need. There is no need to wean during treatment for depression. In fact, continuing breastfeeding may help in recovery, particularly when exclusively breastfeeding. Because breastfeeding downregulates the inflammatory and stress responses, and upregulates the oxytocin response, it is an important mechanism that protects mental health and lowers the risk of depression.[1,3-6] However, breastfeeding problems, particularly pain, can increase the risk of depression because these problems upregulate the stress and inflammatory responses.[6,7] Depression is too serious to ignore or not treat. There are many nonpharmacologic treatments for depression, and most antidepressants are compatible with breastfeeding.

I. Introduction

A. Mental disorders, such as depression, PTSD, and anxiety disorders, increase the risk of breastfeeding cessation.[8] As such, recognizing these disorders and making appropriate referrals are within the purview of lactation specialists.

B. Exclusive breastfeeding may protect mental health because it downregulates the stress and inflammatory response systems, upregulates oxytocin, and improves sleep. Exclusive breastfeeding results in a significantly lower risk of depression than does mixed feeding and formula feeding.[6,9,10]

C. Many postpartum depression organizations indicate that 10 to 15 percent of birth parents will be depressed after having a baby.[11] Recent studies reveal that this estimate is accurate for middle-class white women, but it substantially underestimates the risk for other groups. The percentage of depression in higher-risk groups can be as high as 40 to 60 percent.[1]

D. The Centers for Disease Control and Prevention indicates that postpartum depression is less likely to be diagnosed and treated in young women, as well as African American, Hispanic, and other nonwhite women.[12]

E. Symptoms of depression include moods of sadness, anhedonia, sleep difficulties unrelated to infant care, fatigue, inability to concentrate, hopelessness, and thoughts of death. For a diagnosis of major depressive disorder, these symptoms must be present for at least 2 weeks.[13]

F. A handy checklist for identifying parents' mental status is presented in **TABLE 18-1**.

G. There are many effective complementary and integrative nonpharmacological treatments for depression that are evidence based and effective, even for major depression.[1]

H. Only one treatment for depression is contraindicated for breastfeeding parents: the monoamine oxidase inhibitor (MAOI) class of antidepressants. All other treatments for depression are compatible with breastfeeding.[1,14]

CLINICAL TIP

Depression may manifest as somatic complaints or severe fatigue. These symptoms are more socially acceptable than depression in many cultures. Another possible indication of depression is increased use of healthcare services for the parent or baby

Sleep difficulties can indicate possible depression. The number of minutes that it takes to fall asleep is an important predictor of depression and is a nonintrusive way to ask about it. Those who take more than 25 minutes to fall asleep are at high risk for depression.[10,15,16]

II. International Incidence and High-Risk Populations

A. Depression is quite common in parents of young children. A study of 86,957 U.S. women, who were either pregnant or had a child up to 12 years of age, found that depression was common. The highest risk of depression was during the first year of parenthood. By the time their children were 12 years old, 39 percent of mothers and 21 percent of fathers had been depressed.[17]

TABLE 18-1 Mental Status Checklist	
Element	**Observations**
General Observations	Appearance, clothing, hygiene
Behavior	Movements appropriate to setting Over-activity or lethargy
Speech	Rate, intelligibility, volume, quality, quantity
Attitude	Cooperative, indifferent, hostile
Mood	Ecstatic, stable, depressed, grieving
Affect	Congruent with words and topic
Thought Content	Evidence of present time focus, coherent Delusional statements or reference to hallucinations[a] Statements of intended self-harm or harm to others[a]
Intellect	Evidence of understanding the situation and information presented Ability to communicate Cultural and language differences
Insight	Ability to understand and use information effectively
Memory	Long-term and short-term memory Impact of any prescribed medications on memory

[a]Requires immediate referral to psychiatric or crisis services.

This checklist is to be used as a guide to gathering information during an interaction with a client to casually assess mental status. It is to be used only to recognize symptoms or interactions that require referral and not for mental health diagnosis. Consider the client's social and cultural background as well as the setting when assessing mental status.

Data from American Psychiatric Association. *Diagnostic and Statistical Manual of Mental Disorders.* 5th ed. Arlington, VA: American Psychiatric Association; 2013.[13]

B. Three studies from Turkey found that 14 to 15 percent of mothers had postpartum depression.[18-20]
C. A longitudinal study of 1,507 mothers from Australia, who were followed from 3 months to 4 years postpartum, found that 31 percent of mothers were depressed in the first 4 years of parenthood. The risk factors for depression included young maternal age, stressful life events, adversity, intimate partner violence, and low income.[21]
D. Two studies from Korea found high rates of depression. In one study, 49 percent of mothers were depressed.[22] In the second study, 41 percent were depressed during pregnancy, and 61 percent were depressed at 4 weeks postpartum.[23] A study from Vietnam found that 16 to 20 percent of new mothers were depressed.[24]
E. A meta-analysis of eight studies of immigrant, asylum-seeking postnatal women in Canada found that up to 42 percent were depressed.[25] Another meta-analysis of 24 studies from multiple countries ($N = 13,749$) found that 20 percent of immigrants had postpartum depression, which was lower than previous studies found, but it was still twice the rate of native-born mothers.[26]

III. Causes of Depression

A. The inflammatory response system is the physiological mechanism underlying depression.
1. Researchers in the field of psychoneuroimmunology have found that inflammation is involved in the pathogenesis of depression.[1,27-29]
2. All types of physical and psychological stress increase the risk of depression in nonpostpartum samples, and also in new parents. Although the types of stressors vary, the underlying physiologic

mechanism in response to these stressors is the same: an upregulation of the stress response, including an increase in proinflammatory cytokines.[3] Proinflammatory cytokines are messenger molecules of the immune system that increase inflammation.

3.   The puerperal period is an especially vulnerable time because inflammation levels rise significantly during the last trimester of pregnancy, which carries the highest risk for depression. Moreover, common experiences of new parenthood, such as sleep disturbance, postpartum pain, and psychological trauma, also increase inflammation.[1,30]

4.   To understand the role of inflammation in depression, it is helpful to first review the normal physiologic response to stress. Human bodies have a number of interdependent mechanisms that are designed to preserve our lives when we are faced with a threat[1,31]:

   a.   The sympathetic nervous system responds by releasing catecholamines (norepinephrine, epinephrine, and dopamine).

   b.   The hypothalamic–pituitary–adrenal (HPA) axis also responds; the hypothalamus releases corticotrophin-releasing hormone (CRH); the pituitary releases adrenocorticotrophin hormone (ACTH); and the adrenal cortex releases cortisol, a glucocorticoid.

   c.   The immune system responds by increasing the production of proinflammatory cytokines, which increase systemic inflammation. Cytokines are proteins that regulate immune response. Proinflammatory cytokines help the body heal wounds and fight infection by stimulating an inflammatory response. These inflammatory molecules are measured in the plasma. In depressed people, inflammation is increased, including high levels of proinflammatory cytokines and acute-phase proteins, such as C-reactive protein (CRP), which is a physiologic response to chronic distress. Inflammation levels can be 40 to 50 percent higher in depressed people than in their nondepressed counterparts.[32,33]

   d.   The proinflammatory cytokines that researchers identified most consistently as being elevated in depression are interleukin-1β (IL-1), interleukin-6 (IL-6), and tumor necrosis factor-alpha (TNFα).[28,29]

5.   Breastfeeding specifically downregulates the stress response and lowers ACTH, cortisol,[34] and inflammation.[35] This is likely one way that breastfeeding decreases the risk for depression. The downregulation is thought to have a survival advantage because it facilitates milk production, energy conservation, and attachment to the baby.[36]

B.   Stressors that increase inflammation and depression risk can be physical or psychological. The stress response is the same whether the stressors are physical or psychological. Three stressors—sleep disturbance, pain, and psychological trauma—are particularly relevant to new parents.

1.   Sleep disturbance:

   a.   The relationship between sleep disturbance and depression is bidirectional; that is, sleep disturbances can cause depression, and depression causes sleep disturbances.[16]

   b.   Even short periods of disrupted sleep can wreak havoc on physical health. Sleep disturbances increase inflammatory responses and, if chronic, increase the risk of chronic diseases, such as heart disease and metabolic syndrome.[37,38] This is relevant to postpartum depression as well. In one recent study of 479 women, 5 hours of sleep or less per night at 1 year postpartum was associated with higher IL-6 at 3 years postpartum.[39]

   c.   Breastfeeding may protect mental health by improving sleep quality and quantity, including total sleep time and minutes to get to sleep. In a number of recent studies, exclusively breastfeeding parents got more sleep than their mixed- or exclusively formula-feeding counterparts.[9,10,40] Exclusively breastfeeding parents report more total sleep time and fewer minutes to get to sleep. Both of these markers are important predictors of postpartum depression.[41] In addition, exclusively breastfeeding parents report more daily energy, and they rate their physical health more positively than mixed- or formula-feeding parents.[10]

   d.   One study of 2,870 mothers found that disturbed sleep increased the risk for postpartum depression and that not exclusively breastfeeding was a risk factor for both.[9] Another study of 6,410 new mothers found the same effect.[10]

   e.   Breastfeeding increases deeper slow-wave sleep.[42] In a study of 31 women, those who breastfed got an average of 182 minutes of slow-wave sleep. Those in the nonpostpartum control group had an average of 86 minutes. Slow-wave sleep is an important marker of sleep quality, and those with a lower percentage of slow-wave sleep report more daytime fatigue.

f. Supplementing will likely decrease the amount of sleep that a parent gets.[10,40]

g. The protective effects of exclusive breastfeeding is true even when parents have a history of sexual assault. In a study of 6,410 mothers, 994 reported rape or sexual assault.[43] Sexual assault had a pervasive negative effect on sleep and mental health. Exclusive breastfeeding attenuated the negative effects of sexual assault. For example, exclusively mothers with a history of sexual assault (EBF-SA) reported fewer depressive symptoms and less anxiety, and less anger and irritability than those who were mixed or formula feeding and had been sexually assaulted (M- or FF-SA). Further, the EBF-SA mothers reported more total sleep and fewer minutes to get to sleep than the M- or FF-SA mothers. Even with exclusive breastfeeding, there were still effects of sexual assault, but they appeared to be significantly reduced. Mothers who were mixed feeding did not have these same protective effects.

CLINICAL TIP

Fatigue and sleep problems are often overlooked or minimized because they are so common in new parents. But fatigue is often of great concern to parents. If a breastfeeding parent is very fatigued, physical causes, such as anemia, hypothyroidism, or low-grade infection, should be tested and ruled out. Parents may also need help with mobilizing their support network so they can get more rest.

2. Pain:
   a. Postpartum pain can trigger postpartum depression and should be addressed promptly. In a study of 1,288 new mothers, the severity of postpartum pain predicted postpartum depression. Acute pain increased the risk of depression by three times.[44]
   b. Nipple pain is one common type of postpartum pain. In two studies, more than half of new mothers reported nipple pain at 5 weeks[45] and 2 months[46] postpartum, which can also cause postpartum depression. In a study of 2,586 women in the United States, nipple pain at day 1, week 1, and week 2 was associated with depression at 2 months postpartum.[7] However, in those with moderate to severe pain, breastfeeding helped protected their mental health.
   c. Pain and inflammation are mutually upregulatory; that is, pain increases inflammation, and inflammation increases pain. In addition, pain upregulates the stress system, including the sympathetic nervous system, which inhibits oxytocin release and directly contributes to problems with milk ejection.[6,47]
3. Psychological trauma:
   a. Psychological trauma increases the risk for depression, and PTSD and depression are highly comorbid.[48]
   b. Trauma increases inflammation. In the Dunedin Multidisciplinary Health and Development Study, a birth cohort study from Dunedin, New Zealand, childhood maltreatment was related to increased inflammation (CRP) 20 years later. There was a dose–response effect: the more severe the abuse, the higher the level of inflammation.[49] At the 32-year assessment of this same study, those who experienced childhood adversities (low socioeconomic status, maltreatment, or social isolation) had higher rates of major depression, systemic inflammation, and at least three metabolic risk markers.[50]
   c. With regard to new mothers, the most common types of psychological trauma are adverse childhood experiences and trauma related to their birth experience.[51,52] One study from Guatemala found that stressful births delayed lactogenesis II.[53] A study of 5,332 mothers from the United Kingdom found that those who had cesareans or forceps-assisted births were significantly more likely to have breastfeeding difficulties at 3 months postpartum.[54] One qualitative study found that traumatic birth made breastfeeding more difficult for some mothers,[55] but others found that breastfeeding helped mothers heal from traumatic birth.
   d. An adverse childhood experience (ACE) also carries increased risks.
      i. ACEs include childhood physical and sexual abuse, emotional abuse, neglect, witnessing domestic violence between parents or parents and their partners, parental mental illness, substance abuse, and criminal activity.[56]
      ii. These types of experiences are common. In the original paper from an ACE study, which included more than 17,000 patients in the Kaiser Permanente system, 51 percent of patients

had experienced at least one type of ACE.[57] These patients were predominantly middle aged and middle class. This study was the first to connect adversity in childhood to adult physical health problems. Samples with higher-risk populations may have even higher rates of ACEs.

    iii.   Childhood adversities are related to a number of chronic health conditions in adults, including cardiovascular disease, metabolic syndrome, and diabetes.[58]

    iv.   Childhood adversities are related to sleep disturbances[43] and chronic pain syndromes.[59]

    v.   ACEs can affect mothers prenatally and postpartum, most notably by increasing the risk of depression and PTSD. A recent review of 43 studies found that women who were abused as children, or by their partners, had more lifetime depression and more depression during pregnancy and postpartum.[60]

    vi.   Two studies demonstrated that women who had histories of childhood sexual abuse had higher rates of intention to breastfeed; one study included low-income minority women in Baltimore,[61] and the other included a nationally representative sample of U.S. mothers of children under the age of 3.[62] Data from the Survey of Mothers' Sleep and Fatigue, which utilized a sample of 6,410 new mothers from 59 countries, including 994 sexual assault survivors, revealed that sexual assault survivors and nonassaulted women exclusively breastfed at the same rate.[43]

CLINICAL TIP

According to the principles of trauma-informed care, practitioners may need to help modify breastfeeding to make it more comfortable for abuse survivors. However, it is equally important that practitioners do not disempower parents by making decisions for them. Doing so would be paternalistic and not trauma-informed care. For example, do not assume that parents with a history of sexual abuse or assault do not want to breastfeed; it may be a very important goal for them. Find out what parents want to do and empower them to do it. Depending on their experience, some strategies that may make breastfeeding easier include using distraction while breastfeeding (such as reading or watching TV), avoiding nighttime feedings, reducing the amount of skin-to-skin contact, and feeding expressed milk from a bottle. Be flexible and help parents find a way that works best for them. This strategy is effective even if a parent does not reveal a history of abuse but you suspect there was abuse.

---

    e.   A negative birth experience is a form of psychological trauma.

        i.   Birth interventions may be necessary in some cases, but they can have negative consequences. Several birth interventions, such as epidurals and other anesthesia, decrease the rates of exclusive breastfeeding and increase depressive symptoms. In a prospective study of 1,280 mothers from Australia, intrapartum anesthesia was associated with breastfeeding difficulties at 1 week postpartum and cessation at 3 months postpartum.[63] In a survey of 6,410 new mothers, those who had epidurals, postpartum hemorrhage, or postpartum surgery had significantly higher depressive symptoms than those who did not have these interventions or complications, even after controlling for other factors that increase the risk of depression (history of depression or sexual assault, other birth interventions, and low income or education level).[64] Some studies with small samples, however, have not found that epidurals increased breastfeeding problems[65] or depression.[66]

        ii.   In the U.S. Listening to Mothers II Survey, 9 percent of mothers met full criteria for PTSD, and an additional 18 percent scored above the cutoff for posttraumatic stress symptoms following birth.[67] In comparison, 7.5 percent of lower Manhattan, New York, residents met the full criteria for PTSD following the 9/11 terrorist attacks.[68]

        iii.   A study of 933 mothers in Brisbane, Australia, showed similarly high rates.[51] At 6 weeks postpartum, 6.3 percent of participants met the full criteria for PTSD, and 46 percent described their birth as traumatic. They had high rates of depression (47 to 66 percent) and anxiety (58 to 74 percent). This finding is consistent with the trauma literature, which shows that not everyone exposed to a traumatic event develops PTSD, but they may show other symptoms, such as depression and anxiety.[48]

        iv.   Women in countries where birth is treated as a normal event, and who have continuous labor support, have lower rates of PTSD. For example, a prospective study of 1,224 women in

Sweden found that 1.3 percent had birth-related PTSD, and 9 percent described their births as traumatic.[69] Similarly, a study of 907 women in the Netherlands found that 1.2 percent of women had birth-related PTSD, and 9 percent identified their births as traumatic.[70]

    v.   Conversely, women who give birth in countries where the status of women is generally low have higher rates of birth trauma. A study from Iran of 400 women found that 218 participants reported traumatic births at 6 to 8 weeks postpartum, and 20 percent had postpartum PTSD.[71]

CLINICAL TIP

Objective aspects of birth (e.g., cesarean versus vaginal) account for only some reactions. Cesarean birth somewhat increases the risk of having a negative reaction, but that is not always true. Subjective aspects of birth, such as the following, are more likely to lead to a negative assessment of the birth:

- Questioning whether giving birth was dangerous to the parent or the baby
- The ability to feel in control of either the medical situation or oneself during labor
- Feeling supported during labor and birth[1,72]

---

    vi.   Mothers are more vulnerable to PTSD if they have had prior episodes of depression or PTSD, are abuse survivors (which increases the risk of both PTSD and depression), had prior episodes of loss (including childbearing loss), or were depressed during pregnancy.[1]

    vii.   A highly stressful birth may delay lactogenesis II because high cortisol levels suppress prolactin.[53]

    f.   Infant illness, preterm birth, and disability can cause depression in birth parents, particularly if the babies are at high risk for severe illness or death. However, this reaction is often delayed and may not manifest until the babies are out of danger, or even several months after they are discharged.

        i.   A study of 21 mothers of very low birth weight (VLBW) babies in Quebec found that 23 percent were in the clinical range for PTSD at 6 months after NICU discharge.[73] Those with more PTSD symptoms were less sensitive in their interactions with their babies than those with fewer symptoms.

        ii.   A study from Germany of 230 mothers and 173 fathers found that depression scores were 4 to 18 times higher in mothers of VLBW infants, and 3 to 9 times higher in fathers of VLBW infants, compared to parents of full-term infants at 4 to 6 weeks postpartum.[74] The sample included parents of VLBW infants ($N = 111$) and parents of full-term infants ($N = 119$).

IV. Treatment Options

    A.   Recognizing the scope of practice of a lactation consultant without prescription privileges does not encompass prescription of medication, supplements, or exercise, the guidelines below are provided for referral. A variety of treatment options that are effective for postpartum mood disorders are available. All but one of these modalities (MAOI antidepressants) are compatible with breastfeeding, and most can be safely combined. All effective treatments for depression are anti-inflammatory.[1,28]

    B.   Omega-3 fatty acids:

        1.   Dietary alpha linolenic acid (ALA) can be metabolized in the liver to the longer-chain omega-3 fatty acids, eicosapentaenoic acid (EPA), and docosahexaenoic acid (DHA). Only about 10 percent of ALA is converted to these longer-chain fatty acids, so ALA cannot be used as a treatment for depression.

        2.   The long-chain omega-3 fatty acids EPA and DHA have been used successfully both to prevent and treat depression. Both of these are found in fatty fish. Populations with high rates of fish consumption have lower rates of several types of mental illness, including postpartum depression.[1,75]

        3.   EPA is the omega-3 that treats depression because it specifically lowers proinflammatory cytokines and downregulates the stress response.[29,76] The combination of EPA and DHA has been used by itself or in combination with medications. When used with medications, EPA and DHA enhance the effectiveness of the medications. The American Psychiatric Association recognizes EPA as a promising treatment for mood disorders.[77,78] DHA alone does not treat depression, but it seems to play a role in prevention.[79]

4.   A prospective study in western Norway found that low omega-3 levels at 28 weeks' gestation predicted higher levels of depression at 3 months postpartum.[80]

5.   Even in relatively large doses, EPA and DHA are safe during pregnancy and lactation and provide a number of other health benefits for breastfeeding parents, including lowering their risk of heart disease and making them less vulnerable to stress.[81,82]

6.   ALA, the omega-3 in flaxseed and other plant sources, such as walnuts and canola oil, does not prevent or treat depression. ALA is not harmful, and it can be helpful in other ways. But it is metabolically too far removed from EPA to aid in lessening depression by lowering inflammation.

CLINICAL TIP

Doses typically recommended for DHA and EPA are:

- 200 to 400 mg of DHA is the minimum dose for prevention
- 1 gram of EPA is used to treat depression

For safe sources of fish oil products, refer to the United States Pharmacopeial Convention website at http://www.USP.org.

C.   Bright light therapy:
1.   Bright light is an effective treatment for depression. It has been used to treat depression during pregnancy and breastfeeding, although the sample sizes in studies are small.[83]
2.   An illumination level of 10,000 lux for 30 to 40 minutes is the most commonly used dosage. Regular home lighting is not sufficiently bright to alleviate depression. Light therapy first thing in the morning is more effective than light therapy later in the day.[84]

D.   Exercise:
1.   Exercise is as effective as medications for even major depression. Two clinical trials from the Duke University Medical Center compared exercise to sertraline for adults aged 50 to 80 years.[85,86] Both studies found that exercise was as effective as sertraline for major depression.
2.   A recent Cochrane Review of 37 studies on exercise and depression found a moderate effect of exercise for reducing depressive symptoms.[87] Exercise was as effective as psychotherapy in seven trials, and it was as effective as medications in four trials.
3.   Another study randomized mothers to receive a combination of exercise and parenting education ($N = 62$) or education only ($N = 73$) for 8 weeks.[88] Those in the education plus exercise group had a 50 percent reduction in their risk for postpartum depression, and they had significantly lower depression scores and higher well-being scores than those in the education only group.
4.   A review of 17 studies on postpartum depression and exercise found that leisure time physical activity decreased postpartum depressive symptoms.[89]
5.   Exercise lowers inflammation. An overall fitness level lowers the inflammatory response to stress.[90-92]
6.   Exercise at a moderate level is safe during pregnancy and lactation, and it does not decrease milk production or increase lactic acid in the milk.[93,94]

CLINICAL TIP

Most studies that have examined the impact of exercise as a treatment for depression have used aerobic exercise. The recommended amounts are as follows.

For mild to moderate depression:

- Two or three times per week
- Moderate intensity
- 20–30 minutes

For major depression:

- Three to five times per week
- 60 to 85 percent maximal capacity
- 45–60 minutes

One study found that resistance training twice per week was helpful in lowering symptoms.[95]

E.   Psychotherapy:
1.   There are two types of psychotherapy that are effective for depression during pregnancy and lactation: cognitive-behavioral therapy (CBT) and interpersonal psychotherapy (IPT).
2.   The premise of CBT is that depression is caused by distortions in people's beliefs about themselves and the world. By addressing these beliefs, depression diminishes. It is as effective as medications for treating depression and other conditions.[96]
      a.   A study of 105 mothers of preterm infants were assigned to either a 6- or 9-week course of trauma-focused CBT or one education session.[97] Those in the CBT group had lower rates of depression, anxiety, and trauma than those in the one-session group. At 6 months, those in the CBT group showed that the benefits of the program (lower depression, anxiety, and trauma) actually increased for them.
3.   IPT specifically addresses the parents' key relationships and the support they receive from those relationships. It teaches them to identify sources of support and increase the amount of support they receive from existing relationships. It has been used with many high-risk mothers both to prevent and to treat depression during pregnancy and in the postpartum period.[98]
      a.   A study from China compared IPT to usual care for 180 first-time birth mothers.[99] IPT consisted of a 1-hour education session, with one telephone follow-up at 2 weeks postpartum. Those in the IPT group had significantly less depression, more social support, and better maternal role competence at 6 weeks postpartum than those in the usual-care group.

F.   St. John's wort:
1.   The herbal antidepressant St. John's wort is the most widely used antidepressant in the world, and it is highly effective in treating depression. Its standard uses are for mild to moderate depression, but it has been used for major depression as well.
2.   When researchers compared St. John's wort to sertraline and paroxetine, St. John's wort was as effective as the medications, and patients reported fewer side effects.[100,101]
3.   St. John's wort is probably compatible with lactation, with low transfer into milk.[14,102]
4.   Used by itself, St. John's wort has an excellent safety record. It does interact with several types of medications, so parents should always advise their healthcare provider if they are taking it. For example, St. John's wort should not be combined with antidepressants, birth control pills, cyclosporins, antineoplastic agents, HIV medications, and several other classes of medications.[1,103]

G.   Antidepressants:
1.   Most antidepressants are compatible with lactation, but they vary in how much exposure the infant receives.
2.   Tricyclic antidepressants, selective serotonin reuptake inhibitors (SSRIs), and serotonin norepinephrine reuptake inhibitors (SNRIs) are compatible with lactation.[1,14] SSRIs and SNRIs are the most widely used because many consider the side-effect profile to be better. However, the older tricyclic antidepressants are still sometimes used. Within these classes of medications, some have lower transfer rates into milk than others. Resources for current medication recommendations can be found in *Medications and Mothers' Milk*,[14] at the Infant Risk Center website (http://infantrisk.com), and in the LactMed online database (https://toxnet.nlm.nih.gov/newtoxnet/lactmed.htm).
3.   MAOIs are contraindicated during lactation.[14]

▶ Key Points from This Chapter

A.   Depression and related disorders in new parents are common in many countries.
B.   When breastfeeding is going well, it protects mental health because it upregulates the oxytocin system and downregulates the stress and inflammatory response systems. Conversely, breastfeeding problems increase the risk of depression because they upregulate the stress and inflammatory systems and downregulate oxytocin.
C.   There are many effective treatments for depression that are nonpharmacological, and almost all antidepressants are compatible with breastfeeding.

🔍 CASE STUDY

Shelby describes experiences of perinatal anxiety and panic attacks. Breastfeeding was going well and helped to overcome the anxiety disorder, but family members were consistently urging Shelby to wean the baby.

When my first was born, I was completely overwhelmed with the feeling of being the primary caregiver. I had no family or friends in the area, and my partner had to go back to work when our baby was 5 or 6 days old. I had panic attacks, and I felt like there was no way I was up to being the kind of parent our baby deserved. Breastfeeding was going well, though, and it was often the only thing that I felt like I was doing right.

Well-meaning family and friends often tried to suggest that I let my partner give our baby a bottle to reduce the burden on me of providing the care. They also suggested that if we moved our baby out of our bed, I could get more and better sleep, and recover more easily. I knew that being kept close at night helped to make it more OK that I wasn't holding our baby all the time during the day, and also that I was able to get more sleep and rest by breastfeeding in bed. As things started to improve for me hormonally, I was able to look back at the fact that I met our baby's most basic needs, even as I was struggling, and it helped me feel better about myself, which helped my emotional healing. I know that the advice I received came with good intentions, but I was vulnerable then, and I wanted a magic cure to all my problems. I seriously considered sleep training and letting my partner give our baby an occasional bottle of formula, even though it didn't feel right. I am so glad that my partner was strong enough to help me through that horrible time in other ways and always remind me of our child's needs in a kind and loving way.

Questions

1. What were some of the challenges Shelby faced?
2. What types of supports did Shelby have?
3. Was the experience of breastfeeding helpful or not helpful to Shelby?
4. Were the family's and friends' suggestions to wean or give the baby a bottle perceived as helpful to Shelby?

References

1. Kendall-Tackett KA. *Depression in New Mothers.* 3rd ed. Abington, UK: Routledge; 2017.
2. Wouk K, Stuebe AM, Meltzer-Brody S. Postpartum mental health and breastfeeding practices: an analysis using the 2010-2011 Pregnancy Risk Assessment Monitoring System. *Maternal Child Health J.* 2017;21:636-647.
3. Kendall-Tackett KA. A new paradigm for depression in new mothers: the central role of inflammation and how breastfeeding and anti-inflammatory treatments protect maternal mental health. *Int Breastfeeding J.* 2007;2:6.
4. Dennis C-L, McQueen K. The relationship between infant-feeding outcomes and postpartum depression: a qualitative systematic review. *Pediatrics.* 2009;123:e736-e751.
5. Groer MW. Differences between exclusive breastfeeders, formula-feeders, and controls: a study of stress, mood, and endocrine variables. *Biol Nurs Res.* 2005;7:106-117.
6. Uvnas-Moberg K. *Oxytocin: The Biological Guide to Motherhood.* Amarillo, TX: Praeclarus Press; 2015.
7. Watkins S, Meltzer-Brody S, Zolnoun D, Stuebe AM. Early breastfeeding experiences and postpartum depression. *Obstet Gynecol.* 2011;118:214-221.
8. Machado MC, Assis KF, Oliveira FdeC, et al. Determinants of the exclusive breastfeeding abandonment: psychosocial factors. *Revista Saude Publica.* 2014;48:985-994.
9. Dorheim SK, Bondevik GT, Eberhard-Gran M, Bjorvatn B. Sleep and depression in postpartum women: a population-based study. *Sleep.* 2009;32:847-855.
10. Kendall-Tackett KA, Cong Z, Hale TW. The effect of feeding method on sleep duration, maternal well-being, and postpartum depression. *Clin Lactation.* 2011;2:22-26.
11. Ko JY, Rockhill KM, Tong VT, Morrow B, Farr SL. Trends in postpartum depressive symptoms: 27 states, 2004, 2008, and 2012. *MMWR Morbidity Mortality Weekly Rep.* 2017;66:153-158.
12. Centers for Disease Control and Prevention. *Mental Health Among Women of Reproductive Age.* Atlanta, GA: Centers for Disease Control and Prevention; 2015.
13. American Psychiatric Association. *Diagnostic and Statistical Manual of Mental Disorders.* 5th ed. Arlington, VA: American Psychiatric Association; 2013.
14. Hale TW, Rowe HJ. *Medications and Mothers' Milk.* 16th ed. New York, NY: Springer Publishing; 2017.
15. Goyal D, Gay CL, Lee KA. Patterns of sleep disruption and depressive symptoms in new mothers. *J Perinat Neonatal Nurs.* 2007;21:123-129.
16. Posmontier B. Sleep quality in women with and without postpartum depression. *J Obstet Gynecol Neonatal Nurs.* 2008;37:722-737.
17. Dave S, Petersen I, Sherr L, Nazareth I. Incidence of maternal and paternal depression in primary care: a cohort study using a primary care database. *Arch Pediatric Adolesc Med.* 2010;164:1038-1044.

18. Danaci AE, Dinc G, Deveci A, Sen FS, Icelli I. Postnatal depression in Turkey: epidemiological and cultural aspects. *Soc Psychiatry Psychiatr Epidemiol*. 2002;37:125-129.

19. Kirpinar I, Gozum S, Pasinlioglu T. Prospective study of postpartum depression in eastern Turkey: prevalence, socio-demographic and obstetric correlates, prenatal anxiety and early awareness. *J Clin Nurs*. 2010;19:422-431.

20. Turkcapar AF, Kadioglu N, Aslan E, Tunc S, Zayifoglu M, Mollamahmutoglu L. Sociodemographic and clinical features of postpartum depression among Turkish women: a prospective study. *BMC Pregnancy Childbirth*. 2015;5:108.

21. Woolhouse H, Gartland D, Mensah F, Brown SJ. Maternal depression from early pregnancy to 4 years postpartum in a prospective pregnancy cohort study: implications for primary health care. *Br J Obstet Gynecol*. 2015;122:312-321.

22. Lee JY, Hwang JY. A study on postpartum symptoms and their related factors in Korea. *Taiwanese J Obstet Gynecol*. 2015;54:355-363.

23. Park J-H, Karmaus W, Zhang H. Prevalence of and risk factors for depressive symptoms in Korean women throughout pregnancy and in postpartum period. *Asian Nurs Res*. 2015;9:219-225.

24. Murray L, Dunne MP, Vo TV, Anh PNT, Khawaja NG, Cao TN. Postnatal depressive symptoms amongst women in central Vietnam: a cross-sectional study investigating prevalence and associations with social, cultural, and infant factors. *BMC Pregnancy Childbirth*. 2015;15:234.

25. Collins CH, Zimmerman C, Howard LM. Refugee, asylum seeker, immigrant women and postnatal depression: rates and risk factors. *Arch Womens Ment Health*. 2011;14:3-11.

26. Falah-Hassani K, Shiri R, Vigod S, Dennis C-L. Prevalence of postpartum depression among immigrant women: a systematic review and meta-analysis. *J Psychiatr Res*. 2015;70:67-82.

27. Kendall-Tackett KA, ed. *The Psychoneuroimmunology of Chronic Disease*. Washington, DC: American Psychological Association; 2010.

28. Maes M, Yirmyia R, Noraberg J, et al. The inflammatory and neurodegenerative hypothesis of depression: leads for future research and new drug developments in depression. *Metab Brain Dis*. 2009;24:27-53.

29. Kiecolt-Glaser JK, Derry HM, Fagundes CP. Inflammation: depression fans the flames and feast in the heat. *Am J Psychiatry*. 2015;172:1075-1091.

30. Corwin EJ, Pajer K, Paul S, Lowe N, Weber M, McCarthy DO. Bidirectional psychoneuroimmune interactions in the early postpartum period influence risk of postpartum depression. *Brain Behav Immun*. 2015;49:86-93.

31. Kim Y, Ahn S. A review of postpartum depression: focused on psychoneuroimmunological interaction. *Korean J Womens Health Nurs*. 2015; 21(2):106-114.

32. Berk M, Williams LJ, Jacka FN, et al. So depression is an inflammatory disease, but where does the inflammation come from? *BMC Med*. 2013;11:200.

33. Pace TW, Hu F, Miller AH. Cytokine-effects on glucocorticoid receptor function: relevance to glucocorticoid resistance and the pathophysiology and treatment of major depression. *Brain Behav Immun*. 2007;21:9-19.

34. Heinrichs M, Meinlschmidt G, Neumann I, et al. Effects of suckling on hypothalamic-pituitary-adrenal axis responses to psychosocial stress in postpartum lactating women. *J Clin Endocrinol Metab*. 2001;86:4798-4804.

35. Groer MW, Kendall-Tackett KA. *How Breastfeeding Protects Women's Health throughout the Lifespan: The Psychoneuroimmunology of Human Lactation*. Amarillo, TX: Hale Publishing; 2011.

36. Groer MW, Davis MW, Hemphill J. Postpartum stress: current concepts and the possible protective role of breastfeeding. *J Obstet Gynecol Neonatal Nurs*. 2002;31:411-417.

37. McEwen BS. Mood disorders and allostatic load. *Biol Psychiatry*. 2003;54:200-207.

38. Suarez EC, Goforth H. Sleep and inflammation: a potential link to chronic diseases. In: Kendall-Tackett KA, ed. *The Psychoneuroimmunology of Chronic Disease*. Washington, DC: American Psychological Association; 2010:53-75.

39. Taveras EM, Rifas-Shiman SL, Rich-Edwards JW, Mantzoros CS. Maternal short sleep duration is associated with increased levels of inflammatory markers at 3 years postpartum. *Metabolism*. 2011;60:982-986.

40. Doan T, Gardiner A, Gay CL, Lee KA. Breastfeeding increases sleep duration of new parents. *J Perinat Neonatal Nurs*. 2007;21:200-206.

41. Dorheim SK, Bondevik GT, Eberhard-Gran M, Bjorvatn B. Subjective and objective sleep among depressed and non-depressed postnatal women. *Acta Psychiatrica Scandinavia*. 2009;119:128-136.

42. Blyton DM, Sullivan CE, Edwards N. Lactation is associated with an increase in slow-wave sleep in women. *J Sleep Res*. 2002;11:297-303.

43. Kendall-Tackett K, Cong Z, Hale TW. Depression, sleep quality, and maternal well-being in postpartum women with a history of sexual assault: a comparison of breastfeeding, mixed-feeding, and formula-feeding mothers. *Breastfeeding Med*. 2013;8:16-22.

44. Eisenach JC, Pan PH, Smiley R, Lavand'homme P, Landau R, Houle TT. Severity of acute pain after childbirth, but not type of delivery, predicts persistent pain and postpartum depression. *Pain*. 2008;140:87-94.

45. McGovern P, Dowd BE, Gjerdingen D, et al. Postpartum health of employed mothers 5 weeks after childbirth. *Ann Fam Med*. 2006;4:159-167.

46. Ansara D, Cohen MM, Gallop R, Kung R, Kung R, Schei B. Predictors of women's physical health problems after childbirth. *J Psychosom Obstet Gynecol*. 2005;26:115-125.

47. Beilin B, Shavit Y, Trabekin E, et al. The effects of postoperative pain management on immune response to surgery. *Anesth Analg*. 2003;97:822-827.

48. Ruglass L, Kendall-Tackett KA. *The Psychology of Trauma 101*. New York, NY: Springer; 2015.

49. Danese A, Pariante CM, Caspi A, Taylor A, Poulton R. Childhood maltreatment predicts adult inflammation in a life-course study. *Proc Natl Acad Sci USA*. 2007;104:1319-1324.

50. Danese A, Moffitt TE, Harrington H, et al. Adverse childhood experiences and adult risk factors for age-related disease: depression, inflammation, and clustering of metabolic risk factors. *Arch Pediatric Adolesc Med*. 2009;163:1135-1143.

51. Alcorn KL, O'Donovan A, Patrick JC, Creedy D, Devilly GJ. A prospective longitudinal study of the prevalence of post-traumatic stress disorder resulting from childbirth events. *Psychological Med*. 2010;40:1849-1859.

52. Beck CT. Impact of birth trauma on breastfeeding: a tale of two pathways. *Nurs Res*. 2008;57:229-236.

53. Grajeda R, Perez-Escamilla R. Stress during labor and delivery is associated with delayed onset of lactation among urban Guatemalan women. *J Nutr.* 2002;132:3055-3060.

54. Rowlands IJ, Redshaw M. Mode of birth and women's psychological and physical wellbeing in the postnatal period. *BMC Pregnancy Childbirth.* 2012;12:1-11.

55. Beck CT, Watson S. Impact of birth trauma on breast-feeding. *Nurs Res.* 2008;57:228-236.

56. Anda RF, Dong M, Brown DW, et al. The relationship of adverse childhood experiences to a history of premature death of family members. *BMC Public Health.* 2009;9:106.

57. Felitti VJ, Anda RF, Nordenberg D, et al. Relationship of childhood abuse and household dysfunction to many of the leading causes of death in adults. The adverse childhood experiences (ACE) study. *Am J Prev Med.* 1998;14:245-258.

58. Kendall-Tackett KA. *Treating the Lifetime Health Effects of Childhood Victimization.* 2nd ed. Kingston, NJ: Civic Research Institute; 2013.

59. Sachs-Ericsson N, Kendall-Tackett KA, Hernandez A. Childhood abuse, chronic pain, and depression in the national comorbidity survey. *Child Abuse Negl.* 2007;31:531-547.

60. Alvarez-Segura M, Garcia-Esteve L, Torres A, et al. Are women with a history of abuse more vulnerable to perinatal depressive symptoms? A systematic review. *Arch Womens Ment Health.* 2014;17:343-357.

61. Benedict MI, Paine L, Paine L. *Long-Term Effects of Child Sexual Abuse on Functioning in Pregnancy and Pregnancy Outcomes (Final Report).* Washington, DC: National Center of Child Abuse and Neglect; 1994.

62. Prentice JC, Lu MC, Lange L, Halfon N. The association between reported childhood sexual abuse and breastfeeding initiation. *J Hum Lactation.* 2002;18:291-326.

63. Torvaldsen S, Roberts CL, Simpson JM, Thompson JF, Ellwood DA. Intrapartum epidural analgesia and breastfeeding: a prospective cohort study. *Int Breastfeeding J.* 2006;1:24.

64. Kendall-Tackett KA, Cong Z, Hale TW. Birth interventions related to lower rates of exclusive breastfeeding and increased risk of postpartum depression in a large sample. *Clin Lactation.* 2015;6:87-97.

65. Hiltunen P, Raudaskoski T, Ebeling H, Moilanen I. Does pain relief during delivery decrease the risk of postnatal depression? *Acta Obstetrica Gynecologica Scandanavica.* 2004;83:257-261.

66. Ding T, Wang DX, Chen Q, Zhu SN. Epidural labor analgesia is associated with a decreased risk of postpartum depression: a prospecitive cohort study. *Anesth Analg.* 2014;119:383-392.

67. Beck CT, Gable RK, Sakala C, Declercq ER. Posttraumatic stress disorder in new mothers: results from a two-stage U.S. national survey. *Birth.* 2011;38:216-227.

68. Galea S, Vlahov D, Resnick H, et al. Trends of probable post-traumatic stress disorder in New York City after the September 11 terrorist attacks. *Am J Epidemiol.* 2003;158:514-524.

69. Soderquist I, Wijma B, Thorbert G, Wijma K. Risk factors in pregnancy for post-traumatic stress and depression after childbirth. *Br J Obstet Gynecol.* 2009;116:672-680.

70. Stramrood CA, Paarlberg KM, Huis In 't Veld EM, et al. Posttraumatic stress following childbirth in homelike- and hospital settings. *J Psychosom Obstet Gynaecol.* 32:88-97.

71. Modarres M, Afrasiabi S, Rahnama P, Montazeri A. Prevalence and risk factors of childbirth-related post-traumatic stress symptoms. *BMC Pregnancy Childbirth.* 2012;12:88.

72. Kendall-Tackett KA. Childbirth-related posttraumatic stress disorder symptoms and implications for breastfeeding. *Clin Lactation.* 2014;5:51-55.

73. Feeley N, Zelkowitz P, Cormier C, Charbonneau L, Lacroix A, Papgeorgiou A. Posttraumatic stress among mother of very low birthweight infants 6 months after discharge from the neonatal intensive care unit. *Appl Nurs Res.* 2011;24:114-117.

74. Helle N, Barkmann C, Bartz-Seel J, et al. Very low birth-weight as a risk factor for postpartum depression four to six weeks postbirth in mothers and fathers: cross-sectional results from a controlled multicentre cohort study. *J Affective Disord.* 2015;180:154-161.

75. Hibbeln JR. Seafood consumption, the DHA content of mothers' milk and prevalence rates of postpartum depression: a cross-national, ecological analysis. *J Affective Disord.* 2002;69:15-29.

76. Maes M, Christophe A, Bosmans E, Lin A, Neels H. In humans, serum polyunsaturated fatty acid levels predict the response of proinflammatory cytokines to psychologic stress. *Biol Psychiatry.* 2000;47:910-920.

77. Freeman MP, Fava M, Lake J, Trivedi MH, Wisner KL, Mischoulon D. Complementary and alternative medicine in major depressive disorder: the American Psychiatric Association task force report. *J Clin Psychiatry.* 2010;71:669-681.

78. Freeman MP, Hibbeln JR, Wisner KL, et al. Omega-3 fatty acids: evidence basis for treatment and future research in psychiatry. *J Clin Psychiatry.* 2006;67:1954-1967.

79. Kendall-Tackett KA. Long-chain omega-3 fatty acids and women's mental health in the perinatal period. *J Midwifery Womens Health.* 2010;55:561-567.

80. Markhus MW, Skotheim S, Graff IE, et al. Low omega-3 index in pregnancy is a possible biological risk factor for postpartum depression. *PLoS One.* 2013;8:e67617. doi:10.1371/journal.pone.0067617.

81. Dunstan JA, Mori TA, Barden A, et al. Effects of n-3 polyunsaturated fatty acid supplementation in pregnancy on maternal and fetal erythrocyte fatty acid composition. *Eur J Clin Nutr.* 2004;58:429-437.

82. Grandjean P, Bjerve KS, Weihe P, Steuerwald U. Birthweight in a fishing community: significance of essential fatty acids and marine food contaminants. *Int J Epidemiol.* 2001;30:1272-1278.

83. Oren DA, Wisner KL, Spinelli M, et al. An open trial of morning light therapy for treatment of antepartum depression. *Am J Psychiatry.* 2002;159:666-669.

84. Terman M, Terman JS. Light therapy for seasonal and nonseasonal depression: efficacy, protocol, safety, and side effects. *CNS Spectrums.* 2005;10:647-663.

85. Babyak M, Blumenthal JA, Herman S, et al. Exercise treatment for major depression: maintenance of therapeutic benefit at 10 months. *Psychosom Med.* 2000;62:633-638.

86. Blumenthal JA, Babyak MA, Doraiswamy PM, et al. Exercise and pharmacotherapy in the treatment of major depressive disorder. *Psychosom Med.* 2007;69:587-596.

87. Cooney GM, Dwan K, Greig CA, et al. Exercise for depression. *Cochrane Database Syst Rev.* 2013;(9):CD004366. doi:10.1002/14651858 .CD004366.pub6.

88. Norman E, Sherburn M, Osborne R, Galea MP. An exercise and education program improves well-being of new mothers: a randomized controlled trial. *Phys Ther.* 2010;90:348-355.

89. Teychenne M, York R. Physical activity, sedentary behavior, and postnatal depressive symptoms: a review. *Am J Prev Med.* 2013;45:217-227.

90. Starkweather AR. The effects of exercise on perceived stress and IL-6 levels among older adults. *Biol Nurs Res.* 2007;8:1-9.

91. Kiecolt-Glaser JK, Christian L, Preston H, et al. Stress, inflammation, and yoga practice. *Psychosom Med.* 2010;72:113-121.

92. Emery CF, Kiecolt-Glaser JK, Glaser R, Malarky WB, Frid DJ. Exercise accelerates wound healing among health older adults: a preliminary investigation. *J Gerontol: Med Sci.* 2005;60A:1432-1436.

93. Su D, Zhao Y, Binna C, Scott J, Oddy W. Breast-feeding mothers can exercise: results of a cohort study. *Public Health Nutr.* 2007;10:1089-1093.

94. Quinn TJ, Carey GB. Does exercise intensity or diet influence lactic acid accumulation in breast milk? *Med Sci Sports Exerc.* 1999;31:105-110.

95. LeChiminant JD, Hinman T, Pratt KB, et al. Effect of resistance training on body composition, self-efficacy, depression, and activity in postpartum women. *Scand J Med Sci Sports.* 2014;24:414-421.

96. Rupke SJ, Blecke D, Renfrow M. Cognitive therapy for depression. *Am Fam Physician.* 2006;73:83-86.

97. Shaw RJ, St John N, Lilo E, et al. Prevention of traumatic stress in mothers of preterms: 6-month outcomes. *Pediatrics.* 2014;134:e481-e488.

98. Zlotnick C, Miller IW, Pearlstein T, Howard M, Sweeney P. A preventive intervention for pregnant women on public assistance at risk for postpartum depression. *Am J Psychiatry.* 2006;163:1443-1445.

99. Gao L-L, Xie W, Yang X, Chan SW-C. Effects of an interpersonal-psychotherapy-oriented postnatal programme for Chinese first-time mothers: a randomized controlled trial. *Int J Nurs Stud.* 2015;52:22-29.

100. Angheiescu IG, Kohnen R, Szegedi A, Klement S, Kieser M. Comparison of hypericum extract WS 5570 and paroxetine in ongoing treatment after recovery from an episode of moderate to severe depression: results from a randomized multicenter study. *Pharmacopsychiatry.* 2006;39:213-219.

101. Van Gurp G, Meterissian GB, Haiek LN, McCusker J, Bellavance F. St. John's wort or sertraline? Randomized controlled trial in primary care. *Can Fam Physician.* 2002;48:905-912.

102. Klier CM, Schmid-Siegel B, Schafer MR, et al. St. John's wort (*Hypericum perforatum*) and breastfeeding: plasma and breast milk concentrations of hyperforin for 5 mothers and 2 infants. *J Clin Psychiatry.* 2006;67:305-309.

103. Schultz V. Safety of St. John's wort extract compared to synthetic antidepressants. *Phytomedicine.* 2006;13:199-204.

Suggested Reading

American Botanical Council. *The Commission E Monographs*. Austin, TX: American Botanical Council; 2017. http://cms.herbalgram.org /commissione/index.html.

Beck CT, Driscoll JW, Watson S. *Traumatic Childbirth*. Abington, UK: Routledge; 2018.

Hale TW, Rowe HE. *Medications and Mothers' Milk*. 17th ed. New York, NY: Springer; 2017.

Kendall-Tackett KA. *Depression in New Mothers*. 3rd ed. Abington, UK: Routledge; 2017.

Kendall-Tackett KA. *A Breastfeeding-Friendly Approach to Postpartum Depression*. Amarillo, TX: Praeclarus Press; 2015.

Kendall-Tackett KA, Ruglass LM, eds. *Women's Mental Health across the Lifespan*. New York, NY: Routledge; 2017.

Ruglass LM, Kendall-Tackett KA. *Psychology of Trauma 101*. New York, NY: Springer; 2016.

Seng J, Taylor J. *Trauma-Informed Care in the Perinatal Period*. Edinburgh, UK: Dunedin Academic Press; 2015.

Wenzel A. *Anxiety in Childbearing Women: Diagnosis and Treatment*. Washington, DC: American Psychological Association; 2011.

Additional Resources

Association for Behavioral and Cognitive Therapies. www.abct.org.

Breastfeeding Made Simple. Seven Natural Laws for Nursing Mothers. www.breastfeedingmadesimple.com.

Information for Mothers on Postpartum Depression, Trauma, and Treatment Options

International Society of Interpersonal Psychotherapy. www.interpersonalpsychotherapy.org.

National Alliance on Mental Illness. www.nami.org.

National Association of Cognitive-Behavioral Therapists. www.nacbt.org.

Postpartum Support International. www.postpartum.net.

Resources for Those Who May Be Experiencing Prenatal or Postnatal Mood or Anxiety Disorders

Kathleen Kendall-Tackett, PhD, IBCLC, FAPA. Information about depression, sexual abuse, breastfeeding, and other women's issues is presented in articles, video clips, and other educational materials. http://www.kathleenkendall-tackett.com.

United States Pharmacopeial Convention. Information about the quality, safety, and benefit of medicines and foods, including information about specific brands of fish oil products. www.usp.org.

UppityScienceChick.com. http://uppitysciencechick.com.

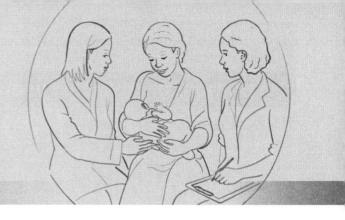

CHAPTER 19

Induced Lactation and Relactation

Virginia Thorley

OBJECTIVES

- Define induced lactation and relactation.
- Discuss the historical basis and cultural issues of induced lactation and relactation.
- List the indications for inducing lactation and relactation.
- Identify infant-related factors that influence the outcome of induced lactation.
- Describe the hormonal and physiological changes required for lactation to occur nonpuerperally.
- Describe physical and other nonpharmaceutical actions that can assist in inducing lactation and relactation.
- Describe the use of medications that are sometimes prescribed to support induced lactation and relactation.
- Describe current evidence on the efficacy and safety of nonpharmaceutical substances that are used as galactagogues.
- Describe the management of induced lactation and relactation.

DEFINITIONS OF COMMONLY USED TERMS

autocrine control The separate control of milk production in each breast in direct response to stimulation and milk removal, rather than dependence on endocrine control.[1]

galactagogue Pharmaceutical or herbal preparation used with the belief that it will increase milk production.

gestational surrogacy The carrying of a pregnancy by another woman on behalf of the intended parents.

(continues)

303

induced lactation The purposeful stimulation of lactation when it was previously absent, usually in the absence of a pregnancy in the months immediately prior to the induction of lactation (nonpuerperally). Also includes adoptive breastfeeding when a parent who is not breastfeeding induces lactation, whether or not having breastfed in the past.[2]

relactation Resumed lactation in a parent who has previously breastfed the same baby (that is, reversing weaning). Also, reestablishing lactation for a biological child the parent has never breastfed following the suppression of lactation postpartum. May also indicate a parent who has lactated in the past and is inducing lactation for another child.[3] The term is used generically for any type of induced lactation,[2] and sometimes includes reversing a significant decrease or lag in milk production.[4,5]

Any use of the term *mother, maternal,* or *breastfeeding* is not meant to exclude transgender or nonbinary parents who may be breastfeeding or providing human milk to their infant.

▶ Overview

Breast development and maturation during pregnancy are the usual precursors to lactation. However, both the historical and the contemporary literature demonstrate that a parent can produce milk without the preparatory effect of pregnancy and birth, that is, nonpuerperally. After breast and nipple stimulation is commenced, the breasts feel full and tender, leading to milk secretion if the stimulation is maintained. Induced lactation and relactation have occurred and continue to occur with an unknown prevalence in indigenous societies,[6,7] in developing countries,[8-10] and in the developed world.[11,12] Nonpuerperal lactation has also been described in animals, both female and male, in response to suckling.[13,14]

Where the society or the family has a strong breastfeeding culture, some parents easily resume lactation after a gap in milk production for a number of reasons, while others induce lactation for a baby not born to them. In 1997, the importance of context in relation to different outcomes in different settings was first raised.[15] Some consider nonpuerperal lactation to be a normal physiological response of the breasts to suckling.[16] Interest in induced lactation and relactation appears to have paralleled the increased interest in breastfeeding in developed countries. Where breastfeeding is accepted as the norm in the social milieu, the normal course of lactation in individual parents may differ from the stereotype of exclusive breastfeeding, followed sequentially by mixed feeding and weaning. Thus, breastfeeding can follow a number of other patterns (see **TABLE 19-1**), with the first weaning followed by one or more episodes of partial or exclusive breastfeeding.[10,17]

I. Research in Relactation and Induced Lactation

A. Most larger observational studies are not recent. The largest is a report of 1,000 consecutive cases of healthy mothers and their biological infants younger than 6 weeks of age in India; 83.4 percent achieved complete relactation, and 8.2 percent achieved partial relactation, within 10 days.[18]

B. A classic study[19] included both relactation and adoptive breastfeeding by 606 U.S. and Canadian women with a wide range of infant and maternal histories; the 366 women who were relactating and the 240 adoptive mothers were also described in separate articles.[20,21] Irrespective of milk yield, two thirds of the women considered the experience to be positive, defining their own success.[20]

C. One retrospective study[22] included 65 adoptive mothers in North America who induced lactation. In another study of Papua New Guinean women,[6] 89 percent of the 27 who completed a lactation induction program achieved adequate lactation and breastfed for 9 months or longer. They included 12 women who had never previously lactated, 11 of whom completed the program and achieved adequate lactation.

D. Most recent reports have comprised single cases or small case series.[23] However, one study[10] reported on successful relactation in 85.8 percent of 381 mothers who had infants aged 2 to 22 weeks and defined success as substantial (partial) or exclusive breastfeeding.

TABLE 19-1 Patterns in Human Lactation

Pattern[a]	Type
EBF → MF → W	Classic physiological breastfeeding pattern after delivery of an infant
MF → W	Initial difficulties followed by weaning
MF → EBF → MF → W	Progression to classic pattern after initial difficulties
EBF → MF → W_n → MF → W	One or more temporary weanings (W_n) followed by relactation[17]
EBF → MF → W → MF → W	Pattern involving relactation
EBF → MF → EBF → MF → W	Pattern involving relactation
MF → W → MF → EBF → MF → W	Pattern involving relactation
MF → W → MF → W	Pattern involving relactation
NBF → MF → EBF → MF → W	Pattern associated with both adoptive breastfeeding and establishing breastfeeding for the parent's biological child who was not initially breastfed
NBF → MF → W	Pattern associated with both adoptive breastfeeding and establishing breastfeeding for the parent's biological child who was not initially breastfed

[a] Patterns: EBF, exclusive breastfeeding; MF, mixed feeding or partial breastfeeding; NBF, never breastfed; W, weaned

E. Since the classic studies and a more recent dissertation,[3,24] most reports of purposeful lactation induction after adoption or gestational surrogacy concern single cases.[25,26]
  1. In 2002, the first known report of lactation induction for a baby born through gestational surrogacy was published.[26]
  2. Recently, a case of lactation induction for preterm twins born of surrogacy was reported, with supplemented breastfeeding achieved.[27]
  3. In both of these reports, galactagogues were used in addition to nonpharmaceutical methods. The Newman-Goldfarb Protocols for Induced Lactation were developed specifically for parents expecting babies via gestational surrogacy or adoption. It involves advanced preparation, with medications and pumping to begin the intended parent's milk production.
F. Rarely have studies randomized mothers to compare groups that use, or do not use, pharmaceutical medications.
  1. One study[28] showed high rates of complete relactation (92 percent) and partial relactation (6 percent) in 50 mothers who were randomized to suckling alone or suckling plus metoclopramide. Both groups received intensive support.
  2. Randomized controlled trials of induced lactation or relactation otherwise are lacking. In some situations, ethical considerations and recruitment would likely prove a barrier to acceptable study design.

II. **Physiological Mechanisms**

A. In the absence of a pregnancy, mammary stimulation triggers the release of prolactin and facilitates proliferation of secretory tissue, enabling milk secretion to occur.[29,30]
B. Suckling or milk expression, or other nipple and areola stimulation, stimulates both prolactin secretion and the release of oxytocin, and it is the most important factor in inducing lactation.[29,31]

C. Milk removal enables milk secretion to continue, through autocrine control of each breast, similar to the maintenance stage of lactation after a birth (lactogenesis III).[1]

D. Confidence building and ongoing support are important to the release of oxytocin by the posterior pituitary because the process can be inhibited by stress.

E. Oxytocin release can become a conditioned response.[32]

III. Inducing Lactation or Relactating

A. Induced lactation and relactation are recommended to prevent or reduce infant mortality and morbidity in humanitarian emergency situations, such as during natural disasters, warfare, or civil strife.[33,34]

B. Some individuals who induce lactation or relactate achieve full milk production, while others are able to breastfeed with supplementation for an extended period of time.[6,8,35]

C. Induced lactation is practiced in numerous cultures.

1. Parents wish to induce lactation for numerous reasons:

    a. To normalize the arrival of a child when adopting or fostering a baby (or a child of any age), or to create the closeness of breastfeeding, sometimes referred to as adoptive breastfeeding.[25,29] The biological mother may breastfeed while the adoptive parent is establishing lactation.[6]

    b. To simulate the experience of biological parenting and develop a close parent–infant relationship.[36]

    c. To optimize the baby's health or give a debilitated infant a chance at survival (e.g., during a natural disaster).

    d. To nourish an infant if the biological parent is unable to breastfeed.[37]

    e. To create kinship by milk for a child who is fostered or adopted in an Islamic culture, to fully integrate the child into the family.[38-40]

    f. When an adoptive child seeks the comfort of the breast, or the parent (sometimes grandparent) suckles to comfort a distressed child at the breast.[6,41]

    g. To breastfeed a baby born to a gestational surrogate.[3] The gestational surrogate (birth mother) may initially breastfeed while the intended parent is establishing lactation, thus accustoming the child to breastfeeding and providing optimum nutrition.

2. Parents may or may not know when they will receive an adopted child.

    a. It is often difficult to predict the date when the baby will be received,[29] especially with overseas adoptions.

    b. The baby may arrive on short notice, reducing preparation time. Or there may be a longer wait than anticipated.

    c. With the following exceptions, most parents do not receive their adopted babies at or soon after birth:

        i. Following the birth of a baby through a gestational surrogate.

        ii. Traditional adoptions, such as indigenous adoptions or open adoptions within a family.

3. It is helpful to learn about the child's feeding, including the following, prior to placement:

    a. The type of milk the child is being fed at present and whether it is an appropriate choice.

    b. The current feeding method (e.g., wet nursed, fed by bottle, fed by cup).

D. Relactation is practiced for a variety of reasons:

1. To recommence breastfeeding after weaning.

2. To ameliorate an infant health problem, such as the following, that occurred after early weaning:

    a. Diarrheal disease, other illnesses, malnutrition, or constipation.[10,42]

    b. Proven or suspected intolerance or allergy to artificial baby milks.

3. When the situation that led to weaning, or failure to initiate breastfeeding, has been overcome or ameliorated.

4. Breast or nipple conditions,[43,44] illness, or separation of the dyad.[23,42]

5. Unsupportive hospital practices that impacted breastfeeding initiation in the postnatal period or led to early replacement feeding.[45,46]

6. Infant conditions such as prematurity,[5] oral–facial anomalies,[42] malnutrition,[30] severe gastroenteritis and dehydration,[45] or hospitalization.[10]

7. The child wishes to resume breastfeeding following weaning.[12,15]

IV. Parent Expectations and Support

A. Ascertain the parent's expectations and how breastfeeding success is defined.
   1. Emphasize the breastfeeding relationship, facilitated by skin-to-skin contact, and realistic levels of achievement.[25]
   2. Determine the parent's expectations about the ability to produce milk.
      a. Success is best defined as how the parent feels about the experience, irrespective of the milk yield.[17]
      b. Avoid suggesting a specific time frame because of individual variation and the numerous parent and baby factors involved.[42]
      c. Some parents will achieve exclusive breastfeeding or breastmilk feeding,[25,35] while others will not and will need reassurance that there are different kinds of success.
   3. Explain that two partners are involved: the parent and the baby. Focus on having the baby learn to accept and actively suckle the breast, and encourage realistic levels of achievement in a positive manner.
B. Provide counseling and support to parents.
   1. Ascertain and build on the parent's level of breastfeeding confidence.[47] Low confidence, lack of support, and infrequent suckling have been associated with poorer outcomes in adoptive parents.[8]
   2. Provide regular telephone or online video contact through a service such as Skype, which may be appropriate forms of professional support.[46]
   3. Explore cultural factors, recognizing that cultural context is important to the quality of support and expectations.[40,48,49]
      a. Identify any cultural or community barriers to breastfeeding, such as beliefs about modesty and the ability to breastfeed away from home.
      b. Assess the family's support system.
      c. Explore any religious beliefs regarding breastmilk and breastfeeding that affect family relationships (milk kinship), including relationships of this baby.
   4. Ensure that there is adequate support.
      a. Provide appropriate and intensive support from a knowledgeable healthcare worker.[10,42] Parents need support, encouragement, and appropriate information from a lactation consultant or other healthcare professionals, with an emphasis on confidence building.[10,18,25]
      b. Facilitate support from professional and lay sources, including psychological support and household assistance from the other parent or partner and the family.[10,18,25,46]
      c. Help adoptive parents find an online support group for adoptive breastfeeding parents to help normalize the experience.
      d. Parents may receive little support or outright discouragement from adoption agencies, centers for surrogate parenting, family members, and friends.
   5. Encourage building the trust of the baby, especially an older baby, before offering the breast.[11,41] The breast can become a place of comfort where the baby feels safe.
   6. In one case study,[27] visualization of effective breastfeeding was used in conjunction with other stimuli.
   7. Finding the time to achieve milk production can be challenging with competing demands of other children, existing health concerns, or employment.[50]
   8. See **BOX 19-1** for tips in counseling parents who are inducing lactation or relactating.

BOX 19-1 Clinical Implications of Counseling

- Counseling and ongoing support are especially valuable when inducing lactation or relactating.
- Optimal support involves both professional and lay input.
- Proactive support, such as contacting the parent regularly instead of waiting for a call, is recommended.
- Information and support are available from websites that are specific to adoptive breastfeeding and relactation.

V. History and Assessment

A. Explore the parent's reproductive history.
1. The number and duration of pregnancies and births, and how long ago they occurred, can be a factor. One study[3] found a positive association between peak milk volume and at least one birth, compared to pregnancy alone.
2. A history suggestive of infertility, hormonal imbalance, polycystic ovary syndrome, assisted conception technology, thyroid or pituitary disorders, or physical anomalies may impact success with achieving milk production.
3. Provide anticipatory guidance about possible menstrual cessation or irregularities resulting from establishing lactation.
B. Inquire about previous breastfeeding experience.
1. Assess the parent's level of knowledge about breastfeeding management.
2. Determine how many children were breastfed and the length of time for each.
   a. In the largest American study,[21] individuals who never lactated experienced more difficulty with inducing milk flow. In a case series,[6] there was no disadvantage.
   b. If the previous breastfeeding experience was with an adopted baby, counsel the parent that the experience with another adopted baby may be different.
3. If the mother has breastfed, be aware of the following factors:
   a. Explore any previous breastfeeding difficulties and whether they were resolved.
   b. If weaning preceded a wish to relactate, ask about the reason for weaning and the age of the child.
   c. Determine the length of time since previous breastfeeding occurred.
      i. A short lactation gap has been positively associated with a high percentage of milk flow and exclusive breastfeeding in relactating mothers.[10,45]
      ii. An observational study of 1,000 mothers with lactation gaps of 1 to 45 days reported relactation in 97.6 percent of the mothers within 10 days, with 83.4 percent completely meeting their infants' needs.[18]
      iii. A longer lactation gap is usually associated with a longer time to achieve milk production,[42,45,51] although study authors differ in their definition of *longer*.
      iv. The literature is divided on the significance of the gap in lactation; infant factors may be more of an influence. A long lactation gap, even months or years, has not been an obstacle in other reports.[6,42]
C. Explore the infant's current health status, including the following:
1. Birth details (e.g., vaginal, forceps, vacuum extraction, cesarean, birth asphyxia).
2. Health history, current growth, developmental status, prematurity, tongue tie, other oral anomalies, hypertonic bite, developmental lag, neurological issues, and whether the infant is strong enough to suckle.
3. Factors that may positively or negatively impact efforts to breastfeed (e.g., an irritable, inconsolable baby).[52]
D. Assess the breasts and nipples. (See Chapter 20, *Breast Pathology.*)
1. Assess the physical characteristics of the breasts that may make inducing milk production a greater challenge.[53,54]
2. Assess the size and shape of the nipples and areolae for factors that may affect the baby's latch and the positioning of the baby at the breast.
3. Be alert to nipple and breast changes, including fullness, and address any nipple or breast pain.

VI. Initiating Milk Production

A. Assist with encouraging the infant to suckle at the breast.
1. If relactation is initiated by an older baby or a child who is an experienced breastfeeder[12] and who is eating semisolid complementary foods daily, little assistance may be required other than reassurance.
2. Early rejection of the breast need not mean the baby will always refuse.
3. Age can be a factor in a baby's acceptance of breastfeeding.

a. The older the child is when introduced to the breast, the greater the possibility of unwillingness to suckle, unless the child is being breastfed by the biological mother or a foster mother at the time of adoption or has previously been breastfed.

b. Newborns and babies younger than 8 weeks are most likely to suckle willingly.[20] This may be because sucking is initially reflexive, and it changes to a voluntary action by about 3 months of age.[55]

c. Infants older than 2 months may resist or respond negatively when put to the breast.[20] Some infants may require techniques similar to those that help resolve breast refusal. (See Chapter 16, *Breastfeeding and Growth: Birth through Weaning.*)

d. Babies older than 6 months are likely to require patience in the gradual process of introducing the breast, with the need to first establish trust.[41]

e. In babies older than 9 months, their personality may influence their willingness to accept breastfeeding attempts. In the case of adoption, high-quality foster care prior to adoption (versus negative care with little physical contact) may be an influence.[11]

f. Children, including toddlers, who have previously breastfed may seek the breast of their own accord.[12,41]

B. Optimize the baby's willingness to go to the breast.

1. Begin skin-to-skin contact when the baby is not showing hunger cues and is still sleepy.

2. Put the baby to the breast while sleepy and not fully awake, and use other techniques associated with breast refusal. Early breast refusal is not predictive; infants who initially reject the breast may later learn to accept it.[20] (See Chapter 16, *Breastfeeding and Growth: Birth through Weaning,* for techniques to encourage a reluctant baby to breastfeed.)

3. Avoid all practices that limit the close body contact and very frequent suckling that support relactation and induced lactation. This includes rigid timing of feeding attempts and separation of the parent and baby, including in a baby carriage or buggy.

4. Encourage optimal latch and breastfeeding techniques to maximize stimulation and milk removal.[18,56]

5. Discontinue the use of bottles and pacifiers so that all suckling is done at the breast.[9,21] Use a feeding tube, syringe, or cup to provide supplements.[37]

6. Dropping milk onto the areola may encourage the baby to suck.[9,57] Doing this to reward each suck can encourage further sucking and reduce frustration.[36]

7. A feeding tube can be used to provide a flow of milk while the baby suckles at the breast.[30,42] (See Chapter 24, *Breastfeeding Devices and Topical Treatments.*)

a. Whether the device is purchased or homemade, it stimulates the breasts and provides a breastfeeding experience for the baby; at the same time, it eliminates the use of bottle nipples.

b. While they learn to use the device, parents benefit from both professional and partner support.[58]

C. Assist with breast stimulation in preparation for breastfeeding.

1. Nipple and breast stimulation may help with the development and maturation of breast tissue prior to breastfeeding[21,30] and for maintaining lactation.

2. In the case of adoption, nipple stimulation every 3 to 4 hours through gentle stroking and rolling can begin about 4 weeks prior to receiving the baby.[29] Breast massage and the application of warmth are also useful.[29]

3. Many parents have achieved milk production by suckling the baby intensively at the breast, usually with, but sometimes without, manual stimulation of the breast and nipples.[17,18,42] The baby suckling at the breast may be the sole or main stimulus.[10,33]

4. Some researchers found no difference in relactation outcomes between mothers who used only breast and nipple hyperstimulation (very frequent suckling) and those who used metoclopramide (a galactagogue) in addition to frequent suckling.[51,59]

5. Back massage, up and down both sides of the spinal column, has been used to enhance oxytocin release in conjunction with stimulation of the breasts and nipples.[42]

D. Assist with milk expression.

1. Milk expression sessions may start with only a few minutes, according to comfort, and build up to a maximum of 15 to 25 minutes.

a. Express as frequently as a newborn would breastfeed (8 to 12 times per 24 hours),[37] with one or more expressions at night.

b. Express at least six times per 24 hours, for 15 minutes per breast.[25]

2. Simultaneous bilateral pumping with a portable hospital-grade electric pump saves time, compared to other pumping options. There is no difference in milk yield for simultaneous bilateral pumping versus single sequential pumping.[60]

3. Teach and assess the parent's ability to hand express.[61]

   a. Manual expression has been shown to extract colostrum more effectively than a hospital-grade breast pump alone in postnatal women.[56,62]

   b. Manual expression is appropriate for the low volume of fluid in the early stages of inducing lactation so that none is wasted on pump surfaces.

4. After the child accepts the breast, expressing can be gradually discontinued and replaced with frequent suckling. Monitor the child's growth, as well as urinary and fecal output. (See Chapter 16, *Breastfeeding and Growth: Birth through Weaning.*)

E. Galactagogues may assist with the initiation of milk production.

1. Healthcare providers are frequently asked for information about the use of galactagogues to increase milk production. They may recommend specific pharmaceutical or botanical medications for this purpose despite the lack of strong evidence about the efficacy and safety of many products.[63-66] (See Chapter 22, *Low Milk Production and Infant Weight.*)

2. Galactagogues are sometimes used to assist with inducing lactation.[6,35] They are appropriately used only after optimizing the infant's latch and the parent's expression technique for breast stimulation and milk removal.

3. Parents have induced lactation or relactation through breast stimulation alone;[8,48] however, in a contemporary Western context, it is common to use hormonal medications and domperidone.[3] (See Chapter 5, *Lactation Pharmacology.*)

4. Instead of using galactagogues, many parents have induced lactation or relactation solely by expressing or by putting their baby to the breast, or combining this with nipple and breast stimulation.[8,10]

F. Hormonal medications are sometimes used to assist with inducing lactation for an adopted child.[6,35]

1. Estrogen and progesterone in an oral contraceptive pill should be started as many weeks as possible before the adoption.[6,23,25] Breastfeeding or expressing begins when the oral contraceptive pill is discontinued.

   a. Caution is advised because of the potential risk of venous thrombosis associated with high doses of estrogen, or estrogen combinations, and older age.[67] Ongoing medical supervision is essential.

   b. Parents who plan to induce lactation for infants born through gestational surrogacy are typically older than 35 years, and they may be older than 40 years or even much older.[68,69]

   c. Parents with a history of venous thrombosis should avoid hormone treatment.[70] The risk of venous thrombosis may be increased with long-distance air travel, which is a factor if the child is adopted from overseas.

2. The hormone oxytocin stimulates the milk ejection reflex by acting on receptors in the breast. It stimulates the contraction of the myoepithelial cells surrounding the alveoli and forces the milk out.[1] (See Chapter 6, *Breast Anatomy and Milk Production.*)

   a. Synthetic oxytocin, usually administered as an intranasal spray, has been used to help milk ejection.

   b. Suckling or other nipple stimulation and skin-to-skin contact cause the release of oxytocin from the hypothalamus without using pharmaceuticals.[1,70]

   c. Synthetic forms of oxytocin should be used only after milk is present and it has been determined that the milk ejection reflex is ineffective.

   d. Intranasal spray should be limited to the first week postpartum.[71] In induced lactation, it is reasonable to extrapolate this to the first week after milk is present beyond a few drops, although this has not been studied.

   e. Oxytocin intranasal spray is not likely to affect milk yield because this is not its purpose.[72]

VII. When Milk Production Begins

A. Some parents may not have breast secretions prior to putting the baby to the breast.

B. Parents who have previously breastfed are more likely to have colostrum or milk after manual or mechanical stimulation, although the difference is not always significant.

C.   The first drops of liquid in the absence of a baby can be expected after a few days to a few weeks of preparation.
  1.   According to case reports, the secretion may initially be yellow or gold and colostrum-like, and it can continue for days or longer before becoming opaque.[23,26]
  2.   With tandem breastfeeding (continuing to breastfeed an older baby along with a new baby), milk is already available. Anecdotally, it may change to colostrum, though studies have yet to be conducted.[23]
  3.   If the baby is suckling effectively, milk may be evident earlier, but there is wide individual variation. Consequently, it is advisable to not provide an estimate for how long this will take.
D.   Teach parents to recognize the signs of milk transfer. (See Chapter 13, *Facilitating and Assessing Breastfeeding Initiation*.)
  1.   Numerous case series and case studies have noted normal infant growth on human milk produced after induced lactation[6] or relactation,[8,10,46] including weight-for-age growth in three infants of HIV-infected mothers who had never breastfed prior to relactating.[50]
  2.   Relactation has been used to correct poor growth in weaned infants.[17]

VIII.   Milk Composition Following Induced Lactation and Relactation

A.   Milk composition following induced lactation has been shown in bovine and rat species to be similar to milk produced after pregnancy and delivery.[37]
B.   Few studies have focused specifically on the nutritional and immunological composition of milk produced in induced lactation or relactation.
  1.   Investigations of the milk composition of adoptive mothers involve only a handful of cases.
  2.   Biochemical research on milk composition after induced lactation is still very limited and contradictory because the methodologies differ.
    a.   A pilot study examined the milk of two women who had induced lactation without a pregnancy and who provided weekly samples for 2 months.[73] The concentrations of total protein, secretory immunoglobulin A, lactoferrin, and lysozyme were similar or greater, compared to the mature milk after giving birth.
    b.   In one case report, the biological mother secreted colostrum for 2 weeks after beginning relactation at 9 weeks postpartum.[23] Additionally, her sister, while breastfeeding the biological mother's child along with her own infant and a toddler, produced a colostrum-like milk for 1 month.
    c.   These reports differ from two small case series of adoptive mothers who reported the absence of a colostral stage, and protein values that approximated those of transitional milk, indicating there is individual variation.[74,75]

IX.   Feeding the Baby

A.   Supplementation is essential for the baby's well-being while milk production is being established or reestablished.
  1.   Insufficient milk for the baby's needs may necessitate continued supplementation. Worry about the baby getting enough milk or self-doubt can lead to stress, and reassurance is needed that continued supplements are commonly required.
  2.   If banked human milk is not available, artificial formula should be continued. Mixed feeding with artificial formula or age-appropriate complementary foods may be an achievable goal.
B.   A combination of supplementation methods has been used.[4]
  1.   Eliminating or decreasing the use of bottles and artificial nipples (including pacifiers), and putting the child to the breast frequently, will help increase milk production.[37]
    a.   In a study of 381 cases, establishing milk production for infants who had previously been supplemented with bottles took longer than for those fed with other devices.[10]
    b.   A number of papers report that infant refusal was overcome by frequent suckling in which bottle use was avoided and supplementation was done at the breast, including the drop-and-drip technique.[20]
    c.   In an Egyptian study, bottle feeding of expressed milk failed to address breast refusal for 30 percent of the mothers, leading to abandonment of relactation.[46]

    d.   Additional nourishment can be provided with a feeding tube at the breast, or with a cup or syringe after breastfeeding.[37]

    e.   Expressed milk can be given as a drink or mixed in other food, even if the child never accepts suckling at the breast.

    f.   If the baby is accustomed to being bottle fed with a fast flow, introduce bottle nipples with a slower flow to accustom the baby to receiving milk more slowly.

    g.   If a bottle is preferred, teach the parent how to pace the feeds and pause several times. (See Chapter 24, *Breastfeeding Devices and Topical Treatments,* for a discussion of paced bottle feeding and devices discussed in this section.)

2.   The use of a supplemental feeding tube at the breast provides both breast stimulation and food for the baby.

    a.   The baby uses one type of oral motor action, reducing any potential confusion between the breast and the bottle.

    b.   A temporary supplementer is easy to make at home; commercially available supplementers are also available.

3.   A small, soft feeding cup, syringe, or local equivalent can be used for supplements. Teach the parent to cup-feed the baby in an upright position.

    a.   Offer the supplement only after the baby has suckled at the breast.

    b.   Offer the supplement after every second feed, provided the breastfeedings are every 2 hours or more frequently.

    c.   Feed the baby exclusively on the breast at night, if the breastfeeding parent and baby are sleeping in close proximity so feeding can occur as needed.

C.   Decreasing supplementation requires regular contact with relevant members of the healthcare team (lactation consultant, physician, child health nurse) for guidance.

1.   Use the infant's output and growth as guides for decreasing supplements and other foods as appropriate.

2.   Do not keep the baby hungry in an attempt to encourage suckling at the breast. This is counterproductive because the baby becomes weak and less effective at suckling.

3.   To ensure adequate nutrition, do not dilute the supplementary milk or restrict the amounts of supplements.

4.   If the baby's output lessens or if the growth rate falters, temporarily increase the supplement.

5.   Replace milk expression with additional breastfeeds; however, expression after some feeds may be necessary for additional stimulation if the baby is weak and suckles poorly.

6.   Gradually reduce the use of galactagogues, if any are used.

7.   Some babies will require supplementation for the duration of breastfeeding (see **BOX 19-2**).

BOX 19-2 Evidence-Informed Practice: Herbal Medications and Dietary Supplements

- Herbal and dietary supplements are commonly recommended to breastfeeding parents by healthcare practitioners, despite the lack of strong evidence.[64]
- Most information is anecdotal and consists of case reports or listings of commonly used herbs and foods and their usual dosages. For most of these substances there is only weak evidence of their safety and efficacy as galactagogues.[76]
- Poor methodology, wide inconsistency in what is measured, and small numbers of participants limit the value of most existing studies.[64-66]
- In the absence of well-conducted randomized controlled trials, the placebo effect of specific herbal medications and supplementary foods used as galactagogues cannot be ruled out.[56]
- Many cultures believe that specific herbal or dietary supplements, or increasing fluid intake, will stimulate milk production, but evidence to support this claim is either conflicting or lacking.
- Literature reviews that source only English-language studies may miss information that is available elsewhere.
- Well-designed randomized controlled trials are needed to investigate the effects of herbal and dietary supplements on milk production so lactation professionals can make evidence-based recommendations.[56,64,66]
- Future research should include parents of normal babies born at term, not only preterm babies.

▶ **Key Points from This Chapter**

A.   Investigate the causes of breastfeeding cessation and ascertain if they have been treated or eliminated.

B.   Provide appropriate counseling and ongoing professional and lay support to the parent.

C.   Eliminate bottles and pacifiers (dummies, soothers).

D.   While additional nutrition is needed, supplement the baby in ways other than by bottle.

E.   Supplements may continue to be needed to provide adequate hydration and growth.

F.   Provide manual stimulation to the breasts and nipples, beginning with about 3 times per day, increasing to 8 to 12 times or the age-appropriate number of times that an infant would breastfeed in 24 hours.

G.   In the absence of the baby (e.g., if the baby is hospitalized), manual stimulation should include breast massage, nipple stimulation, and hand expression.

H.   Industrial quality electric breast pumps, if available, may be used to stimulate the breasts after colostrum or milk is present.

I.   The best stimulation is the suckling of a well-attached baby at the breast.

🔍 *CASE STUDY*

Caroline breastfed five biological children for more than 12 months each; the last child breastfed for 2 years. At age 50, Caroline adopted a newborn after a 9-year lactation gap. This was an open adoption within the extended family, and Caroline had a positive support network of family members and professionals.

Ten weeks before the baby's anticipated birth, Caroline started taking domperidone, herbal medications (fenugreek, blessed thistle), and the dietary supplements brewer's yeast and Super B. Two weeks later, Caroline began hand expressing and pumping, and she applied a wheat hot pack to her breasts before pumping. She expressed four or five times per day, then increased expression to six or seven times, along with nipple stimulation many times per day and breast massage three times per day. Sticky yellow colostrum soon appeared. Caroline reported feeling emotionally down, which has been noted anecdotally, although there is no evidence from studies. Six days before she received the baby, her daily milk yield was 35 mL from six expressions. Better results were reported from hand expression than with two electric pumps. Caroline preferred to start with a smaller electric pump and then switch to hand expression.

Caroline first breastfed the baby girl immediately after delivery in a private hospital. She roomed in with the birth mother and baby, and she reported feeling very confident, with strong support from family members, friends, hospital staff members, and a bright, inquisitive baby. Her breasts began filling with milk on the second day at the hospital. Caroline breastfed first, then used a supplemental tube with a bottle and breastfed again. At 11 days, the baby had gained 330 g (11.6 oz), followed by a gain of 550 g (19.4 oz) in the next 2 weeks. There was one night feed, consisting of breastfeeding plus a supplement of 50 mL. Caroline continued to take domperidone and the other tablets. The duration of substantial breastfeeding was 3 months. At 4 months, the baby was bottle fed but kept going to the breast for comfort. Caroline was pleased with the outcome because she enjoyed breastfeeding and had established a close bond with her adopted baby.

Questions

1.   What does this case teach with regard to arbitrary age limits for women to induce lactation?
2.   Which of the methods used to stimulate lactation before receiving the baby were evidence based?
3.   How did Caroline's sources of support impact her outcome?
4.   Caroline considered her outcome to be successful. How did she measure her success?

References

1.   Lee S, Kelleher SL. Biological underpinnings of breastfeeding challenges: the role of genetics, diet, and environment on lactation physiology. *Am J Physiol Endocrinol Metab.* 2016;311(2):E405-E422.

2.   Thorley V. *Relactation and Induced Lactation: Bibliography and Resources.* Rev ed. Brisbane, Australia: Virginia Thorley; 2010.

3.   Goldfarb L. *An Assessment of the Experiences of Women Who Induced Lactation.* Cincinnati, OH: Union Institute and University; 2010.

4.   de Aquino R, Osorio M. Relactation, translactation, and breast-orogastric tube as transition methods in feeding preterm babies. *J Hum Lactation.* 2009;25(4):420-426.

5.   Dehkhoda N, Valizadeh S, Jodeiry B, Hossein M. The effect of an educational and supportive relactation program on weight gain of preterm infants. *J Caring Sci.* 2013;2(2):99-103.

6.   Nemba K. Induced lactation: a study of 37 non-puerperal mothers. *J Trop Pediatr.* 1994;40:240-242.

7. Slome C. Non-puerperal lactation in grandmothers. *J Pediatr*. 1956;49:550-552.
8. Abejide O, Tadese M, Babajide D, et al. Non-puerperal induced lactation in a Nigerian community. Case reports. *Ann Trop Paediatr*. 1997;17:109-114.
9. Lakhkar B. Breastfeeding in adopted babies. *Indian Pediatr*. 2000;37:1114-1116.
10. Tomar R. Initiation of relactation: an army hospital based study of 381 cases. *Int J Contemp Pediatr*. 2016;3:635-638.
11. Australian Breastfeeding Association. *Breastfeeding: Relactation and Adoption*. 3rd ed. Melbourne, Australia: Australian Breastfeeding Association; 2015.
12. Phillips V. Relactation in mothers of children over 12 months. *J Trop Pediatr*. 1993;39:45-47.
13. Anonymous. Chemistry, pharmacy, and material medica: analysis of milk taken from a he-goat. *Lancet*. 1845;45(1115):38.
14. Archer M. Coming to grips with male nipples. *Aust Nat Hist*. 1990;23:494.
15. Thorley V. Relactation: what the exceptions can tell us. *Birth Issues*. 1997;6:24-29.
16. Mobbs G, Babbage N. Breast feeding adopted children. *Med J Aust*. 1971;2(8):436-437.
17. Marquis G, Diaz J, Bartolini R, et al. Recognizing the reversible nature of child-feeding decisions: breastfeeding, weaning and relactation patterns in a shanty town community of Lima, Peru. *Soc Sci Med*. 1998;47:645-656.
18. Banapurmath S, Banapurmath S, Kesaree N. Initiation of lactation and establishing relactation in outpatients. *Indian Pediatr*. 2003;40:343-347.
19. Auerbach K. Extraordinary breast feeding: relactation/induced lactation. *J Trop Pediatr*. 1981;27(1):52-55.
20. Auerbach K, Avery J. Relactation: a study of 366 cases. *Pediatrics*. 1980;65:236-242.
21. Auerbach K, Avery J. Induced lactation: a study of adoptive nursing and counseling in 240 women. *Am J Dis Child*. 1981;135:340-343.
22. Hormann E. Breastfeeding the adopted baby. *Birth Fam J*. 1977;4:165-172.
23. Muresan M. Successful relactation—a case study. *Breastfeeding Med*. 2011;6(8):233-239.
24. Goldfarb L. Results of a survey to assess the experiences of women who induce lactation. *J Hum Lactation*. 2012;28(1):83-84.
25. Szucs K, Axline S, Rosenman M. Induced lactation and exclusive breast milk feeding of adopted premature twins. *J Hum Lactation*. 2010;26(3):309-313.
26. Goldfarb L. The premature infant: a mother's perspective. Canadian Breastfeeding Foundation website. https://www.canadianbreastfeedingfoundation.org/basics/mothers_story_basics.shtml. Published 2002. Accessed September 15, 2017.
27. Farhadi R, Philip R. Induction of lactation in the biological mother after gestational surrogacy of twins: a novel approach and review of literature. *Breastfeeding Med*. 2017;12(6):373-376.
28. Seema, Patwari A, Satyanarayana L. Relactation: an effective intervention to promote exclusive breastfeeding. *J Trop Pediatr*. 1997;43:213-216.
29. Wittig S, Spatz D. Induced lactation: gaining a better understanding. *Maternal Child Nurs (MCN)*. 2008;33(2):76-81.
30. World Health Organization. *Infant and Young Child Feeding: Model Chapter for Textbooks for Medical and Allied Health Professionals*. Geneva, Switzerland: World Health Organization; 2009.
31. Zinaman M, Hughes V, Queenan J, et al. Acute prolactin and oxytocin response and milk yield to infant suckling and artificial methods of expressing in lactating women. *Pediatrics*. 1992;89:437-440.
32. Lawrence RA, Lawrence RM. Psychological impact of breastfeeding. In: Lawrence RA, Lawrence RM, eds. *Breastfeeding: A Guide for the Medical Profession*. 8th ed. Philadelphia, PA: Elsevier; 2016:194-213.
33. Branca F, Schultink W. Breastfeeding in emergencies: a question of survival. World Health Organization website. http://www.who.int/mediacentre/commentaries/breastfeeding-in-emergencies/en. Published May 20, 2016. Accessed October 14, 2017.
34. Carothers C, Gribble K. Infant and young child feeding in emergencies. *J Hum Lactation*. 2014;30(3):1-4.
35. Flores-Anton B, Garcia-Lara N, Pallas-Alonso C. An adoptive mother who became a human milk donor. *J Hum Lactation*. 2017;33(2):419-421.
36. Biervliet F, Maguiness S, Hay D, Killick S, Atkins S. Induction of lactation in the intended mother of a surrogate pregnancy. *Hum Reprod*. 2001;16:581-583.
37. Hormann E, Savage F. *Relactation: Review of Experience and Recommendations for Practice*. Geneva, Switzerland: World Health Organization; 1998.
38. Saari Z, Yusof F. Motivating factors to breastfeed an adopted child in a Muslim community in Malaysia. *Jurnal Teknologi*. 2015;74(1):205-214.
39. Thorley V. Milk siblingship, religious and secular: history, applications, and implications for practice. *Women Birth*. 2014;27:e16-e19.
40. Thorley V. Milk kinship and implications for human milk banking: a review. *Womens Health Bull*. 2016;3(3):e36897.
41. Gribble K. Mental health, attachment and breastfeeding: implications for adopted children and their mothers. *Int Breastfeeding J*. 2006;1(5). https://doi.org/10.1186/1746-4358-1-5
42. Agarwal S, Jain A. Early successful relactation in a case of prolonged lactation failure. *Indian J Pediatr*. 2010;77(2):214.
43. Kesaree N, Banapurmath C, Banapurmath S, Shamanur K. Treatment of inverted nipples using a disposable syringe. *J Hum Lactation*. 1993;9:27-29.
44. Wilson-Clay B. Case report of methicillin-resistant *Staphylococcus aureus* (MRSA) mastitis with abscess formation in a breastfeeding woman. *J Hum Lactation*. 2008;24(3):326-329.
45. De N, Pandit B, Mishra S, et al. Initiating the process of relactation: an institute based study. *Indian Pediatr*. 2002;39:173-178.
46. Abul-Fadi A, Kharbouch I, Fikry M, Adel M. Testing communications models for relactation in an Egyptian setting. *Breastfeeding Med*. 2012;7(4):248-254.
47. Persad M, Mensinger J. Maternal breastfeeding attitudes: association with breastfeeding intent and socio-demographics among urban primiparas. *J Community Health*. 2008;33(2):52-60.
48. Gribble K. The influence of context on the success for adoptive breastfeeding: developing countries and the west. *Breastfeeding Rev*. 2004;12(1):5-13.
49. Thorley V. Induced lactation and context. *Breastfeeding Rev*. 2004;12(3):27.
50. Nyati I, Kim H-Y, Gogo A, Violari A, Gray G. Support for relactation among mothers of HIV-infected children: a pilot study in Soweto. *Breastfeeding Med*. 2014;9:450-457.

51. Lakhkar B, Shenoy V, Bhaskaranand N. Relactation—Manipal experience. *Indian Pediatr.* 1999;36:700-703.

52. Lommen A, Brown B, Hollist D. Experimental perceptions of relactation: a phenomenological study. *J Hum Lactation.* 2015;31(3):495-503.

53. Arbour M, Kessler J. Mammary hypoplasia: not every breast can produce sufficient milk. *J Midwifery Womens Health.* 2013;58:457-461.

54. Duran M, Spatz D. A mother with glandular hypoplasia and a late preterm infant. *J Hum Lactation.* 2011;27:394-397.

55. Walker M. *Breastfeeding Management for the Clinician.* Sudbury, MA: Jones and Bartlett Publishers; 2006.

56. Academy of Breastfeeding Medicine Protocol Committee. ABM clinical protocol no. 9: use of galactogogues in initiating or augmenting the rate of maternal milk secretion (first revision January 2011). *Breastfeeding Med.* 2011;6:41-49.

57. Kesaree N. Drop and drip method. *Indian Pediatr.* 1993;30:277-278.

58. Borucki L. Breastfeeding mothers' experiences using a supplemental feeding tube device: finding an alternative. *J Hum Lactation.* 2005;21(4):429-438.

59. Banapurmath C, Banapurmath S, Kesaree N. Initiation of relactation. *Indian Pediatr.* 1993;30:1329-1332.

60. Becker G, Cooney F, Smith H. Methods of milk expression for lactating women. *Cochrane Database Syst Rev.* 2011;12:CD006170. doi:10.1002/14651858.CD006170.pub3.

61. Glynn L, Goosen L. Manual expression of breast milk. *J Hum Lactation.* 2005;21(2):184-185.

62. Ohyama M, Watabe H, Hayasaka Y. Manual expression and electric pumping in the first 48h after delivery. *Pediatr Int.* 2010;52:39-43.

63. Bazzano A, Littrell L, Brandt A, Thibeau S, Threimer K, Theall K. Health provider experiences with galactagogues to support breastfeeding. *J Multidisciplinary Healthcare.* 2016;9:623-630.

64. Schaffir J, Czapla C. Survey of lactation instructions on folk traditions in breastfeeding. *Breastfeeding Med.* 2012;17(4):230-233.

65. Mortel M, Mehta S. Systematic review of the efficacy of herbal galactogogues. *J Hum Lactation.* 2013;29(2):154-162.

66. Budzynska K, Gardner Z, Dugoua J-J, Low Dog T, Gardiner P. Systematic review of breastfeeding and herbs. *Breastfeeding Med.* 2012;7(7):489-503.

67. Oladapo O, Fawole B. Treatments for suppression of lactation. *Cochrane Database Syst Rev.* 2012;9:CD005937. doi:10.1002/14651858 .CD005937.pub3.

68. Arvidsson A, Johnsdottir S, Essen B. Views of Swedish commissioning parents relating to the exploitation discourse in using transnational surrogacy. *PLOS One.* 2015;10(5):e0126518. doi:10.1371/journal.pone.0126518.

69. Dar S, Lazar T, Swanson S, et al. Assisted reproduction involving gestational surrogacy: an analysis of the medical, psychosocial and legal issues: experience from a large surrogacy program. *Hum Reproduction.* 2015;30(2):345-352.

70. Martinelli I, Taiolo E, Battaglioli T, et al. Risk of venous thromboembolism after air travel: interaction with thrombophilia and oral contraceptives. *Arch Intern Med.* 2003; 163(22): 2771-2774. doi:10.1001/archinte.163.22.2771.

71. Hale T, Rowe H. *Medications and Mothers' Milk.* 17th ed. New York, NY: Springer Publishing Company; 2017.

72. Fewtrell M, Loh K, Blake A, et al. Randomised double blind trial of oxytocin nasal spray in mothers expressing breast milk for preterm infants. *Arch Dis Child.* 2006;91:F169-F174.

73. Perrin M, Wilson E, Chetwynd E, Fogelman A. A pilot study of the protein composition of induced nonpuerperal human milk. *J Hum Lactation.* 2015;31:166-171.

74. Kulski J, Hartmann P, Saint W, et al. Changes in milk composition of nonpuerperal women. *Am J Obstet Gynecol.* 1981;139:597-604.

75. Kleinman R, Jacobson L, Hormann E, Walker W. Protein values of milk samples from mothers without biologic pregnancies. *J Pediatr.* 1980;97:612-615.

76. Nice F. Selection and use of galactogogues. *Infant Child Adolesc Nutr.* 2015;7(4):192-194.

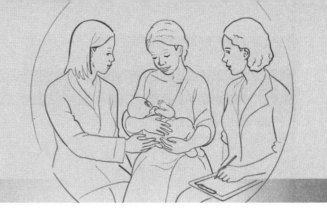

CHAPTER 20

Breast Pathology

Pamela D. Berens

OBJECTIVES

- Assess the breasts for growth, past surgery, anatomical challenges, nipple structure, and variations.
- Implement a breast assessment prior to conception, during pregnancy, and after birth to assess for adequate function.
- Manage pathological conditions of the breast, including painful or damaged nipples, blocked ducts, engorgement, mastitis, and yeast infection.
- Assess the breasts to determine if changes are consistent with adequate lactation function.
- Provide information and strategies to prevent and resolve nipple damage.
- Provide information and strategies to prevent and resolve engorgement, blocked ducts, and mastitis.

DEFINITIONS OF COMMONLY USED TERMS

allodynia Pain sensitization (increased responsiveness) following normally nonpainful and often repetitive stimulation.
ankyloglossia Tongue-tie; an unusually short, thick, or tight band of tissue that tethers the bottom of the tongue to the floor of the mouth and restricts the tongue's range of motion.
areola The pigmented portion of the breast surrounding the nipple.
axilla Armpit.
Cooper's ligaments Fibrous bands that fix the breast to underlying pectoral fascia.
eczema Skin condition characterized by itching; typically occurs in response to a topical irritant.
erythema Abnormal redness in the skin.
exudate Fluid that extrudes or seeps out of injured tissue.
fissure A division, split, or grove in tissue (in lactation, the term specifically refers to the nipple).
fluctuant Subject to change, variable, movable, compressible.
inferior pedicle technique Breast reduction surgery in which some portion of the breast remains intact.
mastitis Inflammation of the breast.
Montgomery glands Sebaceous glands within the areola, surrounding the nipple.
nipple bleb A small white spot on the tip of the nipple that looks like a tiny, milk-filled blister.

(continues)

DEFINITIONS OF COMMONLY USED TERMS   *(continued)*

nipple translocation Surgery in which the nipple is removed, the breast tissue is reduced, and the nipple is reattached.
plugged duct Localized area of milk stasis, with distension of the breast tissue.
psoriasis Skin condition with clearly demarcated plaques.
vesicle A small fluid-filled sac or blister.

Any use of the term *mother, maternal,* or *breastfeeding* is not meant to exclude transgender or nonbinary parents who may be breastfeeding or providing human milk to their infant.

▶ Overview

The medical term for the breast is *mammary gland,* which comes from the Latin word *mamma,* meaning "the breast." The breast provides both nutrition and nurturing. The lactation consultant requires a basic understanding of the structures and functions of the breast to provide proper breastfeeding management guidelines and to troubleshoot problems. This chapter provides information about breast conditions and complications that may arise during lactation. Assessment features and information about management options are discussed, and medications for the treatment of pathologic breast conditions are presented. Medications must be recommended by healthcare professionals who are licensed to prescribe.

I. Breast Evaluation and Variations in Exam

A. Properly addressing breast pathology requires knowledge of normal breast anatomy and physiology. In cases of difficulty with breastfeeding, it is important to assess the breast to provide guidance. Due to the sensitive nature of examining the breasts, always obtain permission prior to doing any breast examination. (See Chapter 6, *Breast Anatomy and Milk Production,* for a detailed description of normal breast development.)

B. The majority of women will notice a change in the size of their breasts starting early in pregnancy. Further enlargement is often noticed in the immediate postpartum period.[1,2]

  1. When assessing concerns about the potential for milk production, it may be helpful to ask if there was a noticeable change in breast size during pregnancy and after birth. The presence of breast growth is reassuring. There is great variation in breast size and shape, and these do not usually affect breast function.

  2. Much of breast size is a reflection of adipose (fat) tissue, not the functional milk-producing portion of the breast. The breast tissue may extend into the axilla, or armpit. This variation is normal, although in some cases severe engorgement of the axillary breast tissue may be painful and may cause a parent to seek care.

  3. It is normal for there to be minor differences in breast size, with the left breast often larger than the right. Minor differences in breast size (1 bra cup size or less) are common and do not cause concern. Severe asymmetry in breast size may be an indicator of abnormal breast development and warrants concern if insufficient milk production is noted.

C. The breast forms along the embryologic milk line, which extends from the axilla to the groin.

  1. Approximately 2 to 6 percent of women have accessory mammary tissue.[1]

  2. Polythelia refers to accessory nipple tissue, and polymastia refers to accessory breast tissue.

D. The breast is fixed to the underlying pectoral fascia by fibrous bands (Cooper's ligaments).

  1. Weakening of the bands may result in breast sagging.

  2. Sagging may occur because of breast changes during pregnancy and does not affect lactation.

E. There is great diversity in the size of the nipple and areola.

  1. A normal nipple protrudes from the areola.

    a. During embryologic development, the future lactiferous ducts open into an epithelial pit. When the underlying tissue proliferates, it causes the pit to evert.[3]

    b. Inverted nipples result when the epithelial pit fails to evert.

    c.   Nipples that appear flattened may not actually be inverted. When compression is applied behind the areola, a nipple that is truly inverted will invert further, whereas a flattened nipple will protrude.

  2. It is important to assess the nipple for any lesions, which may suggest infection or trauma. Nipple fissuring is suggestive of suboptimal latch and should prompt further observation and assessment of infant feeding (or pumping, if applicable) to explore a potential source of trauma.

F.   Montgomery glands are ductal openings of lactiferous and sebaceous glands that appear on the areola.

  1. These often become more prominent in pregnancy and lactation, and they may be of concern to a new parent.

  2. Some secretion from these glands may occur. This is normal physiology, and no special care is required.

  3. In rare circumstances, these glands can become obstructed and painful. Warm compresses may provide relief. Infection or cellulitis can rarely occur, which might require antibiotics.

G.   Prior breast surgery should be explored by both detailed history and examination.

  1. Attention should be given to the location of scars. Those in the periareolar region are most concerning for potential insufficient milk production.[3]

  2. Breast biopsy scars are typically small and can be either in the periareolar region or elsewhere on the breast.

  3. Parents who have had breast biopsies for benign disease can usually breastfeed successfully.

  4. Breast augmentation can be performed using a variety of incisions for implant placement.

    a.   Implants can be placed via laparoscopic tunneling from the periumbilical region, so there are no visible breast scars. More commonly, breast implants are placed from incisions in the axilla or inframammary fold (under the breast), or periareolar incisions are used.

    b.   One study comparing women with periareolar verses inframammary implants did not find a statistically significant difference between groups in breastfeeding success. The study found a rate of breastfeeding difficulties similar to those noted in women without breast augmentation.[4]

    c.   Inquire about breast augmentation because there may be implants because of developmental failure if there is no underlying breast tissue, although this is rare. Most breast implants are placed for cosmetic reasons, and in these cases there is typically sufficient breast tissue. Silicone implants are not a contraindication to breastfeeding.[5,6]

  5. Breast reduction surgery can be performed with a number of different techniques.

    a.   One technique involves nipple translocation, in which the nipple is removed, the breast tissue is reduced, and the nipple is reattached. In this procedure, there is a circumferential periareolar incision. All ducts and nerves to the nipple are severed. With this procedure milk may still exit the nipples, presumably due to recanalization.

    b.   Another common way to perform breast reduction is with the inferior pedicle technique. During this procedure, some portion of the breast remains intact. An inferior pedicle reduction can be identified by surgical scars around the edges of the areola and an additional scar line extending downward from the inferior areola at the midbreast.

    c.   Breast reduction is routinely associated with decreased milk production, although breastfeeding is possible with prior breast reduction. Research on breastfeeding in women with prior breast reduction did not find differences in lactation success related to which pedicle technique was used for reduction or the amount of tissue removed.[7-9] Women who underwent the nipple translocation technique were not included in these studies.

    d.   In studies of lactation in women with prior breast reduction, a lack of breastfeeding support is frequently reported as a cause of not breastfeeding.[7,9] Lactation consultants should ensure that parents with breast reduction communicate their surgery to the infant's healthcare provider. The pediatrician, family physician, or other healthcare provider should also closely monitor infant growth and milk transfer due to the risk of insufficient milk production.

H.   Observation of the breast in all four quadrants should include the following:

  1. Divide the breast in four quadrants for observation by visualizing a horizontal line and a vertical line that intersect at the center of the nipple.

    a.   Document findings according to observations noted in the upper outer, upper inner, lower outer, and lower inner quadrants.

b. Note any significant breast asymmetry, wide spacing of nipples or breast tissue, nipples or areola that appear disproportionately large in relation to the breasts, visible scars, piercings, or skin retraction.

c. Some parents may not mention prior breast surgery because they are not aware of its potential impact on lactation. Also, they may not realize that previous injury to the chest area can affect lactation.

2. Observing the breast can be very important in assessing infection.

a. Mastitis typically results in breast erythema and cellulitis (swelling) overlying the affected portion of the breast.

b. Early mastitis may have a subtle color change, so it may be useful to gently touch and release the skin in the suspected area.

c. A red color that blanches upon release suggests erythema; this may be more difficult to assess in darker-skinned parents.

d. Warmth of the overlying skin can be useful in assessing for infection.

II. Palpation

A. In addition to observation and evaluation for color change and warmth, palpating the breast will assess for any masses that could result from a plugged duct or an abscess.

B. When evaluating breast masses, it is useful to document the size, location, and mobility of the mass in addition to noting if the mass is tender and if it changes after feeding. Parents with persistent breast masses during lactation should be referred to an appropriate healthcare provider for further evaluation.

C. Palpation of the breast can be useful in assessing tissue. Breasts that are widely spaced, tube shaped, severely asymmetric, or have scant palpable tissue can be concerning for insufficient glandular tissue and possible low milk production and poor infant growth.[10] Physical examination of the breast alone is not highly predictive of low milk production.

III. Breastfeeding Complications and Breast Pathology

A. Nipple pain is a common reason why many women may cease breastfeeding earlier than their intended goals for duration.[11]

1. There are many causes of nipple pain.[11]

a. During early breastfeeding, some degree of breast discomfort is common.

b. The Infant Feeding Practices Study II found that 73 percent of breastfeeding mothers experienced pain on the first day of breastfeeding. Additionally, 86 percent of women noted pain into the second week of breastfeeding, although only 34 percent rated the pain as 5 or more on a 10-point scale.[12]

c. It is unclear why so many breastfeeding parents notice initial pain, but it is likely that hormones and trauma related to learning correct latch and positioning of the infant are contributors.

2. Trauma to the nipples worsens pain and predisposes the parent to other complications. Pain that persists past the first few weeks of breastfeeding deserves further evaluation by an experienced lactation professional. Optimizing latch and positioning remains the mainstay of nipple pain management.

3. The Infant Feeding Practices Study II of 1,323 mothers who stopped breastfeeding within the first month postpartum, 29 percent reported pain, and 37 percent reported sore, cracked, or bleeding nipples.[13] Research suggests that nipple pain and trauma are associated with early breastfeeding termination and postpartum depression.[14,15]

4. If parents are pumping or manually expressing milk, it is important to assess their technique. For those who are pumping, assessing for proper use of the pump and the fit of pump flanges is important because a poorly fitting flange will traumatize the nipple and areolar skin.[16]

B. Treatment for nipple pain is essential to promote effective breastfeeding.

1. A 2014 Cochrane Review regarding the management of nipple pain found four trials of "good quality" that looked at the use of glycerin pads, lanolin, expressed breastmilk, and all-purpose nipple ointment (a combination of topical antibiotic, antifungal, and steroids).[17] The review concluded that there is

insufficient evidence to support a particular treatment. It also found that pain improved by 7 to 10 days postpartum, regardless of intervention.

2. When evaluating persistent pain, it is important to conduct a careful assessment and take a careful history, including a detailed breastfeeding history.

   a. The history should include the following:

      i. When the pain began and the nature and details of when the pain occurs.

      ii. History of medical and pregnancy complications.

      iii. History of prior breastfeeding experiences, if applicable.

      iv. History about the infant.

   b. The assessment should include the following:

      i. Examination of the breasts.

      ii. Examination of the infant's oral anatomy and a suck assessment.

      iii. Observation of a breastfeeding session (or pumping or manual expression, if applicable).

3. Other causes of persistent pain include nipple damage and trauma, dermatologic conditions, infections, vasospasm, pain syndromes (allodynia), and breast drainage issues such as plugged ducts and oversupply.[11]

   a. Nipple trauma or fissuring.

      i. This is most likely due to poor latch or positioning, which should be assessed and optimized. If the fissures are persistent or have yellow crusting, a superficial bacterial infection should be suspected.

      ii. An infection can be treated with a topical mupirocin or bacitracin ointment. These ointments may be blotted off prior to the next feeding and are compatible with breastfeeding.[18] The recommendation for topical medications must come from a healthcare provider who is licensed to prescribe medications.

   b. Ankyloglossia

      i. Inspect the infant's mouth for ankyloglossia (tongue-tie) or short lingual frenulum (lip-tie).

      ii. If these conditions occur in conjunction with persistent nipple trauma or pain, consider referring the infant to a trained professional for a frenulotomy.[19] (See Chapter 3, *Infant Anatomy and Physiology for Feeding*, for a detailed discussion about ankyloglossia.)

   c. Nipple trauma and pain may result from pumping or manual expression.

      i. Parents who are pumping their breasts and have pain should be assessed to assure the pump flanges fit correctly. Pain can also result from pumping at inappropriate intervals or with the suction set too high.

      ii. Occasionally parents may massage their breasts or manually express milk in an overly vigorous way, which causes pain due to bruising and trauma.

   d. Dermatologic conditions may cause discomfort.

      i. Eczema (atopic dermatitis) is characterized by itching and may vary in appearance. Acute eczema may have vesicles with exudate and crusting, whereas chronic lesions are typically dry and scaly. Skin thickening may occur due to persistent scratching.

      ii. Eczema typically occurs in response to an irritant that is often topical. A detailed history should be taken to identify any potential triggers for the eczema; avoiding the triggers often resolves the condition.

      iii. Psoriasis appears as clearly demarcated plaques that may have overlying scale. There is often a history of psoriasis elsewhere on the body.

      iv. It may be helpful to apply an emollient. If the symptoms persist, the parent should be referred to a healthcare provider who may prescribe a topical steroid. These topical agents are typically compatible with breastfeeding; any excess should be blotted off the nipple prior to breastfeeding.[18]

      v. A healthcare provider may also prescribe or recommend a nonsedating antihistamine, such as loratadine or cetirizine, that may be beneficial for itching. These medications are also compatible with breastfeeding.[18]

      vi. A distinct, persistent dermatologic lesion on the nipple or areola, without other features of eczema or psoriasis, should prompt a visit to the parent's healthcare provider for further evaluation.

    e.   Herpes simplex virus (HSV) can affect breastfeeding.[20]

        i.   HSV typically presents as a cluster of small vesicles that later burst and leave ulcers. These lesions are extremely painful.

        ii.   HSV-1 is most commonly responsible for oral lesions, and HSV-2 typically causes genital lesions. However, both viruses can present in either location.

        iii.   HSV can cause lesions on the breast. Oral and genital lesions do not preclude breastfeeding, but they do require meticulous hygiene and good hand washing to avoid spreading the virus to the infant.

        iv.   HSV lesions on the breast require temporary cessation of breastfeeding on the affected breast due to the risk of spreading the virus to the infant.[21] Milk from the affected breast should not be given to the infant because of risk of contamination. It is important to prevent contact between the infant and HSV lesions because a life-threatening infection can occur in the newborn.

        v.   Oral medications for HSV, such as acyclovir or valacyclovir, are prescribed to treat and prevent infection. These medications are typically compatible with breastfeeding.[18]

    f.   Herpes zoster can also affect breastfeeding.

        i.   Herpes zoster is caused by reactivation of the varicella-zoster virus (VZV), which causes chickenpox.

        ii.   Initial infection with VZV causes chickenpox, which typically produces vesicles that are very pruritic, or itchy. These vesicles later become pustular and then form a crust.

        iii.   Mothers with acute chickenpox at the time of birth should be separated from their infants because the infection is spread by respiratory contact or contact with lesions.

        iv.   Any lesions involving the breast could contaminate milk.

        v.   VZV vaccination is available for infants older than 1 year of age. Vaccination after exposure to the virus is typically effective in preventing disease due to a long incubation period.

        vi.   Reactivation of VZV results in shingles or herpes zoster. This is a localized skin infection characterized by a painful, vesicular rash that occurs in a linear pattern along dermatomes. These lesions form a crust in 7 to 10 days, then it is no longer contagious.

        vii.   If a shingles outbreak is remote from the breast, covering the lesions, practicing good hygiene, and diligent hand washing should prevent transmission, and breastfeeding can continue.[21] However, if the shingles outbreak involves the breast, nipple, or areola, breastfeeding should be temporarily avoided on the affected breast, and milk from that breast should be discarded.

    g.   Vasospasm is another potential cause of nipple pain.

        i.   Vasospasm typically results in shooting, burning, or spasming pain associated with blanching and color change of the nipple. The onset of symptoms may be sudden.

        ii.   The nipple appears pale due to limited blood flow. This is followed by a bluish discoloration due to lack of oxygen, then it turns to a red color with reperfusion. Cold exposure may trigger the symptoms.

        iii.   Parents may have a history of Raynaud phenomenon, or they may note similar symptoms in their fingers or toes with cold exposure. Visualizing the nipple color changes associated with pain is typically diagnostic.

        iv.   The initial treatment includes keeping the breasts warm, applying warm compresses immediately after breastfeeding, and avoiding cold. A medication such as nifedipine may be prescribed for more severe cases.[22]

    h.   Allodynia is a condition in which pain sensitization (increased responsiveness) follows normally nonpainful and often repetitive stimulation. Even light touch is perceived as pain.

        i.   Parents with allodynia may note sensitivity to their bra or clothing. It is useful to explore any history the parent may have of chronic pain disorders, fibromyalgia, or other painful condition.[23]

        ii.   Over-the-counter pain medications, such as ibuprofen, may be useful in managing symptoms. If this is not successful, a referral to an experienced healthcare provider for further evaluation may be needed.

i.   Plugged ducts, engorgement, and oversupply can result in breast and nipple pain. Pain may be due to breast distension and inflammation associated with these conditions, in addition to subsequent difficulty these conditions may cause with infant latch and milk transfer.

j.   An overproduction of milk and an overactive milk ejection reflex may cause the infant to pinch the nipple to reduce flow, causing pain and trauma.

C.   Engorgement can interfere with the infant's ability to latch and transfer milk.

1.   Swelling and distension of the breasts in early lactation is common.

a.   Engorgement is caused by increased vascular flow, tissue edema, and the onset of copious milk production (lactogenesis II) that may exceed the infant's ability to extract the milk.[24]

b.   When this occurs, compression of the blood vessels and milk ducts can worsen the engorgement.

2.   It is not uncommon for the parent to experience a low-grade fever, but fevers of 101°F or higher should prompt an investigation for infection and a referral to the parent's healthcare provider. Infections can occur in either breast or in another location, such as the uterus, perineum, or surgical incision if the baby was delivered by cesarean section.

3.   Primary engorgement occurs with the onset of lactogenesis II. This is typically 3 to 5 days after delivery, although it may be delayed for an additional 1 to 2 days with cesarean delivery.

a.   According to information from the Infant Feeding Practices Study II, 36 percent of mothers experienced engorgement during the first week postpartum.[12]

b.   The most effective management for primary engorgement is proactive avoidance. Having a person who is knowledgeable about breastfeeding evaluate the feeding frequency, latch, and milk transfer early during lactation can avoid severe engorgement.

4.   Secondary engorgement occurs later during established lactation. This occurs due to a mismatch of milk production and removal. Possible causes include the following:

a.   Excessive pumping.

b.   Intentional or unintentional change in feeding intervals.

c.   Infant illness, such as an upper respiratory illness, that adversely affects the infant's ability to remove milk.

d.   Latch difficulties.

5.   Engorgement can lead to problems with latch due to difficulties infants can have in attaching to an engorged breast.

a.   This may lead to a cycle of worsening engorgement due to poor milk removal.

b.   Engorgement can also lead to mastitis.

6.   Treatment for engorgement includes adequate milk removal.

a.   Massaging the breasts prior to and during feeding, or pumping the breasts, may be helpful. If the infant is unable to latch, pumping for a brief period to extend the nipple can be helpful.

b.   Reverse pressure softening of the nipple can be useful in resolving periareolar edema to improve latch. This involves using gentle pressure toward the chest wall, moving outward from the base of the nipple through the areolar edge, to soften 1 to 2 inches around the nipple base.[24]

c.   Therapeutic breast massage was investigated in a trial.[25] The technique described for engorgement includes alternating fingertip massage from the areola toward the armpit, with reverse pressure softening within the areola.

d.   Nonsteroidal anti-inflammatory drugs, such as ibuprofen, are important to minimize pain from engorgement because pain can interfere with milk letdown. Any recommendations for medications must come from a healthcare provider who is licensed to prescribe medicine.

e.   It is important for the parent to alternate feeding positions and to feed, pump, or manually express frequently to keep the breasts well drained. Some parents find that a warm shower prior to feeding helps soften the breasts, although this may not be culturally appropriate or practical for some parents.

f.   A 2016 Cochrane Review found 13 trials involving 919 women that assessed treatments such as cabbage leaves, acupuncture, ultrasound, gua sha scraping, warm and cold packs, massage, and medicinal treatments. The studies were found to be of low quality and high risk for bias. The review found that there is currently insufficient evidence to recommend any particular therapy, and further research is needed.[26]

D. Plugged ducts can be painful and lead to a breast infection.

    1. A plugged duct is a localized area of milk stasis with distension of the involved mammary tissue. The parent often notes a palpable lump or knot in the breast, which sometimes might decrease in size with milk removal. With plugged ducts, there is an absence of systemic symptoms that indicate infection (i.e., no fever or redness).

    2. Predisposing factors for plugged ducts are similar to those for engorgement. They may occur after missed feedings, prolongation of feeding intervals, or poor infant latch or attachment.

        a. Parents with very abundant milk production may be at risk for plugged ducts.

        b. Another risk factor for plugged ducts could be pressure against a portion of the breast (e.g., a poorly fitting or overly restrictive bra).

    3. The treatment for plugged ducts includes frequent breastfeeding, being sure to adequately drain that portion of the breast.

        a. Moist heat prior to feeding and gentle massage of the affected area during feedings may be helpful.

        b. Alternating the feeding position to place the infant's chin or nose in line with the plugged area may optimize milk extraction.

        c. Lecithin 1,200 mg three times daily has been suggested for recurrent plugged ducts, although rigorous scientific investigation of this therapy has not been performed.[27]

        d. Therapeutic breast massage has been suggested for treating plugged ducts, although the specific technique for plugged ducts is different.

        e. Hand expression between the areola and the plugged duct can be effective. Start near the nipple, move outward, then stroke the breast from the plugged duct toward the areola.[25]

        f. If the suspected plugged duct does not resolve within approximately 72 hours, a referral for further evaluation should be considered to exclude other possible reasons for the lump.

E. Nipple blebs, or milk blebs, sometimes occur in association with plugged ducts so an inquiry should be made regarding both.

    1. A milk or nipple bleb appears as a small white spot on the tip of the nipple.

        a. It looks like a tiny, milk-filled blister and appears at a discrete nipple pore on the nipple tip.

        b. A blister on the nipple can occasionally be mistaken for a milk bleb. Blisters typically result from trauma, so latch and positioning should be assessed.

    2. Data supporting the effectiveness of treatment options is limited.

        a. The initial therapy should be to optimize latch and positioning to ensure good breast drainage and reduce trauma, which may cause inflammation.

        b. If the parent has incidentally noted the bleb and is not in pain or does not notice any difficulty from the bleb, provide assurance that it does not pose a problem.

        c. One investigator examined tissue biopsies from milk blebs and found an inflammatory response in the specimens.[28] Based on this finding, the use of topical steroids directly on the bleb may be beneficial.

        d. Rarely, a referral to an experienced professional for unroofing, or opening, persistent blebs may be considered if the parent continues to be in pain. The parent should be discouraged from unroofing the milk blebs due to the risk for infection and the potential trauma caused by unroofing, which may worsen the inflammatory response.

F. *Candida* infections are relatively common and can affect breastfeeding for both parent and infant.

    1. There is controversy regarding the diagnosis of candidal infections of the breast.

        a. In immunocompetent people, a superficial candidal infection can involve skin in other areas of the body, such as the mucous membranes of the vagina, and in skin folds, such as those on the vulva and under the breasts.

        b. *Candida albicans* causes most clinical infections.

        c. If the breast or nipple remains moist and warm, a superficial candidal infection of the breast can occur.

        d. This infection is typically red and may have satellite lesions on the periphery of the redness.

        e. Infants may have a similar-appearing diaper rash that is caused by *Candida*.

        f. *Candida* is a normal organism that can be cultured from normal healthy tissue from skin, mucous membranes, and the gastrointestinal tract.

       g.   Superficial contamination of the breast is noted in breastfeeding parents.[29] The superficial infection occurs when *Candida* becomes overgrown and causes symptoms such as itching and burning.

       h.   Invasive candidal infections are rare in immunocompetent adults.

  2.   Newborn infants can get oral thrush or a candidal infection of the oral mucous membranes.

       a.   This is characterized by white plaques on the inner cheeks, palate, or tongue. A white appearance of the tongue or cheeks may be a tongue coated with milk rather than thrush. White plaques that are persistent and cannot be wiped off are more indicative of thrush.

       b.   The infant's mouth can be treated with a nystatin suspension or a miconazole gel. Oral topical medications require a prescription from the infant's healthcare provider. Treatment of the infant does not mandate treatment of the asymptomatic parent.

  3.   Risk factors for *Candida* include conditions that may lead to an overgrowth of yeast.

       a.   *Candida* thrives in a warm, moist environment, so objects that keep the breast unusually warm and moist can predispose the parent to infection. These objects include breastfeeding pads with plastic backing that limits airflow or a bra made from material other than cotton.

       b.   Antibiotics increase the risk of candidal infections by killing normal competing bacteria, thus allowing the yeast to overgrow.

       c.   Diabetes is a significant risk factor for candidal infection.

       d.   Other risk factors include the use of steroids, immunosuppressant medications, and immune deficiency diseases.

  4.   A suspected superficial candidal infection can be treated with a dilute solution of gentian violet (less than 0.5 percent aqueous solution) applied for not more than 7 days.

       a.   Longer durations and higher doses have been associated with ulcerations.

       b.   Parents should be warned that gentian violet dyes anything it contacts, so caution should be used.

       c.   Topical antifungal ointments or creams, such as miconazole or clotrimazole, can be applied to the affected area. These medications are poorly absorbed orally. Excessive amounts should be blotted off the breast prior to feeding, but meticulous removal is not indicated because it can cause further nipple trauma and these medications are compatible with breastfeeding.[18]

       d.   Oral fluconazole can be prescribed if the parent has difficulty complying with topical therapy. An antifungal medication such as fluconazole 200 mg once followed by 100 mg for 7 to 10 days is sufficient therapy.[11] Larger doses used for more extended periods of time are not supported by scientific evidence, and further investigation about the etiology of the parent's symptoms should be undertaken.

       e.   Fluconazole should not be used with domperidone, erythromycin, or other medications that prolong the cardiac QT interval as a potential side effect.[30]

  5.   The association of *Candida* with nipple and breast pain in a normal-appearing nipple remains controversial.

       a.   Some authors have suggested that candida may be responsible for deep, shooting pain in the breast.[29] Studies to support *Candida* as a causative organism in such cases have varied findings.[31-35]

       b.   When nipple trauma or fissuring is present, research suggests that a bacterial infection is more likely and may benefit from topical antibiotics.[36-37]

       c.   Other recent research suggests that deep shooting breast pains may result from a subacute bacterial infection or possibly a biofilm (a group of microorganisms in which cells stick to each other and often to a surface).[37,38] Further research in this area is needed.

G.   Mastitis is an inflammatory condition of the breast.[39]

  1.   The affected portion of the breast becomes painful, red, and swollen.

       a.   Most infections affect one breast.

       b.   Fever is common with mastitis, and other flu-like symptoms, such as muscle aches, headache, fatigue, and nausea, may occur.

       c.   The frequency of mastitis in breastfeeding women varies across studies from 9 to 20 percent.[40,41] This variation may be related to different diagnostic criteria and severity of symptoms used by the researchers.

2. Predisposing factors for mastitis include nipple damage, overproduction, plugged ducts, engorgement, and use of a nipple shield.[42,43]
   a. The infection appears to be more common in first-time parents and in those who have previously experienced mastitis.
   b. Some research suggests that the use of manual breast pumps may increase the risk for mastitis.[40]
3. The treatment of early mastitis includes rest, fluid, and frequent and thorough breast drainage.[43]
   a. It is important to try to identify why the mastitis occurred and correct any predisposing factors so it is less likely to persist or recur.
   b. If nipple trauma is present, attention should be given to optimizing latch.
   c. If engorgement is present, the focus should be on draining the breast and avoiding abrupt changes in breastfeeding frequency.
   d. If symptoms worsen or are unresolved after 12 to 24 hours of conservative measures, consideration should be given to starting antibiotics.
   e. Parents with more severe symptoms or high fever should start antibiotics promptly and are not ideal candidates for an attempt at conservative measures.
   f. Prompt referral to the patient's healthcare provider within 24 hours of symptom onset is essential.
4. Nonsteroidal anti-inflammatory drugs, such as ibuprofen, should be used to treat mastitis pain.
   a. Pain can inhibit the letdown reflex and limit breast drainage, which can worsen mastitis.
   b. During an episode of mastitis, the milk is not harmful to a full-term, healthy infant.
   c. Weaning during mastitis can increase the risk for developing a breast abscess.
5. The most common organisms that cause mastitis include *Staphylococcus aureus* (both methicillin sensitive and resistant strains), *Streptococcus* species (groups A and B), and *Escherichia coli*.
   a. First-line antibiotics include a penicillinase-resistant penicillin, such as dicloxacillin 500 mg four times daily for 10 to 14 days. The optimal duration of treatment has not been adequately studied.
   b. First-generation cephalosporin antibiotics, such as cephalexin, are also reasonable options.
   c. For parents with severe penicillin allergy, clindamycin 300 mg four times daily can be used.
   d. If the parent is allergic to all these choices, a milk culture may be beneficial to ensure that the infection responds to the prescribed antibiotic.
6. Possible reasons for hospital admission due to mastitis include the following:
   a. A parent who is extremely ill and needs supportive care.
   b. An infection that has not responded to oral antibiotics.
   c. An unclear source of the infection or an uncertain diagnosis.
   d. A parent who is too ill to tolerate oral medications.
   e. Cases where there is a high suspicion for a breast abscess, which depends on the available outpatient support for managing a breast abscess.
7. A milk culture should be considered for mastitis if the condition does not respond to antibiotics; if the parent is not directly breastfeeding (so the organism did not come from the infant's nose or mouth) or was recently hospitalized; if the infant is ill or in a neonatal intensive care unit; if the parent has multiple allergies to antibiotics and an unusual antibiotic is chosen for treatment; or if the parent has recurrent episodes of mastitis.
   a. If a culture is performed, the nipple and areola should be cleansed prior to collecting the milk specimen, and the parent should avoid touching the nipple during milk collection to limit contamination.
   b. A small amount of milk is expressed and discarded.
   c. If sterilized pump parts are available, a pumped sample can be collected in a sterile container. If sterilized pump parts are not available, milk can be manually expressed into a sterile collection cup (such as used for sterile urine cultures) without touching the nipple to the inner portion of the collection cup.
   d. The milk culture is not anticipated to be sterile.
   e. The purpose of the culture is to assure that a resistant organism is not found, which would require changing antibiotics.
   f. If the mastitis does not respond to therapy or resistance to the initially prescribed antibiotic is suspected, the healthcare provider may choose a different antibiotic that is expected to be

effective against a methicillin-resistant staphylococcus infection; such antibiotics include trimethoprim–sulfamethoxazole. If a culture and sensitivity test are performed, the bacteria isolated will determine the most specific and effective antibiotic therapy.

    g.   Knowing the antibiotic resistance in your community can help direct the need for culture and antibiotic therapy.

8.   Recent studies suggest that the use of probiotics may be helpful in managing early mastitis.[42,45] Specifically, a probiotic containing *Lactobacillus fermentum* and *Lactobacillus salivarius* may be beneficial.[44] More research about this type of therapy is needed.

9.   Recurrent mastitis requires investigation into the cause of recurrence.

    a.   Questions to consider include the following:

        i.   Was the initial episode of mastitis incompletely treated?

        ii.   Did the symptoms resolve, and did the parent stop the therapy early?

        iii.   Was the initial antibiotic choice inadequate to treat the infection?

        iv.   Did the infection resolve, but the underlying predisposing factor persisted so the infection recurred (such as continued nipple trauma or poor breast drainage)?

        v.   Does the parent continue to have an overproduction of milk?

    b.   It is important to note if the recurrence is in the same breast and the same portion of the breast as the prior episode of mastitis.

        i.   Recurrence in the same position suggests a structural problem localized to that aspect of the breast.

        ii.   Recurrence in different breasts suggests a milk production or drainage issue.

    c.   If the parent is pumping, it is important to evaluate the pump as a potential site of contamination.

        i.   Is the pump being cleaned properly?

        ii.   Are all pump parts correctly maintained?

        iii.   What hygiene and cleaning practices is the parent using?

    d.   For recurrent infections, a midstream milk culture should be performed. The use of antibiotics for a more prolonged course, such as 2 to 3 weeks, may be needed. To minimize concerns about an antibiotic-resistant organism, it may be advisable to choose a different antibiotic than was used to treat the initial infection if the recurrences are frequent.

    e.   It is important to stress compliance with medication and to minimize any predisposing factors.

    f.   A breast examination to evaluate for any structural abnormalities or masses in the breast is needed if the recurrence involves the same aspect of the breast as the prior infection.

H.   A breast abscess is a localized collection of pus in the breast tissue.

1.   Breast abscess symptoms

    a.   The symptoms are very similar to the symptoms of mastitis (fever, pain, flu-like symptoms, muscle aches, fatigue, and breast redness), with the additional finding of a fluctuant mass in the breast.

    b.   Symptoms can be localized to the abscess in the breast if the infection is well encapsulated.

    c.   A diagnosis can typically be made by physical examination, although ultrasound can be useful to evaluate the size of the abscess and to help with drainage.

2.   An Australian survey of women 6 months postpartum found that approximately 3 percent of women with mastitis developed a breast abscess. Of all women who completed the survey, 14.5 percent were treated with antibiotics for at least one episode of mastitis.[47]

3.   Predisposing factors for developing a breast abscess include those that increase the risk of mastitis (nipple trauma, inadequate breast drainage, primiparity, and prior history of mastitis).

4.   Additionally, delayed or inadequate treatment of mastitis increases the likelihood of a breast abscess.

5.   Breast abscesses are commonly caused by *S. aureus* (either methicillin-sensitive or resistant strains).

    a.   Culturing the breast abscess fluid can be helpful to ensure antibiotic sensitivity.

    b.   A study of women who were hospitalized at two urban centers for a breast abscess found a 63 percent rate of methicillin-resistant *S. aureus*.[48]

6.   The initial management of breast abscess by performing serial ultrasound guided aspirations and using antibiotics is frequently successful and avoids the more interventional incision and drainage.[49,50]

    a.   Multiple studies report successful management of breast abscesses using antibiotics and serial breast abscess aspirations.[51] The success rate of abscess aspiration for lactational breast abscess is 82 to 97 percent.[52,53]

    b.   Studies have employed different techniques and frequencies for aspirations. Some have suggested aspirations as often as every 2 to 3 days, and others suggest every 4 to 7 days. The number of follow-up aspirations required for resolution ranged between one and four.

    c.   Some suggest placing a drainage catheter for abscesses larger than 3 cm, but others do not.[49-52]

    7.   Incision and drainage, in addition to antibiotics, may be required for abscesses larger than 10 cm or those that fail management with serial aspirations.

        a.   Incision and drainage are more likely to be associated with hospitalization, longer healing time, use of packing, pain, worse cosmetic result, and disruption of breastfeeding.

        b.   Using smaller incisions and drains may limit these disadvantages.

        c.   Milk fistula formation can be a rare complication of incision and drainage (5 to 12 percent).[54] It is more likely with the use of a periareolar incision and with larger, central, and deeper abscesses. In this situation, milk continues to drain through the surgical incision during lactation. This can be managed by occluding the incision site with something that can collect the leaked milk during feedings.

    8.   Effective pain management should be employed during the treatment of breast abscess.

        a.   Pain can inhibit the letdown reflex and result in concerns about milk production.

        b.   Nonsteroidal anti-inflammatory drugs, such as ibuprofen, can be given.

        c.   Parents who require incision and drainage may need narcotics for pain control.

    9.   During treatment of a breast abscess, feeding from the unaffected breast can continue.

        a.   Feeding from the affected breast depends on the clinical situation, method of drainage, breast anatomy, and location of the abscess.

        b.   In one study, continued breastfeeding was more likely when the women were managed with needle aspiration, compared to incision and drainage.[48]

I.   Breast masses

    1.   Breast masses that occur during lactation should be evaluated.

        a.   Although breast masses may be related to lactation (such as a plugged milk duct, lactating adenoma, or breast abscess), other masses can occur during lactation.

        b.   Breast cancer is rare in breastfeeding women. On average, women with pregnancy-associated breast cancer (breast cancer that occurs during pregnancy, within 1 year of delivery, or during lactation) are aged 32 years.[55] A delay in diagnosis has been reported in pregnant and breastfeeding women; therefore, it is important that lactating parents who have a breast mass that does not resolve after 72 hours seek additional care to assess if the mass is benign.[56,57]

    2.   If a persistent breast mass is noted in a lactating parent, it can be safely evaluated while breastfeeding continues.

        a.   Ultrasound is the preferred initial imaging technique for breastfeeding parents. Ultrasound can determine if the mass is cystic or solid. Solid masses can be evaluated with a biopsy without weaning.

        b.   Mammography can be performed on breastfeeding parents.

            i.   Mammography does not adversely affect the milk.

            ii.   The parent should pump or breastfeed prior to the mammogram so the breast is well drained to assist with optimal visualization.

            iii.   A normal mammogram result is not a sufficient evaluation for a breast mass; a breast ultrasound should also be performed.

        c.   An MRI can be performed on breastfeeding parents. When a mammogram or an MRI is performed, it is important that the radiologist be aware that the parent is breastfeeding for a more accurate interpretation of the test.

        d.   Breastfeeding can continue even if an excisional biopsy of a mass is required.

▶ Key Points from This Chapter

    A.   In the majority of diseases and illnesses, both acute and chronic, breastfeeding is not contraindicated.

    B.   The major concern for the healthcare provider, and often the parent, is whether treatment of the condition is compatible with breastfeeding.

    C.   Individualized lactation support is key to supporting parents and breastfeeding infants.

🔍 CASE STUDY

Cassidy is breastfeeding Andrew, a full-term, healthy infant, who is now 6 weeks old. Cassidy contacts you for assistance due to pain in the upper, outer aspect of the right breast. The pain was first evident after waking up early this morning and has continued to worsen. Cassidy has no other complaints. Breastfeeding is now going well after initial painful nipples and nipple trauma due to problems with latch in the first few weeks. Cassidy saw a lactation consultant, who helped with the latch, and the nipples have since healed. Milk production is good and Andrew has gained weight well. In fact, Cassidy has more milk than needed for feedings and pumps and stores the extra milk. Last night was the first time Andrew slept 5 consecutive hours (feedings had usually been every 3 to 4 hours at night).

On evaluation, you notice that Cassidy does not have a fever, the nipples are normal appearing, there is no nipple trauma, and there is no breast erythema. The painful area of the right breast is full and tender to touch. You observe a feeding and notice that Andrew latches well. The painful area is somewhat softer after the feeding, but the breast is not fully drained and the area remains tender. You suggest warm compresses prior to feeding, gentle massage of that area of the breast toward the nipple, and frequent feedings with positioning of the infant to drain that portion of the breast well. You also suggest that Cassidy avoid any abrupt changes in feeding frequency and return for another visit if the pain does not improve in 48 to 72 hours.

Questions

1. What risk factors for plugged ducts does Cassidy exhibit?
2. What other physical exam findings should you look for when assessing for breast pain?
3. What characteristics suggest that Cassidy does not currently have mastitis and need antibiotic therapy?
4. What would make you more concerned about mastitis?
5. Why is it important for Cassidy to follow up if things are not better in the next few days?

References

1. Lawrence RA, Lawrence RM. *Breastfeeding: A Guide for the Medical Profession.* 8th ed. Philadelphia, PA: Elsevier Saunders Mosby; 2016.
2. Hale TW, Hartmann P. *Textbook of Human Lactation.* Amarillo, TX: Hale Publishers; 2007.
3. Neifert M, DeMarzo S, Seacat J, Young D, Leff M, Orleans M. The influence of breast surgery, breast appearance, and pregnancy-induced breast changes on lactation sufficiency as measured by infant weight gain. *Birth.* 1990;17(1):31-38.
4. Semple JL. Breast-feeding and silicone implants. *Plast Reconstr Surg.* 2007;120(7 suppl 1):123S-128S.
5. Semple JL, Lugowski SJ, Baines CJ, Smith DC, McHugh A. Breast milk contamination and silicone implants: preliminary results using silicon as a proxy measurement for silicone. *Plast Reconstr Surg.* 1998;102(2):528-533.
6. Lund HG, Turkle J, Jewell ML, Murphy DK. Low risk of skin and nipple sensitivity and lactation issues after primary breast augmentation with form-stable silicone implants: follow-up in 4927 subjects. *Aesthetic Surg J.* 2016;36(6):672-680.
7. Thibaudeau S, Sinno H, Williams B. The effects of breast reduction on successful breastfeeding: a systematic review. *J Plast Reconstr Aesthetic Surg.* 2010;63(10):1688-1693.
8. Chiummariello S, Cigna E, Buccheri EM, Dessy LA, Alfano C, Scuderi N. Breastfeeding after reduction mammaplasty using different techniques. *Aesthetic Plast Surg.* 2008;32(2):294-297.
9. Kraut RY, Brown E, Korownyk C, et al. The impact of breast reduction surgery on breastfeeding: systematic review of observational studies. *PloS One.* 2017;12(10):e0186591.
10. Neifert MR, Seacat JM, Jobe WE. Lactation failure due to insufficient glandular development of the breast. *Pediatrics.* 1985;76(5):823-828.
11. Berens P, Eglash A, Malloy M, Steube AM, Academy of Breastfeeding Medicine. ABM clinical protocol #26: persistent pain with breastfeeding. *Breastfeed Med.* 2016;11(2):46-53.
12. Centers for Disease Control and Prevention. Infant Feeding Practices Study II and its year six follow up: results. Centers for Disease Control and Prevention website. www.cdc.gov/ifps/results/ch2/table 2-37.htm. Updated April 25, 2017. Accessed September 1, 2017.
13. Li R, Fein SB, Chen J, Grummer-Strawn LM. Why mothers stop breastfeeding: mothers' self-reported reasons for stopping during the first year. *Pediatrics.* 2008;122(suppl 2):S69-S76.
14. Amir LH, Dennerstein L, Garland SM, Fisher J, Farish SJ. Psychological aspects of nipple pain in lactating women. *J Psychosom Obstet Gynecol.* 1996;17(1):53-58.
15. Watkins S, Meltzer-Brody S, Zolnoun D, Stuebe A. Early breastfeeding experiences and postpartum depression. *Obstet Gynecol.* 2011;118(2 pt 1):214-221.
16. Eglash A, Malloy ML. Breastmilk expression and breast pump technology. *Clin Obstet Gynecol.* 2015;58(4):855-867.
17. Dennis CL, Jackson K, Watson J. Interventions for treating painful nipples among breastfeeding women. *Cochrane Database Syst Rev.* 2014;12:CD007366. doi:10.1002/14651858.CD007366.pub2.
18. Hale TW, Rowe HE. *Medications and Mothers' Milk 2017.* New York, NY: Springer Publishing Company; 2017.
19. O'Shea JE, Foster JP, O'Donnell CP, et al. Frenotomy for tongue-tie in newborn infants. *Cochrane Database Syst Rev.* 2017;3:CD011065.
20. Barrett ME, Heller MM, Fullerton Stone H, Murase JE. Dermatoses of the breast in lactation. *Dermatologic Therapy.* 2013;26(4):331-336.
21. Hale TW, Berens PD. *Clinical Therapy in Breastfeeding Patients.* 3rd ed. Amarillo, TX: Hale Publishing; 2010.

22. Barrett ME, Heller MM, Stone HF, Murase JE. Raynaud phenomenon of the nipple in breastfeeding mothers: an underdiagnosed cause of nipple pain. *JAMA Dermatol.* 2013;149(3):300-306.

23. Amir LH, Jones LE, Buck ML. Nipple pain associated with breastfeeding: incorporating current neurophysiology into clinical reasoning. *Australian Family Physician.* 2015;44(3):127-32.

24. Berens P, Brodribb W, Academy of Breastfeeding Medicine. ABM clinical protocol #20: engorgement, revised 2016. *Breastfeed Med.* 2016;11(4):159-163.

25. Witt AM, Bolman M, Kredit S, Vanic A. Therapeutic breast massage in lactation for the management of engorgement, plugged ducts, and mastitis. *J Hum Lactation.* 2016;32(1):123-131.

26. Mangesi L, Zakarija-Grkovic I. Treatments for breast engorgement during lactation. *Cochrane Database Syst Rev.* 2016;6:CD006946.

27. Scott CR. Lecithin: it isn't just for plugged milk ducts and mastitis anymore. *Midwifery Today Int Midwife.* 2005;Winter(76):26-27.

28. O'Hara MA. Bleb histology reveals inflammatory infiltrate that regresses with topical steroids; a case series [platform abstract]. *Breastfeed Med.* 2012;7(suppl 1):2.

29. Amir LH, Pakula S. Nipple pain, mastalgia and candidiasis in the lactating breast. *Aust N Z J Obstet and Gynaecol.* 1991;31(4):378-380.

30. Goldstein EJ, Owens Jr RC, Nolin TD. Antimicrobial-associated QT interval prolongation: pointes of interest. *Clin Infect Dis.* 2006;43(12):1603-1611.

31. Morrill JF, Heinig MJ, Pappagianis D, Dewey KG. Risk factors for mammary candidiasis among lactating women. *J Obstet Gynecol Neonatal Nurs.* 2005;34(1):37-45.

32. Amir LH, Donath SM, Garland SM, et al. Does *Candida* and/or *Staphylococcus* play a role in nipple and breast pain in lactation? A cohort study in Melbourne, Australia. *BMJ Open.* 2013;3(3):e002351.

33. Betzold CM. Results of microbial testing exploring the etiology of deep breast pain during lactation: a systematic review and meta-analysis of nonrandomized trials. *J Midwifery Womens Health.* 2012;57(4):353-364.

34. Hale TW, Bateman TL, Finkelman MA, Berens PD. The absence of *Candida albicans* in milk samples of women with clinical symptoms of ductal candidiasis. *Breastfeed Med.* 2009;4(2):57-61.

35. Andrews JI, Fleener DK, Messer SA, Hansen WF, Pfaller MA, Diekema DJ. The yeast connection: is *Candida* linked to breastfeeding associated pain? *Am J Obstet Gynecol.* 2007;197(4):424-e1–424-e4.

36. Thomassen P, Johansson VA, Wassberg C, Petrini B. Breast-feeding, pain and infection. *Gynecol Obstet Invest.* 1998;46(2):73-74.

37. Mediano P, Fernández L, Jiménez E, et al. Microbial diversity in milk of women with mastitis: potential role of coagulase-negative staphylococci, viridans group streptococci, and corynebacteria. *J Hum Lactation.* 2017;33(2):309-318.

38. Jiménez E, Arroyo R, Cárdenas N, et al. Mammary candidiasis: a medical condition without scientific evidence? *PLOS One.* 201;12(7):e0181071.

39. Amir LH, Academy of Breastfeeding Medicine Protocol Committee. ABM clinical protocol #4: mastitis, revised March 2014. *Breastfeed Med.* 2014;9(5):239-243.

40. Amir LH, Forster DA, Lumley J, McLachlan H. A descriptive study of mastitis in Australian breastfeeding women: incidence and determinants. *BMC Public Health.* 2007;7(1):

41. Foxman BL, D'Arcy H, Gillespie B, Bobo JK, Schwartz K. Lactation mastitis: occurrence and medical management among 946 breastfeeding women in the United States. *Am J Epidemiol.* 2002;155(2):103-114.

42. Mediano P, Fernández L, Rodríguez JM, Marín M. Case–control study of risk factors for infectious mastitis in Spanish breastfeeding women. *BMC Pregnancy and Childbirth.* 2014;14(1):195.

43. Cullinane M, Amir LH, Donath SM, et al. Determinants of mastitis in women in the CASTLE study: a cohort study. *BMC Fam Pract.* 2015;16(1):181.

44. Arroyo R, Martín V, Maldonado A, Jiménez E, Fernández L, Rodríguez JM. Treatment of infectious mastitis during lactation: antibiotics versus oral administration of lactobacilli isolated from breast milk. *Clin Infect Dis.* 2010;50(12):1551-1558.

45. Jiménez E, Fernández L, Maldonado A, et al. Oral administration of *Lactobacillus* strains isolated from breast milk as an alternative for the treatment of infectious mastitis during lactation. *Appl Environ Microbiol.* 2008;74(15):4650-4655.

46. Amir LH, Griffin L, Cullinane M, Garland SM. Probiotics and mastitis: evidence-based marketing? *Int Breastfeed J.* 2016;11:19.

47. Amir LH, Foster D, McLachlan H, Lumley J. Incidence of breast abscess in lactating women: report from an Australian cohort. *BJOG.* 2004;111(12):1378-1381.

48. Berens P, Swaim L, Peterson B. Incidence of methicillin-resistant *Staphylococcus aureus* in postpartum breast abscesses. *Breastfeed Med.* 2010;5(3):113-115.

49. Irusen H, Rohwer AC, Steyn DW, Young T. Treatments for breast abscesses in breastfeeding women. *Cochrane Database Syst Rev.* 2015;8:CD010490.

50. Trop I, Dugas A, David J, et al. Breast abscesses: evidence-based algorithms for diagnosis, management, and follow-up. *Radiographics.* 2011;31(6):1683-1699.

51. Christensen AF, Al-Suliman N, Nielson KR, et al. Ultrasound-guided drainage of breast abscesses: results in 151 patients. *Br J Radiol.* 2005;78:186-188.

52. Dixon JM. Outpatient treatment of non-lactational breast abscesses. *Br J Surg.* 1992;79(1):56-57.

53. Karstrup S, Solvig J, Nolsøe CP, et al. Acute puerperal breast abscesses: US-guided drainage. *Radiology.* 1993;188(3):807-809.

54. Larson KE, Valente SA. Milk fistula: diagnosis, prevention, and treatment. *Breast J.* 2016;22(1):111-112.

55. Van den Rul N, Han SN, Van Calsteren K, Neven P, Amant F. Postpartum breast cancer behaves differently. *Facts Views Vis.* 2011;3(3):183.

56. Callihan EB, Gao D, Jindal S, et al. Postpartum diagnosis demonstrates a high risk for metastasis and merits an expanded definition of pregnancy-associated breast cancer. *Breast Cancer Res Treat.* 2013;138(2):549-559.

57. Lyons TR, Schedin PJ, Borges VF. Pregnancy and breast cancer: when they collide. *J Mammary Gland Biol Neoplasia.* 2009;14(2):87-98.

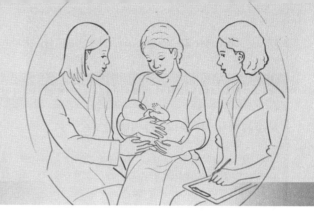

CHAPTER 21

Newborn Challenges: Hyperbilirubinemia and Hypoglycemia

Sahira Long
Michal Young

OBJECTIVES

- Recognize the common symptoms of hypoglycemia in the newborn period.
- Identify infants who are at greater risk of developing neonatal hypoglycemia.
- Identify strategies that can help establish normoglycemia.
- Provide information regarding the management of hypoglycemia in the breastfed infant.
- Recognize the common types of jaundice in the newborn period.
- Identify infants who are at greater risk of developing neonatal hyperbilirubinemia.
- Recognize the importance of preventing and detecting kernicterus.
- Provide information regarding the management of jaundice in the breastfed infant.

DEFINITIONS OF COMMONLY USED TERMS

hyperbilirubinemia An elevated level of bilirubin in a neonate's blood. A sign of elevated bilirubin levels is jaundice, or yellowing of the skin and whites of the neonate's eyes.
hypoglycemia A whole blood glucose value that is less than 45 mg/dL.
infants with perinatal stress Infants with a 5 minute Apgar score of less than 5. This score lets the healthcare team know how well the baby is doing outside the womb.
kernicterus A disorder due to severe jaundice in the newborn. Deposition of the pigment bilirubin in the brain, which causes damage to the brain, potentially leading to sensorineural hearing loss, upward gaze palsy, dental enamel dysplasia, cerebral palsy, and cognitive impairment. Also called bilirubin encephalopathy.

(continues)

large for gestational age (LGA) An infant with a birth weight that is greater than the 90th percentile for gestational age.

low birth weight Infants born weighing less than 2,500 grams (5 pounds, 8 ounces).

pathologic jaundice A condition that occurs within 24 hours after birth, with a rapidly rising total serum bilirubin concentration (increase of more than 5 mg/dL per day) and a total serum bilirubin level higher than 17 mg/dL in a full-term newborn.

phototherapy A treatment for reducing high bilirubin levels in which the infant's dermal and subcutaneous bilirubin absorb light waves, which convert the bilirubin into a more easily excreted form. In the standard form of phototherapy, the baby lies in a bassinet or enclosed plastic crib (incubator) and is exposed to a type of fluorescent light that is absorbed by the baby's skin, also called ultraviolet (UV) light therapy.

physiologic jaundice A condition caused by the breakdown of red blood cells (which release bilirubin into the blood) and the immaturity of the newborn's liver (which cannot effectively metabolize bilirubin and prepare it for excretion into the stool and urine).

preterm An infant born earlier than 37 completed weeks of gestation.

small for gestational age (SGA) An infant with a birth weight that is less than the 10th percentile for gestational age.

transcutaneous bilirubin (TcB) A screening tool used to assess bilirubin levels in infants.

Any use of the term *mother*, *maternal*, or *breastfeeding* is not meant to exclude transgender or nonbinary parents who may be breastfeeding or providing human milk to their infant.

▶ Overview

Glucose is an obligate metabolic fuel for the brain. The brain has a unique dependence on glucose, but it cannot synthesize glucose or store it. Therefore, the brain requires a continuous supply of glucose from the circulation. Current evidence does not support a specific concentration of glucose that can definitively indicate irreversible neurologic damage.[1-3]

However, because glucose is the preferred brain fuel, it is important to have a practical approach to anticipate the risk of hypoglycemia and prevent it as best as possible in the newborn. Research during the past 50 years has identified what is considered transient hypoglycemia, which occurs in normal-term infants. It corrects itself over the first few hours after birth through metabolism of fats, proteins, and ketones to make glucose.[4] That work indicates the resilience of a normal newborn. In earlier years, the practice was to separate mothers and babies, but better practices today note that routine separation is unwarranted, and early feedings should begin within an hour after birth. Adhering to this new and better practice should help decrease the incidence of hypoglycemia.

Jaundice is the yellow discoloration of an infant's skin, mucous membranes, or the sclera of the eyes. This yellow discoloration is due to elevated bilirubin levels in an infant's bloodstream. Bilirubin is formed by the breakdown of heme present in hemoglobin, myoglobin, cytochromes, catalase, peroxidase, and tryptophan pyrrolase. Jaundice occurs when bilirubin builds up in the newborn's bloodstream faster than the liver can break it down and excrete it through the baby's stool.[5]

These two clinical concerns, hypoglycemia and jaundice, can have adverse outcomes for a newborn infant. Therefore, it is important to screen for them when indicated and treat as appropriate.

I. Normal Glucose Regulation in the Newborn

A. Glycogen reserves that are available for conversion to glucose during the immediate neonatal period are laid down during the later part of the third trimester.

B. Glucose is the primary nutrient for brain metabolism, and the placentally derived supply terminates at birth.

C. Newborns have a greater demand for glucose than children and adults because of their large brain-to-body weight.

D. Preterm infants have an even greater demand for glucose and have limited to absent glycogen reserves, depending on their gestational age at birth.

E. Neonatal physiology is a factor in glucose levels.
   1. At birth, there is a transition period as glucose homeostasis is established by the infant. The net effect is mobilization of glycogen and fatty acids.
   2. The collective activities that maintain glucose homeostasis are called counterregulation, and they consist of the following:
      a. Glycogenolysis: Mobilization and release of glycogen from body stores to form glucose.
      b. Gluconeogenesis: Production of glucose by the liver and kidneys from noncarbohydrate substrates, such as fatty acids and amino acids.
   3. After 12 hours, the baby is dependent on glucose made from dietary intake of milk components (20 to 50 percent) and gluconeogenesis to maintain blood glucose (galactose, amino acids, glycerol, and lactate), as well as free fatty acids from fat stores and milk.
   4. Human milk is more ketogenic than formula, enabling a breastfed baby to create high levels of alternative fuels until the milk production increases sufficiently to draw on milk components for glucose synthesis.
   5. High levels of ketone bodies enable breastfed babies to demonstrate lower measured blood glucose levels but still maintain the optimal production of brain fuels.
   6. Glycogen stores are converted to glucose (glycogenolysis), rapidly depleting glycogen stores over the first hours of life; liver glycogen stores are 90 percent depleted by 3 hours and are gone by 12 hours.
   7. Fat metabolism provides glucose substrate beginning at 2 to 3 days of age.

II. Risk Factors and Clinical Signs for Hypoglycemia

A. Routine screening and monitoring of blood glucose concentration is not indicated in healthy term newborns after a normal pregnancy and delivery. The blood glucose concentration should be measured in term infants who are known to be at risk or who are clinically symptomatic.[1,2]
B. Some infants with hypoglycemia may be asymptomatic; however, common symptoms of neonatal hypoglycemia include the following:
   1. Jitteriness.
   2. Tremors.
   3. Feeding intolerance (poor suck or refusal to feed).
   4. Seizures.
   5. Apnea, bradycardia, or both.
   6. Hypotonia (lethargy), listlessness, or limpness.
   7. Hypothermia; temperature instability.
   8. Respiratory distress, including grunting and tachypnea or apnea.
   9. High-pitched cry.
   10. Irritability.
   11. Cyanosis.
C. Infants who may be at risk for developing neonatal hypoglycemia include the following:
   1. Small for gestational age.
   2. Large for gestational age.
   3. Low birth weight infants.
   4. Infants born to mothers who have pregestational or gestational diabetes.
   5. Preterm infants.
   6. Infants with perinatal stress.
   7. Discordant twin (smaller twin's weight is 10 percent less than larger twin's).
   8. Infants experiencing cold stress.
   9. Infants exposed to mediations during labor that are known to cause decreased blood sugar (e.g., oral hypoglycemics, terbutaline, or propranolol).
   10. Infants with clinical evidence of wasting of fat or muscle bulk.
   11. Any infant that is not feeding well.

III. Testing Methods

A. Bedside glucose reagent test strips are inexpensive and practical. However, they are not reliable because they have a significant variance from true blood glucose levels, especially at low glucose concentrations.[1]

B. Bedside glucose tests done on a warmed heel may be used for screening. However, laboratory levels sent stat (immediate determination, without delay) must confirm the results before a diagnosis of hypoglycemia can be made, especially in infants with no clinical signs.[1]

IV. General Glucose Management Recommendations for All Term Newborns

A. Early and exclusive breastfeeding meets the nutritional and metabolic needs of healthy, term newborn infants.
1. Routine supplementation is unnecessary.
2. Initiate breastfeeding within 30 to 60 minutes of birth and continue on demand.
3. Facilitate skin-to-skin contact.
4. Feedings should be frequent, 10 to 12 times per 24 hours in the first few days after birth.
5. Feedings should be assessed for adequacy of latch and to ensure effectiveness.

B. Blood glucose screening and testing is performed only on at-risk infants or infants with clinical signs.
1. Routine monitoring of blood glucose in all term newborns is unnecessary and may be harmful.
2. At-risk infants should be screened for hypoglycemia, with a frequency and duration related to the specific risk factors of the individual infant (see **FIGURE 21-1**).
3. Monitoring continues until normal prefeed levels (glucose greater than 45 mg/dL) are consistently obtained.
4. Bedside glucose screening tests must be confirmed by formal laboratory testing. However, treatment should not be delayed while waiting for a serum glucose result.

V. Management of Documented Hypoglycemia in the Breastfed Infant

A. Infants with no clinical signs should be monitored.
1. Continue breastfeeding approximately every 1 to 2 hours, or feed 1 to 5 mL/kg of expressed milk or substitute nutrition.
2. Recheck the blood glucose concentration before subsequent feedings until the value is acceptable and stable (i.e., greater than or equal to 45 mg/dL).
3. Avoid forced feedings.
    a. If the glucose level remains low (less than 45 mg/dL) despite feedings, begin intravenous glucose therapy.
    b. Breastfeeding may continue during intravenous glucose therapy.
    c. Carefully document the infant's response to treatment.

B. Infants with clinical signs or blood glucose levels less than 20 to 25 mg/dL require intervention.
1. Initiate intravenous 10 percent glucose solution with a minibolus (i.e., 2 mL/kg of 10 percent dextrose in water).
2. Do not rely on oral or enteral feeding to correct extreme or clinically significant hypoglycemia.
3. The blood glucose level in infants who have had clinical signs should be maintained at more than 45 mg/dL (more than 2.5 mmol/L).
4. Adjust the intravenous infusion rate based on the infant's blood glucose level.
5. Encourage frequent breastfeeding.
6. Monitor the blood glucose levels before feedings while weaning off the intravenous treatment until the values stabilize off intravenous fluids.
7. Carefully document the response to treatment.

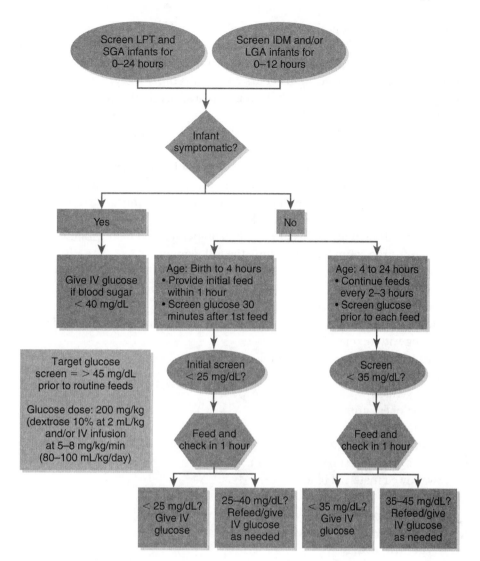

FIGURE 21-1 Screening and management of postnatal glucose homeostasis in late preterm (LPT) and term small for gestational age (SGA), infant of diabetic mother (IDM), or large for gestational age (LGA) infants.

Data from Adamkin DH, American Academy of Pediatrics, Committee on Fetus and Newborn. Clinical report--postnatal glucose homeostasis in late-preterm and term infants. *Pediatrics*. 2011;127:575-579. © Sahira Long, MD, FAAP and Michal Young, FAAP.

VI. Hyperbilirubinemia

A. Approximately 60 percent of full-term infants and 80 percent of preterm infants develop jaundice within several days of birth.[5]

1. Fortunately, there are elaborate physiologic mechanisms for bilirubin detoxification and disposition, which, although immature, usually work sufficiently so that most infants do not require treatment.

2. There are clinical situations that increase the risk for elevated bilirubin levels.

B. Because of the risk for neurotoxicity, all infants are required to have an objective bilirubin assessment within 48 hours of birth.[5,6,7]

1. Although a visual assessment is helpful, differences in pigmentation can sometimes challenge a clinician's assessment.

2. An objective assessment, either by serum levels or transcutaneous bilirubin (TcB), is the best way to determine levels and hence document infants who may be at risk for a rapid rise of levels, which can place the infant at risk for adverse outcomes.

3. TcB levels may be lower or higher than serum levels; thus, a correlation should be made between TcB levels and serum bilirubin levels in the laboratory being used.

C. Bilirubin exists in two forms in the bloodstream[8]:
1. Conjugated (direct) bilirubin occurs when bilirubin is attached to glucuronide by an enzymatic process in the liver. Elevated levels are not neurotoxic but may be indicative of a more serious illness (e.g., hepatitis).
2. Unconjugated (indirect) bilirubin occurs when bilirubin is not yet attached to a glucuronide in the liver. Elevated levels of this form of bilirubin can cause neurotoxicity, also known as bilirubin-induced neurologic dysfunction (BIND).
   a. Acute manifestations of BIND include lethargy, hypotonia, opisthotonos, seizures, high-pitched cry, poor feeding, and loss of the Moro (startle) reflex.
   b. Kernicterus is diagnosed when there are chronic and permanent symptoms of BIND. These symptoms include sensorineural hearing loss, upward gaze palsy, dental enamel dysplasia, cerebral palsy, and cognitive impairment. The infants most at risk for developing kernicterus are those who are preterm and sick.
D. The risk factors for developing neonatal hyperbilirubinemia include the following:
1. Maternal or intrapartum factors include the following:
   a. Maternal diabetes.
   b. Poor breastmilk transfer or low breastfeeding volumes.
   c. Asian or Hispanic ancestry.
   d. Blood group incompatibilities, or other hemolytic diseases (e.g., G6PD deficiency).
   e. Sibling with neonatal jaundice.
2. Newborn factors include the following:
   a. Sepsis.
   b. Male gender.
   c. Cephalohematoma.
   d. Prematurity.
   e. Trisomy 21/Down syndrome.
   f. Upper gastrointestinal obstruction.
   g. Swallowed maternal blood.
   h. Acidosis.
   i. Polycythemia.
   j. Delayed bowel movements.
   k. Hypothyroidism.

VII. Common Types of Jaundice

A. Physiologic jaundice is a condition caused by the breakdown of red blood cells (which release bilirubin into the blood) and the immaturity of the newborn's liver (which cannot effectively metabolize bilirubin and prepare it for excretion into the urine).
1. About 60 percent of term infants and 80 percent of preterm infants who have jaundice usually experience physiologic jaundice.
2. It is usually seen at 2 to 5 days of age, when there is usually a peak bilirubin concentration of 5 to 12 mg/dL.
3. Several factors that contribute to the development of physiologic jaundice are depicted in **FIGURE 21-2**[9]:
   a. Unconjugated hyperbilirubinemia during the first week of life.
   b. Decreased activity of the conjugating enzyme.
   c. Short life span of the infant's red blood cells.
B. Pathologic jaundice develops in the first 24 hours of life. Jaundice that occurs during this time frame is always pathologic.
1. Features of pathologic jaundice include the following:
   a. Total serum bilirubin greater than 12 mg/dL in a term infant.
   b. Conjugated bilirubin greater than 2 mg/dL or greater than 20 percent of the total bilirubin level.
   c. Total serum bilirubin rate of rise greater than 5 mg/dL per day.
   d. Persistence of jaundice beyond 10 to 14 days.
2. Pathologic jaundice usually occurs in infants with a family history of hemolytic disease. The presence of any additional signs or symptoms, such as concomitant hepatomegaly, splenomegaly, failure of

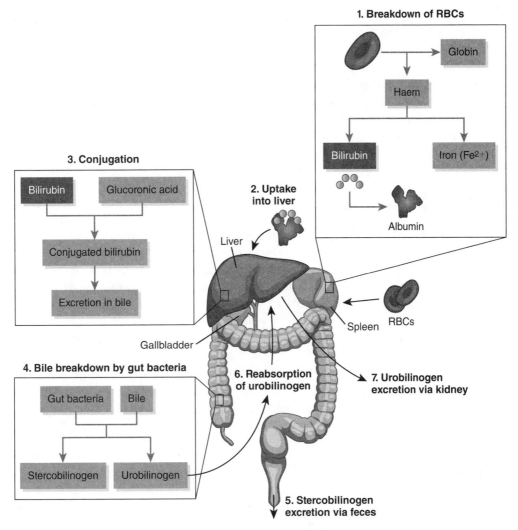

FIGURE 21-2 Bilirubin metabolism.

Data from University of Bristol. Blackboard online jaundice seminar. Part 1 - bilirubin metabolism. https://www.ole.bris.ac.uk/bbcswebdav/institution/Faculty%20of%20Health%20Sciences/MB%20ChB%20Medicine/Year%203%20Medicine%20and%20Surgery%20-%20Hippocrates/Abdomen%20-%20Jaundice%20core%20topic/part_1__bilirubin_metabolism.html. Accessed March 10, 2018.

phototherapy, vomiting, lethargy, apnea, bradycardia, or excessive weight loss, can be indicative of potential underlying disease.

3. Pathologic jaundice causes include septicemia, biliary atresia, hepatitis, galactosemia, hypothyroidism, cystic fibrosis, congenital hemolytic anemia, and drug-induced hemolytic anemia.

4. Although there is no consensus on the current terminology that is best to describe them, there are two major categories of pathologic jaundice that are associated with breastfeeding. An effort is being made to move away from the historical terminology that tends to fault breastfeeding because breastfeeding, per se, has not been proven to be the cause of either.

    a. Prolonged jaundice associated with breastfeeding is also known as prolonged unconjugated hyperbilirubinemia or breastmilk jaundice.

        i. It has been speculated that breastmilk inhibits uridine glucuronosyltranferase, although the exact mechanism has not been identified.

        ii. This type of jaundice is seen in up to 2 percent of breastfed full-term infants after day 7 of life (usually presents in week 2).

        iii. During weeks 2 to 4, bilirubin levels up to 30 mg/dL can be seen. These levels gradually decrease as breastfeeding continues, with a more rapid decrease noted when formula is substituted for 12 to 24 hours as a treatment.

        iv. When breastfeeding interruption is selected as the treatment course, it can be resumed without the return of hyperbilirubinemia.

    b.   Suboptimal intake jaundice has historically been referred to as breastfeeding jaundice, which is an inaccurate term to describe the underlying cause of insufficient feedings.

        i.   When the quantity of milk consumed is low, infants do not have bowel movements as fast, so the body reabsorbs bilirubin through increased enterohepatic circulation, causing it to build up.

        ii.   Increased unconjugated bilirubin is typically seen because bilirubin must be unconjugated to be reabsorbed.

        iii.   Focused parental support to provide early and frequent breastfeeding increases the number and volume of feeds and a resultant decrease in bilirubin levels as stooling increases.

VIII. Tests to Evaluate Jaundice

A.   When there is concern for pathologic jaundice, tests should be performed.[10,11]

B.   The following tests may be useful to help identify the cause:

    1.   Blood smear may show hemolysis in cases where indirect bilirubin alone is elevated.

    2.   Coombs test is used to distinguish between immune mediated hemolytic disorders (ABO incompatibility) and non-immune-mediated hemolytic disorders, including glucose-6-phosphate dehydrogenase (G6PD) deficiency and hereditary spherocytosis.

    3.   Liver function, alkaline phosphatase, bile acids, and sweat tests may identify a diagnosis if direct bilirubin is elevated.

    4.   Sepsis work-up (complete blood count and blood culture) is indicated in any jaundiced neonate with fever, hypotension, and tachypnea.

    5.   Maternal–fetal ABO and Rh incompatibilities (maternal and infant blood groups and types) may identify immune-related hyperbilirubinemia.

IX. Differential Diagnosis

A.   Within 24 hours, assess for hemolysis (ABO–Rh isoimmunization or hereditary spherocytosis).

B.   Within 48 hours, assess for the following:

    1.   Hemolysis.

    2.   Infection.

    3.   Physiologic jaundice.

C.   After 48 hours, assess for the following:

    1.   Infection.

    2.   Hemolysis.

    3.   Suboptimal intake jaundice.

    4.   Congenital malformation (biliary atresia).

    5.   Hepatitis.

X. Medical Management

A.   Usually no treatment is indicated in physiologic jaundice. However, early and frequent breastfeeding or human milk feeds may help keep bilirubin levels lower.

B.   When indicated, treatment should be initiated for any underlying infectious causes.

C.   Phototherapy, or ultraviolet (UV) light therapy, is indicated when bilirubin levels are greater than 15 to 20 mg/dL, regardless of cause. UV light converts the skin bilirubin (isomerization) into a more easily excreted form.

    1.   Phototherapy is typically used for unconjugated hyperbilirubinemia.

    2.   During phototherapy, infants should be unclothed with their eyelids shielded. Care must be taken to ensure that hydration is maintained.

    3.   Phototherapy can be delivered in two forms, overbed lights or fiber-optic blankets.

        a.   Both forms of phototherapy can be used in the nursery or in the hospital room.

      b.   Phototherapy lights can be used only in the hospital where there are professionals trained to assess dehydration.

      c.   Phototherapy blankets can be used at home, but only under close monitoring (e.g., daily hydration and weight checks).

    4.   Phototherapy lights are preferred for efficient management of significant hyperbilirubinemia. The number of lights used for phototherapy (i.e., single, double, or triple banks) increases the isomerization and also the risk for dehydration.

    5.   Phototherapy blankets are often used to augment phototherapy lights or when bilirubin levels are near the threshold for initiating phototherapy and trending down toward normal.

D.   Specific nomograms exist to govern when UV light therapy is indicated. BiliTool (http://bilitool.org) is an online risk assessment tool based on the American Academy of Pediatrics hour-specific nomogram that aids clinicians in identifying risks toward the development of hyperbilirubinemia.[11]

E.   Exchange transfusion may be indicated in very severe cases of hyperbilirubinemia when there has been no improvement with conservative measures. There are risks associated with exchange transfusion, including air embolism, volume imbalance, anemia, polycythemia, blood pressure fluctuation, infection, and necrotizing enterocolitis.[5,8,10]

XI. Breastfeeding Management of the Jaundiced Infant During Phototherapy [5,7,10,12]

A.   Explain to parents the reason for the jaundiced color and the implications related to breastfeeding.

B.   Teach parents how to determine whether their infant is feeding effectively.

C.   Provide written information regarding the clinical indicators of sufficient intake and infant danger signals.

D.   Assist the breastfeeding parent with techniques for the stimulation of milk production if a supplement is required.

    1.   Feed the baby frequently and effectively.

    2.   Express the breasts through hand or mechanical expression as an adjunct if supplementation has been recommended.

E.   Advocate for the avoidance of separating the dyad, if possible.

F.   Work with the clinician to develop a feeding plan that is individualized to the dyad's particular need.

G.   Provide a feeding diary to record feedings, supplement amounts, and infant output.

H.   Ensure the parents understand the importance of close follow-up.

XII. Evaluation of Successful Resolution of Hyperbilirubinemia

A.   Normal infant weight gain should occur, with 15 to 30 grams of weight gain per day after the onset of copious milk production.

B.   The onset of effective feeding will result in appropriate stooling for a baby with suboptimal intake jaundice. As stooling increases, the bilirubin level will decrease. There may be a rapid fall in the bilirubin level if effective feeding is established within 12 to 24 hours, which might eliminate the need for medical therapy.

C.   Milk production will develop normally, or improve if it had been insufficient, as evidenced by infant weight, hydration, and stool patterns and the ability to decrease or eliminate supplements.

D.   The breastfeeding relationship will be maintained and strengthened based on the previous parameters.

E.   Failure of the infant to improve within 12 to 24 hours indicates other underlying problems and a need for reappraisal of the infant by the clinician. Further exploration of reasons for insufficient milk production may also be indicated.

▶ Key Points from This Chapter

A.   Early, frequent, and exclusive breastfeeding meets the needs of healthy term infants.

B.   Routine screening and supplementation are not necessary and may harm the normal establishment of breastfeeding. However, at-risk infants should be screened for hypoglycemia, followed up as needed, and treated with supplementation or IV glucose if there are clinical signs or the expected blood glucose levels are not reached.

C. Helping parents continue to breastfeed or provide expressed milk should be the continuing focus in helping babies whose birth is complicated by hypoglycemia or hyperbilirubinemia.

D. Clinical jaundice is seen in almost all newborns and is usually benign. However, because of the risk for neurotoxicity, all infants are required to have an objective bilirubin assessment within 48 hours of birth.

🔍 CASE STUDY 1

Baby boy James was delivered via normal spontaneous vaginal delivery to 32-year-old Hailey, whose pregnancy was complicated with gestational diabetes that was poorly controlled on glyburide. At birth, James weighed 3,950 g (8 pounds, 11 ounces). Hailey had indicated a desire to breastfeed James. Her two previous children had not been breastfed; she produced milk and chose not to use it. James's initial glucose check at 1 hour of age was 33 mg/dL; there were no obvious symptoms.

Questions

1. Which of the following actions would you take and why?
   A. Give James approximately 15 mL of formula and repeat the glucose check in 30 minutes.
   B. Ask if James's heel was warmed before the test was done. If not, warm the heel and repeat the test immediately.
   C. Have Hailey breastfeed James now and repeat the test in 30 minutes.
   D. Start an IV and give a glucose bolus.
2. How long should glucose checks be done on James?
   A. Every 6 hours for 24 hours.
   B. Before each feeding for 24 hours.
   C. Repeat only if James becomes symptomatic.
   D. There is no reason to repeat any checks.
3. What follow-up will you recommend to Hailey?

Answers to multiple choice questions: 1, C and 2, B.

🔍 CASE STUDY 2

Demitrius was delivered via normal spontaneous vaginal delivery at 39.2 weeks to 34 year-old Sandra, a gravida 2 para 2 African American woman with blood type O positive. At birth, Demitrius weighed 3,170 g (6 pounds, 15.8 ounces). Sandra was positive for Group B Streptococcus but received adequate treatment during labor. The infant's initial serum bilirubin level at 24 hours of age was 7. 4/0.4 mg/dL and his blood type was O positive, Coombs negative. Demitrius's older sibling was born at 38.1 weeks and was small for gestational age at 2,528 g (5 pounds, 9 ounces). Her bilirubin peaked at 12 mg/dL and she did not require phototherapy. Demitrius had a TcB level done at 36 hours of 11.4. This was repeated via his serum and he was discharged home after the 48-hour serum bilirubin level returned at 9.8/0.4 mg/dL. His discharge weight was 2,995 g (6 pounds, 9.6 ounces).

The next day, he was seen by his primary care pediatrician. He weighed 2,835g (7 pounds, 6 ounces). Sandra reported trouble latching during breastfeeding but noted that Demitrius had 8 wet diapers and 4 bowel movements during the previous 24 hours. He was also evaluated by a lactation consultant. His bilirubin level was checked during his pediatrician visit at 70 hours of life via serum and the result was 16.8/0.4 mg/dL. The pediatrician instructed Sandra to pump breastmilk at the end of breastfeeding and supplement with pumped breastmilk after feedings at least 8–12 times per day. Phototherapy was not ordered, but Sandra was instructed to bring Demitrius back daily to evaluate bilirubin levels. Demitrius's bilirubin level peaked at 18.5/0.6 mg/dL on day 4 of life and decreased to 11.2/0.3 mg/dL on day 10 of life. No phototherapy was ordered, but a G6PD screen was ordered and returned negative on day 7 of life.

Questions

1. What risk factors for jaundice does Demitrius have?
2. Why was phototherapy not ordered for Demitrius?
3. What guidance would you give Sandra for pumping and supplementing Demitrius with her own breastmilk?
4. Describe the importance of obtaining serum bilirubin levels to assess hyperbilirubinemia rather than relying on physical assessment.

References

1. Wight N, Marinelli KA, Academy of Breastfeeding Medicine. ABM clinical protocol #1: guidelines for blood glucose monitoring and treatment of hypoglycemia in term and late-preterm neonates, revised 2014. *Breastfeed Med.* 2014;9(4):173-179.
2. Cornblath M, Reisner SH. Blood glucose in the neonate and its clinical significance. *N Engl J Med.* 1965;273:378-381.
3. Dalgiç N, Ergenekon E, Soysal S, Koç E, Atalay Y, Gücüyener K. Transient neonatal hypoglycemia—long-term effects on neurodevelopmental outcome. *J Pediatr Endocrinol Metab.* 2002;15:319-324.
4. de Rooy L, Hardin J. Nutritional factors that affect the postnatal metabolic adaptation of full term and small and large for gestational age infants. *Pediatrics.* 2002;109(3):E42.
5. Flaherman VJ, Maisels MJ, Academy of Breastfeeding Medicine. ABM clinical protocol #22: guidelines for management of jaundice in the breastfeeding infant 35 weeks or more gestation, revised 2017. *Breastfeed Med.* 2017;12(5):250-257. https://doi.org/10.1089/bfm.2017.29042.vjf.
6. American Academy of Pediatrics, American College of Obstetricians and Gynecologists. Care of the newborn. In: *Guidelines for Perinatal Care.* 7th ed. Elk Grove, IL: American Academy of Pediatrics; 2012:265-320.
7. Maisels MJ. Managing the jaundiced newborn: a persistent challenge. *CMAJ.* 2015;187(5):335-343.
8. Kliegman R, Stanton B, St Geme JW III, Schor NF, Behrman RE. *Nelson Textbook of Pediatrics.* 20th ed. Philadelphia, PA: Elsevier; 2016.
9. University of Bristol. Blackboard online jaundice seminar. Part 1 - bilirubin metabolism. https://www.ole.bris.ac.uk/bbcswebdav/institution/Faculty%20of%20Health%20Sciences/MB%20ChB%20Medicine/Year%203%20Medicine%20and%20Surgery%20-%20Hippocrates/Abdomen%20-%20Jaundice%20core%20topic/part_1__bilirubin_metabolism.html. Accessed March 10, 2018.
10. Lauer BJ, Nancy ND. Hyperbilirubinemia in the newborn. *Pediatr Rev.* 2011;32(8):341-349.
11. American Academy of Pediatrics Subcommittee on Hyperbilirubinemia. Management of hyperbilirubinemia in the newborn infant 35 or more weeks of gestation. *Pediatrics.* 2004;114(4):297-316.
12. Gourley GR, Li Z, Kreamer BL, Kosorok MR. A controlled, randomized, double-blind trial of prophylaxis against jaundice among breastfed newborns. *Pediatrics.* 2005;116(2):385-391.

Additional Resources

Academy of Breastfeeding Medicine Protocols. http://www.bfmed.org/protocols.
BiliTool. http://bilitool.org.

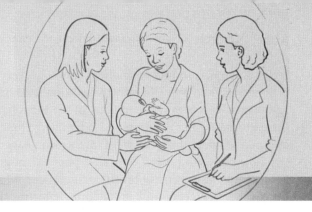

CHAPTER 22

Low Milk Production and Infant Weight

Kathleen L. Hoover
Lisa Marasco

OBJECTIVES

- Differentiate between infant and maternal contributions to infant poor weight gain.
- Describe the indicators and potential causes of low milk production.
- Develop appropriate management strategies for an infant with a weight gain problem.
- List options for increasing the rate of milk production.

DEFINITIONS OF COMMONLY USED TERMS

calibration of milk production The breast's adjustment of the rate of milk synthesis to match the infant's needs.
delayed lactation When the initiation of copious milk production takes longer than 72 hours. Also called delayed onset of lactation or delayed secretory activation.
incomplete lactogenesis Failure to reach full milk production despite effective, frequent breastfeeding.
primary lactation problems Poor milk synthesis due to maternal physiological issues.
secondary lactation problems Inadequate milk production due to outside interferences.

Any use of the term *mother*, *maternal*, or *breastfeeding* is not meant to exclude transgender or nonbinary parents who may be breastfeeding or providing human milk to their infant.

▶ Overview

Healthy breastfed infants grow robustly in the first few months following birth.[1] Deviations from this normal pattern merit evaluation. Inadequate weight gain in the breastfed infant occurs mainly in infants younger than 6 months. Newborns dehydrate quickly, so it is imperative that they be assessed frequently in the early days.[2] An infant who is not doing well should be followed carefully every few days until the weight gain is appropriate. Failure to thrive is dangerous and requires early recognition and corrective action. Failure to thrive beyond 1 month of age is often associated with organic conditions of the birth parent or infant,[3,4] but it can also be due to mismanagement of breastfeeding. After the problem is identified, clinicians have a responsibility to provide effective lactation support and to document the recovery of infants who have failed to gain weight or have lost excessive weight.

Low milk production can cause poor infant growth and continues to be the major reason given worldwide for the discontinuation of breastfeeding.[5] Poor infant growth can lead to poor feeding at the breast and a further decrease in the rate of milk production, reflecting the interdependent nature of the breastfeeding relationship and what has been referred to as the "mother–baby dance" (see *Additional Resources*). Whether the problem is perceived or real, getting to the root of the issue is crucial for the baby's appropriate weight gain.

Solving the riddle of poor infant growth and low milk production starts with deciphering the causes so a targeted strategy can be formulated. The timing of the onset of a problem coupled with the elapsed time to identify the issues and implement necessary changes contribute to the outcome. When milk production has been robust, course corrections are more likely to yield good responses. When milk production has been suppressed in the early days or weeks, there may be more difficulty with increasing production, even when all variables are successfully addressed. Clinicians need to consider all of these variables as they counsel parents about their options.

I. Identifying the Causes for Weight Gain Issues

A.   Listen to the whole story first, then take a detailed history to collect information regarding the problem.
1.   Screen the infant's health and analyze the infant's weight history based on World Health Organization (WHO) growth velocity charts. (See *Additional Resources* later in this chapter for a link to the WHO charts.)
a.   Determine whether the baby is fed exclusively at the breast or is also being supplemented. If the baby is being supplemented, determine the amount and type of supplementation (expressed milk versus other milk) and include this as part of the weight analysis.
b.   Assess the big picture. Was the weight gain within expected parameters? What role did supplementation play in this gain? Did the baby leave a significant amount of milk in the breast?
2.   Screen the parent's health, including reproductive and pregnancy history, and examine the breasts. Are there any risk factors for lactation problems?
B.   Observe one or more feedings to assess latch and milk transfer. (See Chapter 13, *Facilitating and Assessing Breastfeeding Initiation*, for a feeding assessment and signs of milk transfer.)
C.   If there is a problem, take the following steps:
1.   First and foremost, make sure the baby is adequately fed; this may require supplementation.
2.   Second, try to determine the root cause, or causes, of the low milk production.
a.   Has the problem been present since birth? If no, when did it become apparent?
b.   Screen for breastfeeding management problems.
c.   Screen for primary factors related to the parent.
d.   If milk remained in the breast after the feeding, determine the cause for the baby's inability to remove milk.
3.   Support milk production as needed and address the problem as soon as possible (see **FIGURE 22-1**).

II. Poor Growth in Breastfed Babies

A.   Watch for red flags indicating weight loss in newborns (first 28 days).
1.   Fluids received during labor may artificially increase the birth weight.[6] The baby's day 2 weight may be more appropriate for calculating weight loss because the baby may have been experiencing diuresis of extra fluids during the first 24 hours.[7]
2.   Transition stools should appear by day 3 to 4 with the onset of lactogenesis.
a.   Stools that have not turned yellow by day 5 indicate that the baby is not taking in enough milk. The cause may be either a delay in the onset of copious milk production or an impairment in the baby's ability to transfer sufficient milk.[8]
b.   A lack of stools or persistent dark stools should trigger an immediate, careful evaluation.

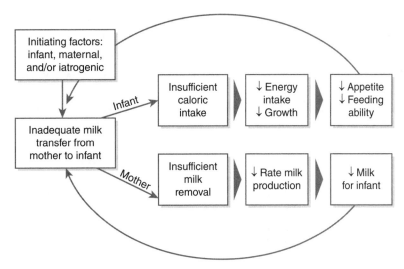

FIGURE 22-1 Interdependent factors influencing maternal milk production and infant growth.

© Christina M. Smilie, MD, IBCLC, FAAP, FABM.

   3.   Further investigation is warranted for any baby who has failed to regain birth weight by one week.
        a.   A baby who lost significant weight but is now gaining it back does not need immediate assistance but should be followed to ensure continued progress.
        b.   Chronically underfed babies who are not gaining become weak, ineffective feeders and may lose their appetite and feed sleepily. This can lead to inadequate milk transfer that can compromise milk production. These babies require assistance to gradually take in more milk and begin regaining weight.
   4.   Be alert for clinical signs of dehydration (e.g., poor skin turgor, dry mucous membranes in the mouth, scant or concentrated urine, urate crystals in the diaper past the first 2 days, or sunken fontanelle).
        a.   When an infant has no urine output in any given 24-hour period, or in the case of weight loss greater than 12 percent, the baby should be immediately seen by a healthcare provider for further testing.
        b.   Careful rehydration should commence right away, followed by an investigation into the contributing factors.[9]

B.   Be alert to red flags for failure to thrive.
   1.   Failure to thrive is defined by any of the following[10 (pp 344-345)]:
        a.   Infant continues to lose weight beyond 10 days after birth.
        b.   Infant does not regain birth weight by 3 weeks of age.
        c.   Infant gains at a rate below the 10th percentile for weight beyond 1 month of age.
        d.   Infant drops more than two standard deviations from a previously stable weight curve.
   2.   Infants who fail to thrive may have one or more of the following characteristics:
        a.   Apathetic or weak cry.
        b.   Poor muscle tone and skin turgor.
        c.   Concentrated and scant urine; urate crystals presenting after 2 days.
        d.   Infrequent and small bowel movements; newborns may still be passing black, tarry meconium stools into week 2.
        e.   Very sleepy with infrequent feedings; parents may misinterpret their low energy as being good babies.
        f.   Constantly fussy with frequent feedings.
        g.   Poor, erratic, or no weight gain.
        h.   Swallow only with the milk ejection reflex or have sporadic swallowing.
        i.   Too weak to take in enough milk by breast or bottle; require gentle prodding to gradually take more.

C.   Watch for other red flags and causes of poor weight gain.
   1.   In infants between the ages of 2 weeks and 3 months, the situation must be assessed when weight gain is less than 200 grams per week. For infants older than 3 months, the minimum acceptable gain is lower. Use the WHO growth charts to help determine when a baby is in trouble. (See *Additional Resources* later in this chapter.)
   2.   Older babies may be skinny but still alert and happy, leading parents to believe all is well. Yet these babies may constantly have their hands in their mouth (a feeding cue).
   3.   The baby may have an impaired suck due to conditions such as tongue mobility restriction.
   4.   The baby may demonstrate self-limiting feeding behaviors secondary to painful experiences, such as reflux, allergies, illness, or responding to high milk flow.
   5.   The overuse of pacifiers can mask infant feeding cues and reduce milk intake.
   6.   A deficiency of vitamin B12 in the milk, due to a lack in the parent's diet, can lead to poor growth and brain damage in a breastfed baby.[11] See **TABLE 22-1**.

TABLE 22-1 Infant Factors That May Contribute to Slow Weight Gain and Low Milk Production

Factor	Effect
Alterations in oral and facial anatomy	Alterations—such as ankyloglossia,[11] cleft lip, cleft of hard or soft palate,[12] or facial or other congenital anomalies—may contribute to poor sucking ability and thus inadequate milk intake.
Suck impairment	A baby with an impaired suck of any etiology will not remove milk well, which can cause poor milk production. Research shows that babies with higher suction pressure stimulated higher prolactin surges, and their mothers reported better milk production. Mothers of infants with lower suction pressure had smaller prolactin surges and were more likely to report problems with milk production.[13]
Peripartum factors affecting suck	Cesarean delivery, labor medications, epidural analgesia, forceps, and vacuum extraction can affect brain function, state control, and anatomical structures and nerves that may lead to ineffective milk transfer.[14]
Neurological problems; muscle tone issues; airway restrictions; or sensory integration problems	Hypotonia, hypertonia, neurologic pathology or physiology may interfere with the performance, strength, or stamina of the structures involved in the suck, swallow, and breathe cycle. Tracheomalacia and laryngomalacia are two conditions that affect the airway. Infants affected with sensory integration problems may not feed well, leading to poor breast stimulation, reduced milk removal, and decreased milk production.[15]
High energy requirements	Cardiac defects often put an infant at risk for poor growth because of the combination of low endurance for feeding and high metabolic demands. Respiratory involvement (bronchopulmonary dysplasia) and metabolic disorders can create a need for increased caloric intake. Some conditions require volume restrictions that place limits on intake, so high-calorie breastmilk is needed.
Gestational age	Infants born preterm, late preterm, postterm, small for gestational age, with intrauterine growth restriction, and large for gestational age may lack mature feeding skills and have difficulty with sucking or feeding stamina.
Syndromes; illnesses; infections; injuries; allergies; and gastrointestinal, metabolic or malabsorption problems	Chromosomal defects—such as trisomy 21 (Down syndrome), cystic fibrosis, infections or sepsis, infant botulism, injuries (e.g., nuchal cord, fractured clavicle, repeated heel sticks, scalp or brain bleeds from vacuum or forceps extraction, meconium aspiration, or deep suctioning), atopic dermatitis,[16] or growth faltering—may be apparent in the early months. Gastroesophageal reflux disease, or other conditions that limit intake, can affect nutrient absorption or metabolism. Pyloric stenosis, hypoxia, and syndromes such as Pierre Robin, DiGeorge, Turner, and Rett can also affect infant growth.

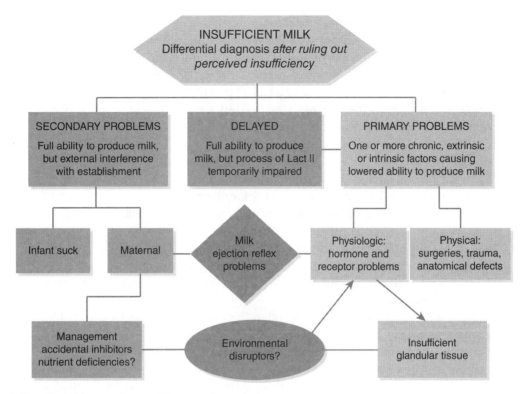

FIGURE 22-2 Differential diagnosis for insufficient milk production.

Lisa Marasco, © 2017.

III. Unsubstantiated Low Milk Production

A. Parents often misjudge their milk production, based on infant behavior or personal experiences, and may perceive insufficiency when there is actually plenty of milk.[12] This is referred to as "perceived insufficient milk production."

B. The belief that milk production is insufficient to meet the baby's needs may lead to the introduction of unnecessary supplementation, less feeding at the breast, and ultimately a decrease in the rate of milk production.

C. After ruling out perceived insufficiency, the clinician needs to determine the cause for insufficient milk production. The cause may be secondary (due to external issues), delayed lactogenesis II, or a primary maternal problem (see **FIGURE 22-2**). These are explored in the next sections.

IV. Secondary Causes for Insufficient Milk Production

A. Secondary causes for insufficient milk production include one or more forces that interfere with the normal process of breastfeeding, resulting in a lower calibration of milk production.[9] Individuals with secondary causes begin with the potential for full milk production.

B. Iatrogenic factors in the process of treating a parent or baby for a condition can result in a negative impact on lactation.

   1. Formula supplementation, sometimes suggested for neonatal hyperbilirubinemia or hypoglycemia, can disrupt frequent breastfeedings.

   2. Delays in the initiation of breastfeeding for any reason, or any interruption of breastfeeding, can impair early milk production.[13]

   3. Suboptimal hospital practices may place restrictions on the length or frequency of feedings. The family may then interpret their baby's normal desire to feed longer or more frequently as a sign that the colostrum is not enough for the baby, leading to supplementation.

4. Encouraging families to send the baby to the nursery at night can lead to formula supplementation. Infants then become dissatisfied with the smaller volume of colostrum, starting a downward spiral of supplementation and down regulation of milk production.

5. Parents may delay feedings or milk expression because they are uncomfortable doing so in front of visitors and hospital personnel due to a lack of privacy.

6. Errant instructions to discontinue breastfeeding because of medications or anesthesia, without compensatory milk removal, will decrease production.

C. Failure to understand the concept of demand and supply may lead to choices that can unwittingly undermine milk production.

1. When the baby is unable to feed directly at the breast, failure to remove milk as often as the baby would normally feed will decrease the rate of milk production.

2. Failure to remove residual milk when the baby is not feeding effectively will decrease the rate of production.

3. Pain from latch or birth sequelae can lead parents to delay or skip feedings.

4. Prolonged, unrelieved breast engorgement leads to cessation of lactation.[14]

5. Combining breastfeeding with formula feeding compromises milk production, especially in the early postpartum period.[15]

6. Scheduled feedings or sleep training often impose longer intervals than babies would normally adopt for feedings.

7. Working parents may not express milk as often as their baby feeds at home.[16]

8. A parent of a preterm baby might not express milk to the peak level, but only to the transient limited needs of the small baby at the time, causing a lowered calibration of milk yield.

D. Nipple anomalies (e.g., large, long, meaty, or flat) can affect a baby's ability to latch or remove milk effectively, thereby reducing milk production.[17-19]

E. Unsupervised use of, or inappropriate reliance on, nipple shields (especially in the absence of efforts to protect milk production with hand expression or pumping) may lead to lower milk production when the baby is not able to remove milk efficiently or stimulate the breast effectively.[20]

F. Suboptimal milk expression methods and equipment can negatively impact milk production when they are used in place of breastfeeding.[21]

1. Parents who combine manual expression along with pumping produce more milk than those who use only one expression method.[22]

2. Parents of preterm infants who use electric pumps with specialized expression patterns have greater cumulative milk outputs than those who use pumps with standard patterns.[23]

G. Some medications can reduce milk production.

1. Pseudoephedrine, a nasal decongestant for colds and allergies, has a suppressive effect on lactation, causing a lowered calibration of milk yield.[24]

2. First-generation antihistamines (diphenhydramine, chlorpheniramine) administered in high dosages by injection may have an inhibitory effect on lactation.[25]

3. Hormonal birth control (oral, injectable, implants, transdermal patch, vaginal ring, or emergency contraceptives) or other hormone treatments should be avoided until at least 6 weeks postpartum.[26-29]

    a. Estrogen has a stronger inhibitory effect in the early postpartum months, making combined hormonal contraception riskier.[31]

    b. Progesterone is less risky but still may reduce milk production in the early weeks and months.[32,33]

4. Prolactin-inhibiting dopaminergic drugs, such as levodopa (for Parkinson disease), bromocriptine, cabergoline, lisuride, ergonovine, and methylergonovine, can inhibit lactation.[25]

5. Bupropion (an antidepressant and smoking deterrent medication) and aripiprazole and promethazine (antipsychotics that do not antagonize dopamine) have been reported to suppress lactation in a few mothers.[25,34]

H. Cigarette smoking reduces milk volume and the duration of lactation.[35]

I. Nutritional factors in the maternal diet may cause insufficient milk.

1. A deficiency of certain lactation-critical nutrients may contribute to lactation failure.[36] These include zinc,[37] iodine,[38] iron,[39,40] and protein.[41-43]

2. Eating disorders are associated with shorter duration of lactation, yet this cause is often misattributed generically to "insufficient milk."[44,45]
    a. Anorexia nervosa during pubertal breast development can cause a reduction of the fat pad and subsequent breast shrinkage.[46] Current anorexia may result in inadequate nutrition or body fat from which nutrients are drawn.
    b. The active binge and purge cycle of bulimia can cause lower prolactin levels; the implications are unknown.[47]
3. A severe restriction of food intake during pregnancy or lactation, especially if the energy intake drops below 1,500 kcal daily on a regular basis, may cause milk production problems.[48,49]
4. Gastric bypass surgery is associated with lactation problems.[50] Individuals who have had this surgery should eat at least 65 grams of protein daily and will need extra vitamin B12.[51]

J. Any time the milk ejection reflex is chronically impaired, poor milk removal can lead to down regulation of milk production. Inhibiting factors can be psychological, hormonal, or physical. They include stress, thyroid dysfunction,[52] and cigarette smoking.[53] Obese mice have demonstrated a poor milk ejection reflex and lactation failure.[54]

K. Other possible inhibitors of milk production include a new pregnancy; ingesting large amounts of anti-galactagogue herbs such as sage, parsley, and mint; and high doses of vitamin B6 (pyridoxine).[25]

V. Delayed Lactogenesis II as a Cause of Insufficient Milk Production

A. Delayed lactogenesis, also called delayed onset of lactation or delayed secretory activation, is defined as the onset of copious milk production beyond 72 hours.[19]
1. Mothers with delayed onset of lactation have the ability to produce sufficient milk for the baby. The problem is temporary and usually self-resolves with improved breastfeeding management.[55]
2. Incomplete lactogenesis II is differentiated from delayed onset of lactation in that full copious milk production is never reached, despite appropriate management. This results in chronic suboptimal milk production.[56]
3. When the onset of lactation takes longer than 72 hours, the long-term survival rate of breastfeeding drops below that of individuals with a normal onset.[57] Prompt assistance is critical to the potential for full milk production.

B. A variety of risk factors can cause delayed lactation.[55]
1. Primiparous mothers are at higher risk of experiencing delayed lactation, likely because they are establishing prolactin receptors for the first time.[58]
2. Factors surrounding the birth can affect the onset of lactation, including the following:
    a. Stress during labor.[58]
    b. Prolonged stage 2 of labor (greater than 1 hour).[19]
    c. Labor analgesics and anesthesia.[59,60]
    d. Significant edema of extremities, such as swollen legs and ankles, especially when pregnancy edema worsens after delivery or edema develops for the first time after birth.[6,61]
    e. Cesarean birth (especially when urgent[62]), the use of forceps, or vacuum delivery.
    f. Augmentation of labor with synthetic oxytocin administration during labor,[19,63] although the studies are conflicting.[64]
3. Preterm labor treatments and preterm birth increase the risk for delayed onset of lactation. The potential causes include the following:
    a. Beta-agonist tocolytics, such as terbutaline.[59,65]
    b. Corticosteroid treatment prior to delivery.[65]
    c. Delayed and inadequate milk removal when the baby is not at the breast.[67]
    d. Stress related to the preterm experience.[62,68]
4. Selective serotonin reuptake inhibitor (SSRI) antidepressants during pregnancy can affect the onset of lactation.[59,69]
5. Retained placental tissue may continue to issue progesterone and interfere with full milk production until the tissue passes or is removed.[70] Treatments such as methylergonovine maleate, a vasoconstrictor

used to treat postdelivery hemorrhaging, can inhibit lactation, either temporarily during short-term use or more seriously if used long-term.[34]

6. Gestational ovarian theca lutein cysts—a condition that causes high testosterone levels during pregnancy—will delay secretory activation.[71]

   a. In some cases, the cysts may also cause virilization (balding, deepening of the voice, facial or abdominal hair growth, pimples on the face or back, or enlargement of the clitoris).

   b. High testosterone gradually resolves on its own days to weeks after birth. With continued breast stimulation, full milk production may eventually be achieved.

VI. Primary Physical Causes of Insufficient Milk Production

A. Breast anatomy variations, anomalies, or other physically damaging events can chronically limit the secretory capacity of the breast.

B. Breast surgery, such as augmentation and reduction, carries the risk of disrupting nerves and ducts and interfering with lactation. The longer the time since the surgery, the better the chance for ducts to recanalize and nerves to reinnervate.[72,73]

C. Primary hypoplasia, a condition of insufficient glandular tissue, results in suboptimal milk production ranging from mild to severe.[74] It is loosely defined as insufficient lactation tissue to produce enough milk to support adequate infant growth and development, if all other factors are normal.[75]

   1. Insufficient glandular tissue is not always visually evident, but is usually more evident on palpation. Some breasts present with normal dimensions, but their appearance suggests a failure to respond normally to pregnancy hormones.[76]

   2. Risk factors for poor lactation related to insufficient glandular tissue include the following:

      a. Interbreast spacing greater than 1.5 inches (3.8 cm).

      b. Lack of significant visible veining on the breasts.

      c. Stretch marks (striae) on the breast in the absence of growth.

      d. Higher hypoplasia breast type; severity increases from 1 to 4[77] (**FIGURE 22-3**).

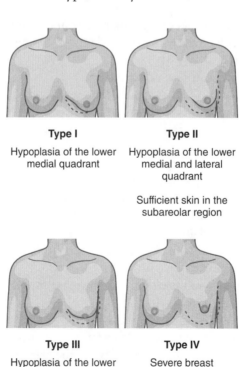

Type I
Hypoplasia of the lower medial quadrant

Type II
Hypoplasia of the lower medial and lateral quadrant

Sufficient skin in the subareolar region

Type III
Hypoplasia of the lower medial and lateral quadrant

Skin deficiency in the subareolar region

Type IV
Severe breast constriction

Minimal breast base

FIGURE 22-3 Classification of tuberous breast deformity.

3. Insufficient glandular tissue poses a high risk for losing even the small amount of milk a mother may be producing. It is very important to assess milk transfer and residual milk (removed by pump). If the baby leaves behind more than a negligible amount of milk, expressing after feedings is crucial to protect milk production.[30]

D. A number of damaging events can impair milk production.

1. Mastitis, including subclinical mastitis, can cause a drop in milk production when gap junctions temporarily open to clear out the infection.[78] This usually reverses within a few days.

   a. In some anecdotal cases, abscesses and mastitis have damaged lactation tissue permanently, limiting milk production.[79]

   b. Trauma or other insults to the breast, such as radiation,[80] burns, repeated chest X-rays, or chemotherapy for breast cancer, can disrupt mammary development and lactation potential.[81,82]

2. Spinal cord injuries can potentially inhibit milk production.

   a. The breast is innervated through thoracic vertebrae T3 to T6; if damage occurs at T6 or above, lactation may be affected.[83]

   b. Lactation often falters around 3 months after a spinal cord injury. A report of three cases suggests that aiding milk ejection via visualization or synthetic oxytocin spray may help sustain lactation.[84]

3. Endocrine disruptors, or chemicals that interfere with hormones, can inhibit mammary development or milk production in humans and other mammals. These include, but are not limited to, TCDD, bisphenol A, PCBs, and polycyclic aromatic hydrocarbons.[36,76,85-87]

4. Pregnancy complications, such as placental insufficiency, can negatively affect mammary development during pregnancy,[88] although the breasts can continue to grow after birth with sufficient breastfeeding stimulation.

5. When delivery occurs between 22 and 34 weeks, breast development may or may not be sufficiently complete for full lactation at the time of birth.[89]

VII. Primary Physiological Causes of Insufficient Milk Production

A. Physiological conditions may limit the secretory capacity of the breast. Some primary factors (e.g., parent's age, weight, diabetes) have previously been categorized as risk factors for delayed lactation. However, these tend to result in incomplete lactogenesis and longer-term suppression of lactation, leading to premature weaning.

B. Older parents (defined variously as ranging from 30 to 40 years) are at greater risk of producing less milk or not exclusively breastfeeding.[61,90] The reasons are not clear and may be multifactorial.

C. A history of hypertension or pregnancy-induced hypertension is associated with a higher risk of suboptimal lactation.[90,91]

D. Obesity, defined as body mass index greater than 27 kilograms per meter squared, is associated with a higher risk for poor lactation onset[19,61,92-94] and inadequate milk production.[95,96]

E. Excessive weight gain during pregnancy is associated with greater difficulty in initiating and sustaining lactation.[97]

F. Insulin dysregulation of any type can potentially interfere with mammary development or milk synthesis.[98,99] Poor metabolic control increases the risk of delayed lactation in primiparous mothers,[100] and the overall lactation duration decreases as the severity of diabetes increases.[101]

1. Type 1 insulin-dependent diabetes mellitus may cause a delayed onset of lactation for up to 24 hours. Milk production may continue to struggle if the condition is unstable.[102]

2. Insulin resistance, including non-insulin-dependent Type 2 diabetes mellitus and gestational diabetes mellitus, is associated with more difficulty in initiating and sustaining lactation.[103,104] Insulin treatment during pregnancy multiplies the risk for lactation problems.[105,106]

   a. Elevated values for hemoglobin A1c, body mass index, oral glucose tolerance test, and subscapular thickness are associated with shorter lactation duration.[107]

   b. Infants born to women with gestational diabetes mellitus have less mature sucking patterns and do not remove milk as efficiently as their unaffected counterparts.[108]

   c. Treatment with metformin, an insulin-sensitizing drug, has reportedly helped increase milk production modestly in some women with polycystic ovarian syndrome.[109] In a recent study, mothers with low milk production and at least one sign of insulin resistance who started taking metformin sustained their milk production level or had slight increases, while those taking placebo suffered further declines.[110]

G. Thyroid dysfunction may affect both oxytocin and prolactin. Human research is scarce, but animal studies elucidate the likely pathways of disturbance.[38,52,86] Subclinical or borderline thyroid dysfunction may present first as a lactation problem.[52,111]

   1. In rat studies, hypothyroidism induced during pregnancy negatively affects prolactin and oxytocin release and also inhibits prolactin signaling through decreased prolactin receptors, resulting in premature involution of the mammary gland.[112,113] Only small studies and case reports document the same impact on human mothers.[111,114]

   2. Hyperthyroid pregnant rats have accelerated mammary development and early onset of lactation. However, there is impairment in oxytocin and milk ejection, as well as lipid metabolism.

      a. The more severe the hyperthyroid state during pregnancy, the more severe the impairment of oxytocin, resulting in early onset of lactation with quick engorgement, milk stasis, possible mastitis, and eventual involution.[115]

      b. Later-onset hyperthyroidism can stimulate hyperlactation.[38,52,116]

   3. Postpartum thyroiditis is a transient condition occurring anytime in the first year after birth.

      a. It may begin as hyperthyroid and then swing to hypothyroid, or it may occur as hyperthyroid or hypothyroid alone.

      b. Postpartum thyroiditis is often not caught until the hypothyroid stage when milk production is more likely to decline.[111,117,118]

   4. Milk production is not likely to improve with normal measures if an underlying thyroid problem is not addressed. Healthcare professionals should consider lactation problems as a symptom when interpreting laboratory results and determining treatments.[119]

H. Prolactin is essential to the start-up and maintenance of milk production; problems with prolactin secretion result in poor or no lactation.

   1. Low baseline prolactin can be the simple result of infrequent milk removal or breast stimulation.

      a. It also may develop as the result of poor prolactin surges secondary to other conditions, such as obesity[120] or poor infant suck.[121]

      b. Primary low prolactin is considered rare.

      c. Mothers with a family history of alcoholism had lower prolactin responses to suckling, and their infants fed more frequently than mothers without this family history.[122]

   2. If baseline prolactin is low, increasing prolactin should result in higher milk production. If additional breast stimulation is not sufficient, drugs such as domperidone, metoclopramide, and sulpiride can stimulate the pituitary to release more prolactin.

I. Hypopituitarism results in loss of prolactin secretion, with resulting failure of lactation. The causes include prior radiation to the brain, Sheehan syndrome,[123,124] and empty sella syndrome.[125]

J. Individuals with Sjögren syndrome may have poor milk production that, in some cases, responds favorably to hydroxychloroquine therapy.[10,126]

K. Hypertension and pregnancy-induced hypertension are associated with lactation problems. HELLP syndrome (hemolysis, elevated liver enzymes, low platelets) is a severe form of this condition.[127]

L. Hyperandrogenism, an excess of male hormones, is a risk factor for lactation problems.[128]

M. Women with a history of infertility, especially those requiring assisted reproductive technology to achieve a successful pregnancy, have more difficulty with lactation and do not breastfeed as long as controls.[86,129] Polycystic ovarian syndrome is the leading cause of infertility in women; it can cause low progesterone, insulin resistance, elevated estrogen, or hyperandrogenism, all of which have the potential to negatively affect lactation[98,130-132] (see **FIGURE 22-4**).

VIII. Management of Low Milk Production and Poor Weight Gain

A. The first step in assessing how to manage concerns about low milk production or poor weight gain is to gauge the adequacy of the baby's overall weight gain and rate of growth. Most babies will fall between the 25th and 75th percentiles. If growth falls below the 25th percentile, further investigation into factors related to the parent versus infant is warranted.

SCREENING FOR MILK PRODUCTION PROBLEMS

Mother: Secondary

- Poor latch, struggles from start
- Poor breast/ mouth fit
- Firm, inelastic breast tissue
- Infrequent feeds (< 8x/24 hours)
- Restricted/scheduled feeding times
- Infrequent pumping sessions _____
- Chronic incomplete breast drainage
- Reliance on poor quality breast pump
- Breast infection
- Smokes cigarettes or uses tobacco products
- Medications _____
- Hormonal birth control started: _____
  - ○ Pill   ○ Patch   ○ IUD   ○ Injection
- Herbs, teas _____
- Eating disorder _____
- Poor nutrition or < 1,500kcals/day
- Deficiency zinc, iodine, iron, calcium, protein
- Gastric bypass surgery: when? _____
- New pregnancy

Mother: Delayed/Suppressed Lactation

- Milk in > 72 hours _____
- Difficult birth/stress/urgent c-section
- Swelling after birth (edema)
- Hypertension
- Overweight/obese or excess pregnancy gain
- GDM/TI/T2 Diabetes/Metabolic Syndrome
- Insulin treatment of T2 or GDM during pregnancy
- Advanced Maternal Age
- Severe PP bleeding/hypotensive/anemia
- Placental problems during pregnancy/delivery
- Retained placental tissue
- Placenta accreta, increta, percreta
- Gestational ovarian theta-lutein cyst
- SSRIs in late pregnancy or early pp
- Corticosteroids for prem labor 3–9 d prior to birth
- Prenatal tocolytics (for preterm contractions)
- B-6 for hyperemesis-dose & duration? _____

Mother: Other Primary

- Breast surgery: augmentation, reduction, other
- Breast or cranial radiation, or chemotherapy
- Blunt trauma to chest or burn wounds
- Spinal cord injury, accidents (nerves)
- Obstructed ducts or nipple pores
- Previous severe mastitis or abscess
- History of Infertility or PCOS
- Obesity, excessive pregnancy weight gain _____
- Diabetes T1, T2, Insulin Resistance
- Thyroid dysfunction (hypo/hyper, or PP)
- Hyperandrogenism/clinical or lab
- Low baseline prolactin
- Other _____

Maternal Red Flag Risk Factors

- Failed oral glucose tol test or elevated A1C
- Early return of menses
- Chronic breast inflammation
- Family hx alcoholism
- History of autoimmune condition
- History of hyperprolactinemia: tx? _____
- Exposure to hormonal disruptors-when?

Mother: IGT Risk Factors

- Breast type (Huggins):   1   2   3   4
- Unusual breast shape _____
- Distance between breasts > 1.5"
- Significant asymmetry of breasts
- Prenatal breast growth? ○ None   ○ A little   ○ A lot
- Postpart breast growth? ○ None   ○ A little   ○ A lot
- Stretch marks with little breast growth
- Scant veining
- Bulbous areola
- Sparse palpable glandular tissue
- Masculine body shape
- Late breast development
- Obese/insulin resistant prior to puberty
- Hormonal birth control before breasts fully developed

Mother: Milk Ejection

- History of abuse
- Recent traumatic event or birth
- Post-traumatic stress disorder or bfg pain
- Weak infant suck
- Breast surgery, especially peri-areolar
- Spinal cord injury
- Alcohol or cigarettes
- Thyroid problems, especially hyperthyroid

Baby:

- Weak suction or slips off a lot
- Suck/swallow/breathe difficulties
- Stridor (squeaking)
- High or low muscle tone
- Torticollis (head pulls to one side)
- Small or Large for gestational age baby
- Very receding chin
- Hard/soft/submucosal cleft palate
- Bubble palate
- Restrictive lingual frenulum/tongue-tie
- Restrictive maxillary frenum/lip-tie
- Clicking, tongue retracting or thrusting
- Cardiac or respiratory problems

FIGURE 22-4 Screening tool for investigating low milk production.

TABLE 22-2 Adaptation of WHO Weight Velocity in Grams per Day Standards for the Rate of Weight Gain over the First 60 Days of Life for Exclusively Breastfed Infants Born at 37+ Weeks' Gestation Who Were Enrolled in the WHO Growth Reference Study, All Birth Weights Combined

Age (n)	Centile	Girls (g/day)	Boys (g/day)
0–7 days	Median	14	21
	25th	0	0
	10th	−14	−21
	5th	−29	−36
	(n)	(384)	(384)
7–14 days	Median	29	36
	25th	14	19
	10th	0	0
	5th	−7	−7
	(n)	(382)	(381)
14–28 days	Median	39	40
	25th	32	32
	10th	25	25
	5th	21	21
	(n)	(441)	(417)
28–42 days	Median	35	40
	25th	27	32
	10th	21	25
	5th	18	21
	(n)	(441)	(417)
42–60 days	Median	29	34
	25th	22	28
	10th	18	22
	5th	15	18
	(n)	(440)	(416)

Data from World Health Organization. *WHO Child Growth Standards: Growth Velocity Based on Weight, Length and Head Circumference: Methods and Development.* Geneva, Switzerland: World Health Organization; 2009.

B. Data from the WHO show that most infants gain rapidly in the first 2 months, slowing down thereafter.
 1. **TABLE 22-2** provides a detailed view of the velocity of growth during the first 2 months. Note that in the first week of life, babies who fall below the 25th percentile are still losing weight. The general expectation is that babies will gain at the median rate or higher.
 2. **TABLE 22-3** provides the larger picture of total weight gain per month by percentiles. The majority of infants fall between the 25th and 75th percentiles.
 3. These tables provide the practical data behind the WHO growth curves and complement their use. See Additional Resources for links to the growth curves.
C. If the baby is not gaining weight appropriately, consider the following actions:
 1. Massage the breasts before breastfeeding to trigger faster milk ejection and increase the cream content of the milk to help fuel faster weight recovery.[133,134]

TABLE 22-3 Adaptation of WHO 1-Month Weight Increments (Total Grams Gained per Month) Simplified Field Tables, Birth to 12 months by Percentiles

Interval	Girls					Boys				
	5th	25th	50th	75th	95th	5th	25th	50th	75th	95th
0–4 wks	446	697	879	1068	1348	460	805	1023	1229	1509
4wks–2mo	578	829	1011	1198	1476	713	992	1196	1408	1724
2–3 mo	369	571	718	869	1094	446	658	815	980	1228
3–4 mo	259	448	585	726	937	285	476	617	764	985
4–5 mo	172	355	489	627	833	194	383	522	666	883
5–6 mo	93	271	401	537	739	103	287	422	563	773
6–7 mo	37	214	344	480	684	42	223	357	496	706
7–8 mo	−2	178	311	450	659	−1	181	316	457	671
8–9 mo	−40	139	273	412	623	−36	148	285	429	646
9–10 mo	−70	110	245	385	598	−66	120	259	405	627
10–11 mo	−89	95	233	378	598	−89	100	243	394	623
11–12 mo	−102	88	232	383	612	−106	91	239	397	635

Data from World Health Organization. *WHO Child Growth Standards: Growth Velocity Based on Weight, Length and Head Circumference: Methods and Development*. Geneva, Switzerland: World Health Organization; 2009.

CLINICAL TIP

Much has been researched and written about the normal needs and intakes of infants. When it comes to undernourished babies, however, we have only clinical experience and expert opinion to support common strategies regarding appropriate amounts for supplementation. There are conflicting thoughts on whether allowing babies to gain weight rapidly to catch up to their expected weight could result in a permanently higher demand and a heightened risk for childhood obesity. Research into the long-term growth outcomes of previously compromised babies is needed to provide a firm basis for recommendations of how much milk is needed in the context of fueling necessary growth without overfeeding or underfeeding babies.

2. Increase the number of effective breastfeedings and verify that the baby is removing milk.
3. Ensure that the baby feeds on both breasts at each feeding.
4. If the baby is sleepy or not sucking actively, use breast compression to increase the milk flow and encourage more drinking.
5. Avoid bottles, pacifiers, and nipple shields unless clinically indicated. Supervise their use and devise a plan to withdraw these interventions when they are no longer necessary. Sleepy babies may temporarily need a high-flow method to take in enough calories so they can build up energy for improved feeding skills.
6. Remind the parent to practice good self-care, such as rest, drink plenty of fluids, and eat a balanced diet with plenty of protein.[17,135]

D.   Supplementary feeding might be necessary.[136]

1.   Temporary or permanent supplementation may be required for recovery from malnutrition and is ideally achieved with human milk feedings. The first choice should be the parent's expressed milk.

2.   Ideally, give only human milk in the first 6 months; however, formula supplements may be required if the milk production is insufficient and a safe source of donor human milk is not available.

3.   In some cases, high-calorie weaning foods may be introduced earlier than 6 months, in addition to breastfeeding, as an alternative to formula.[137]

4.   Recommendations about the types and methods of supplemental feedings depend on the parent's motivation and condition (physical and emotional), as well as the availability of human milk banks.[136] Provide as close to a breastfeeding relationship as possible; ideally, offer supplements after the breast, although some babies may need to be supplemented first and breastfed second. (See Chapter 31, *Expression and Use of Human Milk.*)

5.   If extra milk is available, expressed hindmilk can be used as a high-calorie supplement.[138] An alternative is to skim the cream layer from extra milk that has been allowed to settle and separate.

6.   Supplementation of babies who are not feeding, or are not feeding effectively, at the breast in the first 4 days after birth (assuming eight feeds per 24 hours):[136]

a.   24 hours from birth: 2–10 mL per feed is the normal volume per feed.

b.   24–48 hours from birth: 5–15 mL per feed is the normal volume per feed.

c.   48–72 hours from birth: 15–30 mL per feed is the normal volume per feed.

d.   72–96 hours from birth: 30–60 mL per feed is the normal volume per feed.

7.   The infant's intake begins to stabilize after the first week. From 1 month to 6 months, most babies take in approximately 750–900 milliliters (26–32 ounces) per 24 hours, rising approximately 120 milliliters (4 ounces) from the 1st month to the 6th month.[139-141]

8.   When supplementation is required for babies aged 1 week to 6 months, the starting amount depends on the situation. Supplementation should be adjusted according to the results. For example, for a baby who has been just maintaining weight, or losing weight, start with at least 30–60 milliliters (1–2 ounces) per feeding, and offer more if the baby will take it.

a.   Many underfed babies cannot take much at the start and may need coaxing. As they take in more calories, however, their energy should increase, along with their appetite. They may even start asking for larger amounts, which should be given. This increase is usually temporary until they catch up to where they should be.[142] See **FIGURE 22-5**, **FIGURE 22-6**, **FIGURE 22-7**, and **FIGURE 22-8**.

b.   Often a baby who has been gaining weight slowly will have the energy to take 60 milliliters or more after each breastfeeding and will quickly reach the appropriate growth curve.

c.   A baby whose weight has maintained or dropped may not have the energy at first to take more than 20–30 milliliters per feeding, even though the baby's caloric needs are greater. A few days of coaxing an increased intake will boost the baby's energy for better feeding and increased appetite to drive catch-up growth.

d.   The amount of milk a baby needs daily to regain weight and then grow appropriately varies depending on the caloric value of the milk, the baby's sex, and the baby's individual metabolic needs. Most babies need additional milk for only a few days. Recheck the baby's weight after 2–4 days to confirm that the trend has reversed.[142]

E.   Improved milk production starts with optimal positioning and good milk transfer.

1.   Teach parents how to position their baby at the breast, what constitutes an effective latch, and how to know when the baby is swallowing milk. (See Chapter 13, *Facilitating and Assessing Breastfeeding Initiation.*)

a.   Nipple pain during a feeding can indicate that the baby is not positioned effectively, not latched optimally, or is not sucking correctly.

b.   Any of these factors increase the likelihood of low milk transfer, less milk removed from the breast, and less milk synthesized.[143]

2.   Teach parents infant behavioral feeding cues and encourage them to feed the baby when they observe feeding readiness. (See the discussion of feeding cues in Chapter 13, *Facilitating and Assessing Breastfeeding Initiation.*)

3.   If the infant has neuromuscular central nervous system disorders, a consultation with an occupational therapist may be necessary to assist in the selection of an optimal feeding method to facilitate full feedings.

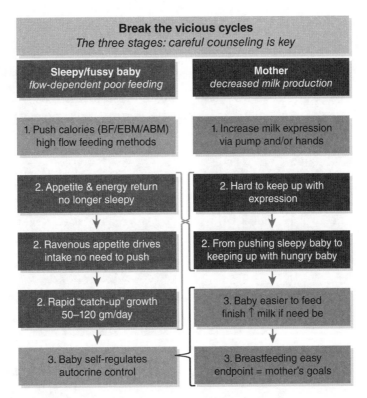

FIGURE 22-5 Break the vicious cycles overview.
© Christina M. Smilie MD, IBCLC, FAAP, FABM.

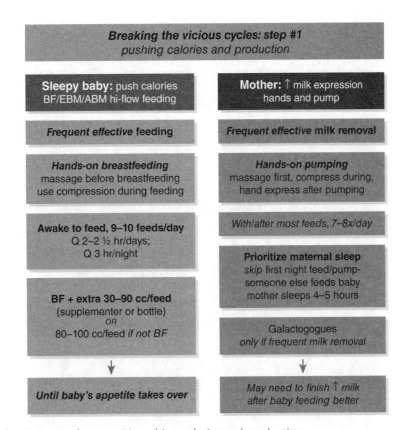

FIGURE 22-6 Breaking the vicious cycles: step #1 pushing calories and production.
© Christina M. Smilie MD, IBCLC, FAAP, FABM.

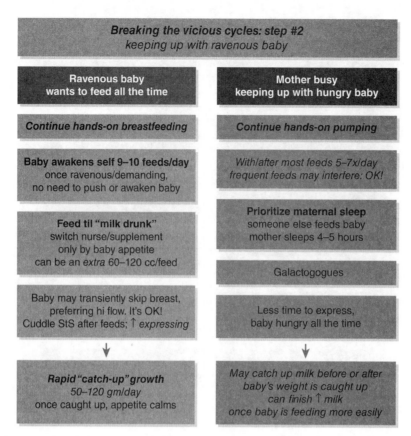

FIGURE 22-7 Breaking the vicious cycles: step #2 keeping up with ravenous baby.

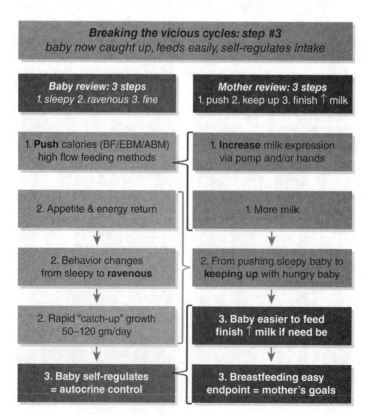

FIGURE 22-8 Breaking the vicious cycles: step #3 baby caught up.

F. There may be underlying conditions that intefere with milk production, such as maternal thyroid dysfunction and metabolic problems. Refer to an appropriate healthcare provider for screening and treatment.

G. If the baby is not able to remove milk effectively or if there are maternal problems, additional milk expression may be necessary to protect or increase milk production.

1. Hand expression is usually the most effective method in the first 48 hours or until lactogenesis II. Beyond this time, the milk volume is greater when an electric breast pump is used, and it is optimal when pumping is combined with hand expression.[22,144,168]

2. Breast massage[134] and the application of warmth to the breasts[145,146] prior to expressing help increase milk yield.

3. Holding the baby skin-to-skin, prior to or during milk expression, can increase the amount of milk removed.[147]

4. To avoid being excessively time-consuming, breastfeeding, supplementation, and expression preferably should take no longer than 1 hour altogether. This may need to be further condensed to breastfeeding or expressing during the middle of the night to allow for sufficient rest.

    a. The goal of postfeed expression is to remove residual milk and provide a strong stimulus to encourage greater milk production.

    b. Encourage milk expression immediately or as soon as baby is settled. Parents who wait longer for the purpose of increasing the yield end up removing some of baby's next meal, and then must feed the milk back to satisfy hunger. This is an unnecessary extra step.

    c. Power pumping, which involves short, very frequent pumping sessions for 1 to 2 days, has been successful in some cases for increasing milk production.

IX. Additional Therapies to Increase Milk Production

A. Pharmacologic galactagogues (substances that stimulate milk production) may be helpful when corrective measures are not enough.

1. No drug is manufactured specifically for the purpose of increasing milk production. In the United States, all drugs that are prescribed as galactagogues are used off label; that is, they have not been reviewed or approved by the U.S. Food and Drug Administration for that purpose.

2. Medications that are commonly used include the following.[148] (See Chapter 5, *Lactation Pharmacology*, for further information about these drugs.)

    a. Domperidone (Motilium) is used for the treatment of certain gastrointestinal disorders and increases milk production without the side effects of metoclopramide.[149,150]

        i.   The dosages vary worldwide, typically 10 to 20 milligrams, three to four times daily.[34,151]

        ii. Domperidone is available over the counter in some countries and by prescription only in others.

        iii. A healthcare provider should be consulted first, especially if there is a history of cardiac problems or prolonged QT intervals.[152-154]

    b. Metoclopramide (Reglan and Maxeran) is a similar drug that also stimulates lactation by increasing serum prolactin.

        i.   Depression and anxiety are possible side effects, and more serious acute symptoms have also been reported.

        ii. Parents with a history of depression are not good candidates for this medication.

        iii. The most common dosage is 10–15 milligrams three times daily.[149,155]

    c. Sulpiride, an antipsychotic drug, is used in some African and South American countries to stimulate or induce lactation. It also works by increasing serum prolactin levels.

        i.   The typical dosage is 50 milligrams two to three times daily.[156,157]

        ii. Although studies have reported only some mild side effects,[155] there is the potential for more serious problems, such as extrapyramidal symptoms and acute dystonic reactions, similar to metoclopramide.

B. Botanical (plant-based) galactagogues have been used for millennia to support and increase milk production; they are controversial in the Western world.[148,158-160]

1. Currently there is limited formal research to validate the effectiveness of botanical galactagogues. A Cochrane Review found "very low quality" evidence for the efficacy of oral galactagogues in mothers of full-term, healthy infants, noting that all included studies favored the galactagogue over placebo.[161]

2. When they are effective, galactagogues work only in conjunction with good breastfeeding management (i.e., frequent and effective milk removal).

3. The quality of these agents can vary among manufacturers.

4. The dosages are largely anecdotal, due to the lack of formal testing.

5. Parents considering the use of botanical galactagogues should be provided with available evidence-based resources regarding the impact of the supplement on milk production and any potential effect on the baby. Lactation consultants should record all relevant information, refer to other experts as needed, and work collaboratively with healthcare providers.[162]

C. Oxytocin nasal spray has been used to stimulate milk production via a stronger milk ejection reflex for better milk removal.[163,164]

1. Conflicting research has cast doubt on the usefulness of oxytocin to improve lactation.[165] This therapy can be effective regardless of whether a problem with milk ejection is physical or psychological.

2. Oxytocin nasal spray is not available commercially; it typically must be compounded. The recommended dosage is one spray in one or both nostrils 2 to 3 minutes before breastfeeding or expressing for no longer than 2 days. Each 1 milliliter dose contains oxytocin 40 USP units.

D. Complementary therapies are used in conjunction with mainstream therapies and may address an underlying problem in a way that standard treatment does not.

1. Imagery, relaxation, hypnosis, music, and biofeedback have helped some parents increase milk output.[166-168]

2. Acupuncture, acupressure, and reflexology[169-171] have been used in China for low milk production since AD 256 and are reportedly most effective if started within 20 days of birth. Milk production can start to increase as soon as 2 to 4 hours following treatment or as late as 72 hours; the faster the response, the better the outcome.[172]

3. Chiropractic adjustments have helped correct some subluxations that interfered with lactation nerve pathways.[173]

4. Placentophagy, the practice of ingesting one's own placenta, has been claimed to help with milk production by some and to hinder it by others. The preparation of the placenta, the amount ingested, and the timing of the ingestion are all variables of unknown significance to the outcomes. Existing evidence is of low quality, with mixed results.[174]

5. Homeopathic remedies for milk production are individualized for each parent after a root cause assessment by a homeopathic practitioner.[175]

CLINICAL TIP

Lactation consultants routinely encounter scenarios for which there is insufficient research to guide clinical strategies and recommendations. Healthcare providers are often not willing to treat based on theories alone, frequently leaving parents without answers. Researchers need to turn their attention to these numerous "unsolved mysteries of the human mammary gland"[86] and more funding needs to be allocated to study this important phenomenon.

▶ Key Points from This Chapter

A. Insufficient milk production is the most common reason for parents to supplement or wean prematurely.

B. Undernourished and malnourished infants need enough calories per day to help them return to the energy level that allows them to maintain adequate growth. Some babies may demand more than typical amounts until they catch up.

C. It is important to determine whether the factors that led to a growth crisis relate to the parent, the baby, or both. The cause may be multifactorial and may be iatrogenic.

D. After the baby's growth has been addressed, the parent will need help in developing a strategy to increase milk production. This will include addressing causative issues and may also require compensatory milk removal if the baby is not able to remove milk adequately.

🔍 CASE STUDY

Shawna, gravida 2 para 2, presented at 16 days postpartum with an uncomplicated pregnancy, vaginal birth, and a healthy baby. The baby's birth weight was 3,146 g (6 lb 15 oz). At 15 days old the baby weighed 2,777 g (6 lb 2 oz), which was an 11.7 percent weight loss. The chief complaints were nipple pain and low milk production.

History: At age 14 Shawna was diagnosed with Hodgkin disease. A large tumor was removed from the chest with subsequent radiation treatment from the chin to the waist. Shawna also had a history of irregular menstrual cycles and hypothyroidism. There were no breast changes during either pregnancy, and the breasts were very small with scant veining. Thyroid function remained stable after the first birth and was well-controlled during this pregnancy, though it had not been checked postpartum. There was very little milk with the first baby. Shawna had seen a lactation consultant and used a rented electric pump, but was never able to produce much milk for the first child.

Infant and feeding assessment: The baby appeared to have an effective suck at the breast but transferred only 8 g (0.3 oz) of milk after a 20-minute feeding. When an at-breast supplementer was added, the baby transferred 90 mls (3 oz) over the next 20 minutes.

Shawna had small but normal-appearing breasts that did not exhibit growth during pregnancy, a history of radiation exposure to the breast, and a past history of very little milk despite pumping. Therefore, the lactation consultant concluded that the radiation treatment damaged the milk-making tissue and permanently impaired the ability of the breasts to make milk. The low thyroid history was another red flag and potential contributor to be explored, but the cancer treatment was the most likely cause of Shawna's inability to produce sufficient milk for optimal infant growth.

Given the history and assessment, the pediatrician recommended that the baby be fed formula. The question then became whether the baby would be fed by bottle or at the breast with a supplementer. After further discussion, Shawna decided to supplement at the breast and discontinue pumping.

Questions

1. What was the differential diagnosis for Shawna's low milk production?
2. What information led to the elimination of the other possibilities?
3. Do you feel that the decision to discontinue pumping efforts would make a difference in the outcome? Why or why not?
4. What emotions might Shawna be experiencing by the end of the consult? How would you address them?

References

1. Dewey KG, Heinig MJ, Nommsen LA, Peerson JM, Lonnerdal B. Growth of breast-fed and formula-fed infants from 0 to 18 months: the DARLING study. *Pediatrics.* 1992;89(6 pt 1):1035-1041.
2. Unver Korgali E, Cihan MK, Oguzalp T, Sahinbas A, Ekici M. Hypernatremic dehydration in breastfed term infants: retrospective evaluation of 159 cases. *Breastfeed Med.* 2017;12:5-11.
3. Emond A, Drewett R, Blair P, Emmett P. Postnatal factors associated with failure to thrive in term infants in the Avon longitudinal study of parents and children. *Arch Dis Child.* 2007;92(2):115-119.
4. Lukefahr JL. Underlying illness associated with failure to thrive in breastfed infants. *Clin Pediatr (Phila).* 1990;29(8):468-470.
5. Newby RM, Davies PS. Why do women stop breast-feeding? Results from a contemporary prospective study in a cohort of Australian women. *Eur J Clin Nutr.* 2016;70(12):1428-1432.
6. Chantry CJ, Nommsen-Rivers LA, Peerson JM, Cohen RJ, Dewey KG. Excess weight loss in first-born breastfed newborns relates to maternal intrapartum fluid balance. *Pediatrics.* 2011;127(1):e171-e179.
7. Noel-Weiss J, Woodend AK, Peterson WE, Gibb W, Groll DL. An observational study of associations among maternal fluids during parturition, neonatal output, and breastfed newborn weight loss. *Int Breastfeed J.* 2011;6:9.
8. Nommsen-Rivers LA, Heinig MJ, Cohen RJ, Dewey KG. Newborn wet and soiled diaper counts and timing of onset of lactation as indicators of breastfeeding inadequacy. *J Hum Lactation.* 2008;24(1):27-33.
9. Neifert MR. Prevention of breastfeeding tragedies. *Pediatr Clin North Am.* 2001;48(2):273-297.
10. Lawrence RA, Lawrence RM. *Breastfeeding: A Guide for the Medical Profession.* 8th ed. Philadelphia, PA: Elsevier; 2016.
11. Kaska L, Kobiela J, Abacjew-Chmylko A, et al. Nutrition and pregnancy after bariatric surgery. *ISRN Obes.* 2013;2013:492060. doi: 10.1155/2013/492060.
12. Gatti L. Maternal perceptions of insufficient milk supply in breastfeeding. *J Nurs Scholarsh.* 2008;40(4):355-363.
13. Parker LA, Sullivan S, Krueger C, Mueller M. Association of timing of initiation of breastmilk expression on milk volume and timing of lactogenesis stage II among mothers of very low-birth-weight infants. *Breastfeed Med.* 2015;10(2):84-91.
14. Marti A, Feng Z, Altermatt H, Jaggi R. Milk accumulation triggers apoptosis of mammary epithelial cells. *Eur J Cell Biol.* 1997;73(2):158-165.

15. Holmes AV, Auinger P, Howard CR. Combination feeding of breast milk and formula: evidence for shorter breast-feeding duration from the national health and nutrition examination survey. *J Pediatr.* 2011;159(2):186-191.

16. Mohrbacher N. The magic number and long-term milk production. *Clin Lactation.* 2011;2(1):15-18.

17. Wilson-Clay B, Hoover K. *The Breastfeeding Atlas.* 6th ed. Austin, TX: LactNews Press; 2017.

18. Caglar MK, Ozer I, Altugan FS. Risk factors for excess weight loss and hypernatremia in exclusively breast-fed infants. *Braz J Med Biol Res.* 2006;39(4):539-544.

19. Dewey KG, Nommsen-Rivers LA, Heinig MJ, Cohen RJ. Risk factors for suboptimal infant breastfeeding behavior, delayed onset of lactation, and excess neonatal weight loss. *Pediatrics.* 2003;112(3 pt 1):607-619.

20. Walker M. Nipple shields: what we know, what we wish we knew, and how best to use them. *Clin Lactation.* 2016;7(3):100-107.

21. Meier PP, Patel AL, Hoban R, Engstrom JL. Which breast pump for which mother: an evidence-based approach to individualizing breast pump technology. *J Perinatol.* 2016;36(7):493-499.

22. Morton J. The importance of hands. *J Hum Lactation.* 2012;28(3):276-277.

23. Meier PP, Engstrom JL, Janes JE, Jegier BJ, Loera F. Breast pump suction patterns that mimic the human infant during breastfeeding: greater milk output in less time spent pumping for breast pump-dependent mothers with premature infants. *J Perinatol.* 2012;32(2):103-110.

24. Hale T, Ilett K, Hartmann P, et al. Pseudoephedrine effects on milk production in women and estimation of infant exposure via human milk. *Adv Exp Med Biol.* 2004;554:437-438.

25. Anderson PO. Drugs that suppress lactation, part 2. *BreastfeedMed.* 2017;12(4):199-201.

26. Berens P, Labbok M. ABM clinical protocol #13: contraception during breastfeeding, revised 2015. *Breastfeed Med.* 2015;10(1):3-12.

27. Lopez LM, Grey TW, Stuebe AM, Chen M, Truitt ST, Gallo MF. Combined hormonal versus nonhormonal versus progestin-only contraception in lactation. *Cochrane Database Syst Rev.* 2015;3:CD003988. doi:10.1002/14651858.CD003988.pub2.

28. Pieh Holder KL. Contraception and breastfeeding. *Clin Obstet Gynecol.* 2015;58(4):928-935.

29. Sridhar A, Salcedo J. Optimizing maternal and neonatal outcomes with postpartum contraception: impact on breastfeeding and birth spacing. *Matern Health Neonatol Perinatol.* 2017;3:1.

30. Duran MS, Spatz DL. A mother with glandular hypoplasia and a late preterm infant. *J Hum Lactation.* 2011;27(4):394-397.

31. Tepper NK, Phillips SJ, Kapp N, Gaffield ME, Curtis KM. Combined hormonal contraceptive use among breastfeeding women: an updated systematic review. *Contraception.* 2016;94(3):262-274.

32. Brownell EA, Fernandez ID, Howard CR, et al. A systematic review of early postpartum medroxyprogesterone receipt and early breastfeeding cessation: evaluating the methodological rigor of the evidence. *Breastfeed Med.* 2011;7(1):10-18.

33. Betzold C, DeNicola G. Progestin-only contraception during lactation: a re-analysis. *Breastfeed Med.* 2010;5(6):339.

34. Hale T, Rowe H. *Medications and Mothers' Milk.* 17th ed. New York, NY: Springer Publishing Company; 2017.

35. Napierala M, Mazela J, Merritt TA, Florek E. Tobacco smoking and breastfeeding: effect on the lactation process, breast milk composition and infant development. A critical review. *Environ Res.* 2016;151:321-338.

36. Lee S, Kelleher SL. Biological underpinnings of breastfeeding challenges: the role of genetics, diet, and environment on lactation physiology. *Am J Physiol Endocrinol Metab.* 2016;311(2):E405-E422.

37. Scheplyagina LA. Impact of the mother's zinc deficiency on the woman's and newborn's health status. *J Trace Elem Med Biol.* 2005;19(1):29-35.

38. Speller E, Brodribb W. Breastfeeding and thyroid disease: a literature review. *Breastfeed Rev.* 2012;20(2):41-47.

39. Rioux FM, Savoie N, Allard J. Is there a link between postpartum anemia and discontinuation of breastfeeding? *Can J Diet Pract Res.* 2006;67(2):72-76.

40. Salahudeen MS, Koshy AM, Sen S. A study of the factors affecting time to onset of lactogenesis-II after parturition. *J Pharm Res.* 2013;6(1):68-72.

41. Achalapong J. Effect of egg and milk supplement on breast milk volume at 48 and 72 hours postpartum: a randomized-controlled trial. *Thai J Obstet Gynaecol.* 2016;24(1):20-25.

42. Edozien JC, Khan MAR, Waslien CI. Human protein deficiency: results of a Nigerian village study. *J Nutr.* 1976;106(3):312-328.

43. Torris C, Thune I, Emaus A, et al. Duration of lactation, maternal metabolic profile, and body composition in the Norwegian EBBA I-study. *Breastfeed Med.* 2013;8(1):8-15.

44. Torgersen L, Ystrom E, Haugen M, et al. Breastfeeding practice in mothers with eating disorders. *Matern Child Nutr.* 2010;6(3):243-252.

45. Kimmel MC, Ferguson EH, Zerwas S, Bulik CM, Meltzer-Brody S. Obstetric and gynecologic problems associated with eating disorders. *Int J Eat Disord.* 2016;49(3):260-275.

46. Javed A, Lteif A. Development of the human breast. *Semin Plast Surg.* 2013;27(1):5-12.

47. Monteleone P, Brambilla F, Bortolotti F, Ferraro C, Maj M. Plasma prolactin response to D-fenfluramine is blunted in bulimic patients with frequent binge episodes. *Psychological Med.* 1998;28(4):975-983.

48. Motil KJ, Sheng HP, Montandon CM. Case report: failure to thrive in a breast-fed infant is associated with maternal dietary protein and energy restriction. *J Am Coll Nutr.* 1994;13(2):203-208.

49. Dewey KG, McCrory MA. Effects of dieting and physical activity on pregnancy and lactation. *Am J Clin Nutr.* 1994;59(2):446S-452S.

50. Caplinger P, Cooney AT, Bledsoe C, et al. Breastfeeding outcomes following bariatric surgery. *Clin Lactation.* 2015;6(4):144-152.

51. Stefanski J. Breastfeeding after bariatric surgery. *Todays Dietitian.* 2006;January:47-50.

52. Marasco L. The impact of thyroid dysfunction on lactation. *Breastfeeding Abstracts.* 2006;25(2):9-12.

53. Napierala M, Merritt TA, Mazela J, et al. The effect of tobacco smoke on oxytocin concentrations and selected oxidative stress parameters in plasma during pregnancy and post-partum—an experimental model. *Hum Exp Toxicol.* 2017;36(2):135-145.

54. Kamikawa A, Ichii O, Yamaji D, et al. Diet-induced obesity disrupts ductal development in the mammary glands of nonpregnant mice. *Dev Dyn.* 2009;238(5):1092-1099.

55. Hurst N. Recognizing and treating delayed or failed lactogenesis II. *J Midwifery Womens Health.* 2007;52(6):588-594.

56. Nommsen-Rivers LR, Riddle S, Thompson A, Ward L, Wagner E, Woo JG. Metabolic syndrome severity score identifies persistently low milk output. *Breastfeed Med.* 2017;12(suppl):S22.

57. Hruschka DJ, Sellen DW, Stein AD, Martorell R. Delayed onset of lactation and risk of ending full breast-feeding early in rural Guatemala. *J Nutr.* 2003;133(8):2592-2599.

58. Dimitraki M, Tsikouras P, Manav B, et al. Evaluation of the effect of natural and emotional stress of labor on lactation and breast-feeding. *Arch Gynecol Obstet.* 2015;293(2):317-328.

59. Anderson PO. Drugs that suppress lactation, part 1. *Breastfeed Med.* 2017;12(3):1-3.

60. Lind JN, Perrine CG, Li R. Relationship between use of labor pain medications and delayed onset of lactation. *J Hum Lactation.* 2014;30(2):167-173.

61. Nommsen-Rivers LA, Chantry CJ, Peerson JM, Cohen RJ, Dewey KG. Delayed onset of lactogenesis among first-time mothers is related to maternal obesity and factors associated with ineffective breastfeeding. *Am J Clin Nutr.* 2010;92(3):574-584.

62. Zhu P, Hao J, Jiang X, Huang K, Tao F. New insight into onset of lactation: mediating the negative effect of multiple perinatal biopsychosocial stress on breastfeeding duration. *Breastfeed Med.* 2013;8:151-158.

63. Garcia-Fortea P, Gonzalez-Mesa E, Blasco M, Cazorla O, Delgado-Rios M, Gonzalez-Valenzuela MJ. Oxytocin administered during labor and breast-feeding: a retrospective cohort study. *J Matern Fetal Neonatal Med.* 2014;27(15):1598-1603.

64. Fernández-Cañadas Morillo A, Marín Gabriel MA, Olza Fernández I, et al. The relationship of the administration of intrapartum synthetic oxytocin and breastfeeding initiation and duration rates. *Breastfeed Med.* 2017;12:98-102

65. Bjelakovic L, Trajkovic T, Kocic G, et al. The association of prenatal tocolysis and breastfeeding duration. *Breastfeed Med.* 2016;11(10):561-563.

66. Henderson J, Hartmann P, Newnham J, Simmer K. Effect of preterm birth and antenatal corticosteroid treatment on lactogenesis II in women. *Pediatrics.* 2008;121(1):192-100.

67. Cregan MD, de Mello TR, Hartmann PE. Pre-term delivery and breast expression: consequences for initiating lactation. *Adv Exp Med Biol.* 2000;478:427-428.

68. Zanardo V, Gambina I, Begley C, et al. Psychological distress and early lactation performance in mothers of late preterm infants. *Early Hum Dev.* 2011;87(4):321-323.

69. Marshall AM, Nommsen-Rivers LA, Hernandez LL, et al. Serotonin transport and metabolism in the mammary gland modulates secretory activation and involution. *J Clin Endocrinol Metab.* 2010;95(2):837-846.

70. Neifert MR, McDonough SL, Neville MC. Failure of lactogenesis associated with placental retention. *Am J Obstet Gynecol.* 1981;140(4):477-478.

71. Betzold CM, Hoover KL, Snyder CL. Delayed lactogenesis II: a comparison of four cases. *J Midwifery Womens Health.* 2004;49(2):132-137.

72. Andrade RA, Coca KP, Abrao AC. Breastfeeding pattern in the first month of life in women submitted to breast reduction and augmentation. *J Pediatr (Rio J).* 2010;86(3):239-244.

73. Filiciani S, Siemienczuk GF, Nardin JM, et al. Cohort study to assess the impact of breast implants on breastfeeding. *Plast Reconstr Surg.* 2016;138(6):1152-1159.

74. Cassar-Uhl D. *Finding Sufficiency: Breastfeeding with Insufficient Glandular Tissue.* Amarillo, TX: Praeclarus Press LLC; 2014.

75. Neifert MR, Seacat JM, Jobe WE. Lactation failure due to insufficient glandular development of the breast. *Pediatrics.* 1985;76(5):823-828.

76. Guillette EA, Conard C, Lares F, Aguilar MG, McLachlan J, Guillette LJ Jr. Altered breast development in young girls from an agricultural environment. *Environ Health Perspect.* 2006;114(3):471-475.

77. Huggins K, Petok ES, Mireles O. Markers of lactation insufficiency. In: Auerbach, KG, ed. *Current Issues in Clinical Lactation.* Sudbury, MA: Jones and Bartlett; 2000:25-35.

78. Fetherston CM, Lai CT, Hartmann PE. Relationships between symptoms and changes in breast physiology during lactation mastitis. *Breastfeed Med.* 2006;1(3):136-145.

79. Fetherston CM, Wells JI, Hartmann PE. Severity of mastitis symptoms as a predictor of C-reactive protein in milk and blood during lactation. *Breastfeed Med.* 2006;1(3):127-135.

80. Stopenski S, Aslam A, Zhang X, Cardonick E. After chemotherapy treatment for maternal cancer during pregnancy, is breastfeeding possible? *Breastfeed Med.* 2017;12:91-97.

81. Dow KH, Harris JR, Roy C. Pregnancy after breast-conserving surgery and radiation therapy for breast cancer. *J Natl Cancer Inst Monogr.* 1994(16):131-137.

82. Leal SC, Stuart SR, Carvalho HdA. Breast irradiation and lactation: a review. *Expert Rev Anticancer Ther.* 2013;13(2):159-164.

83. Halbert LA. Breastfeeding in the woman with a compromised nervous system. *J Hum Lactation.* 1998;14(4):327-331.

84. Cowley KC. Psychogenic and pharmacologic induction of the let-down reflex can facilitate breastfeeding by tetraplegic women: a report of 3 cases. *Arch Phys Med Rehabil.* 2005;86(6):1261-1264.

85. Kasper N, Peterson KE, Zhang Z, et al. Association of bisphenol A exposure with breastfeeding and perceived insufficient milk supply in Mexican women. *Matern Child Health J.* 2016;20(8):1713-1719.

86. Marasco LA. Unsolved mysteries of the human mammary gland: defining and redefining the critical questions from the lactation consultant's perspective. *J Mammary Gland Biol Neoplasia.* 2015;19(3-4):271-288.

87. Romano ME, Xu Y, Calafat AM, et al. Maternal serum perfluoroalkyl substances during pregnancy and duration of breastfeeding. *Environ Res.* 2016;149:239-246.

88. O'Dowd R, Kent J, Mosely J, Wlodek M. Effects of uteroplacental insufficiency and reducing litter size on maternal mammary function and postnatal offspring growth. *Am J Physiol Regul Integr Comp Physiol.* 2008;294(2):R539-R548.

89. Cregan M. Complicating influences upon the initiation of lactation following premature birth. *J Hum Lactation.* 2007;23(1):77.

90. Murase M, Nommsen-Rivers L, Morrow AL, et al. Predictors of low milk volume among mothers who delivered preterm. *J Hum Lactation.* 2014;30(4):425-435.

91. Hall RT, Mercer AM, Teasley SL, et al. A breast-feeding assessment score to evaluate the risk for cessation of breast-feeding by 7 to 10 days of age. *J Pediatr.* 2002;141(5):659-664.

92. Rasmussen KM, Hilson JA, Kjolhede CL. Obesity as a risk factor for failure to initiate and sustain lactation. *Adv Exp Med Biol.* 2002;503:217-222.

93. Lovelady CA. Is maternal obesity a cause of poor lactation performance? *Nutr Rev.* 2005;63(10):352-355.

94. Hilson JA, Rasmussen KM, Kjolhede CL. High prepregnant body mass index is associated with poor lactation outcomes among white, rural women independent of psychosocial and demographic correlates. *J Hum Lactation.* 2004;20(1):18-29.

95. Turcksin R, Bel S, Galjaard S, Devlieger R. Maternal obesity and breastfeeding intention, initiation, intensity and duration: a systematic review. *Matern Child Nutr.* 2014;10(2):166-183.

96. Lepe M, Bacardi Gascon M, Castaneda-Gonzalez LM, Perez Morales ME, Jimenez Cruz A. Effect of maternal obesity on lactation: systematic review. *Nutr Hosp.* 2011;26(6):1266-1269.

97. Haile ZT, Chavan BB, Teweldeberhan A, Chertok IR. Association between gestational weight gain and delayed onset of lactation: the moderating effects of race/ethnicity. *Breastfeed Med.* 2017;12:79-85.

98. Riddle SW, Nommsen-Rivers LA. A case control study of diabetes during pregnancy and low milk supply. *Breastfeed Med.* 2016;11(2):80-85.

99. Riddle SW, Nommsen-Rivers LA. Low milk supply and the pediatrician. *Curr Opin Pediatr.* 2017;29(2):249-256.

100. Nommsen-Rivers LA, Dolan LM, Huang B. Timing of stage II lactogenesis is predicted by antenatal metabolic health in a cohort of primiparas. *Breastfeed Med.* 2012;7(1):43-49.

101. Soltani H, Arden M. Factors associated with breastfeeding up to 6 months postpartum in mothers with diabetes. *J Obstet Gynecol Neonatal Nurs.* 2009;38(5):586-594.

102. Hartmann P, Cregan M. Lactogenesis and the effects of insulin-dependent diabetes mellitus and prematurity. *J Nutr.* 2001;131(11):3016S-3020S.

103. Nommsen-Rivers LA, Riddle SA, Thompson A, Ward L, Wagner E. Milk production in mothers with and without signs of insulin resistance. *FASEB J.* 2017;31:650-659.

104. Haile ZT, Oza-Frank R, Azulay Chertok IR, Passen N. Association between history of gestational diabetes and exclusive breastfeeding at hospital discharge. *J Hum Lactation.* 2016;32(3):36-43.

105. Herskin CW, Stage E, Barfred C, et al. Low prevalence of long-term breastfeeding among women with type 2 diabetes. *J Matern Fetal Neonatal Med.* 2016;29(15):2513-8.

106. Matias SL, Dewey KG, Quesenberry CP Jr, Gunderson EP. Maternal prepregnancy obesity and insulin treatment during pregnancy are independently associated with delayed lactogenesis in women with recent gestational diabetes mellitus. *Am J Clin Nutr.* 2014;99(1):115-121.

107. Glover AV, Berry DC, Schwartz TA, Stuebe AM. The association of metabolic dysfunction with breastfeeding outcomes in gestational diabetes. *Am J Perinatol.* 2018. [Epub ahead of print]. doi:10.1055/s-0038-1626713.

108. Bromiker R, Rachamim A, Hammerman C, Schimmel M, Kaplan M, Medoff-Cooper B. Immature sucking patterns in infants of mothers with diabetes. *J Pediatr.* 2006;149(5):640-643.

109. Biloš LSK. Polycystic ovarian syndrome and low milk supply: is insulin resistance the missing link? *Endocr Oncol Metab.* 2017;3(2):49-55.

110. Nommsen-Rivers L, Thompson A, Riddle S, Ward L, Wagner E, King E. A preliminary randomized trial of metformin to augment low supply (MALMS). *Breastfeed Medicine.* 2017;12(suppl):S22-S23.

111. Stein M. Failure to thrive in a four-month-old nursing infant. *Dev Behav Ped.* 2002;23(4):S69-S73.

112. Campo Verde Arbocco F, Sasso CV, Actis EA, Caron RW, Hapon MB, Jahn GA. Hypothyroidism advances mammary involution in lactating rats through inhibition of PRL signaling and induction of LIF/STAT3 mRNAs. *Mol Cell Endocrinol.* 2016;419:18-28.

113. Hapon MB, Simoncini M, Via G, Jahn GA. Effect of hypothyroidism on hormone profiles in virgin, pregnant and lactating rats, and on lactation. *Reproduction.* 2003;126(3):371-382.

114. Buckshee K, Kriplani A, Kapil A, Bhargava VL, Takkar D. Hypothyroidism complicating pregnancy. *Aust N Z J Obstet Gynaecol.* 1992;32(3):240-242.

115. Varas SM, Munoz EM, Hapon MB, Aguilera Merlo CI, Gimenez MS, Jahn GA. Hyperthyroidism and production of precocious involution in the mammary glands of lactating rats. *Reproduction.* 2002;124(5):691-702.

116. Trimeloni L, Spencer J. Diagnosis and management of breast milk oversupply. *J Am Board Fam Med.* 2016;29(1):139-142.

117. Pereira K, Brown AJ. Postpartum thyroiditis: not just a worn out mom. *J Nurs Pract.* 2008;4(3):175-182.

118. Stagnaro-Green A. Clinical review 152: postpartum thyroiditis. *J Clin Endocrinol Metab.* 2002;87(9):4042-4047.

119. Alexander EK, Pearce EN, Brent GA, et al. 2017 guidelines of the American Thyroid Association for the diagnosis and management of thyroid disease during pregnancy and the postpartum. *Thyroid.* 2017;27(3):315-389.

120. Rasmussen K, Kjolhede C. Prepregnant overweight and obesity diminish the prolactin response to suckling. *Pediatrics.* 2004;113(5):1388.

121. Zhang F, Xia H, Shen M, et al. Are prolactin levels linked to suction pressure? *Breastfeed Med.* 2016;11(9):461-468.

122. Mennella JA, Pepino MY. Breastfeeding and prolactin levels in lactating women with a family history of alcoholism. *Pediatrics.* 2010;125(5):e1162-e1170.

123. Dökmetas HS, Kilicli F, Korkmaz S, Yonem O. Characteristic features of 20 patients with Sheehan's syndrome. *Gynecol Endocrinol.* 2006;22(5):279-283.

124. Gei-Guardia O, Soto-Herrera E, Gei-Brealey A, Chen-Ku CH. Sheehan's syndrome in Costa Rica: clinical experience on 60 cases. *Endocr Pract.* 2011;17(3):337-344.

125. Okada K, Ishikawa S, Saito T, Kumakura S, Sakamoto Y, Kuzuya T. A case of partial hypopituitarism with empty sella following normal course of pregnancy and delivery. *Endocrinol Jpn.* 1986;33(1):117-123.

126. Revai K, Briars L, Cochran K. Poster abstracts #13 case series of Sjögren's syndrome and poor milk supply. *Breastfeed Med.* 2010;5(6):333.

127. Leeners B, Rath W, Kuse S, Neumaier-Wagner P. Breast-feeding in women with hypertensive disorders in pregnancy. *J Perinat Med.* 2005;33(6):553-560.

128. Carlsen SM, Jacobsen G, Vanky E. Mid-pregnancy androgen levels are negatively associated with breastfeeding. *Acta Obstet Gynecol Scand.* 2010;89(1):87-94.

129. Cromi A, Serati M, Candeloro I, et al. Assisted reproductive technology and breastfeeding outcomes: a case-control study. *Fertil Steril.* 2015;103(1):89-94.

130. Marasco L, Marmet C, Shell E. Polycystic ovary syndrome: a connection to insufficient milk supply? *J Hum Lactation.* 2000;16(2):143-148.

131. McGuire E, Rowan M. PCOS, breast hypoplasia and low milk supply: a case study. *Breastfeed Rev.* 2015;23(3):29-32.

132. Vanky E, Isaksen H, Moen MH, Carlsen SM. Breastfeeding in polycystic ovary syndrome. *Acta Obstet Gynecol Scand.* 2008;87(5): 531-535.

133. Foda MI, Kawashima T, Nakamura S, Kobayashi M, Oku T. Composition of milk obtained from unmassaged versus massaged breasts of lactating mothers. *J Pediatr Gastroenterol Nutr.* 2004;38(5):484-487.

134. Bowles BC. Breast massage: a "handy" multipurpose tool to promote breastfeeding success. *Clin Lactation.* 2011;2(4):21-24.

135. Buntuchai G, Pavadhgul P, Kittipichai W, Satheannoppakao W. Traditional galactagogue foods and their connection to human milk volume in Thai breastfeeding mothers. *J Hum Lactation.* 2017;33(3):552-559.

136. Kellams A, Harrel C, Omage S, Gregory C, Rosen-Carole C. ABM clinical protocol #3: supplementary feedings in the healthy term breastfed neonate, revised 2017. *Breastfeed Med.* 2017. 12: 188-198.

137. Eidelman AI, Schanler RJ. American Academy of Pediatrics policy statement: Breastfeeding and the use of human milk. *Pediatrics.* 2012;129(3):e827-e841.

138. Meier PP. Supporting lactation in mothers with very low birth weight infants. *Pediatr Ann.* 2003;32(5):317-325.

139. Kent JC, Mitoulas L, Cox DB, Owens RA, Hartmann PE. Breast volume and milk production during extended lactation in women. *Exp Physiol.* 1999;84(2):435-447.

140. Kent JC, Mitoulas LR, Cregan MD, Ramsay DT, Doherty DA, Hartmann PE. Volume and frequency of breastfeedings and fat content of breast milk throughout the day. *Pediatrics.* 2006;117(3):e387-e395.

141. Nielsen SB, Reilly JJ, Fewtrell MS, Eaton S, Grinham J, Wells JC. Adequacy of milk intake during exclusive breastfeeding: a longitudinal study. *Pediatrics.* 2011;128(4):e907-e914.

142. Powers NG. How to assess slow growth in the breastfed infant. Birth to 3 months. *Pediatr Clin North Am.* 2001;48(2):345-363.

143. McClellan H, Geddes D, Kent J, Garbin C, Mitoulas L, Hartmann P. Infants of mothers with persistent nipple pain exert strong sucking vacuums. *Acta Paediatr.* 2008;97(9):1205-1209.

144. Morton J, Hall JY, Wong RJ, Thairu L, Benitz WE, Rhine WD. Combining hand techniques with electric pumping increases milk production in mothers of preterm infants. *J Perinatol.* 2009;29(11):757-764.

145. Kent JC, Geddes DT, Hepworth AR, Hartmann PE. Effect of warm breastshields on breast milk pumping. *J Hum Lactation.* 2011;27(4):331-338.

146. Yigit F, Cigdem Z, Temizsoy E, et al. Does warming the breasts affect the amount of breastmilk production? *Breastfeed Med.* 2012;7(6):487-488.

147. Acuna-Muga J, Ureta-Velasco N, de la Cruz-Bertolo J, et al. Volume of milk obtained in relation to location and circumstances of expression in mothers of very low birth weight infants. *J Hum Lactation.* 2014;30(1):41-46.

148. Bunik M, Chantry CJ, Howard CR, et al. ABM clinical protocol #9: use of galactogogues in initiating or augmenting the rate of maternal milk secretion (first revision January 2011). *Breastfeed Med.* 2011;6(1):41-49.

149. Ingram J, Taylor H, Churchill C, Pike A, Greenwood R. Metoclopramide or domperidone for increasing maternal breast milk output: a randomised controlled trial. *Arch Dis Child Fetal Neonatal Ed.* 2012;97(4):F241-F245.

150. Osadchy A, Moretti ME, Koren G. Effect of domperidone on insufficient lactation in puerperal women: a systematic review and meta-analysis of randomized controlled trials. *Obstet Gynecol Int.* 2012;2012:642893. doi:10.1155/2012/642893.

151. Knoppert DC, Page A, Warren J, et al. The effect of two different domperidone doses on maternal milk production. *J Hum Lactation.* 2013;29(1):38-44.

152. Buffery PJ, Strother RM. Domperidone safety: a mini-review of the science of QT prolongation and clinical implications of recent global regulatory recommendations. *N Z Med J.* 2015;128(1416):66-74.

153. Grzeskowiak LE, Amir LH. Pharmacological management of low milk supply with domperidone: separating fact from fiction. *Med J Aust.* 2015;202(6):298.

154. Grzeskowiak LE, Amir LH. Use of domperidone to increase breast milk supply: further consideration of the benefit-risk ratio is required. *J Hum Lactation.* 2015;31(2):315-316.

155. Zuppa A, Sindico P, Orchi C, Carducci C, Cardiello V, Romagnoli C. Safety and efficacy of galactogogues: substances that induce, maintain and increase breast milk production. *J Pharm Pharm Sci.* 2010;13(2):162-174.

156. Ylikorkala O, Kauppila A, Kivinen S, Viinikka L. Sulpiride improves inadequate lactation. *Br Med J (Clin Res Ed).* 1982;285(6337):249-251.

157. Aono T, Aki T, Koike K, Kurachi K. Effect of sulpiride on poor puerperal lactation. *Am J Obstet Gynecol.* 1982;143(8):927-932.

158. Abascal K, Yarnell E. Botanical galactagogues. *Altern Complement Ther.* 2008;14(6):288-294.

159. Mortel M, Mehta SD. Systematic review of the efficacy of herbal galactogogues. *J Hum Lactation.* 2013;29(2):154-162.

160. Zapantis A, Steinberg JG, Schilit L. Use of herbals as galactogogues. *J Pharm Pract.* 2012;25(2):222-231.

161. Foong SC, Tan ML, Marasco LA, Ho JJ, Foong WC. Oral galactogogues for increasing breast-milk production in mothers of non-hospitalised term infants. *Cochrane Database Syst Rev.* 2015;4: CD011505. doi:10.1002/14651858.CD011505.

162. International Board of Lactation Consultant Examiners. *Scope of practice for International Board Certified Lactation Consultant (IBCLC) Certificants.* Published September 15, 2012. Accessed November 29, 2017, from International Board of Lactation Consultant Examiners website: https://iblce.org/wp-content/uploads/2017/05/scope-of-practice.pdf.

163. Renfrew MJ, Lang S, Woolridge M. Oxytocin for promoting successful lactation. *Cochrane Database Syst Rev.* 2000;2:CD000156.

164. Ruis H, Rolland R, Doesburg W, Broeders G, Corbey R. Oxytocin enhances onset of lactation among mothers delivering prematurely. *Br Med J (Clin Res Ed).* 1981;283(6287):340-342.

165. Fewtrell MS, Loh KL, Blake A, Ridout DA, Hawdon J. Randomised, double blind trial of oxytocin nasal spray in mothers expressing breast milk for preterm infants. *Arch Dis Child Fetal Neonatal Ed.* 2006;91(3):F169-F174.

166. Demirci JR, Bare S, Cohen SM, Bogen DL. Feasibility and acceptability of two complementary and alternative therapies for perceived insufficient milk in mothers of late preterm and early term infants. *Altern Complement Ther.* 2016;22(5):196-203.

167. Keith DR, Weaver BS, Vogel RL. The effect of music-based listening interventions on the volume, fat content, and caloric content of breast milk-produced by mothers of premature and critically ill infants. *Adv Neonatal Care.* 2012;12(2):112-119.

168. Becker GE, Smith HA, Cooney F. Methods of milk expression for lactating women. *Cochrane Database Syst Rev.* 2016;9:CD006170. doi:10.1002/14651858.CD006170.pub5.

169. Esfahani MS, Berenji-Sooghe S, Valiani M, Ehsanpour S. Effect of acupressure on milk volume of breastfeeding mothers referring to selected health care centers in Tehran. *Iran J Nurs Midwifery Res.* 2015;20(1):7.

170. Neri I, Allais G, Vaccaro V, et al. Acupuncture treatment as breastfeeding support: preliminary data. *J Altern Complement Med.* 2011;17(2):133-137.

171. Tipping L, Mackereth PA. A concept analysis: the effect of reflexology on homeostasis to establish and maintain lactation. *Complement Ther Nurs Midwifery.* 2000;6(4):189-198.

172. Clavey S. The use of acupuncture for the treatment of insufficient lactation (Que Ru). *Am J Acupunct.* 1996;24(1):35-46.

173. Vallone S. The role of subluxation and chiropractic care in hypolactation. *J Clin Chiroprac Pediatr.* 2007;8(1-2):518-524.

174. Cole M. Placenta medicine as a galactogogue: tradition or trend? *Clin Lactation.* 2014;5(4):116-122.

175. Hatherly P. *The Homeopathic Physician's Guide to Lactation.* Chapel Hill, Australia: Luminoz Pty Ltd; 2004.

Additional Resources

Kellams A, Harrel C, Omage S, Gregory C, Rosen-Carole C, Academy of Breastfeeding Medicine. ABM clinical protocol #3: supplementary feedings in the healthy term breastfed neonate, revised 2017. *Breastfeeding Med.* 2017;12(3). http://www.bfmed.org/Media/Files/Protocols /Protocol%203%20Supplementation%20English%20Version.pdf.

Penn State Hershey Medical Center. NEWT: Newborn Weight Tool. https://www.newbornweight.org.

Smillie CM. Baby-Led Breastfeeding . . . The Mother-Baby Dance [DVD]. Los Angeles, CA: Geddes Productions, LLC; 2007. http://www .geddesproduction.com/breast-feeding-baby-led.php.

World Health Organization. Child Growth Standards: Weight Velocity. http://www.who.int/childgrowth/standards/w_velocity/en/.

World Health Organization. Growth Curves, Length/Height for Age, Female. http://www.who.int/childgrowth/standards/sft_lhfa_girls_p/en/.

World Health Organization. Growth Curves, Length/Height for Age, Male. http://www.who.int/childgrowth/standards/sft_lhfa_boys_p/en/.

World Health Organization. Growth Curves, Weight for Age, Female. http://www.who.int/childgrowth/standards/chts_wfa_girls_p/en/.

World Health Organization. Growth Curves, Weight for Age, Male. http://www.who.int/childgrowth/standards/chts_wfa_boys_p/en/.

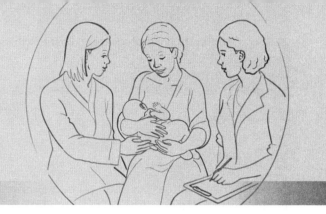

CHAPTER 23

Breastfeeding and Infant Birth Injury, Congenital Anomalies, and Illness

Catherine Watson Genna

OBJECTIVES

- Discuss how congenital anomalies, neurologic impairments, illness, and birth trauma can affect early breastfeeding.
- List strategies for assisting these infants with initiating and maintaining breastfeeding.

DEFINITIONS OF COMMONLY USED TERMS

birth trauma Injury or damage of the tissues or organs of a newborn that were sustained during labor and delivery.
congenital anomaly A physical or structural malformation or disease that developed in utero.
inborn errors of metabolism A congenital disorder resulting from genetic defects that lead to enzyme deficiency. Some enzyme deficiencies impair the infant's ability to break down and metabolize various nutrients, or they result in a buildup of toxins.
neurologic impairment A deficit related to any disorder of the nervous system from infection or structural, biochemical, or electrical abnormalities.

Any use of the term *mother*, *maternal*, or *breastfeeding* is not meant to exclude transgender or nonbinary parents who may be breastfeeding or providing human milk to their infant.

▶ Overview

A number of conditions presenting at birth or shortly thereafter can have a significant impact on the initiation and duration of breastfeeding. Some of these conditions are temporary, whereas others remain for a lifetime. Compromised infants especially benefit from the provision of breastmilk or breastfeeding. For the few infants who cannot feed at the breast, the provision of breastmilk can and should continue as long as possible. Feeding problems may be the first sign or symptom of a medical condition or infant insult. Parents of these infants can experience an enormous range of emotions. They might be frightened, frustrated, anxious, fatigued, angry, or depressed. Their emotional well-being should not be neglected in the flurry of activity surrounding the baby.

I. Postmature Infants

A.   A postmature infant is a fully mature infant born after the onset of the 42nd week of gestation, having remained in utero beyond the time of optimal placental function.

B.   Aging of the placenta and reduced placental function impair nutrient and oxygen transport to the fetus, placing the fetus at risk for a lower tolerance to the stresses of labor and delivery, including hypoxia.
1.   In response to hypoxia, meconium might be passed, increasing the risk for meconium aspiration.
2.   Amniotic fluid might be decreased, increasing the risk for meconium aspiration and umbilical cord compression.

C.   If the placenta continues to function well, the infant might become large for gestational age, which increases the risk for shoulder dystocia and possible fractured clavicle.

D.   Postmature infants are characterized by the following:
1.   Loss of weight in utero.
2.   Dry, peeling skin that appears to hang as a result of losing subcutaneous fat and muscle mass.
3.   A wrinkled, wide-eyed appearance.
4.   Lack of vernix caseosa (the waxy or cheese-like substance coating the newborn's skin; composed of sebum and skin sloughed in utero).
5.   Reduced glycogen stores in the liver.

E.   These infants might be at higher risk for hypoglycemia as a result of low glycogen reserves. Skin-to-skin contact from birth and early, frequent breastfeeding, or feeding of colostrum if not latching, can help maintain blood glucose levels.[1,2]

F.   These infants might feed poorly, appear lethargic, and require considerable incentives to sustain suckling. Incentives include the following:
1.   Alternate massage and breast compression.
2.   Expressed colostrum.
3.   Skin-to-skin contact (because their body temperature is quite labile).
4.   Avoidance of crying episodes, which can further drop their blood glucose levels.

II. Birth Trauma

A.   Forceps use might result in small areas of ecchymosis (bruising) on the sides of the face where the blades were placed. Forceps use can also cause neurological injuries.
1.   Trauma to the facial nerves can occur. Any muscles innervated by these nerves might be temporarily hypotonic, making latching and sucking difficult. Observe for asymmetric movement of the mouth, drooping mouth, or a drooping eyelid.
2.   Forceps, vacuum, and especially failure of one followed by use of the other, can result in shoulder dystocia and brachial plexus injury, causing paralysis or weakness of the hand or arm.[3] These injuries can interfere with stable positioning and normal manual nipple seeking, stimulating, and shaping behaviors at the breast.[4]

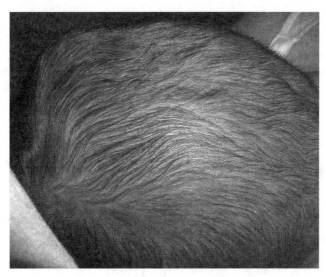

FIGURE 23-1 Cephalhematoma in newborn.
© Catherine Watson Genna, BS, IBCLC.

B.   Vacuum-assisted deliveries can pose an increased risk of cranial hemorrhage in term and preterm infants, as can vacuum or forceps use during labor or cesarean birth during labor.[5-8]

1.   Extracranial hemorrhage is bleeding between the skin and cranial bone.

   a.   Caput succedaneum (hemorrhagic edema of the soft tissues of the scalp) usually resolves within the first week of life.

   b.   Cephalhematoma is bleeding that is contained within the subperiosteal space, preventing it from crossing suture lines (see **FIGURE 23-1**).

   c.   Subgaleal hemorrhage can represent a significant blood loss to the infant.

      i.   It presents as a fluctuant area of the scalp, sometimes increasing in size to the point of blood dissecting into the subcutaneous tissue of the back of the neck.[9]

      ii.   These infants need special help in positioning to keep pressure off the hemorrhagic area.

      iii.   Some infants feed poorly or not at all until some of the hemorrhage has resolved, increasing the risk of high bilirubin levels as the body breaks down the red blood cells and recycles the hemoglobin.

2.   Intracranial hemorrhage is not visible externally.

   a.   The infant might present with common signs, such as sleepiness, feeding intolerance, apnea, and decreased muscle tone.[8]

   b.   Subdural (cerebral) hemorrhage is the most common intracranial hemorrhage resulting from a traumatic delivery.[10] The incidence of subarachnoid hemorrhage increases more after vacuum deliveries than forceps deliveries, and both types of delivery carry a higher incidence than unassisted vaginal deliveries.[11] Intraventricular hemorrhages are more likely after forceps birth but are also increased in vacuum deliveries.[11]

   c.   Some of the signs and symptoms become evident following discharge. Infants who have a history of vacuum extraction and demonstrate lethargy, feeding problems, hypotonia, increased irritability, diffuse swelling of the head, and pallor need immediate follow-up care.[12]

   d.   The abilities to suck, swallow, breathe, and root are sensitive to neurologic insults.[13] Feeding difficulties are more likely in infants delivered via vacuum or forceps.[11]

   e.   Intradural and subdural hemorrhages are associated with a heightened risk of hypoxic–ischemic encephalopathy.[14]

   f.   Infants with intracranial hemorrhage might be treated therapeutically with hypothermia,[15] which precludes direct breastfeeding during treatment.

      i.   Trophic feedings of colostrum can be given during hypothermia.[16]

      ii.   Parents should be assisted with manual expression of colostrum within the first hour after delivery and with an electric breast pump if possible.[17,18]

    C.   A fractured clavicle can occur with a large for gestational age infant or with malpresentations of the infant.

        1.   The infant might display a decreased movement of the arm or distress with arm movements. The arm and shoulder are immobilized, and special positioning might be needed for breastfeeding.

        2.   Some infants are not diagnosed until after discharge when certain positions are associated with crying. Using the clutch hold or placing the infant on the unaffected side at each breast might be helpful.

III. Fetal Distress and Hypoxia–Ischemia (Decreased Blood Flow and Oxygen)

    A.   Infants can be compromised in utero by maternal or fetal infectious illness, rapid changes in blood pressure, energy failure from mitochondrial disorders, or maternal cardiopulmonary collapse.

    B.   During delivery, insufficient placental reserve, umbilical cord compression, or umbilical cord prolapse may occur.

    C.   Newborns are vulnerable to brain cell death from hypoxia–ischemia.

        1.   *Neonatal encephalopathy* is the current term for altered level of consciousness, seizures, apnea, and reduced brain stem function, including impaired feeding ability.

            a.   A blood pH lower than 7.0 and a base deficit at birth indicate an acute hypoxic–ischemic event. Normal pH of newborns is 7.26 to 7.30.

            b.   Recovery begins after 3 to 4 days. Some infants remain compromised and may develop cerebral palsy or other neurologic deficits.

            c.   Low Apgar scores combined with an inability to suck that requires tube feeding are the most sensitive indicators of later disability; additional indicators are seizures and the need for mechanical ventilation.[19]

            d.   Hypoxia decreases the motility of the gut and reduces the gut-stimulating hormones.

            e.   These infants might have a depressed suck that is not well coordinated with the swallow, and they may have difficulty bottle feeding.

        2.   Colostrum is very important to these infants because their gastrointestinal tract might have suffered hypoxic damage.

            a.   Colostrum should be expressed and used as soon as the infant can tolerate feedings by mouth. Parents should frequently hand express or pump during this time.

            b.   Infants can safely receive small-volume colostrum feeds during hypothermia treatment.

        3.   Breastfeeding interventions are similar to those for infants who have Down syndrome.

            a.   A supplementer device, cup, or other feeding device might initially be needed until the infant's feeding skills recover.

            b.   Milk expression will be necessary when the infant is unable to remove milk.[20]

            c.   A hypotonic (low muscle tone) infant might breastfeed better in a clutch hold with the trunk stabilized against the parent's side or prone on a semireclined parent.[21]

            d.   A hypertonic (high muscle tone) infant should be held in a flexed, well-supported position to reduce the overall extensor patterning. Preparatory handling (such as gentle rocking) can reduce tone.

            e.   Cheek and jaw support (Dancer hand) will help with maintaining the latch.

        4.   These infants have increased effort of feeding, fatigue easily, and may require very short, frequent feedings.

        5.   Recovery usually proceeds for many months, and infants who cannot breastfeed at birth may develop the skills later, especially if oral motor therapy is provided and attempts at the breast continue.

IV. Neurologic Disorders

    A.   Infants who have neurologic impairments often have extremely complex needs.

        1.   The infant's nervous system can be damaged, abnormally developed, immature, or temporarily incapacitated from insults such as intrauterine infection, asphyxia, sepsis, trauma, or drugs.

2. Infants can have an absent or depressed rooting response, gag reflex, sucking reflex, or difficulty swallowing (dysphagia).

3. Giving a bottle to an infant who is to be breastfed provides inconsistent sensory input that additionally disorganizes the nervous system.

B. There may be a depressed or absent suck reflex with limited response to stimulation of the palate and tongue. These infants might also have decreased muscle tone.

1. A weak or poorly sustained sucking reflex denotes an oral musculature that has been weakened to the point of an inability to sustain a rhythmic suck.

2. The rhythm is interrupted by irregular pauses and sometimes lacks the 1:1 suck-to-swallow ratio.

3. Adequate negative intraoral pressure is not generated, causing the nipple to fall out of the mouth.

4. The lips do not form a complete seal.

5. The hypotonic tongue might remain flat and not cup around the breast.

C. Uncoordinated sucking includes a mistiming of the component muscle movements of the suck–swallow–breathe cycle (abnormal kinematics).

1. There may be extraneous movements of the mouth, head, or neck. Supportive techniques can help reduce abnormal movements and provide stability for oral structures during feeding.[22]

2. The infant might have difficulty organizing feeding behaviors and initiating sucking. Gentle organizing input before feeds improves feeding.[23]

3. Hypersensitivity or hyposensitivity might be seen in other areas of the body.[24]

4. There may be dysfunctional tongue movements and uncoordinated swallowing, increasing the risk of aspiration. Positioning modifications can improve swallowing during breastfeeding.[22]

V. Inborn Errors of Metabolism

A. Galactosemia.

1. Galactosemia is caused by a deficiency of the enzyme galactosyl-1-phosphate uridylyltransferase (GALT), causing an inability in the infant to metabolize galactose.

2. Infants can have severe and persistent jaundice, vomiting, diarrhea, electrolyte imbalance, cerebral involvement, cataracts, and weight loss.

3. These infants are weaned from the breast to a lactose- and galactose-free formula.

4. Duarte galactosemia is a condition in which low but functional levels of GALT allow breastfeeding to continue.[25] Despite slightly elevated levels of galactose breakdown products in blood and urine, developmental outcomes are not improved by restricting lactose intake during the first year of life.[26,27]

B. Phenylketonuria (PKU).

1. PKU is the most common of the amino acid metabolic disorders.

   a. It is an autosomal recessive, inherited disorder in which the amino acid phenylalanine accumulates because of the absence or reduced activity of the enzyme phenylalanine hydroxylase, which converts phenylalanine to tyrosine for further breakdown.

   b. Newborn screening for PKU is done in all 50 U.S. states and in more than 30 other countries.

2. Infants need some phenylalanine.

   a. Infants who have PKU can continue to breastfeed when a balance is maintained between the use of a phenylalanine-free formula and breastmilk.[28]

   b. Human milk has lower levels of phenylalanine than standard commercial formulas do, and infants with PKU who are breastfed (along with phenylalanine-free formula) have lower blood levels of phenylalanine.[29,30]

   c. The amount of phenylalanine-free formula and breastmilk can be calculated by weight, age, blood levels, and the need for growth, and the amount is adjusted weekly.

   d. Another approach is to feed the infant 10 to 30 milliliters of the special formula followed by breastfeeding.

   e. As long as phenylalanine levels are properly maintained, the exact calculations of breastmilk and formula might not need to be made.

   f. Breastmilk might be more than half the diet, improving the infant's exposure to the trophic (tissue building), immune, and immunomodulating functions of breastfeeding.

3. Breastfeeding before diagnosis and dietary intervention has been shown to produce a 14-point higher IQ than in infants who are artificially fed before diagnosis.[31]

4. Supplementation of BH4 (tetrahydrobiopterin, a phenylalanine hydroxylase cofactor) increases the amount of phenylalanine (and human milk) that is tolerated in some individuals with PKU.[32]

5. Challenges for breastfeeding infants with PKU include the following[33]:

    a. Maintaining milk production in the context of constantly changing amounts of milk the infant can consume.

    b. Difficulties integrating pumping into the added work of caring for the child.

    c. Issues with nipple confusion when using a bottle to feed the phenylalanine-free formula.

C. Other inborn errors of metabolism.

1. Infants with metabolic disorders are at risk of failure to thrive, neurologic injury, acid–base balance disturbances, and other life-threatening complications if not identified and treated.

    a. Many infants require dietary supplements to help circumvent a blocked metabolic pathway or reduce the levels or toxicity of products of abnormal metabolism.

    b. If they can safely consume lactose and intact protein, they can at least partially breastfeed.

    c. Mothers require assistance with maintaining milk production during initial stabilization and metabolic crises when infants are temporarily unable to feed.

2. Breastfeeding is recommended as the source of intact protein for infants with maple syrup urine disease as long as they can be appropriately monitored.[34]

3. Breastfeeding should be encouraged for infants with glutaric aciduria (a deficiency of glutaryl-CoA dehydrogenase, an enzyme needed for lysine breakdown).[35] Parents need an emergency plan to reduce protein foods (including human milk) by 50 percent and increase other calories when the infant receives immunizations or becomes ill.[35]

4. Infants with mild urea cycle disorders or organic acidemias may be able to exclusively breastfeed with good metabolic control.[36,37] There were fewer hospitalizations and infections in breastfed infants with organic acidemias.[38]

5. Infants with one of several rare amino acid or protein metabolism disorders have been successfully breastfed along with the provision of powdered amino acid supplements mixed with human milk by bottle, feeding tube, or breastfeeding supplementer.[36,37]

VI. Other Genetic and Congenital Disorders

A. Cystic fibrosis (CF).

1. CF is a congenital disease involving a generalized dysfunction of exocrine glands resulting from a mutation in the gene coding for the CF transmembrane conductance regulator protein.

2. The glands produce abnormally thick and sticky secretions that block the flow of pancreatic digestive enzymes (proteases and lipase), clog hepatic ducts, and affect the movement of the cilia in the lungs.

3. Increased sodium chloride in the child's sweat is frequently the first indicator of the condition; the infant tastes salty when nuzzled.

4. Another early indicator of CF is intestinal obstruction or ileus. The meconium blocks the small intestine, resulting in abdominal distension, vomiting, and failure to pass stools (resulting in the failure to gain weight).

5. Infants who have CF produce normal amounts of gastric lipase, which, when combined with lipase in milk, enhances fat absorption.

6. Breastfed infants with CF are less likely to need intravenous antibiotics and have improved lung function.[39]

7. Breastfed infants with CF can present with protein malnutrition (edema) and reduced weight gain but may escape the characteristic infections, confounding diagnosis.

    a. Pancreatic enzymes can be given to the infant to improve protein metabolism.[40]

    b. Daily oral vitamin K supplements can reduce bleeding risk.[41]

8. Breastfeeding is recommended for infants with CF.[42] Breastfed infants with CF retain normal gut flora longer, which is associated with later time to first exacerbation.[43]

9. Infants with CF are at risk of failure to thrive due to increased energy expenditure.

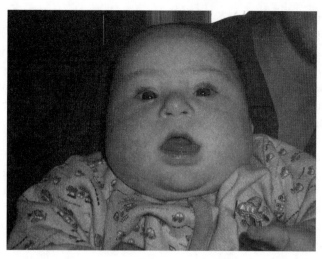

FIGURE 23-2 Infant with Down syndrome. Note hypotonia and small mandible that increase tongue protrusion.

© Catherine Watson Genna, BS, IBCLC.

     a.   This is principally from increased work of breathing, malabsorption due to pancreatic enzyme dysfunction and fat loss in the intestines, and poor appetite secondary to gastroesophageal reflux and gastrointestinal pain.[42]

     b.   Short, frequent breastfeeds with enzyme and fat-soluble vitamin supplements help compensate for these difficulties.

B.   Down syndrome.

   1.   Down syndrome results from an extra chromosome 21 (trisomy 21).

   2.   Common characteristics that relate to feeding in infants with Down syndrome include the following:

     a.   A flaccid tongue that appears too large for the mouth as a result of reduced growth of the mandible (lower jaw) (see **FIGURE 23-2**).

     b.   Generalized hypotonia, including the oral musculature.

     c.   Heart defects (50 percent incidence) that decrease aerobic capacity for feeding and might require surgery.

     d.   Laryngomalacia, tracheomalacia, or bronchomalacia that destabilize the airway and further stress respiratory function. Some infants have multiple airway anomalies.

     e.   Incomplete development of the gastrointestinal tract. Vomiting can be the first sign of an intestinal blockage in infants.

     f.   Hyperbilirubinemia is common in newborn infants with Down syndrome.

     g.   Infants with Down syndrome have increased susceptibility to infection.

     h.   Possible depressed sucking reflex, a weak suck, or both may be present.

   3.   Some infants have no problem sucking, while others might exhibit initial sucking difficulties.

   4.   The Dancer hand position may stabilize the jaw and support the masseter muscles, which decreases the intraoral space and enhances the generation of negative pressure.[44] (See Figure 13-7 in Chapter 13, *Facilitating and Assessing Breastfeeding Initiation.*)

     a.   The breast is supported by the third, fourth, and fifth fingers so the webbing between the thumb and index finger forms a U-shaped cup that the infant's chin rests on.

     b.   The thumb and index finger support the cheeks and produce gentle traction toward the corner of the lips.

   5.   The infant should be in a quiet–alert state to feed.

   6.   The infant might need hindmilk supplementation to gain weight and may benefit from the use of a supplementer at the breast or chest to deliver it.

   7.   Feeding in a prone or semiprone position on a recliner can help gravity stabilize the infant.

   8.   Do not overly flex or extend the infant's head because occiptoatlantal or atlatoaxial instability (lax connection between the base of the skull and upper spine, or between the first two cervical vertebrae, respectively) occurs in 10 to 20 percent of children with Down syndrome. Abnormal movement may trap and injure the spinal cord. This same concern applies to infants with certain forms of dwarfism.

C. Gastrointestinal tract disorders.
   1. Esophageal atresia (EA) is a congenital defect of the esophagus.
      a. In most cases of EA, the upper esophagus does not connect with the lower esophagus and stomach. The condition may be associated with other birth defects.
      b. Tracheoesophageal fistula (TEF) is a common variation of EA that occurs when the esophagus communicates with the trachea. It occurs in 1 of every 3,000 to 5,000 live births.
      c. EA is usually detected in the first few hours of life and is considered a surgical emergency.
      d. The symptoms can include excess amniotic fluid during pregnancy and difficulties with feeding, such as coughing, spilling fluid from the lips, gagging, choking, and cyanosis.
      e. There is no research to justify test feeds of sterile or glucose water to diagnose TEF or EA. Water or low-chloride fluids in the neonatal airway have the potential to cause prolonged apnea.[45]
   2. Gastroesophageal reflux (GER) is persistent, nonprojectile regurgitation (spitting up) after feeds.
      a. It can be mild and self-limiting, requiring no modifications or interventions.
      b. It can be more severe, with worsening regurgitation and weight gain or weight loss problems.
      c. GER can present as follows:
         i. Fussiness at the breast as the stomach contents contact the lower section of the esophagus.
         ii. It might be more apparent in certain side-lying positions at the breast.
         iii. Parents might report increased fussing at the breast, arching off or pulling away from the breast, or crying until the infant is placed upright.
         iv. The infant mouths refluxed milk between feedings (cud chewing).
         v. Upper respiratory infections and congestion may occur from chronic aspiration of refluxing fluid (ascending aspiration).
         vi. Feeding refusal is common.
         vii. Micro- and macroaspiration or nasopharyngeal reflux (entry of milk into the nose from the mouth) may manifest as nasal congestion that increases throughout the feeding, with coughing or wheezing during or between feeds.[46] Aspiration can also be precipitated by high milk flow or the infant's inability to properly coordinate sucking, swallowing, and breathing.
      d. Parents are encouraged to continue breastfeeding.[47,48]
         i. Feed with the infant in an upright position (in clutch hold, or straddled across the lap, or diagonal with parent reclining).
         ii. Feed on one breast at each feeding to keep from overdistending the stomach, and feed frequently.
         iii. Keep the infant upright for 10 to 20 minutes after feedings.
      e. Reflux needs to be differentiated from hyperlactation with overfeeding or lactose overload.
         i. Generally, if the infant is gaining rapidly, has signs of gut irritation and rapid intestinal transit time (green, mucousy stools), and is fussy, hyperlactation might be responsible.
         ii. Reducing milk production by gradually increasing the amount of time before changing breasts is generally successful (block feeding).[49,50]
         iii. Clinicians have anecdotally reported that brief breast massage immediately before feeding helps dislodge fat globules from the duct walls and release them back into the milk to improve the lactose–fat balance in dyads with hyperlactation.
         iv. Reducing milk production by gradually increasing the amount of time before changing breasts is generally successful if massage is insufficient. Clinicians refer to this as block feeding.[49]
      f. If the reflux is associated with esophageal irritation or respiratory complications, the infant might undergo diagnostic tests and be placed on medication. Acid blocking medication is often ineffective to prevent reflux complications in young infants.[51]
   3. Pyloric stenosis is a stricture or narrowing of the pylorus (muscular tissue controlling the outlet of the stomach), caused by muscular hypertrophy.
      a. This hypertrophy might be felt as an olive-shaped mass in the infant's lower abdomen.
      b. It usually occurs between the 2nd and 6th week of life, although it can occur any time after birth. It is more common in formula-fed than breastfed infants.[52-54]

   c. Vomiting is characteristic. It is intermittent at first and progresses to after every feeding, and becomes projectile in nature. Usually the infant is voraciously hungry at first then begins to refuse feeds.
   d. Dehydration, electrolyte imbalance, and weight loss can occur in extreme situations.
   e. If the infant does not outgrow the condition or if it is severe, surgery can be performed after rehydration and correction of electrolyte balance.
      i. Infants can resume breastfeeding as tolerated when awake and stable after surgery.[55,56]
      ii. Positioning the infant upright in a straddle position helps avoid stress on the incision.
D. Congenital heart defects are the most common types of birth defects in newborns.
   1. Congenital heart defects are seen along a continuum from mild with no symptoms to severe with cyanosis, rapid breathing, shortness of breath, and lowered oxygen levels (desaturation) that requires surgical correction.
   2. Cardiac disease is not a medical indication to interrupt or cease breastfeeding.[57]
   3. Congenital heart disease increases vulnerability to necrotizing enterocolitis,[58] increasing the importance of breastfeeding in this population.
   4. Feeding at the breast presents less work for the infant, keeps oxygen levels higher than with bottle feeding, and keeps heart and respiratory rates stable when the infant is at the breast.[59]
   5. Unrestricted breastfeeding on cue results in the best growth in affected infants.[60]
   6. An infant who has more serious heart involvement might be unable to sustain sucking at the breast or might need to pause frequently to rest. If intake is inadequate, the infant will not gain weight or will exhibit weight loss.
   7. Infants with untreated cardiac disease often have increased caloric requirements, which normalize after corrective surgery.[61,62]
   8. Infant behavior and symptoms may be described in the following ways[63]:
      a. Able to sustain sucking for only short periods of time.
      b. Pulling off the breast frequently.
      c. Turning blue around the lips (circumoral cyanosis).
      d. Rapid breathing, panting, or breathlessness; rapid heart rate.
      e. Sweating while at the breast.
      f. Need for very frequent feedings.
      g. Vomiting after feeding.
   9. If surgery is planned, it is typically scheduled after the infant reaches a predetermined weight or age.
   10. Feeding modifications are similar to those for preterm infants or those with respiratory disorders.[64-66]
      a. Small, frequent, unilateral feeds might be necessary.
      b. Upright or prone feeding positions improve coordination of swallowing and breathing.
   11. If additional calories are needed, consider hindmilk supplementation at the breast with a supplementer device or breast massage before breastfeeding.
   12. Infants with congenital heart disease benefit from immediate skin-to-skin contact if they are sufficiently stable, with developmental care and team care that includes lactation consultants.[67-69]
E. Respiratory disorders can impact an infant's ability to feed effectively.
   1. Common features of respiratory disorders include the following:
      a. Increased effort of breathing leaves less energy for feeding.
      b. Increased baseline respiratory rate reduces the amount of swallowing that can be done because swallowing inhibits breathing.[70]
      c. Short sucking bursts are typical signs of respiratory disorders.
   2. Types of respiratory disorders include the following:
      a. In laryngomalacia the epiglottis lacks normal stiffness, neural innervation,[71] muscle tone, or sensorimotor integration.[72]
         i. The epiglottis collapses into the airway on inspiration, causing inspiratory stridor, suprasternal retractions, and increased work of breathing, particularly during crying, feeding, and supine positioning.
         ii. The laryngeal vestibule itself may be overly small or high or low tone, creating difficulty with breathing and feeding. The pharynx may be low tone, creating problems with the smooth coordination of the epiglottis and larynx during the protection phase of the cycle.

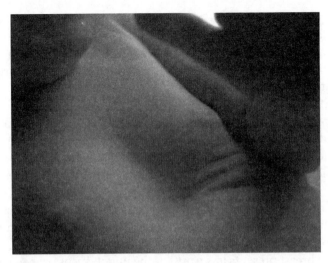

FIGURE 23-3 Sternal and substernal retraction due to tracheomalacia.
© Catherine Watson Genna, BS, IBCLC.

    iii.   Laryngomalacia is associated with increased risk of dysphagia (abnormal swallowing), regardless of severity.[73]

    iv.   Laryngomalacia is strongly associated with GER because of increased pressure on the lower esophageal sphincter.

    v.   Head extension and prone positioning during feeding reduce airway resistance. Short frequent feeds may be necessary to prevent failure to thrive.[74]

    vi.   Laryngomalacia generally peaks at age 6 months. It is thought to resolve by age 18 to 24 months as the neck elongates and structures become anatomically separated. However, it can persist and cause laryngeal obstruction in adolescents during exercise.[75]

  b. Tracheomalacia increases the work of respiration and feeding.

    i.   Cartilage rings in the trachea may be malformed and are insufficiently stiff so that rapid airflow during expiration (also inspiration in newborns) causes a partial collapse of the trachea.[76]

    ii.   Tracheomalacia can be seen as sternal retraction and heard as stridor (see **FIGURE 23-3**).

    iii.   The strategies described above for laryngomalacia are also helpful.

    iv.   Tracheomalacia is outgrown in the first year or two of life.

  c. Laryngeal webs are a persistence of tissue in the lumen of the airway.

    i.   Laryngeal webs can cause significant respiratory distress.

    ii.   Infants with laryngeal webs may have great difficulty feeding. Very careful pacing of feeding is necessary to prevent hypoxia.

  d. Laryngeal clefts are openings of variable size and position between the larynx and the esophagus.

    i.   Laryngeal clefts result in stridor or aspiration during feeding.[77]

    ii.   Laryngeal clefts interfere with normal functioning in all phases of swallowing: oral phase, swallow initiation, and pharyngeal phase (predisposing to laryngeal penetration and aspiration).[78]

    iii.   Laryngeal clefts usually require repair (surgery or gel foam injections) to allow the infant to feed safely, although some affected infants breastfeed well in upright or prone positions.

    iv.   Laryngeal clefts can be comorbid with tracheobronchomalacia or tracheoesophageal fistula.[79]

  e. Vocal fold paresis or paralysis

    i.   Weakness (paresis) or paralysis of a vocal cord is usually unilateral from injury to the vocal fold or its nerve supply. It can be congenital or result from recurrent laryngeal nerve injury during cardiovascular surgery.[80]

    ii.   An infant with vocal cord paresis or paralysis may have a hoarse or weak cry.

    iii.   If the cord is unable to close well, it will reduce airway protection on the affected side.

    iv.   Infants will usually coordinate swallowing and breathing better if the weak or paralyzed cord is oriented upward.

        f. Velopharyngeal insufficiency or incompetence
- i. This condition is characterized by hypoplasia or dysfunction of the soft palate or pharyngeal constrictor muscles that prevent milk from entering the nasopharynx, sometimes resulting from submucosal cleft palate.
- ii. Nasal regurgitation, harsh respiration in feeding pauses, apnea from milk in the nasopharynx, and feeding resistance can be consequences of velopharyngeal incompetence.
- iii. Careful pacing and upright positioning (straddle) may help infants have less nasopharyngeal reflux (flow of milk into the nose during feeding).

        g. Cardiorespiratory disorders
- i. Cardiorespiratory disorders create tension between the infant's needs for food and oxygen.
- ii. Short, frequent feedings reduce fatigue and oxygen debt, which can exacerbate dysphagia.
- iii. Prone feeding positions with mild head extension can improve the infant's ability to coordinate swallowing and breathing.
- iv. Infants with cardiac malformations may feed better in upright positions.
- v. Flow during breastfeeding can be reduced by prepumping the breast or using manual pressure to block milk ducts.

   3. General breastfeeding implications for respiratory disorders include the following:
- a. Very careful pacing of the feed (making sure the infant can control the speed of milk flow), head extension to reduce airway resistance to airflow,[74,81] prone feeding positions (with parent reclined), and more frequent feedings are generally helpful. Pressing on the breast to block some ducts can also reduce the flow.[82]
- b. Growth should be monitored closely, and expressed milk should be provided by slow-flow methods if the infant is unable to meet the needs at the breast.

VII. Acute and Systemic Illness

A. Illness can reduce appetite, causing transient growth flattening or even weight loss.
1. Breastfed infants maintain their energy intake from human milk, protecting them against growth failure during illness.[83]
2. Infants receive active and passive immunity through human milk, including leukocytes[84] and immunomodulators.[85]
3. Lactoferrin and secretory immunoglobulin A (sIgA) are both present in breastmilk and provide immune protection to infants. Lactoferrin levels in the milk are higher in the month before and the month after an infant's illness. Higher sIgA levels in the milk are associated with less incidence of illness.[86]

B. Gastroenteritis can be a serious illness in infants and young children.
1. It is particularly important to maintain breastfeeding during diarrhea and vomiting to prevent dehydration.
2. Oral rehydration can be used with breastfeeding if needed.

C. Respiratory infections can increase the work of breathing and make breastfeeding more difficult for infants.
1. Infants with nasal congestion may come on and off the breast to mouth breathe during feedings. Sterile saline nasal spray may reduce the nasal blockage and can be used before feeding.
2. Infants with lower respiratory infections may use shorter sucking bursts during feeding. Parents can be counseled to offer very frequent feeds.
3. Prone feeding positions with mild head extension improve the infant's ability to coordinate swallowing and breathing when it is stressed by respiratory illness.

D. Otitis media, or middle ear infections, are one of the most common illnesses in infants.
1. Ear infections are painful and are common causes of breastfeeding strikes. Positioning changes to avoid pressure on the affected ear may allow the infant to feed more comfortably.
2. Exclusive or predominant breastfeeding is protective against otitis media in the early years of life.[87,88]

E. Candidiasis is the result of an overgrowth of *Candida* species, or yeast.
1. Breastfeeding infants may develop painful white plaques on the oral mucosa.
2. Oral candidiasis may be comorbid with diaper rash, typically with red, shiny skin that becomes friable (weakened) and cracks or peels.

3. Oral candidiasis can be difficult to treat because the plaques contain biofilms that protect the yeasts from medication. Topical medication should be used for twice the time it takes to eliminate symptoms.[89]

4. Gentian violet (especially when dissolved in alcohol) can cause painful mouth and throat lesions in infants and should be used only under medical supervision.[90]

5. Studies isolating *Candida* from painful nipples vary in their findings. They are more likely to be positive when molecular techniques are used instead of microbiological cultures.[91]

6. Pacifiers and bottle nipples may need to be disinfected in bleach solution daily to avoid recontamination.[92]

F. Allergy symptoms in infants have a wide presentation from changes in stools, vomiting, skin rashes, and respiratory symptoms ranging from nasal congestion to coughing, to respiratory distress.

1. Lactation consultants should recognize common symptoms of allergic disorders and assist with elimination diets and protection of milk production in rare cases when bowel rest is necessary.

2. The management strategies will depend on the type of allergy.

   a. Allergic proctocolitis causes bloody stools with mucous in infants who are generally growing well. Removal of the allergen from the infant's diet, and sometimes the mother's diet, resolves symptoms in 48 to 72 hours. The symptoms can also be associated with a subclinical infection and will resolve with time.[93]

   b. Food protein-induced enterocolitis syndrome causes severe vomiting 1 to 3 hours after ingestion, and diarrhea 2 to 10 hours after ingestion, and is rare in exclusively breastfed infants.
      i. Infants may become lethargic and hypotensive.[94]
      ii. The offending food needs to be avoided only if it triggers symptoms in their infant.[95]

   c. Eosinophilic gastroenteritis can cause altered gastrointestinal permeability and protein loss, leading to peripheral and periorbital edema and growth failure.
      i. Avoidance of the allergen involved generally resolves the condition.[96]
      ii. CF in the breastfed infant can present with the same symptoms.

   d. Eczema (atopic dermatitis) risk is increased if solids are delayed past 9 months of life.
      i. Broken skin allows allergens to enter and provoke allergic sensitization.
      ii. The severity of eczema predicts food and respiratory allergy in exclusively breastfed children.[97]
      iii. Treating the eczema, and careful washing after eating and before handling the infant, may help avoid allergies.

   e. Introducing small amounts of solids while continuing breastfeeding improved tolerance in small studies of peanuts and eggs.[98,99] Further studies are needed to help find the right balance between protecting breastfeeding and preventing allergies.[100]

▶ Key Points from This Chapter

A. Infants with alterations to health or anatomy may have specific feeding difficulties that are amenable to alterations in breastfeeding management or, conversely, may require milk expression and alternate feeding.

B. Infants with painful birth injuries require careful positioning to avoid pressure on the lesion.

C. Neurological disabilities lead to poorer coordination and speed of motor movements and increased risk of dysphagia. Supportive techniques may improve functioning.

D. Breastfeeding (full or partial with the addition of medical formula) is appropriate and beneficial for infants with many metabolic disorders. Classic galactosemia is one notable exception.

E. Ill infants especially need the immune properties in human milk.

🔍 CASE STUDY

Shawna brought 4-day-old Braden to see you because of a sudden reluctance to breastfeed after she achieved lactogenesis II. Braden's father states that Braden will only sleep when held upright, and he cries when laid down on his back. Shawna's breasts are slightly engorged. After therapeutic breast massage, some manual expression, and reverse pressure softening, Braden is put on Shawna's chest and self-attaches. As soon as the milk ejection reflex occurs, Braden

CASE STUDY *(continued)*

begins to squeak on inspiration (inspiratory stridor). He swallows only three times before coming off the breast and coughing. You encourage Shawna to cuddle Braden against her shoulder for a few minutes until his breathing rate slows and the stridor stops, and then try again. Braden returns to the breast and sucks and swallows with a return of the stridor, sucking and swallowing an average of three times between respiratory pauses. Braden's hands and feet become mildly cyanotic (blue).

Your further assessment reveals suprasternal and sternal retractions with inspiratory stridor when Braden is supine. These improve when Braden calms down or is laid on his side. Braden feeds better, with less stridor and agitation, when Shawna reclines and Braden is prone on Shawna with his head extended, or when Braden is straddling her thigh facing her in a semisitting position.

Questions

1. So far, what does this history make you suspect?
2. What might you further assess in this infant?
3. Why might this condition have manifested at this time?
4. What positions and other breastfeeding modifications might help this infant to feed more effectively?
5. What interventions are generally contraindicated by this history?
6. What information will you communicate with the infant's primary healthcare provider?
7. What is the most likely condition causing these difficulties?
8. What other recommendations would be helpful for this family?

References

1. Tozier PK. Colostrum versus formula supplementation for glucose stabilization in newborns of diabetic mothers. *J Obstet Gynecol Neonatal Nurs.* 2013;42(6):619-628.
2. Rollins K. There's nothing sweeter than mom's own milk. *J Obstet Gynecol Neonatal Nurs.* 2013;42(suppl 1):S104.
3. Brimacombe M, Iffy L, Apuzzio JJ, et al. Shoulder dystocia related fetal neurological injuries: the predisposing roles of forceps and ventouse extractions. *Arch Gynecol Obstet.* 2008;277(5):415-422.
4. Genna CW, Barak D. Facilitating autonomous infant hand use during breastfeeding. *Clin Lactation.* 2010;1(1):15-20.
5. Ng PC, Siu YK, Lewindon PJ. Subaponeurotic haemorrhage in the 1990s: a 3-year surveillance. *Acta Paediatr.* 1995;84(9):1065-1069.
6. Ali UA, Norwitz ER. Vacuum-assisted vaginal delivery. *Rev Obstet Gynecol.* 2009;2(1):5.
7. Åberg K, Norman M, Ekéus C. Preterm birth by vacuum extraction and neonatal outcome: a population-based cohort study. *BMC Pregnancy Childbirth.* 2014;14(1):42.
8. Towner D, Castro MA, Eby-Wilkens E, Gilbert WM. Effect of mode of delivery in nulliparous women on neonatal intracranial injury. *N Engl J Med.* 1999;341(23):1709-1714.
9. Cavlovich FE. Subgaleal hemorrhage in the neonate. *J Obstet Gynecol Neonatal Nurs.* 1995;24(5):397-405.
10. Steinbach MT. Traumatic birth injury-intracranial hemorrhage. *Mother Baby J.* 1999;4:5-14.
11. Wen SW, Liu S, Kramer MS, et al. Comparison of maternal and infant outcomes between vacuum extraction and forceps deliveries. *Am J Epidemiol.* 2001;153(2):103-107.
12. Davis DJ. Neonatal subgaleal hemorrhage: diagnosis and management. *Can Med Assoc J.* 2001;164(10):1452-1453.
13. Katz-Salamon M, Allert K, Bergström BM, Ericsson K, Hesser U, Forssberg H. Perinatal risk factors and neuromotor behaviour during the neonatal period. *Acta Paediatr.* 1997;86(S419):27-36.
14. Scheimberg I, Cohen MC, Vazquez RE, et al. Nontraumatic intradural and subdural hemorrhage and hypoxic ischemic encephalopathy in fetuses, infants, and children up to three years of age: analysis of two audits of 636 cases from two referral centers in the United Kingdom. *Pediatr Dev Pathol.* 2013;16(3):149-159.
15. Jacobs SE, Berg M, Hunt R, Tarnow-Mordi WO, Inder TE, Davis PG. Cooling for newborns with hypoxic ischaemic encephalopathy. *Cochrane Database Syst Rev.* 2013;1;CD003311. doi:10.1002/14651858.CD003311.pub3.
16. Thyagarajan B, Tillqvist E, Baral V, Hallberg B, Vollmer B, Blennow M. Minimal enteral nutrition during neonatal hypothermia treatment for perinatal hypoxic-ischaemic encephalopathy is safe and feasible. *Acta Paediatr.* 2015;104(2):146-151.
17. Parker LA, Sullivan S, Krueger C, Mueller M. Association of timing of initiation of breastmilk expression on milk volume and timing of lactogenesis stage II among mothers of very low-birth-weight infants. *Breastfeed Med.* 2015;10(2):84-91. doi:10.1002/14651858 .CD003311.pub3.
18. Lussier MM, Brownell EA, Proulx TA, et al. Daily breastmilk volume in mothers of very low birth weight neonates: a repeated-measures randomized trial of hand expression versus electric breast pump expression. *Breastfeed Med.* 2015;10(6):312-317.
19. Moster D, Lie RT, Markestad T. Joint association of Apgar scores and early neonatal symptoms with minor disabilities at school age. *Arch Dis Child Fetal Neonatal Ed.* 2002;86(1):F16-F21.
20. Kellams A, Harrel C, Omage S, Gregory C, Rosen-Carole C, Academy of Breastfeeding Medicine. ABM clinical protocol #3: supplementary feedings in the healthy term breastfed neonate, revised 2017. *Breastfeed Med.* 2017;12(4):188-198.

21. McBride MC, Danner SC. Sucking disorders in neurologically impaired infants: assessment and facilitation of breastfeeding. *Clin Perinatol.* 1987;14(1):109-130.
22. Genna CW, Fram JL, Sandora L. Neurological issues and breastfeeding. In: Genna CW, ed. *Supporting Sucking Skills in Breastfeeding Infants.* 3rd ed. Burlington, MA: Jones & Bartlett Learning; 2017:305.
23. Medoff-Cooper B, Rankin K, Li Z, Liu L, White-Traut R. Multi-sensory intervention for preterm infants improves sucking organization. *Adv Neonatal Care.* 2015;15(2):142.
24. Genna CW. *Supporting Sucking Skills in Breastfeeding Infants.* 3rd ed. Burlington, MA: Jones & Bartlett Learning; 2017.
25. Schmidt D, Beebe R, Berg-Drazin P. Galactosemia and the continuation of breastfeeding with variant form. *Clin Lactation.* 2013;4(4):148-154.
26. Ficicioglu C, Hussa C, Gallagher PR, Thomas N, Yager C. Monitoring of biochemical status in children with Duarte galactosemia: utility of galactose, galactitol, galactonate, and galactose 1-phosphate. *Clin Chem.* 2010;56(7):1177-1182.
27. Ficicioglu C, Thomas N, Yager C, et al. Duarte (DG) galactosemia: a pilot study of biochemical and neurodevelopmental assessment in children detected by newborn screening. *Mol Genet Metab.* 2008;95(4):206-212.
28. van Rijn M, Bekhof J, Dijkstra T, Smit PG, Moddermam P, van Spronsen FJ. A different approach to breast-feeding of the infant with phenylketonuria. *Eur J Pediatr.* 2003;162(5):323-326.
29. Duncan LL, Elder SB. Breastfeeding the infant with PKU. *J Hum Lactation.* 1997;13(3):231-235.
30. O'Sullivan E, Boyle F, Mehta S, Kearney J. Breastfeeding improves biochemical control in children with phenylketonuria. *FASEB J.* 2013;27(suppl 1):622-630.
31. Riva E, Agostoni C, Biasucci G, et al. Early breastfeeding is linked to higher intelligence quotient scores in dietary treated phenylketonuric children. *Acta Paediatr.* 1996;85(1):56-58.
32. Hennermann JB, Bührer C, Blau N, Vetter B, Mönch E. Long-term treatment with tetrahydrobiopterin increases phenylalanine tolerance in children with severe phenotype of phenylketonuria. *Mol Genet Metab.* 2005;86:86-90.
33. Banta-Wright SA, Kodadek SM, Steiner RD, Houck GM. Challenges to breastfeeding infants with phenylketonuria. *J Pediatr Nurs.* 2015;30(1):219-226.
34. Frazier DM, Allgeier C, Homer C, et al. Nutrition management guideline for maple syrup urine disease: an evidence-and consensus-based approach. *Mol Genet Metab.* 2014;112(3):210-217.
35. Kölker S, Christensen E, Leonard JV, et al. Diagnosis and management of glutaric aciduria type I–revised recommendations. *J Inherit Metab Dis.* 2011;34(3):677.
36. Huner G, Baykal T, Demir F, Demirkol M. Breastfeeding experience in inborn errors of metabolism other than phenylketonuria. *J Inherit Metab Dis.* 2005;28(4):457-465.
37. MacDonald A, Depondt E, Evans S, Daly A, Hendriksz C, Saudubray JM. Breast feeding in IMD. *J Inherit Metab Dis.* 2006;29(2-3):299-303.
38. Gokcay G, Baykal T, Gokdemir Y, Demirkol M. Breast feeding in organic acidaemias. *J Inherit Metab Dis.* 2006;29(2):304-310.
39. Parker EM, O'Sullivan BP, Shea JC, Regan MM, Freedman SD. Survey of breast-feeding practices and outcomes in the cystic fibrosis population. *Pediatr Pulmonol.* 2004;37(4):362-367.
40. Cannella PC, Bowser EK, Guyer LK, Borum PR. Feeding practices and nutrition recommendations for infants with cystic fibrosis. *J Amer Diet Assoc.* 1993;93(3):297-300.
41. Cottam ST, Connett GJ. Routine use of daily oral vitamin K to treat infants with cystic fibrosis. *Paediatr Respir Rev.* 2015;16:22-24.
42. Haller W, Ledder O, Lewindon PJ, Couper R, Gaskin KJ, Oliver M. Cystic fibrosis: an update for clinicians. Part 1: nutrition and gastrointestinal complications. *J Gastroenterol Hepatol.* 2014;29(7):1344-1355.
43. Hoen AG, Li J, Moulton LA, et al. Associations between gut microbial colonization in early life and respiratory outcomes in cystic fibrosis. *J Pediatr.* 2015;167(1):138-147.
44. Danner SC. Breastfeeding the neurologically impaired infant. *NAACOGS Clin Issu Perinat Womens Health Nurs.* 1992;3(4):640-646.
45. Thach BT. Reflux associated apnea in infants: evidence for a laryngeal chemoreflex. *Am J Med.* 1997;103(5):120S-124S.
46. Catto-Smith AG. Gastroesophageal reflux in children. *Aust Fam Physician.* 1998;27:465-473.
47. Boekel S. *Gastroesophageal Reflux Disease (GERD) and the Breastfeeding Baby.* Raleigh, NC: International Lactation Consultant Association; 2000.
48. Vandenplas Y, Rudolph CD, Di Lorenzo C, et al. Pediatric gastroesophageal reflux clinical practice guidelines: joint recommendations of the North American Society for Pediatric Gastroenterology, Hepatology, and Nutrition (NASPGHAN) and the European Society for Pediatric Gastroenterology, Hepatology, and Nutrition (ESPGHAN). *J Pediatr Gastroenterol Nutr.* 2009;49(4):498-547.
49. van Veldhuizen-Staas CG. Overabundant milk supply: an alternative way to intervene by full drainage and block feeding. *Int Breastfeed J.* 2007;2(1):11.
50. Trimeloni L, Spencer J. Diagnosis and management of breast milk oversupply. *J Am Board Fam Med.* 2016;29(1):139-142.
51. Hegar B, Vandenplas Y. Gastroesophageal reflux: natural evolution, diagnostic approach and treatment. *Turk J Pediatr.* 2013;55(1):1.
52. Osifo DO, Evbuomwan I. Does exclusive breastfeeding confer protection against infantile hypertrophic pyloric stenosis? A 30-year experience in Benin City, Nigeria. *J Trop Pediatr.* 2008;55(2):132-134.
53. Pisacane A, De Luca U, Criscuolo L, et al. Breast feeding and hypertrophic pyloric stenosis: population based case-control study. *BMJ.* 1996;312(7033):745-746.
54. Krogh C, Biggar RJ, Fischer TK, Lindholm M, Wohlfahrt J, Melbye M. Bottle-feeding and the risk of pyloric stenosis. *Pediatrics.* 2012;130(4):e943-e949.
55. Hall NJ, Pacilli M, Eaton S, et al. Recovery after open versus laparoscopic pyloromyotomy for pyloric stenosis: a double-blind multicentre randomised controlled trial. *Lancet.* 2009;373(9661):390-398.
56. Wheeler RA, Najmaldin AS, Stoodley N, Griffiths DM, Burge DM, Atwell JD. Feeding regimens after pyloromyotomy. *Br J Surg.* 1990;77(9):1018-1019.
57. Barbas KH, Kelleher DK. Breastfeeding success among infants with congenital heart disease. *Pediatr Nurs.* 2004;30(4):285.

58. Fisher JG, Bairdain S, Sparks EA, et al. Serious congenital heart disease and necrotizing enterocolitis in very low birth weight neonates. *J Am Coll Surg.* 2015;220(6):1018-1026.

59. Marino BL, O'Brien P, LoRe H. Oxygen saturations during breast and bottle feedings in infants with congenital heart disease. *J Pediatr Nurs.* 1995;10(6):360-364.

60. Combs VL, Marino BL. A comparison of growth patterns in breast and bottle-fed infants with congenital heart disease. *Pediatr Nurs.* 1992;19(2):175-179.

61. Trabulsi JC, Irving SY, Papas MA, et al. Total energy expenditure of infants with congenital heart disease who have undergone surgical intervention. *Pediatr Cardiol.* 2015;36(8):1670-1679.

62. Irving SY, Medoff-Cooper B, Stouffer NO, et al. Resting energy expenditure at 3 months of age following neonatal surgery for congenital heart disease. *Congenit Heart Dis.* 2013;8(4):343351.

63. Clemente C, Barnes J, Shinebourne E, Stein A. Are infant behavioural feeding difficulties associated with congenital heart disease? *Child Care Health Dev.* 2001;27(1):47-59.

64. da Rosa Pereira K, Firpo C, Gasparin M, et al. Evaluation of swallowing in infants with congenital heart defect. *Int Arch Otorhinolaryngol.* 2015;19(01):55-60.

65. Langston S, Reddy S, Miller DM, Hopkins J. Bridging the divide: breastfeeding infants with congenital heart defects. *Infant Child Adolesc Nutr.* 2011;3(3):140-144.

66. Lambert JM, Watters NE. Breastfeeding the infant/child with a cardiac defect: an informal survey. *J Hum Lactation.* 1998;14(2):151-155.

67. Parker ME, Bradshaw WT. Heart for bonding: a new protocol of care. *Neonat Network.* 2012;31(6):e34.

68. Lucas N. Developmental care in the neonatal unit. *Sri Lanka J Child Health.* 2015;44(1):45-52.

69. Lisanti AJ, Cribben J, Connock EM, Lessen R. Developmental care rounds: an interdisciplinary approach to support developmentally appropriate care of infants born with complex congenital heart disease. *Clin Perinatol.* 2016;43(1):147-156.

70. Glass RP, Wolf LS. Incoordination of sucking, swallowing, and breathing as an etiology for breastfeeding difficulty. *J Hum Lactation.* 1994;10(3):185-189.

71. Munson PD, Saad AG, El-Jamal SM, Dai Y, Bower CM, Richter GT. Submucosal nerve hypertrophy in congenital laryngomalacia. *Laryngoscope.* 2011;121(3):627-629.

72. Landry AM, Thompson DM. Laryngomalacia: disease presentation, spectrum, and management. *Int J Pediatr.* 2012;2012:753526.

73. Simons JP, Greenberg LL, Mehta DK, Fabio A, Maguire RC, Mandell DL. Laryngomalacia and swallowing function in children. *Laryngoscope.* 2016;126(2):478-484.

74. Wolf LS, Glass RP. *Feeding and Swallowing Disorders in Infancy: Assessment and Management.* Tucson, AZ: Therapy Skill Builders; 1992.

75. Hilland M, Røksund OD, Sandvik L, et al. Congenital laryngomalacia is related to exercise-induced laryngeal obstruction in adolescence. *Arch Dis Child.* 2016;101(5):443-448.

76. Wiatrak BJ. Congenital anomalies of the larynx and trachea. *Otolaryngolog Clin North Am.* 2000;33(1):91-110.

77. Chien W, Ashland J, Haver K, Hardy SC, Curren P, Hartnick CJ. Type 1 laryngeal cleft: establishing a functional diagnostic and management algorithm. *Int J Pediatr Otorhinolaryngol.* 2006;70(12):2073-2079.

78. Strychowsky JE, Dodrill P, Moritz E, Perez J, Rahbar R. Swallowing dysfunction among patients with laryngeal cleft: more than just aspiration? *Int J Pediatr Otorhinolaryngol.* 2016;82:38-42.

79. Rahbar R, Rouillon I, Roger G, et al. The presentation and management of laryngeal cleft: a 10-year experience. *Arch Otolaryngol Head Neck Surg.* 2006;132(12):1335-1341.

80. Sachdeva R, Hussain E, Moss MM, et al. Vocal cord dysfunction and feeding difficulties after pediatric cardiovascular surgery. *J Pediatr.* 2007;151(3):312-315.

81. Ardran GM, Kemp FH. The mechanism of changes in form of the cervical airway in infancy. *Med Radiogr Photogr.* 1967;44(2):26-38.

82. Genna CW, Sandora L. Breastfeeding: normal sucking and swallowing. In: Genna CW, ed. *Supporting Sucking Skills in Breastfeeding Infants.* 3rd ed. Burlington, MA: Jones & Bartlett Learning; 2017:1-43.

83. Brown KH, Stallings RY, de Kanashiro HC, de Romana GL, Black RE. Effects of common illnesses on infants' energy intakes from breast milk and other foods during longitudinal community-based studies in Huascar (Lima), Peru. *Am J Clin Nutr.* 1990;52(6):1005-1013.

84. Hassiotou F, Hepworth AR, Metzger P, et al. Maternal and infant infections stimulate a rapid leukocyte response in breastmilk. *Clin Transl Immunology.* 2013;2(4):e3.

85. Riskin A, Almog M, Kessel A. Changes in immunomodulatory constituents of human milk in response to active infection in the nursing infant. *Pediatr Res.* 2011;71(2):220-225.

86. Breakey AA, Hinde K, Valeggia CR, Sinofsky A, Ellison PT. Illness in breastfeeding infants relates to concentration of lactoferrin and secretory immunoglobulin A in mother's milk. *Evol Med Public Health.* 2015;2015(1):21-31.

87. Bowatte G, Tham R, Allen KJ, et al. Breastfeeding and childhood acute otitis media: a systematic review and meta-analysis. *Acta Paediatr.* 2015;104(S467):85-95.

88. Brennan-Jones CG, Eikelboom RH, Jacques A, et al. Protective benefit of predominant breastfeeding against otitis media may be limited to early childhood: results from a prospective birth cohort study. *Clin Otolaryngol.* 2017;42(1):29-37.

89. Darwazeh AM, Darwazeh TA. What makes oral candidiasis recurrent infection? A clinical view. *J Mycol.* 2014;2014:758394.

90. Douvoyiannis M, Swank C. The worst thrush I have ever seen. *Pediatr Emerg Care.* 2016;32(9):614-615.

91. Amir LH, Donath SM, Garland SM, et al. Does *Candida* and/or *Staphylococcus* play a role in nipple and breast pain in lactation? A cohort study in Melbourne, Australia. *BMJ Open.* 2013;3(3):e002351. http://dx.doi.org/10.1136/bmjopen-2012-002351.

92. Sachdeva SK, Dutta S, Sabir H, Sachdeva A. Oral thrush in an infant: a case report with treatment modalities. *Pediatr Dent Care.* 2016;1(107):2.

93. Maloney J, Nowak-Wegrzyn A. Educational clinical case series for pediatric allergy and immunology: allergic proctocolitis, food protein-induced enterocolitis syndrome and allergic eosinophilic gastroenteritis with protein-losing gastroenteropathy as manifestations of non-IgE-mediated cow's milk allergy. *Pediatr Allergy Immunol.* 2007;18(4):360-367.

94. Arvola T, Ruuska T, Keränen J, Hyöty H, Salminen S, Isolauri E. Rectal bleeding in infancy: clinical, allergological, and microbiological examination. *Pediatrics.* 2006;117(4):e760-768.

95. Järvinen KM, Nowak-Węgrzyn A. Food protein-induced enterocolitis syndrome (FPIES): current management strategies and review of the literature. *J Allergy Clin Immunol Pract.* 2013;1(4):317-322.

96. Pesonen M, Kallio MJ, Ranki A, Siimes MA. Prolonged exclusive breastfeeding is associated with increased atopic dermatitis: a prospective follow-up study of unselected healthy newborns from birth to age 20 years. *Clin Exp Allergy.* 2006;36(8):1011-1018.

97. Flohr C, Perkin M, Logan K, et al. Atopic dermatitis and disease severity are the main risk factors for food sensitization in exclusively breastfed infants. *J Invest Dermatol.* 2014;134(2):345-350.

98. Du Toit G, Roberts G, Sayre PH, et al. Randomized trial of peanut consumption in infants at risk for peanut allergy. *N Engl J Med.* 2015;372(9):803-813.

99. Natsume O, Kabashima S, Nakazato J, et al. Two-step egg introduction for prevention of egg allergy in high-risk infants with eczema (PETIT): a randomised, double-blind, placebo-controlled trial. *Lancet.* 2017;389(10066):276-286.

100. Abrams EM, Greenhawt M, Fleischer DM, Chan ES. Early solid food introduction: role in food allergy prevention and implications for breastfeeding. *J Pediatr.* 2017;184:13-18.

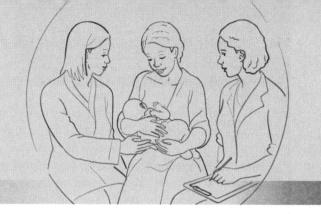

CHAPTER 24

Breastfeeding Devices and Topical Treatments

Vergie I. Hughes
Kathleen Donovan

OBJECTIVES

- Describe the appropriate use of breastfeeding devices.
- State the advantages and drawbacks of specific devices.
- Recommend and teach parents how to use appropriate breastfeeding devices to remedy specific breastfeeding problems.

DEFINITIONS OF COMMONLY USED TERMS

complementary feeding A feeding in addition to breastfeeding.
milk ejection reflex The release of milk in response to breast stimulation. Also called letdown reflex or milk release.
nonnutritive sucking Infant sucking without nutrition; pacifier use to increase physiologic stability and nutrition in preterm infants.
philtrum Area of skin above the upper lip.
postmenstrual age The age of an infant from the first day of the last menstrual period to the day of delivery.
supplementary feeding A feeding that replaces a breastfeeding.

Any use of the term *mother*, *maternal*, or *breastfeeding* is not meant to exclude transgender or nonbinary parents who may be breastfeeding or providing human milk to their infant.

▶ Overview

When breastfeeding discomfort occurs or when infants have difficulty latching on to the breast or gaining weight, interventions might be necessary to correct the cause. Reports suggest that 36 to 96 percent of breastfeeding mothers report some type of nipple pain in the first days to weeks of breastfeeding.[1] A painful or damaged nipple should never be disregarded.[2] The role of the lactation consultant is to identify potential causes of the problem and to offer intervention options to remedy the situation. Often, refining the breastfeeding technique (e.g., positioning, latch, frequency, and duration) is the first strategy toward resolving problems. When an additional intervention is needed, specific devices, equipment, and topical preparations might be helpful.[3] The goal is to establish breastfeeding or return to direct breastfeeding as soon as possible.

There is little recent research on breastfeeding devices, equipment, and topical treatments. Thus, most of what is taught and practiced is based on the accumulated knowledge and expertise of experienced clinicians. The appropriate and conservative use of breastfeeding devices increases healthcare providers' effectiveness in helping with breastfeeding. The overuse of devices can overwhelm parents and make breastfeeding seem difficult. An understanding of the appropriate use of breastfeeding devices and their potential drawbacks will guide clinicians in making appropriate recommendations to parents.

I. Prevention with Education

A. Anticipatory guidance can help parents avoid many problems that lead to the use of special breastfeeding devices.

1. Actively encourage prenatal education in breastfeeding management to prepare parents for initiating breastfeeding.[4] Correct positioning and latch are the first line of defense in preventing nipple damage. Learning about basic breastfeeding management prenatally will help parents become knowledgeable about breastfeeding techniques[4] and the features of a good latch.[5]

2. Knowledge about variations of nipples and their impact on lactation help identify potential challenges and anticipate solutions.

3. It may be challenging to provide necessary education and anticipatory guidance to some families.

4. Some expectant parents may not realize they need to attend, or may have no access to, prenatal breastfeeding classes.

5. There may be insufficient trained nursing staff or dedicated lactation staff available to actively assist the dyad when the infant begins to breastfeed.

B. Healthcare providers who work with breastfeeding families must provide evidence-informed teaching to their clients.[4] When research is lacking, providers must rely on best practices, based on the knowledge and expertise of experienced clinicians.

C. Actively assisting parents with the first breastfeeding after the infant is delivered will help them begin with sound technique.[5]

II. Nipple Devices

A. Nipple shields are devices placed over the nipple and areola; the infant sucks to pull milk through holes in the tip.

1. There are several types of nipple shields.

a. Nipple shield design has advanced over the years from lead, wax, silver, wood, pewter, and animal skins to rubber, latex, and now silicone.[6]

b. The recommended types of nipple shields are thin silicone devices that allow some tactile stimulation to the nerves of the nipple and areola through the shield.[7] One type covers the entire areola, and other types have a partial cutout or butterfly shape to allow the infant's nose to touch the parent's skin and to smell the areola.

c. Thick rubber or latex shields can reduce milk transfer and promote latex allergy and are not recommended.[8] Bottle nipples placed over the parent's nipple, or nipples attached to a plastic base, are not appropriate for use.[7]

d. The sizes of nipple shields vary with manufacturer.

i. The height of the nipple portion ranges from 16 to 26 mm in various increments.

ii. The width of nipple portion at the base varies from 15.7 to 25.4 mm.

iii. The nipple portion is a conical shape and has one to five holes; milk flows best through nipple shields that have multiple holes.

2. Nipple shields are used for a variety of reasons.
   a. Nipple shields can be useful when the infant has difficulty latching because of flat or inverted nipples and when changes in position and latch techniques are ineffective.[9]
      i. The nipple shield provides shape to a flat or inverted nipple, thereby improving the infant's ability to latch on to a flat nipple or an engorged breast.[10]
      ii. The shield stimulates the infant's palate when the parent's nipples are unable to do so.
      iii. Parents who have a higher body mass index are more likely to have flat nipples and require the use of nipple shields.[11] A nipple shield can help stretch and improve the elasticity of a flat or inverted nipple when the infant sucks strongly over the shield.
   b. Nipple shields are sometimes used when the parent's nipples or areola are very sore, painful, damaged, or infected.[11] However, ascertaining the reason for nipple damage should be attempted first (e.g., correcting the latch).
   c. Nipple shields can reduce pain caused by infants who have excessive suction levels.[12]
   d. Nipple shields may be used when there is nipple confusion or breast refusal and when the parent is at risk for early termination of breastfeeding due to breastfeeding problems.[13]
   e. Occasionally nipple shields are used when the parent has an overactive milk ejection reflex or overproduction of milk and the infant has difficulty handling the milk flow.[14]
   f. Nipple shields can assist with latch when an infant is tongue-tied until treatment can be obtained.
   g. Nipple shields can be useful when the infant has a weak, disorganized, or dysfunctional suck.[15]
   h. Nipple shields may be useful in solving the typical problems of small preterm infants at the breast.
      i. These problems may include failure to latch, sucking for an insufficient length of time, immature feeding behaviors, sluggish or poor suck strength, the infant falling asleep soon after being positioned at the breast, and repeatedly slipping off the nipple.[10]
      ii. Shield use has been demonstrated to increase the volume of milk transfer.[16]
      iii. Preterm infants might need to rely on a shield for longer periods of time (2 to 3 weeks or until term-corrected age).
   i. Nipple shields can be helpful in some circumstances when the infant has certain congenital conditions (e.g., cleft palate, Pierre Robin syndrome, or short frenulum).[7]
   j. Nipple shields can be helpful with upper airway problems such as laryngomalacia and tracheomalacia.[16]
   k. A nipple shield may help keep the infant at the breast during remediation of the problem, which can prevent premature weaning.[8,17]
   l. Nipple shields may be a solution for parents who may not otherwise tolerate the intimacy of breastfeeding.[13]
   m. An experimental use of nipple shields is in development to deliver drug therapy, such as treatment for HIV.[18,19]
3. Positive outcomes from the use of nipple shields include the following:
   a. About 18 percent of mothers experiencing breastfeeding problems in the first weeks postpartum find nipple shields to be useful.[20]
   b. A nipple shield is simple to use and will not overwhelm parents, which can be a problem with gadgets that are difficult to use. Mothers report satisfaction with nipple shield use.[21]
   c. Some parents think their infant learns to breastfeed quicker with a nipple shield.[17]
   d. Prolactin and cortisol levels seem unaffected by the use of thin silicone nipple shields.[6,8] In addition, there is little or no reduction of milk transfer when using thin silicone shields, and infants' weight gain is similar.[6]
   e. There is conflicting research regarding the risk for reduced milk production. Some researchers found a reduction in milk production,[8,10,13,22] but other researchers found no reduction.[6] No difference in weight gain was found over a 2-month period both with and without a shield.[6] The best practice suggests that infants be monitored for weight gain during the initiation and use of a nipple shield.
   f. In preterm infants, an increase in milk intake was found with the use of a nipple shield.[6] The suction created in the nipple shield may allow the milk to be accumulated in the shield tip during pauses in sucking. This milk is then immediately available to the infant when sucking resumes, thus increasing the volume of milk consumed.[6]

g. The use of almost any aid to breastfeeding can reduce a parent's breastfeeding self-efficacy. However, nipple shields were demonstrated to be a positive aid and increased breastfeeding self-efficacy scores when mothers had success using them.[21]

h. Success with a nipple shield may be related to improved milk production, milk release, and the strength of the infant's suck.[10]

4. Clinicians need to recognize precautions for using this device.

a. It may be tempting to use a nipple shield as a quick fix rather than referring the parent to skilled care to resolve problems.

b. A nipple shield can damage nipple tissue if not fitted and applied properly.

c. Infants may learn to associate the smell of the nipple shield with getting milk, reducing the effectiveness of attracting the infant directly to the breast by smell.[10]

d. The edge of the nipple shield may curl and appear to block the infant's nose, causing parents to worry about their infant's ability to breathe. Reassure them that the shield does not interfere with breathing.

e. Applying a nipple shield may require two hands, which makes it difficult while holding the infant.[17]

f. If there is not a good seal, the infant can inadvertently dislodge the shield, making it cumbersome to use.[13]

g. Some parents feel dissatisfaction that there is something between them and the infant and that the shield is not natural.[17]

h. Many clinicians recommend the use of a breast pump after feedings to augment breast stimulation because of reduced stimulation while using a nipple shield. There is conflicting advice regarding this practice; individualize the instructions according to the robustness of milk production.

i. The teat portion of the nipple shield has a different feel and texture than a breast nipple, which accustoms the infant to the feel of a firmer teat. The infant may become dependent on the shield, making the transition to the breast difficult.[10]

j. Parents may begin using a latex shield before seeking professional help, which carries a risk of inducing a latex allergy in the parent or infant.

k. Researchers found differing results on the effect of nipple shield use on breastfeeding duration. One study found a shorter duration of exclusive breastfeeding and a shorter duration of any breastfeeding.[10] Another study found that nipple shield use did not negatively affect the duration of breastfeeding.[11]

5. Teach parents how to use a nipple shield appropriately.

a. When sizing the nipple shield, consider the size of the infant's mouth and the size of the nipple.

i. Smaller sizes are most appropriate for small or preterm infants. Larger sizes are appropriate for term infants depending on the size of the nipple.[14]

ii. The teat height should not exceed the length of the infant's mouth, from the lips to the junction of the hard and soft palates. If the height of the teat is greater than this length, the probability increases that the infant's gum ridges will rest beyond where the tongue should begin to exert its peristaltic motion. This could result in the nipple and areola not being drawn into the teat shaft far enough for compression by the infant's tongue, which will reduce milk transfer.

iii. In some babies, excessive length can trigger a gag reflex and an aversion to feeding. In these cases, recommend using the shortest available teat, with a height less than 2 cm.[14]

iv. Some small shields are not wide enough at the base to accommodate larger nipples. Wide bases might be too large for babies who have small mouths. Compromise to find the best fit for the dyad. Do not force a large nipple into a small shield.

b. To apply the nipple shield, roll the shield back most of the length of the nipple shank and apply it to the breast, unrolling the shield onto the nipple and areola.[7]

i. To ensure the shield remains in place during feeding, moisten the areolar portion of the shield before placing it on the breast (some clinicians use a small amount of breast cream).

ii. Warming the shield under hot running water will increase its pliability.

    c.   If there is pain when the infant sucks on the nipple shield, either the nipple is not deeply positioned into the shield or the shield is too small for the nipple.

       i.   To position the nipple deeper into the nipple shank, warm and stretch the area near the base of the shank with the fingers, and release it when placing the shield over the nipple.

       ii.   The infant can pull the nipple even farther into the shield after several minutes of vigorous sucking.

       iii.   The shield may be prefilled with fluid by using hand expression or a periodontal syringe to give the infant a faster reward.

    d.   Present the nipple shield to the infant as you would a breast nipple, tilting the infant's head back and touching the philtrum first with the nipple to stimulate a wide latch. Then place the infant's lower lip on the lower part of the nipple shield; the upper lip glides over the shield for a deep latch.

    e.   In many cases the shield may be removed when vigorous sucking is achieved, and the infant can quickly be placed directly on the breast before the nipple loses its shape.

    f.   A feeding tube can be used in conjunction with a nipple shield to temporarily increase milk flow.

       i.   When the feeding tube is placed outside the shield, the nipple maintains a good fit inside the shield without air leakage.

       ii.   When the feeding tube is placed inside the shield there may be a loss of suction within the shield, so there is less of a pulling sensation on the nipple. However, it is easier to position both the nipple and the shield in the infant's mouth, and the infant does not feel the additional device.

    g.   Follow-up is essential when a nipple shield is used.

       i.   Provide an instruction sheet and a referral to a community lactation consultant.

       ii.   Ensure that the shield is washed thoroughly, dried, and stored in a clean place until the next use to prevent nipple infection. Parents may wish to have several nipple shields because they are easy to misplace.

       iii.   Monitor the infant's output and weigh the infant often.

       iv.   Assess milk transfer by assessing the suck-to-swallow ratio, performing test weights, and observing milk in the tip of the shield.[7,14]

    h.   Help parents discontinue using the shield.

       i.   The mean duration of use is 14 to 33 days.[6,8,13]

       ii.   When it is determined that the shield can be discontinued, start a feeding with the shield, then remove it. If the infant will not latch, replace the shield, continue with the feeding, and try again at the next feeding.

       iii.   Avoid cutting pieces off the tip of the shield in an attempt to wean the infant because blunt, uncomfortable edges might remain.

       iv.   Infants may refuse the breast without the shield.[10] Increased skin-to-skin contact or breastfeeding while co-bathing may help the process of weaning from the shield.

       v.   In a small percentage of cases a shield is used for the entire duration of breastfeeding without problems.[10]

B.   A breast shell is a two-piece plastic device consisting of a vented dome or cup and a concave back contoured to fit the shape of the breast.

   1.   The shell is placed inside the bra over the nipple and areola.

    a.   Breast shells can provide protection for painful, tender nipples. Most brands have an optional back with a much larger opening to keep the bra off the nipple, which allows air to circulate. This may protect painful nipples by preventing chafing caused by clothing, bras, or breast pads. Air vent holes in the dome allow air to circulate around the nipple. Some brands are constructed with flexible silicone backs for more comfort when worn on larger breasts.

    b.   Breast shells can be used to evert flat or inverted nipples either prenatally or postpartum. To evert a flat nipple, use the back with the small opening. It is just large enough for the nipple to protrude. In theory, the pressure on the areola allows the nipple to protrude. Although most research has found shells to be of little value, one study found that wearing a shell 8 or more hours per day increased the nipple length.[23]

c. Breast shells can be used to reduce areolar edema surrounding the nipple in the early postpartum period[9] and to relieve engorgement by encouraging leaking. Milk that drips into a shell should not be fed to the infant due to the possibility of bacterial contamination.

2. Clinicians need to recognize precautions on the use of this device.

   a. Research on the effectiveness of breast shells is limited and insufficient to guide treatment decisions.

   b. There may be a theoretical risk of stimulating preterm labor contractions when used prenatally. Any nipple manipulation should be discussed with a healthcare provider. Breast shells are generally considered safe in a healthy pregnancy where there is no threat of preterm labor.

   c. Breast shells might cause irritation to the nipple or areola, either from contact with the skin or from moisture buildup in the shell and the resulting skin breakdown.

   d. Some breast shells are obvious under the clothing and may cause embarrassment. Selecting a bra one cup size larger may accommodate the shell. Milk can leak out of some brands of shells when leaning over.

   e. Wearing breast shells may cause plugged ducts and mastitis.[24] In the case of fibrocystic breasts, there may be discomfort from the constant pressure.

   f. Prenatal use of shells may make breastfeeding seem difficult and may discourage women from attempting to breastfeed. However, parents who have flat or inverted nipples may be encouraged by a proactive solution to correct a perceived problem.

3. Teach parents how to use shells appropriately.

   a. Place the shell inside the bra, center the opening over the nipple, and close the bra to hold the shell in place.

   b. Wearing shells for gradually longer periods of time during the day will help parents become comfortable wearing them for extended time periods (e.g., while at work).

   c. Shells should be removed when lying down for naps and at bedtime to avoid duct obstruction.

   d. In hot weather or if moisture builds up, remove the shells and allow the breast to dry before reapplying the shells.

   e. The use of shells in conjunction with lanolin or expressed milk on the nipples may promote healing.[2,25]

C. Silver impregnated medical caps are solid caps worn over the nipple.

1. The device is placed over the nipple, and the bra holds it in place.

2. Caps can be used for healing sore or cracked nipples. Silver ions in the cap make contact with the skin and prevent infection from bacteria and fungi.

3. Caps are intended to be worn continuously, when not breastfeeding, until healing occurs (3 to 15 days).[26]

4. Caps are made from natural material, are recyclable, and are easy to use.

5. Caps may not be available in all geographic areas and can be cost prohibitive.

D. Nipple everters are syringe-like devices that are placed over the nipple with a plunger to gently create suction that pulls the nipple outward.

1. There are several types of nipple everters.

   a. A commercially available everter has a soft, flexible areolar cone[9] (see **FIGURE 24-1**).

   b. A thimble-shaped silicone dome is placed over the nipple prenatally. Suction is generated by pulling on a syringe and sealing off the dome. The device remains in place for extended periods of time.[9]

   c. Another thimble-shaped dome is placed over the nipple and squeezed to apply it over the nipple and draw it out (see **FIGURE 24-2**). It is worn for several hours daily or prior to feedings. This device can be worn under breast shells beginning at the 37th week of gestation. Lanolin may assist with better adherence.[9,27]

   d. A small bulb syringe (like a bicycle horn) is used to pull the nipple out prior to feedings (see **FIGURE 24-3**).[9]

2. A nipple everter is a simple, low-cost device that allows suction control to maintain comfort.

   a. It everts a flat or retracted nipple in the prenatal or postpartum period.

   b. It forms a nipple to make the latch easier for an infant who is having difficulty grasping and holding the nipple.

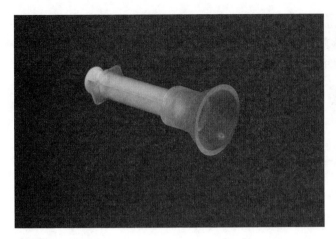

FIGURE 24-1 Everter.

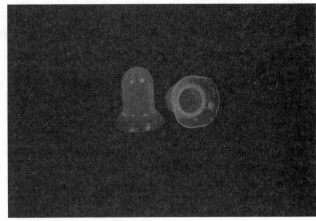

FIGURE 24-2 Supple cup.

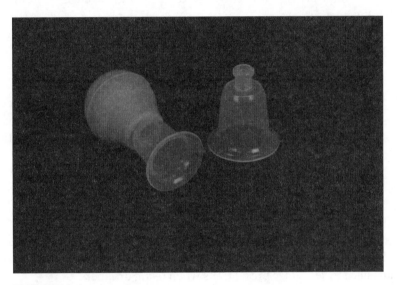

FIGURE 24-3 Latch assist.

3. Clinicians need to recognize precautions for using everters.
   a. There is limited research on the use of nipple everters. However, they are widely marketed to parents and clinicians.
   b. If an everter is used too vigorously or incorrectly, it can cause pain or skin damage.
   c. The nipple might not remain everted long enough for the infant to achieve a latch.
4. Teach parents how to use the device appropriately.
   a. Apply suction to the nipple and hold the everted nipple for about 30 seconds prior to each breastfeeding. Repeat between feedings as necessary.
   b. Assure proper cleaning between uses.

III. Alternative Feeding Devices

Alternative feeding devices may be useful for prefeeding an infant who is reluctant to feed at the breast. These devices may alleviate the initial intense hunger that may cause impatience for an attempted breastfeeding. **BOX 24-1** presents some considerations for selecting an alternative feeding device.

A. Droppers are plastic or glass tubes with a squeeze bulb at one end; some are child sized.
   1. Droppers are a quick way for an infant to receive a small amount of milk while learning to breastfeed, and infants may be more eager to breastfeed because their sucking needs are not met with a dropper.[7]

BOX 24-1 Considerations for Selecting an Alternative Feeding Device

The optimal alternative feeding device has not yet been identified and may vary from infant to infant, parent to parent, and situation to situation. No method is without potential benefits and risks. Consider the following when selecting an alternative feeding device[28]:

- Cost and availability.
- Ease of use and cleaning.
- Potential stress to the infant.
- Whether adequate milk volume can be fed in 20 to 30 minutes.
- Whether the anticipated use is short term or long term.
- Parental preference.
- Expertise of healthcare staff in use of the device.

---

    a.   Droppers may be used with finger feeding to take the edge off hunger before attempting to latch the infant.
       i.   Place the filled dropper along the side of the finger as the infant draws the finger into the mouth.
      ii.   Allow the infant to suck the milk out of the dropper. If the infant is unable to perform this task, one or two drops can be placed on the infant's tongue to initiate swallowing and sucking.
    b.   A dropper can drip milk into the corner of the infant's mouth as an incentive to achieve latch.
       i.   Place the dropper into the corner of the infant's mouth while latching on to the breast.
      ii.   One or two drops of milk can then be placed on the tongue to initiate a swallow followed by a suck.
     iii.   The infant must be alert and have a functioning swallow reflex.
     iv.   Milk should not be squirted into the infant's mouth; it should be dripped at a rate the infant can swallow comfortably.
    c.   A dropper can be used for complementary feeding when the infant's milk intake is not sufficient.
  2.   Droppers avoid the use of artificial nipples and the risk of bottle nipple preference. They are inexpensive and widely available. Droppers are easy to use and easy to teach parents to use.
  3.   Clinicians need to recognize precautions when using droppers.
    a.   There is no research on the use of droppers. However, they are widely used in some parts of the world.
    b.   Droppers can be difficult to clean between uses and must be continually refilled. It is time consuming and messy.
    c.   The infant does not learn to suck unless the dropper is used in conjunction with finger feeding. Sucking on the dropper alone will not teach correct sucking patterns.
B.   Spoons can be used to feed a small amount of colostrum or milk to the infant.
  1.   A common teaspoon, tablespoon, plastic spoon, or medicine spoon with a hollow handle can be used. A commercial spoon-shaped device attached to a milk reservoir is also available. Research on this technique is limited.
  2.   There are several uses for spoon feeding.
    a.   Spoon feeding can be used when breastfeeding is interrupted or when the parent is unavailable for breastfeeding.[29]
    b.   Spoons can be useful to prime the infant for feeding at the breast.
    c.   A spoon may be used to feed the infant colostrum that has been hand expressed or pumped to complement early feedings and prevent hypoglycemia, or it can be used for complementary feeding when breastfeeding is not sufficient.
    d.   A spoon may be used to feed an infant after cleft lip repair if wound dehiscence (opening) is a concern.[30]
  3.   Positive outcomes from the use of spoon feeding include the following:
    a.   Spoons avoid the use of artificial nipples and subsequent bottle nipple preference.[29]
    b.   Spoons can be a temporary aid to initiate breastfeeding for infants who have not latched. Spoon feeding is associated with a shorter subsequent time to full breastfeeding than bottle feeding.[31]

        c. Spoons can administer small volumes (such as colostrum) efficiently. The same muscle groups are involved as with cups and breastfeeding.

        d. Spoons are inexpensive, readily available, and easy to use and clean.

        e. Infants may be more eager to breastfeed because their sucking needs are not met through spoon feeding.

        f. Spoon feeding is safe to use with preterm infants older than 29 weeks postmenstrual age.[32]

   4. Clinicians need to recognize precautions when using spoons.

        a. Spoons hold little volume and must be continually refilled.

        b. Spoon feeding does not teach the infant to suck at the breast because fluid in the mouth is not associated with sucking, and it deprives the infant of normal oral experiences. Spoon feeding does not correct previously learned improper sucking patterns.

        c. Spillage may be a problem. In infants where monitoring volumes consumed is especially important (e.g., preterm infants), the bib can be weighed before and after the feeding to determine the amount of spillage collected in the bib.[33]

   5. Teach parents how to use spoons appropriately.

        a. The infant should be alert and have a functioning swallow reflex.

        b. Position the infant in a semiupright position.

        c. Place the spoon on the infant's lower lip over the tongue. Allow the infant to pace the feeding by sipping or lapping the milk.

        d. Avoid pouring milk into the infant's mouth and observe the infant for signs of milk flow being too fast or too slow.[34]

C. Cups are useful for feeding larger amounts of milk than can be accommodated by a spoon.

   1. A variety of cups can be used.

        a. Cups can vary from common small medicine cups (1 oz or 28–30 mL) to small flexible drinking cups or small 30 mL glasses.

        b. Some commercial cups are available with an extended lip or edge, or a restricted outlet that slows the flow for greater control.

        c. A paladai is a small pitcher-shaped device from India that is similar to a cup but has a long spout. This also allows for more control of feeding and is appropriate for use with infants older than 30 weeks' gestation.[35]

   2. There are a variety of uses for cup feeding.

        a. Cup feeding is preferred by many clinicians as the first choice for an alternative feeding method.[36]

        b. Cups can be used to feed the infant when breastfeeding is interrupted, when the parent is unavailable to breastfeed, or for complementary feeding when breastfeeding is not sufficient.

        c. Cup feeding can be used with both term and preterm infants to avoid bottle nipple preference. Even preterm infants can cup feed easily.

        d. Cup feeding may be useful for feeding infants with cleft lip and palate repair to avoid contact with the surgical site.

        e. Cup feeding is not appropriate for an infant who has recently been extubated, has a poor gag reflex, or has neurological deficits. Delay cup feeding for an infant who is lethargic or having respiratory difficulties.

   3. Cup feeding is well supported in the literature.[37] Positive outcomes from the use of cup feeding include the following:

        a. Because nothing enters the oral cavity, cup feeding avoids potential nipple confusion.

        b. Infants may be more eager to breastfeed because their sucking needs are not met with cup feeding.

        c. When cup feeding is done appropriately, it allows the infant to pace the feeding. If the caregiver provides milk too fast, it dribbles out of the infant's mouth.[28]

        d. Cups are a quick way to supplement or complement breastfeeding. They are inexpensive and widely available.

        e. It is easy to teach parents cup feeding techniques. Cups are the method of choice when cleanliness is suboptimal.[28]

        f. Cup feeding utilizes masseter muscle activity, similar to breastfeeding, moreso than with bottle feeding.[38]

        g. Cup feeding can be useful for helping babies learn to extend their tongues over the lower gum ridge.

      h.   Cup feeding low birth weight infants has been shown to be as safe as bottle feeding, without concerns for physiological decompensation.[39]

      i.   Cup feeding promotes breastfeeding in preterm infants who often have difficulty with breastfeeding or bottle feeding, and it results in fewer desaturation episodes. Preterm infants are more likely to successfully transition to breastfeeding when they are cup fed rather than bottle fed.[37]

      j.   There may be an increased rate of breastfeeding in the hospital, although neonatal intensive care unit (NICU) discharge may be delayed. Cup feeding may also extend the duration of breastfeeding with adequate weight gain.[37]

  4.   Clinicians need to recognize precautions when using cups.

      a.   The cup must frequently be refilled.

      b.   The infant can dribble much milk, reducing intake and risking poor weight gain. If measuring the infant's intake is critical, the bib can be weighed before and after feeding to determine the volume lost.

      c.   The infant does not learn to suck with a cup; therefore, a cup might delay a return to the breast.

      d.   The infant, parents, or healthcare providers can become dependent on use of the cup.

      e.   There is a risk of aspiration (similar to that of bottle feeding) if cup feeding is performed improperly.

  5.   Teach parents how to use cups appropriately.

      a.   Technique is important to avoid pitfalls. The infant should be in a calm, alert state (not sleepy), positioned nearly upright, and wrapped so hands do not bump use of the cup.[34]

      b.   Fill the cup about half full.

      c.   Place the rim of the cup lightly on the infant's lower lip, with the cup tilted just to the point of the milk coming into contact with the upper lip.

      d.   Let the infant pace the feeding by sipping or lapping the milk. Do not pour the milk into the infant's mouth, and do not overwhelm the infant with milk.

      e.   Leave the cup in the same position on the infant's lip during pauses so the infant does not need to continually reorganize the oral conformation. Spillage can be measured by weighing the bib if intake is a concern.[36]

      f.   Demonstrate the technique to the parents or caregiver, and request a return demonstration to assure proper technique.

D.   Syringes can deliver up to 10 mL of milk at a feeding.

  1.   Several types of syringes are used for this type of feeding.

      a.   A periodontal syringe has a curved tip.

      b.   A regular syringe (without a needle) is usually not used because the infant might have difficulty forming a complete seal on the breast or finger with the bulky syringe in place.

      c.   A tuberculin syringe may be used, although the volume is limited.

  2.   There are several uses for syringe feeding.

      a.   Syringe feeding can be used to provide an incentive at the breast to encourage latch, to initiate suckling, or to aid in sustaining the suckling pattern after it has been started.

      b.   It can be used to provide complementary or supplementary feeding while the infant simultaneously sucks on the caregiver's finger.[34]

      c.   A syringe can be used to feed an infant with a cleft palate who is placed in a prone position.[40]

  3.   Positive outcomes from the use of a syringe include the following:

      a.   Using a syringe on the breast or finger avoids the use of artificial nipples and keeps the infant at the breast or on the skin while sucking the finger. Critics suggest that a finger has the same rigid feel as a bottle nipple.[34]

      b.   Syringe feeding provides a source of milk flow that will work to regulate the suck.

      c.   The technique might help improve uncoordinated mouth and tongue movements by encouraging correct tongue peristalsis.

      d.   It is easy to teach parents to use a syringe for feeding.

  4.   Clinicians need to recognize precautions when using syringes.

      a.   Syringe feeding is more intrusive than other alternative feeding methods and may cause aspiration if the caregiver is not mindful of the newborn's capacity to swallow.

      b.   Avoid the tendency to hasten the feeding by pushing the plunger. Allow the infant to withdraw the fluid by sucking.

      c. Supplies might not be readily available in all geographic locations.

      d. Infants can become dependent on the method if it is used exclusively for an extended period of time.

      e. The infant might demonstrate poor jaw excursion while sucking on an adult finger.

      f. Parents with long fingernails may need to cut them or wear gloves during feedings.

      g. Periodontal syringes have a pointed tip that could irritate the infant's mouth if incorrectly placed. Direct the tip of the syringe parallel to the caregiver's finger.

      h. Some professionals have legal concerns about using equipment for a purpose that it was not originally intended for.

5. Teach parents how to use syringes appropriately.[41]

      a. When the infant is feeding at the breast, insert the tip of the syringe just inside the infant's lips at the corner of the mouth.

         i. Give a small bolus of milk (0.25–0.5 mL) when the infant sucks. Because the size of a newborn's typical swallow is 0.6 mL,[42] this volume is safe to prevent aspiration.

         ii. Increase the volume of the bolus as the infant tolerates. Observe the infant carefully to watch for cues that the flow rate is overwhelming or is too slow. This may vary within a feeding or from feeding to feeding.

         iii. Carefully observe the infant to prevent an overwhelming flow rate.

      b. When finger feeding, place the infant in a semiupright position in the caregiver's arms or in an inclined infant seat.

         i. The parents can use a washed finger; healthcare providers should wear a glove.

         ii. Use the finger that is closest in size to the circumference of the parent's nipple.

         iii. Introduce the finger into the infant's mouth with the pad up, enabling the infant to pull the finger back to the junction of the hard and soft palates. If the infant resists, withdraw the finger slightly, pause for the infant to be comforted, then try again.

         iv. Place the periodontal syringe next to the finger, making sure that it is positioned parallel to the finger so it will not poke the infant.

         v. As the infant sucks, reward the correct suckling motions with a small bolus of milk. Increase the size of the bolus as the infant tolerates.

         vi. Request a return demonstration from the parent/caregiver to assure proper technique.

      c. If the infant's tongue lies behind the lower gum ridge, apply slight pressure to the back of the tongue to stroke it gently forward over the lower gum ridge.

      d. The feeding time should take about 15 to 20 minutes or end the feeding when the infant is not alert enough to suck and swallow correctly.

      e. If the infant stops for more than 10 to 20 seconds, arouse the infant by giving a small bolus of milk or stimulate the infant by patting and rubbing the chest, arms, or legs.

      f. If a syringe is being used to entice the infant to the breast, note the following:

         i. Place the infant at the breast when he or she demonstrates a sucking rhythm on the finger.

         ii. A few drops of milk dripped onto the nipple during latch may be enough to direct the infant to the milk source.[43]

E. Tube feeding devices provide supplemental nutrition at the breast.

1. There are several options for tube feeding devices.

      a. Commercially available devices usually consist of a reservoir or container for milk, with one or two thin flexible lengths of tubing attached. The container for milk can be a syringe, a bottle clipped to the parent's shoulder, or a bottle suspended on a cord around the parent's neck. The container might have one or two thin lengths of flexible tubing. Follow the manufacturer's instructions for using larger or smaller tubing sizes.

      b. A device can be made by placing a bottle with a standard artificial nipple on a nearby table and threading a feeding tube through it.

      c. The tubing can be attached with tape to the parent's nipple or areola for supplementing at the breast. The tubing can also be taped to the caregiver's finger for finger feeding.

2. There are several uses for tube feeding.

      a. Tube feeding can provide complementary feeding to an infant at the breast to address low milk production, inefficient suckling, or slow weight gain. It can be used for preterm or neurologically affected infants.[28]

  b. Tube feeding can be used for relactating or inducing lactation.

  c. The tubing can be attached to a finger for others to feed the infant or to prime the infant for going to the breast.

 3. Positive outcomes from the use of tube feeding include the following:

  a. Tube feeding enables the delivery of needed supplements while preserving breastfeeding by maintaining skin-to-skin contact and parental breast stimulation and by not exposing the infant to artificial nipples.[28,44]

  b. Increasing the flow rate at the breast may encourage a reluctant infant to breastfeed and may help improve sucking organization and patterns.

 4. Clinicians need to recognize precautions when using tube feeding.

  a. Tube feeding devices are more intrusive and complex to learn how to use and repeat many times per day. Parents may find it time consuming to clean the equipment after each use. The technique may be rejected by parents.

  b. Feeding tubes may not work with an infant who has ineffective sucking patterns or a weak suck, such as in a preterm infant.

  c. Tube feeding supplies might not be widely available and can be costly for parents to purchase, especially if the supplies need to be replaced.

  d. Infants can become dependent on tube feeding because they can quickly learn to prefer a faster flow rate.

  e. An infant might exhibit shallow jaw excursions while sucking on an adult finger.

  f. Some parents find it awkward at first to get both the tubing and the nipple into the infant's mouth. Do not allow the infant to suck on the tubing like a straw without also latching onto the nipple. Taping the tubing to the breast will facilitate this.

  g. If the milk container is positioned too low or if the tubing is kinked, the infant might not receive milk. The flow should be monitored throughout the feeding. If the milk container is too high, the infant may receive milk without sucking.

  h. Some parents might be allergic to the tape that is used to secure the tubing in place at the breast; consider using paper tape or nonallergenic tapes or dressings. Some parents use small adhesive bandages and thread the tubing under the pad for each feeding; the adhesive part can be left in place.

  i. Expressed milk or infant formula will flow through the tubing, but fortified liquids might not. Shake the liquids well, warm them to help them mix, or use only commercially prepared liquid formula.

 5. Teach parents how to use tube feeding devices appropriately.

  a. Tube feeding on a finger proceeds in a similar manner as syringe feeding.

  b. Tickle the philtrum with your finger until the infant's mouth opens. Place your finger deeply into the infant's mouth to near the juncture of the hard and soft palates. Allow the infant to pull your finger back to near the juncture of the hard and soft palates.[40]

  c. When it is used at the breast, the milk reservoir can be elevated or lowered to control the milk flow. When the fluid level is placed level with the nipple, the milk should flow only when the infant sucks. The infant should suck to pull the milk out and will thereby pace the feeding.[40]

  d. The infant should take in the nipple, areola, and tubing.

   i. The tubing can be taped so it enters the infant's mouth in the corner or under the nipple over the infant's tongue (clinicians recommend the latter technique).

   ii. Placing the tubing so it enters on the roof of the infant's mouth can be irritating to the infant's palate. Position the tube so it will not extend beyond the nipple tip when positioned in the infant's mouth.

  e. Lower the container to increase the flow for small or weaker babies. If the device has two tubes, open the other tube as a vent, use both tubes on one breast, or raise the device higher.[40]

  f. If the device has a choice of tubing sizes, use the largest size for a preterm infant, a disorganized infant, or an infant who needs an easier flow. Advance the infant to the smaller sizes as the sucking becomes more robust.

g. Infants need close follow-up for frequent weight checks while a supplementer is used, and they should be weaned off the device as soon as possible.

h. The flow from the device can be controlled by raising or lowering the milk reservoirs, by using one or both tubes (if provided), by substituting larger or smaller diameter tubing (if provided), or by crimping the tube to stop the flow. If a second tube is provided, it can be used as a vent to increase the flow rate for a weak or neurologically impaired infant.

i. The caregiver may allow the milk to flow at the beginning of the feeding, then turn it off or slow it down considerably after a substantial amount of the feeding has been completed to encourage more vigorous sucking.

   i. Infants are ready to wean from a supplementer when they take a full feed, or nearly full feed, from the breast with the supplementer turned off or kept at a low position so the flow from the supplementer is diminished.

   ii. Doing a test weight can help confirm that the infant has consumed the required amount of milk from the breast.

j. Clean the feeding tube device with hot soapy water, rinse it well, and allow it to dry for the next feeding. Caregivers who use these devices regularly find it handy to have two: one to use while the other is being cleaned. Be sure to flush the tubing with soapy water and clear water, then blow air through the tube to clear it. A curved-tip syringe works well for this.

F. Specially designed bottles, formerly called Haberman Feeders, are available for infants with special needs.

1. Although there is no research on the efficacy of these bottles, they may be useful for preterm infants or those with severe feeding problems, such as in infants with Down syndrome, cleft lip or palate, neurological dysfunction or disorganized sucking, cardiac defects, or cystic fibrosis.

   a. One type of bottle contains a valve and teat mechanism to adjust the milk flow for an infant with a weak suck or an infant who is unable to create an oral seal. Three indicators on the bottle correspond to three flow rates from the slit in the nipple. The nipple portion can be squeezed to provide positive pressure for infants with severe suction deficits.

   b. Similar devices for severe cleft feeding problems are commercially available. They are soft-squeeze bottles and seem to work better than regular bottles for these infants. For infants with cleft palate, the feeder should be placed with the tip under the intact part of the palate and rotated so the longest line is in line with the nose. A rubber-tipped syringe may also be useful for infants with cleft lip and palate.

   c. Various sizes are available for preterm and term infants.

2. A special needs feeder may be effective, in conjunction with advice from an occupational therapist or speech-language therapist, for an infant who is otherwise difficult to feed. If the infant cannot breastfeed at all or needs assistance, the bottle can be carefully squeezed to release a limited volume of milk.

3. Clinicians need to recognize precautions when using special bottles.

   a. Special needs feeders expose the infant to an artificial nipple, which might promote a shallow latch when the infant goes to the breast. It may lead to breast refusal.

   b. Feeders might be difficult to obtain in some geographic areas, and they are more costly than typical bottles.

   c. Special feeders deliver milk to compromised infants, but they do little for normal feeding development.

4. Teach parents how to use special bottles appropriately.

   a. Rest the nipple on the infant's philtrum and allow the infant to draw it into the mouth, if possible.

   b. Gently pull back on the nipple, if needed, to initiate sucking. The teat may be squeezed to assist the milk flow for infants who have a weak suck or are unable to achieve a seal.[43] Slightly pull back on the nipple if it initiates a gag reflex.

   c. One special feeder allows the caregiver to rotate the nipple in the infant's mouth to adjust the rate of flow to meet the needs and capability of the infant. Rotate the feeder to achieve a 1:1:1 (suck–swallow–breathe) ratio.

    G.   Artificial nipples and bottles are used by many parents (see **TABLE 24-1**).

        1.   No artificial nipple precisely mimics the dynamic qualities of the human breast, and no research guides the development of an ideal bottle nipple.[51] Manufacturers' marketing materials or package claims rarely contain objective information,[52] and there are no standards to define the flow rates from nipples.[53]

        2.   Artificial nipples come in a range of materials, shapes, and sizes.

            a.   Artificial nipples are made from silicone rubber or latex rubber. Silicone is more expensive but longer lasting. Latex may become gummy after repeated boiling and can release nitrates (a carcinogen) after repeated boiling.

            b.   Many nipples are round with a straight shank. Some taper to a wider base. Orthodontic nipples have bulb-like tips and narrow shanks. Some have a very wide base designed to encourage a wide latch, which may or may not work depending on how it is used.

            c.   Some nipples require suction only and are designed so compression does not extract milk, while others require compression.

            d.   The types of openings include crosscuts and holes of various numbers and diameters.

                i.   Some nipples have the hole on the top of the shank, rather than the nipple, to avoid milk squirting down the infant's throat.

                ii.   Some nipples are no-drip nipples. Other nipples become no-drip nipples within 5 seconds of turning them over. Nipple dripping is not related to flow.[52]

            e.   Hole size is one of the major determinants of flow rate.

                i.   Crosscut nipples have the fastest flow and are designed for older babies or babies who require thickened milk. Clinicians occasionally recommend thickened feedings for infants with gastroesophageal reflux or infant dysphagia, although this practice is declining.[54]

                ii.   Variations from 2 mL to 85 mL per minute have been observed.[55]

                iii.   Manufacturers claim that nipples have high, medium, and low flow rates, depending on the number of holes and the size of the holes. However, hole diameters can vary among manufacturers and from nipple to nipple from the same manufacturer.[53]

                iv.   Nipples designed for preterm infants are softer and flow more slowly.

            f.   Nipples vary in length.

                i.   Human nipples rest about 5 mm in front of the hard and soft palate juncture during breastfeeding. Ideally, a bottle nipple should also reach this deeply.

                ii.   Long nipples may trigger the gag reflex in some infants.

                iii.   Short nipples may alter tongue movements if they are kept in the front portion of the mouth.

TABLE 24-1 Comparison of Bottle Feeding and Breastfeeding

Bottle Feeding	Breastfeeding
Firm nipple	Soft, amorphous-shaped nipple
Inelastic nipple	Nipple elongates during sucking
Flow begins instantly	Flow is delayed until the milk ejection reflex occurs
Flow is very fast	Flow is slow, faster during the milk ejection reflex
Feeding is very quick	Feeding a newborn may take 30 to 45 minutes
Sucking on bottle creates suction or vacuum	Suckling at breast is peristaltic tongue movement
Tongue is humped in back of mouth	Tongue is forward cupped around the breast

Data from Walker, 2017[29]; Wilson-Clay & Hoover, 2017[34]; Woolridge, 1986[45]; Weber, Woolridge, Baum, 1986[46]; Medoff-Cooper, Bilker, & Kaplan, 2010[47]; Ardran, Kemp, Lind, 1958[48]; Page-Goertz, 2016[49]; Lawrence & Lawrence, 2016.[50]

3. There are some positive uses for bottles with artificial nipples.
    a. Bottles are familiar to parents, and they are easily obtained from grocery and chain store shelves. The feedings can be quick, depending on the flow rate and the baby's sucking ability. Bottles can be useful when parents reject alternative feeding methods.
    b. Some artificial nipples are used in special situations to assist infants in learning sucking patterns.
    c. Bottles may be useful for twins or higher-order multiples who are rotated between breast and bottle feedings.
4. Clinicians need to recognize precautions with the use of bottles and artificial nipples.
    a. Nipple preference can occur, with infants preferring the bottle nipple and rejecting the breast.[56] The shape is different and the consistency is firmer, potentially causing the infant to prefer the stronger stimulus of the artificial nipple.
        i.   There is no way to predetermine which infants are at risk for developing a preference for the bottle nipple.
        ii. Some infants can switch between breast and bottle without apparent difficulty, and others refuse the breast after just one bottle. The term *nipple confusion* has been used to describe when infants are unable to adapt to the different sucking mechanisms necessary to switch between breast and bottle.[56]
    b. Some bottles release milk immediately upon starting a feeding, while breasts take several seconds to several minutes to achieve milk ejection and full flow.
        i.   This is especially likely during the first few days postpartum.
        ii. It is another compelling reason for bottle preference.[56]
        iii. Fast flow can contribute to apnea and bradycardia in preterm or stressed infants. Bottle feeding may pose an aspiration risk because of a too-fast flow.
    c. Different facial muscles are activated during bottle feeding than during breastfeeding. Masseter activity is significantly higher in breastfed newborns than in bottle-fed newborns.[38]
    d. Some bottle nipples encourage infants to close their mouths rather than opening wide, as required for breastfeeding.
        i.   Some infants bite the narrowed neck of some nipples.
        ii. Orthodontic nipples may depress the central grooving of the tongue that naturally occurs in breastfeeding.
        iii. Parents often place the orthodontic nipple so that only the bulb is in the infant's mouth, and the gums are over the narrow neck, resulting in a shallow latch during subsequent breastfeeding.
    e. Depending on the venting mechanism, or the tightness of the collar, many bottles develop an internal vacuum as milk is removed. If this happens, the infant may develop a pattern of releasing the bottle to allow air into it so the flow rate will increase.[51,57]
    f. Parents may begin using latex bottle nipples before seeking help, which places them and the infant at risk for latex allergy.
    g. Parents who rely on bottle feeding, even for a few feedings, may have reduced self-efficacy in their ability to successfully breastfeed.
    h. Bottle feeding may shorten the duration of breastfeeding, but studies have not determined if bottles cause refusal or if they are markers of a different underlying problem.[56]
    i. Bottle-fed infants may not self-regulate volume, leading to obesity.[58,59]
    j. Bottle feeding may lead to excessive weight gain if the baby is offered a fast-flow nipple and an unlimited volume of milk.[60,61]
    k. Bottle feeding can lead to dental caries in infants who are placed in bed with a bottle.
5. There is debate about the preferred type of bottle nipple for a breastfeeding infant.
    a. One opinion recommends a nipple with a long shank, wide base, and slow flow of milk,[28] and it cautions about avoiding a nipple with a straight or narrow base.
    b. A second opinion recommends a nipple with a cylindrical shape (not an orthodontic nipple) and a smooth graduated slope of the nipple from the base to the nipple tip.
    c. A third opinion recommends a nipple shape that allows the infant to obtain a seal, to suck, and to maintain a natural gape similar to breastfeeding.

6. Teach parents how to use bottles appropriately.
    a. Position the infant nearly upright in the caregiver's arms (not in an infant seat). A position that places the infant's cheek against the breast replicates breastfeeding.
    b. Simulate attachment to the breast by resting the nipple on the infant's philtrum. When the infant's mouth opens, tip the nipple deeply into the mouth.
    c. Positioning the bottle horizontally can aid in pacing and lowering the bottle quickly if the milk is flowing too fast for the infant to swallow.[52]
    d. Observe for a good latch on the bottle.[52]
        i. The nipple reaches deeply into the mouth.
        ii. The tongue cups the nipple.
        iii. The lips open widely and rest on a portion of the base.
        iv. The lip forms a complete seal, with no leaking at the corners.
    e. Observe for signs of a milk flow that is too fast or too slow and for stress cues in the infant.
        i. Signs of feeding distress include change of color; tachypnea; nasal flaring; shallow, rapid breathing; high-pitched crowing noise; drooling; gulping; coughing; and choking.
        ii. Other signs of infant distress include squirming; arching; hiccupping; finger splaying; fussiness; looking away; changes in vital signs; and falling asleep.
        iii. Pace the feeding to approximately the same suck–swallow–breathe and pause ratio as in breast-feeding.[52] If the infant drinks too quickly or does not breathe within three to five sucks, keep the baby latched while tipping the bottle down to allow a short break and catch-up breaths.
        iv. Choose a nipple with a slower flow to match the infant's ability to suck, swallow, and breathe.[52]
        v. Mimic breastfeeding patterns of one or two sucks and swallows to one breath, with each cycle of jaw and tongue movement taking about 1.5 seconds.
        vi. If the bottle is removed midfeeding for a break, wait for the infant's cues before offering it again.
        vii. During pacing, the bottle can be lowered so there is no fluid in the nipple until the infant shows readiness, then it can be raised again.
        viii. Pacing is not necessary if the infant is handling the flow rate without evidence of distress.[52]
        ix. For a preterm baby or a baby with respiratory problems, the bottle can be removed from the infant's mouth and rested on the philtrum until the infant shows readiness.
    f. Equalization in air pressure inside and outside the bottle can affect the flow rate from the nipple.
        i. Sometimes this comes from air exchange around the bottle collar or from a hole in the nipple.
        ii. Screwing a collar on too tightly can stop milk flow.
        iii. Mixing brands of bottles and nipples can alter the flow.
        iv. If the nipple collapses or if milk stops flowing, the infant will need to release the bottle to allow air to enter and increase the flow. Infants who transfer this technique to the breast disengage and reattach many times during a feeding.[51]
        v. Bottles that use liners collapse as fluid is removed, so no negative pressure builds up.
    g. Parents who bottle feed more frequently tend to encourage finishing a bottle, even when the infant shows satiety.[62]
    h. When a bottle is offered to a breastfed baby, return the infant to the breast as soon as possible.
        i. If the infant resists, feed with the bottle near the breast.
        ii. Offer the bottle, then the breast; if the infant refuses, begin again with the bottle and repeat the sequence.
        iii. A nipple shield may provide a bridge to breastfeeding because it will give the baby a familiar texture.
    i. Mimic breastfeeding while feeding with a bottle.
        i. Initiate feedings in response to hunger cues, not on a set schedule.
        ii. Hold the infant in an upright position and skin to skin.
        iii. Talk gently and pace the feeding, if necessary, so the infant does not get distressed with the flow rate.
        iv. Maintain eye contact throughout the feeding and do not prop the bottle.
        v. Refrain from distracting activities while feeding, such as cell phone use, talking, napping, and TV watching. Such activities lead to lack of awareness of satiation cues and lack of parental responsiveness.[63] Overfeeding and rapid weight gain in infancy leads to childhood obesity.[64]

      vi.   Switch sides halfway through the feeding.

     vii.   Offer breaks during the feeding, like the ebb and flow of milk ejection.

   viii.   Snuggle and hold the infant, even after nutritive sucking is finished.

     ix.   End the feeding when the infant indicates satiety; do not encourage the infant to finish the bottle.

IV. Pacifiers (Dummies)

A.   A wide variety of pacifier shapes are manufactured; they generally consist of a handle and a nipple-shaped tip connected to a wide guard that rests on the infant's lips.

B.   Despite research linking reduced milk production and shorter duration of breastfeeding, pacifiers are used by 50 to 80 percent of mothers for an average of 13 months.[42]

    1.   Pacifiers are commonly used to soothe a crying infant, to encourage sleepiness, and to stretch out the time between breastfeeding sessions.

    2.   Research has shown a profound positive role of pacifiers in sudden infant death syndrome prevention,[65] and for this reason it is recommended that infants be put to sleep with a pacifier after breastfeeding is well established, at about 3 to 4 weeks of age.[66]

    3.   Pacifiers can provide relief during painful procedures.[67]

    4.   Pacifiers can be useful in a structured program for enhancing sucking function to increase oral tone and improve lip seal on the breast.

    5.   Pacifier use may promote continued breastfeeding among new parents experiencing depressive symptoms.[68]

    6.   Pacifiers can provide nonnutritive sucking practice for preterm infants, especially during tube feedings. Sucking during tube feeding shows decreased intestinal transit time and increased weight gain.[69] Nonnutritive sucking prior to or during tube feedings did not show shorter hospital duration.[70]

    7.   Pacifiers have not been shown to benefit gastroesophageal reflux disease in preterm and low birth weight infants.[71]

C.   Clinicians need to recognize precautions on the use of pacifiers.

    1.   Pacifier use may be a marker for breastfeeding difficulties.[56] The breastfeeding dyad should be evaluated, and intervention should be provided as needed.

    2.   Many studies found an association between pacifier use and shortened duration of breastfeeding.[66] Two recent reviews revealed mixed results.[56,72]

    3.   Newborn infants learn to recognize and prefer their parent's breast through olfactory, tactile, and oral modes by early exclusive exposure. Pacifier use can interfere with the development of this ability.

    4.   When a pacifier is used, the time at the breast is reduced.

    5.   Breastfeeding strengthens the weak oral musculature of infants with Down syndrome, and pacifier use interferes with this process.

    6.   Pacifiers can harbor bacteria, viruses, and yeast, and they can be a vector for biofilm formation and infections.[73]

    7.   The use of a pacifier may cause infant drowsiness and missed feedings, which can contribute to dehydration from postponed feedings.

    8.   Excessive and prolonged use of a pacifier can contribute to changes in dental arch and tooth position, increasing rates of malocclusion and dental problems.[74,75] Prolonged breastfeeding may have a protective effect on malocclusion.[76]

    9.   Pacifier use can result in an increased incidence of otitis media.[69]

  10.   The use of a latex pacifier can increase the risk of latex allergies.

  11.   Pacifiers have been implicated in oral injuries.[77,78]

D.   Teach parents how to use the device appropriately.

    1.   Pacifiers should be avoided until after the first month of life, when breastfeeding is well established.[66]

    2.   Instruct parents in the appropriate selection and use of pacifiers.[79,80]

    3.   Choose a pacifier that is not a potential choking hazard due to the risk of breaking into small parts, or choose a pacifier that is not excessively flexible and could become lodged in the infant's mouth.

    4.   Avoid pacifiers that have a handle because they could be forced into the child's mouth if he or she falls forward.

    5.   Choose a pacifier that has a mouth guard wider than the infant's mouth and has vent holes.

6.   Do not tie the pacifier around the infant's neck, wrist, or crib rung.

7.   Avoid rubber due to possible allergies and phthalates, which are industrial chemicals.

8.   Do not the dip the pacifier in sugar (risk of tooth decay) or honey (risk of *Clostridium botulinum*).[81]

9.   Do not share pacifiers with other children.

10.   Instruct parents in routine cleaning: wash daily, spray with chlorhexidine solution, or boil for 15 minutes. Do not use a microwave, bleach, or a bottle brush that may scratch the surface of the pacifier, thereby harboring more microorganisms.[82]

11.   Discontinue use after all primary teeth have erupted, or by 6 months or 1 year of age.[66,69,79]

V. Infant Scale

A.   There are two types of scales for weighing infants.

1.   A digital scale, with an accuracy within 2 grams, is appropriate for determining milk intake at the breast.[83,84]

2.   A balance scale is useful for serial weights (daily, weekly, monthly) but does not have the accuracy needed for test weights.

B.   Infant scales are used for a variety of reasons.

1.   Scales can determine milk intake at a feeding session (test weight). The amount of milk consumed at the breast can then be used to determine whether supplementation is necessary.

2.   Information gained from test weights can contribute to the decision to discharge a preterm infant from the hospital.

3.   Test weights can validate the adequacy of milk production.[83]

4.   Scales can be used to monitor feeding adequacy and weight gain in compromised infants.[84,85]

C.   Positive outcomes from the use of infant scales include the following:

1.   Test weights are more accurate for determining milk transfer at the breast than observation of a breastfeeding session by a trained observer. Clinical observation of audible swallowing, length of breastfeeding session, and parental perception of breast emptiness are unreliable indicators of intake.

2.   Test weights to determine adequate intake are reassuring to parents of late preterm and preterm infants because the use of scales is not perceived as stressful.[86]

3.   Test weights support the accurate determination of how much supplementation is needed.[84]

4.   Test-weighing the infant prior to hospital discharge is protective to exclusive breastfeeding, but not associated with breastfeeding duration.[87]

D.   Clinicians need to recognize precautions on the use of this device.

1.   Digital scales are expensive and may not be available in all practice settings. They can be rented for home use.

2.   There is a possibility of error if tubing or wires are attached to the infant.

3.   Clinicians disagree about the appropriateness of using test weights.[87,88]

E.   Ensure that the scale is used appropriately.[86]

1.   Place the scale on a flat surface and be sure the leveling bubble is centered.

2.   Periodically check the accuracy of the scale with a reference weight.

3.   If the scale is used by many infants, clean it between uses with a disinfectant solution.

4.   When weighing an infant, ensure that all parameters are the same for the before-feeding weight and the after-feeding weight. Use the same clothing, diaper, and hat, and use the same tubing and wires if the infant is attached to medical equipment.

5.   Do not drape blankets or clothing over the edge of the scale because they can affect its accuracy.

6.   Disconnect any tubing or wires that may be safely disconnected temporarily. Any leads or tubing that cannot be removed can be weighed with the infant. Mark the tubing with tape at the edge of the scale so the exact amount of tubing is weighed both times. Do not lift tubing or leads during weighing because this can lead to error.

7.   Obtain a prefeed weight two times for accuracy.

a.   Remove the infant for feeding.

b.   Reweigh the infant after each breast, if desired, and at the end of the feeding two times for accuracy.

      c.   Determine the weight gain. The weight gain in grams is equal to volume in mL consumed by the infant.

      d.   To get a reliable average of feeding size, do test weights at every feeding for 3 days.[86]

VI. Topical Treatments

A.   Topical treatments can enhance the healing of damaged nipples and promote breastfeeding.

    1.   Many parents discontinue breastfeeding not by choice but because of nipple pain.[5]

      a.   The trauma or pain may present as a lesion, crack, fissure, eroded skin, ulcer, erythema, edema, blister, bleeding, ecchymosis, or the skin looking white or yellow instead of pink.[2]

      b.   This trauma usually happens within the first few days postpartum and should be evaluated by a trained healthcare provider who can provide timely assistance.[5]

    2.   After the trauma has occurred, evidence suggests that there are multiple options to heal the damage.[25]

      a.   Helping the dyad with correct latch and position will decrease overall pain and trauma to the nipple and areola.[89]

      b.   Correcting the position of the infant and the latch will prevent the damage from getting worse.[90]

      c.   Human milk, lanolin, hydrogel pads, breast shells, ointment, olive oil, a nipple shield, and warm compresses are chosen by parents to decrease and heal nipple trauma, although there is little evidence regarding their efficacy.[25]

      d.   Clinicians should help parents discover the cause of the pain and provide appropriate treatment.

    3.   Moist wound healing is the most effective treatment to heal broken skin.

      a.   Creams, ointments, and dressings provide various levels of treatment by keeping the skin moist, preventing scab development, and promoting epithelialization of the wound.

      b.   Repair with moist treatments occurs at twice the rate of dry treatments.[91]

B.   Expressed milk can be used to treat painful and cracked nipples.

    1.   The parent's milk is free and readily available upon massage of the breast. Human milk is a natural remedy with properties that promote wound healing.[25] The use of human milk will decrease the response to inflammation and infection.

      a.   Many factors in human milk protect against tissue damage.

         i.   Factors that protect against infection include secretory immunoglobulin A, immunoglobulin M, immunoglobulin G, lactoferrin, lysozyme, complement component 3, bifida factor, antiviral mucins, oligosaccharides, white blood cells, nucleotides, and xanthine oxidase.[92,93] These factors help the immune system fight against foreign bodies and pathogens.

        ii.   Factors that protect against inflammation include tumor necrosis factor, interleukins, interferon gamma, prostaglandin, alpha-1-antichymotrypsin, alpha-1 antitrypsin, platelet-activating factor acetylhydrolase, and glycopeptides.[92]

      b.   The properties in human milk help stimulate the immune function and growth and development of tissue.[25]

      c.   Human milk has been shown to improve healing within 3 to 6 days.[5,25]

      d.   Some parents may prefer to use remedies other than expressed milk.[25]

    2.   Teach parents how to use their milk appropriately as a topical agent.

      a.   Encourage good hand washing and hygiene.

      b.   Apply a generous amount of expressed milk to the damaged area on the nipple after each feeding or whenever needed.[2]

      c.   Allow the milk to air dry. Use a breast shell over the air-dried milk to enhance healing.[25]

C.   Creams and ointments are used to heal sore and cracked nipples.

    1.   There are several types of creams and ointments.

      a.   Hypoallergenic, medical grade anhydrous, or modified, lanolin has been shown to provide a moist wound healing environment and is the most widely utilized nipple ointment.

         i.   Lanolin is easy to apply, but it remains sticky and messy on both the breast and fingers.[25]

        ii.   One study showed that lanolin use did not decrease pain or nipple trauma, and it did not improve breastfeeding outcomes better than routine postpartum care.[1]

        iii.   One small study showed that lanolin played a role in reducing pain and supporting healing.[94]

b.   Extra virgin olive oil has been shown to have trophic, anti-inflammatory, and antioxidant properties that aid in decreasing pain and increasing healing.[90]

    i.   Olive oil has been shown to prevent skin breakdown, even if the infant is not properly positioned.[90]

    ii.   In one study, olive oil had no adverse effects for mothers and infants when used for up to 6 months.[90]

c.   A moisturizing gel made from peppermint oil shows promise in soothing and healing sore nipples.[95] Peppermint oil contains menthol; in small doses, menthol has been found to be soothing, to have antibacterial properties, and to be safe for babies to ingest.[96,97]

d.   Oil derived from the emu (an Australian bird) has anti-inflammatory properties and enhances wound healing when applied to the nipple.[98,99]

e.   All-purpose nipple ointment contains an antibiotic (to combat bacterial infection), an antifungal (to combat candida infection), and a steroid (to provide pain relief).

    i.   All-purpose nipple ointment aids in the healing of sore nipples.[100]

    ii.   Antifungals are commonly used, often in combination with an antibiotic, for healing nipples.[94]

    iii.   Although all-purpose nipple ointment has become quite popular, research shows it is no more effective than lanolin in reducing pain scores or increasing breastfeeding duration and exclusivity rates at 12 weeks.[5]

f.   Some creams have questionable ingredients and are not recommended. They include vitamin E oil, cocoa butter, Bag Balm, vitamin A and D ointment, petroleum jelly, and baby oil. These agents were found to either not promote moist wound healing or, if ingested, possibly be toxic.

2.   Ensure appropriate use of these agents.

a.   For many years, creams and ointments have been used based on anecdotal reports. The clinician, in consultation with the parents, must use evidence-based research to choose the best remedy for the situation.[25]

b.   Maintain good hand washing and hygiene.

c.   Read all manufacturer directions for use. The correct application of creams and ointments depends on the individual product.[90]

3.   Positive outcomes from the use of topical treatments include the following:

a.   Topical products have been shown to promote healing within 5 to 6 days.[25,90] They may reduce pain and have a soothing effect.[1,90]

b.   They are widely available and inexpensive.[90]

c.   Most do not need to be washed off prior to feedings.[2]

4.   Clinicians need to recognize precautions on the use of topical treatments.

a.   The nipple and areola breathe and perspire like all skin, and the Montgomery glands secrete lubrication that protects the areola and nipple.[4] Creams and ointments decrease the breathing, perspiring, and lubrication of the nipple and areola.[4]

b.   Some products might need to be washed off before each feeding. This can remove moisture from the skin, create further damage, and slow wound healing.[2]

c.   Some combination creams, such as those containing peanut oil, have ingredients that could provoke an allergy in the infant.

d.   Some topical treatments have petroleum bases and other ingredients that could irritate the nipple skin and even clog the pores.[101]

e.   Disruption to the natural environment of the skin, pores, and glands should be considered when choosing a topical cream or ointment.[94]

D.   Commercial dressings are also used for healing nipples.

1.   There are three types of dressings.

a.   Water-based hydrogel dressings are insoluble hydrophilic materials made from synthetic polymers consisting of 70 to 90 percent water. They promote granulation of tissue and epithelium in a moist environment.[102]

  b. Glycerin-based dressings have a humectant that binds and holds moisture. They also demonstrate antibacterial and antifungal qualities.[103] The agent is blended into a dressing with a hydrophilic polymer.

  c. Gel dressings are available in gel, gauze, and precut sheet forms.

 2. Positive outcomes from the use of dressings include the following:

  a. Dressings provide a moist environment for healing and have demonstrated that they heal sore nipples.[94,102]

  b. Hydrogel dressings provide a barrier against contamination and friction to the wound. Their soft elastic property allows for easy application and removal.[102]

  c. Dressings maintain an appropriate wound temperature to increase blood flow to the site.[102]

  d. Hydrogel dressings are nonirritating, soothe irritated tissues, and decrease pain.[94,102]

 3. Clinicians need to recognize precautions on the use of dressings.

  a. They can be expensive to purchase repeatedly.

  b. Hydrogel dressings may increase the risk of wound infection and should not be used if the wound is infected.[2,94] Exudate can accumulate from an infected wound.[94,102]

 4. Teach parents how to use dressings appropriately.

  a. Maintain good hand washing and hygiene.

  b. Read the manufacturer's directions.

  c. Peel the back off the dressing, and apply the dressing directly to the wound.

  d. Remove the dressing during breastfeeding, and reapply between feedings. The breast does not need to be cleaned before breastfeeding.

  e. Dressings can be used for several days if they are rinsed after use and kept in a clean environment when not in use.

  f. Dressings can be chilled when not in use. The chilled dressing is soothing when reapplied.

E. Tea bags are used to heal sore and cracked nipples.

 1. Tea bags are low cost and easily available. A warm tea bag can be applied to sore nipples for 15 minutes after breastfeeding.

  a. Some herbal teas are known to be anti-inflammatory, antimicrobial, and contain healing properties.

  b. Black and green tea bags have been used as cold compresses on nipple trauma. Black tea imparts a bitter taste to the nipple, whereas green tea is much milder and is an antioxidant and anti-inflammatory.

  c. Warm tea compresses bring blood to the area of trauma and aid in healing.

  d. Warm compresses and tea bags decrease pain, compared to no treatment.[94]

 2. Clinicians need to recognize precautions on the use of tea as a topical treatment.

  a. Tea bags should not be the first choice for treatment because they can change the smell and taste of the nipple.

  b. Tea bags may have an astringent effect that can promote more drying and cracking.[104]

  c. The use of tea bags is more of a ritual than a research-based treatment.

▶ Key Points from This Chapter

A. Actively encourage prenatal education in breastfeeding management to prepare parents for initiating breastfeeding.

B. The role of the lactation consultant is to identify potential causes of the problem and to offer intervention options to remedy the situation. Often, refining the breastfeeding technique (e.g., positioning, latch, frequency, and duration) is the first strategy toward resolving problems. The use of breastfeeding devices does not replace guidance from a lactation consultant.

C. When intervention is needed to resolve specific problems, the lactation consultant should be familiar with the scope of devices and topical preparations that might be useful in various situations.

D. A painful or damaged nipple should never be disregarded.

🔍 *CASE STUDY 1*

Jennifer is a 35-year-old primigravida with a history of two miscarriages. She attended birthing and prenatal breastfeeding classes with her husband. She delivered a boy, William, at 40 weeks' gestation by cesarean section after failure to progress. Jennifer held William skin to skin for most of the first day.

At the end of the first day, Jennifer reports that William shows no interest in breastfeeding despite repeated attempts. Jennifer massaged her breasts and expressed colostrum into William's mouth, but William remained unwilling to latch onto the breast. William would suck on Jennifer's finger when offered, but not on the breast. At 24 hours, the hospital nurse instituted supplementation at the breast and a nipple shield. Jennifer began pumping her breasts every 3 hours after feeding attempts. The discharge instructions were to offer the breast first at each feeding. If there was no latch, she was instructed to apply the nipple shield and continue with the feeding.

At the 1-week follow-up visit with the lactation consultant, Jennifer had achieved full milk production and was weaning from the nipple shield. A test weight revealed that William had gained 5 ounces since hospital discharge. Full milk production had begun and her nipples had become more erect due to using the breast pump. The lactation consultant told Jennifer that she was doing everything right and to start weaning from pumping and go to exclusive breastfeeding.

Questions

1. What factors do you think could have affected William's initial disinterest in breastfeeding?
2. Do you think the delay in instituting pumping impacted Jennifer's milk production?
3. What additional remedies other than a nipple shield might have been effective?
4. What suggestions can you offer for weaning from a nipple shield?

🔍 *CASE STUDY 2*

Wanda, who is pregnant with her second baby, was unable to breastfeed her first infant because of flat nipples and meaty, inflexible areolae. She wants to breastfeed this infant and asks what she can do prior to delivery.

Observation and a pinch test reveal flat nipples with nonpliable areolae. Wanda is anxious for assistance and is willing to comply with recommendations. The lactation consultant recommends that she wear devices to pull the nipples out for 2 hours, two times per day, during the last month of pregnancy. Wanda is cautioned to report any increase in prenatal contractions and to also report any changes in nipple erectness. Other recommendations include breastfeeding immediately after delivery using the laid-back position and sandwich hold, continued feedings every 1 or 2 hours as the infant requests, and seeking help from a lactation consultant while in the hospital. Wanda used the nipple devices as recommended without improvement.

Wanda delivered a 6-pound girl at 35 weeks' gestation. She breastfed in the delivery room with limited success because her baby had difficulty latching. The lactation consultant recommended attempting to breastfeed every 1 to 2 hours when the baby exhibits feeding cues and to pump or hand express her breasts after feedings. Wanda is asked to observe her nipples for increased erectness and pliability, to report the volume of milk obtained by pumping, and to feed the expressed milk to the baby by spoon after breastfeeding attempts.

Wanda achieved full milk production, and her infant grew appropriately on breastmilk exclusively. As her infant's volume needs became greater, supplementing with a spoon was not feasible, and Wanda began using a bottle with a medium-based nipple and paced bottle feeding techniques. She continued to use a breast pump and bottle feed her pumped milk for several weeks while continuing to offer her breast. Her breasts softened as milk production became established, and her nipples became more pliable from using the breast pump. As her infant gained strength, Wanda was able to transition to full breastfeeding.

Questions

1. What other remedies could have been offered prenatally to increase the protractility of Wanda's nipples?
2. What impact did having a late preterm infant have on breastfeeding?
3. What other alternative to bottle feeding could have been recommended when spoon feeding was no longer feasible?
4. What tips can you offer for a baby who has been bottle feeding to successfully transition to breastfeeding?
5. What role does parent preference have in selecting appropriate devices to remedy problems?

References

1. Jackson KT, Dennis CL. Lanolin for the treatment of nipple pain in breastfeeding women: a randomized controlled trial. *Matern Child Nutr.* 2017;13(3). doi:10.1111/mcn.12357.

2. Vieira F, Bachion MM, Mota DD, Munari DB. A systematic review of the interventions for nipple trauma in breastfeeding mothers. *J Nurs Scholarsh.* 2013;45(2):116-125.

3. Low K, Otto D. Improving breastfeeding outcomes using appropriate interventions to champion a successful breastfeeding relationship for a mother with flat nipples. *J Obstet Gynecol Neonatal Nurs.* 2013;42(suppl 1):S106.

4. Sasaki BC, Pinkerton K, Leipelt A. Does lanolin use increase the risk for infection in breastfeeding women? *Clin Lactation.* 2014;5(1):28-32.

5. Dennis CL, Jackson K, Watson J. Interventions for treating painful nipples among breastfeeding women. *Cochrane Database Syst Rev.* 2014;12:CD007366.

6. Chow S, Chow R, Popovic M, et al. The use of nipple shields: a review. *Front Public Health.* 2015;3:236.

7. Glover R, Wiessinger D. They can do it, you can help: building breastfeeding skill and confidence in mother and helper. In: Genna CW, ed. *Supporting Sucking Skills in Breastfeeding Infants.* 3rd ed. Burlington, MA: Jones & Bartlett Learning; 2017:113-155.

8. McKechnie AC, Eglash A. Nipple shields: a review of the literature. *Breastfeed Med.* 2010;5(6):309-314.

9. Walker, M. Are there any cures for sore nipples? *Clin Lactation.* 2013;4(3):106-115.

10. Kronborg H, Foverskov E, Nilsson I, Maastrup R. Why do mothers use nipple shields and how does this influence duration of exclusive breastfeeding? *Matern Child Nutr.* 2017;13(1). doi:10.1111/mcn.12251.

11. Ekström A, Abrahamsson H, Eriksson RM, Mårtensson BL. Women's use of nipple shields: their influence on breastfeeding duration after a process-oriented education for health professionals. *Breastfeed Med.* 2014;9(9):458-466.

12. Kent JC, Ashton E, Hardwick CM, et al. Nipple pain in breastfeeding mothers: incidence, causes and treatments. *Int J Environ Res Public Health.* 2015;12(10):12247-12263.

13. Hanna S, Wilson M, Norwood S. A description of breast-feeding outcomes among U.S. mothers using nipple shields. *Midwifery.* 2013;29(6):616-621.

14. Wilson-Clay B, Hoover K. Flat and inverted nipples. In: *The Breastfeeding Atlas.* 6th ed. Manchaca,TX: LactNews Press; 2017:46-53.

15. California Perinatal Quality Care Collaborative. *Care and Management of the Late Preterm Infant Toolkit.* Stanford, CA: California Perinatal Quality Care Collaborative; 2013. https://www.cpqcc.org/sites/default/files/Late%20Preterm%20Infant%20Toolkit%20FINAL%202-13.pdf. Accessed October 4, 2017.

16. Meier PP, Brown LP, Hurst NM, et al. Nipple shields for preterm infants: effect on milk transfer and duration of breastfeeding. *J Hum Lactation.* 2000;16(2):106-114.

17. Flacking R, Dykes F. Perceptions and experiences of using a nipple shield among parents and staff—an ethnographic study in neonatal units. *BMC Pregnancy Childbirth.* 2017;17(1):1.

18. Gerrard SE, Orlu-Gul M, Tuleu C, Slater NK. Modeling the physiological factors that affect drug delivery from a nipple shield delivery system to breastfeeding infants. *J Pharm Sci.* 2013;102(10):3773-3783.

19. Hart CW, Israel-Ballard KA, Joanis CL, et al. Acceptability of a nipple shield delivery system administering antiviral agents to prevent mother-to-child transmission of HIV through breastfeeding. *J Hum Lactation.* 2015;31(1):68-75.

20. Ridgway L, Cramer R, McLachlan HL, et al. Breastfeeding support in the early postpartum: content of home visits in the SILC Trial. *Birth.* 2016;43(4):303-312.

21. Keemer F. Breastfeeding self-efficacy of women using second-line strategies for healthy term infants in the first week postpartum: an Australian observational study. *Int Breastfeed J.* 2013;8(1):18.

22. Perrella SL, Lai CT, Geddes DT. Case report of nipple shield trauma associated with breastfeeding an infant with high intra-oral vacuum. *BMC Pregnancy Childbirth.* 2015;15:155.

23. Chanprapaph P, Luttarapakul J, Siribariruck S, Boonyawanichkul S. Outcome of non-protractile nipple correction with breast cups in pregnant women: a randomized controlled trial. *Breastfeed Med.* 2013;8(4):408-412.

24. Wilson-Clay B, Hoover K. Sore nipples. In: *The Breastfeeding Atlas.* 6th ed. Manchaca,TX: LactNews Press; 2017:54-67.

25. Vieira F, Mota DDCF, Castral TC, Guimarães JV, Salge AKM, Bachion MM. Effects of anhydrous lanolin versus breast milk combined with a breast shell for the treatment of nipple trauma and pain during breastfeeding: a randomized clinical trial. *J Midwifery Womens Health.* 2017. [Epub ahead of print]. doi:10.1111/jmwh.12644.

26. Marrazzu A, Sanna MG, Dessole F, Capobianco G, Piga MD, Dessole S. Evaluation of the effectiveness of a silver-impregnated medical cap for topical treatment of nipple fissure of breastfeeding mothers. *Breastfeed Med.* 2015;10(5):232-238.

27. Bouchet-Horwitz J. The use of supple cups for flat, retracting and inverted nipples. *Clin Lactation.* 2011;2(3):30-33.

28. Kellams A, Harrel C, Omage S, Gregory C, Rosen-Carole C. ABM clinical protocol #3: supplementary feedings in the healthy term breastfed neonate, revised 2017. *Breastfeed Med.* 2017;12:188-198.

29. Walker M. Influence of peripartum factors, birthing practices, and early caretaking behaviors. In: *Breastfeeding Management for the Clinician: Using the Evidence.* 4th ed. Burlington, MA: Jones & Bartlett Learning; 2017:223-301.

30. Augsornwan D, Surakunprapha P, Pattangtanang P, Pongpagatip S, Jenwitheesuk K, Chowchuen B. Comparison of wound dehiscence and parent's satisfaction between spoon/syringe feeding and breast/bottle feeding in patients with cleft lip repair. *J Med Assoc Thai.* 2013;96(suppl 4):S61-S70.

31. Aytekin A, Albayrak EB, Küçükoğlu S, Caner İ. The effect of feeding with spoon and bottle on the time of switching to full breastfeeding and sucking success in preterm babies. *Turk Pediatri Ars.* 2014;49(4):307-313.

32. Genna, CW. *Supporting Sucking Skills in Breastfeeding Infants.* 3rd ed. Burlington, MA: Jones & Bartlett Learning; 2017.

33. Walker M. Beyond the initial 48–72 hours: infant challenges. In: *Breastfeeding Management for the Clinician: Using the Evidence.* 4th ed. Burlington, MA: Jones & Bartlett Learning; 2017:397-484.

34. Wilson-Clay B, Hoover K. Alternative feeding methods. In: *The Breastfeeding Atlas*. 6th ed. Manchaca, TX: LactNews Press; 2017:115-125.

35. Marofi M, Abedini F, Mohammadizadeh M, Talakoub S. Effect of paladay and cup feeding on premature neonates' weight gain and reaching full oral feeding time interval. *Iran J Nurs Midwifery Res*. 2016;21(2):202-206.

36. Nyqvist KH. Breastfeeding preterm infants. In: Genna CW, ed. *Supporting Sucking Skills in Breastfeeding Infants*. 3rd ed. Burlington, MA: Jones & Bartlett Learning; 2017:181-208.

37. Collins CT, Gillis J, McPhee AJ, Suganuma H, Makrides M. Avoidance of bottles during the establishment of breast feeds in preterm infants. *Cochrane Database Syst Rev*. 2016;9:CD005252. doi:10.1002/14651858.CD005252.pub4.

38. França EC, Sousa CB, Aragão LC, Costa LR. Electromyographic analysis of masseter muscle in newborns during suction in breast, bottle or cup feeding. *BMC Pregnancy Childbirth*. 2014;14:154.

39. Dowling DA, Meier PP, DiFiore JM, Blatz M, Martin RJ. Cup-feeding for preterm infants: mechanics and safety. *J Hum Lactation*. 2002;18(1):13-20.

40. Genna CW. The influence of anatomic and structural issues on sucking skills. In: Genna CW, ed. *Supporting Sucking Skills in Breastfeeding Infants*. 3rd ed. Burlington, MA: Jones & Bartlett Learning; 2017:209-267.

41. Oddy WH, Glenn K. Implementing the Baby Friendly Hospital Initiative: the role of finger feeding. *Breastfeed Rev*. 2003;11(1):5-10.

42. Lawrence R, Lawrence R. Practical management of the mother-infant nursing couple. In: *Breastfeeding: A Guide for the Medical Profession*. 6th ed. Philadelphia, PA: Elsevier, Inc. 2016:230-284.

43. Genna CW, Fram JL, Sandora L. Neurological issues and breastfeeding. In: Genna CW, ed. *Supporting Sucking Skills in Breastfeeding Infants*. 3rd ed. Burlington, MA: Jones & Bartlett Learning; 2017:335-397.

44. Penny, F. *Breastfeeding Mother's Use of a Supplemental Feeding Tube Device* [dissertation]. Storrs: University of Connecticut; 2017. http://opencommons.uconn.edu/dissertations/1514. Accessed November 2017.

45. Woolridge MW. The 'anatomy' of infant sucking. *Midwifery*. 1986;2(4):164-171.

46. Weber F, Woolridge MW, Baum JD. An ultrasonographic study of the organization of sucking and swallowing by newborn infants. *Dev Med Child Neurol*. 1986;28(1):19-24.

47. Medoff-Cooper B, Bilker W, Kaplan JM. Sucking patterns and behavioral state in 1- and 2-day-old full-term infants. *J Obstet Gynecol Neonatal Nurs*. 2010;39(5):519-524.

48. Ardran GM, Kemp FH, Lind J. A cineradiographic study of breast feeding. *Br J Radiol*. 1958;31(363):156-162.

49. Page-Goertz S. The ill child: breastfeeding implications. In: Wambach K, Riorden J, eds. *Breastfeeding and Human Lactation*. 5th ed. Burlington, MA: Jones & Bartlett Learning; 2016:717-773.

50. Lawrence R, Lawrence R. Premature infants and breastfeeding. In: *Breastfeeding: A Guide for the Medical Profession*. 8th ed. Philadelphia, PA: Elsevier, Inc. 2016:524-562.

51. Ross E, Fuhrman L. Supporting oral feeding skills through bottle selection. *Perspect Swallow Swallow Disord*. 2015. 24:50-57.

52. Peterson A. Picking bottle nipples for the breastfed baby. The Leaky Boob website. http://theleakyboob.com/2017/02/picking-bottle-nipples-for-the-breastfed-baby/. Published February 24, 2017. Accessed November 10, 2017.

53. McGrattan KE, McFarland DH, Dean JC, Hill E, White DR, Martin-Harris B. Effect of single-use, laser-cut, slow-flow nipples on respiration and milk ingestion in preterm Infants. *Am J Speech Lang Pathol*. 2017;26(3):832-839.

54. Dion S, Duivestein JA, St Pierre A, Harris SR. Use of thickened liquids to manage feeding difficulties in infants: a pilot survey of practice patterns in Canadian pediatric centers. *Dysphagia*. 2015;30(4):457-472.

55. Pados BF, Park J, Thoyre SM, Estrem H, Nix WB. Milk flow rates from bottle nipples used for feeding infants who are hospitalized. *Am J Speech Lang Pathol*. 2015;24(4):671-679.

56. Zimmerman E, Thompson K. Clarifying nipple confusion. *J Perinatol*. 2015;35(11):895-899.

57. Lau C, Fucile S, Schanler RJ. A self-paced oral feeding system that enhances preterm infants' oral feeding skills. *J Neonatal Nurs*. 2015;21(3):121-126.

58. Young, BE, Johnson SL, Krebs NF. Biological determinants linking infant weight gain and child obesity: current knowledge and future directions. *Adv Nutr*. 2012;3(5):675-686.

59. Paul IM, Bartok CJ, Downs DS, Stifter CA, Ventura AK, Birch LL. Opportunities for the primary prevention of obesity during infancy. *Adv Pediatr*. 2009;56:107-133.

60. Ventura AK, Mennella JA. An experimental approach to study individual differences in infants' intake and satiation behaviors during bottle-feeding. *Child Obes*. 2017;13(1):44-52.

61. Li R, Magadia J, Fein SB, Grummer-Strawn LM. Risk of bottle-feeding for rapid weight gain during the first year of life. *Arch Pediatr Adolesc Med*. 2012;166(5):431-436.

62. Ventura AK, Garcia P, Schaffner AA. Associations between bottle-feeding intensity and maternal encouragement of bottle-emptying. *Public Health Nutr*. 2017;12:1-9.

63. Golen RP, Ventura AK. What are mothers doing while bottle-feeding their infants? Exploring the prevalence of maternal distraction during bottle-feeding interactions. *Early Hum Dev*. 2015;91(12):787-791.

64. Golen RB, Ventura AK. Mindless feeding: is maternal distraction during bottle-feeding associated with overfeeding? *Appetite*. 2015;91:385-392.

65. Moon RY, Task Force on Sudden Infant Death Syndrome. SIDS and other sleep-related infant deaths: evidence base for 2016 updated recommendations for a safe infant sleeping environment. *Pediatrics*. 2016;138(5). doi:10.1542/peds.2016-2940.

66. American Academy of Pediatrics. Section on breastfeeding. Breastfeeding and the use of human milk. *Pediatrics*. 2012;129(3):e827-e841.

67. Hall RW, Anand KJ. Pain management in newborns. *Clin Perinatol*. 2014;41(4):895-924.

68. Sipsma HL, Kornfeind K, Kair LR. Pacifiers and exclusive breastfeeding: does risk for postpartum depression modify the association? *J Hum Lactation.* 2017;33(4):692-700.

69. Lubbe W, Ten Ham-Baloyi W. When is the use of pacifiers justifiable in the Baby-Friendly Hospital Initiative context? A clinician's guide. *BMC Pregnancy Childbirth.* 2017;17(130). https://doi.org/10.1186/s12884-017-1306-8.

70. Harding C, Frank L, Van Someren V, Hilari K, Botting N. How does non-nutritive sucking support infant feeding? *Infant Behav Dev.* 2014;37(4):457-464.

71. Psaila K, Foster JP, Pulbrook N, Jeffery HE. Infant pacifiers for reduction in risk of sudden infant death syndrome. *Cochrane Database Syst Rev.* 2017;4:CD011147. doi:10.1002/14651858.CD011147.pub2.

72. Jaafar SH, Ho JJ, Jahanfar S, Angolkar M. Effect of restricted pacifier use in breastfeeding term infants for increasing duration of breastfeeding. *Cochrane Database Syst Rev.* 2016;8:CD007202. doi:10.1002/14651858.CD007202.pub4.

73. da Silveira LC, Charone S, Maia LC, Soares RM, Portela MB. Biofilm formation by *Candida* species on silicone surfaces and latex pacifier nipples: an in vitro study. *J Clin Pediatr Dent.* 2009;33(3):235-240.

74. Gederi A, Coomaraswamy K, Turner PJ. Pacifiers: a review of risks vs benefits. *Dent Update.* 2013;40(2):92-94, 97-98, 101.

75. Lima AA, Alves CM, Ribeiro CC, et al. Effects of conventional and orthodontic pacifiers on the dental occlusion of children aged 24-36 months old. *Int J Paediatr Dent.* 2017;27(2):108-119.

76. Narbutytė I, Narbutytė A, Linkevičienė L. Relationship between breastfeeding, bottle-feeding and development of malocclusion. *Stomatologija.* 2013;15(3):67-72.

77. Tomás CC, Oliveira E, Sousa D, et al. Proceedings of the 3rd IPLeiria's International Health Congress: Leiria, Portugal, 6-7 May 2016. *BMC Health Serv Res.* 2016;16(suppl 3):200.

78. Keim S, Fletcher E, TePoel M, McKenzie L. Injuries associated with bottles, pacifiers, and sippy cups in the United States, 1991-2010. *Pediatrics.* 2012;129(6):1104-1110.

79. Bencosme J. Pacifiers for infants: what nurses need to know. *Nursing.* 2016;46(1):53-54.

80. American Academy of Pediatrics. Pacifiers. AAP website. https://www.aap.org/en-us/about-the-aap/aap-press-room/aap-press-room-media-center/Pages/Pacifiers.aspx. Accessed October 28, 2017.

81. Benjamins LJ, Gourishankar A, Yataco-Marquez V, Cardona EH, de Ybarrondo L. Honey pacifier use among an indigent pediatric population. *Pediatrics.* 2013;131(6):e1838-e1841.

82. Nelson-Filho P, Louvain MC, Macari S, et al. Microbial contamination and disinfection methods of pacifiers. *J Appl Oral Sci.* 2015;23(5):523-528.

83. Froh EB, Hallowell S, Spatz DL. The use of technologies to support human milk and breastfeeding. *J Pediatr Nurs.* 2015;30(3):521-523.

84. Meier P, Patel A, Wright K, Engstrom J. Management of breastfeeding during and after the maternity hospitalization for late preterm infants. *Clin Perinatol.* 2013;40(4):689-705.

85. Thomas J, Marinelli KA, Academy of Breastfeeding Medicine. ABM clinical protocol #16: breastfeeding the hypotonic infant, revision 2016. *Breastfeed Med.* 2016;11(6):112-116.

86. Powers NG. Low intake in the breastfed infant: maternal and infant considerations. In: Wambach K, Riorden J, eds. *Breastfeeding and Human Lactation.* 5th ed. Burlington, MA: Jones & Bartlett Learning; 2016:359-404.

87. Maastrup R, Hansen BM, Kronborg H, et al. Factors associated with exclusive breastfeeding of preterm infants: results from a prospective national cohort study. *PLOS One.* 2014;9(2):e89077. doi:10.1371/journal.pone.0089077.

88. Savenije OEM, Brand PLP. Accuracy and precision of test weighing to assess milk intake in newborn infants. *Arch Dis Child Fetal Neonatal Ed.* 2006;91:F330-F332.

89. Robinson BA, Hartrick Doane G. Beyond the latch: a new approach to breastfeeding. *Nurse Educ Pract.* 2017;26:115-117.

90. Cordero MJ, Villar NM, Barrilao RG, Cortés ME, López AM. Application of extra virgin olive oil to prevent nipple cracking in lactating women. *Worldviews Evid Based Nurs.* 2015;12(6):364-369.

91. CliniMed. Theory of moist wound healing. CliniMed website. http://www.clinimed.co.uk/Wound-Care/Education/Wound-Essentials/Theory-of-Moist-Wound-Healing.aspx. Published 2014. Accessed November 4, 2017.

92. Kim JH, Froh EB. What nurses need to know regarding nutritional and immunobiological properties of human milk. *J Obstet Gynecol Neonatal Nurs.* 2012;41(1):122-137.

93. Jiang M, Zhang F, Tao X. Evaluation of probiotic properties of *Lactobacillus plantarum* isolated from human breast milk. *J Dairy Sci.* 2016;3(99):1736-1746.

94. Buck ML, Amir LH, Donath SM. Topical treatment used by breastfeeding women to treat sore and damaged nipples. *Clin Lactation.* 2015;6(1):16-23.

95. Nice F. Moisturizing gel. Nice Breastfeeding website. www.nicebreastfeeding.com. Published 2016. Accessed October 15, 2017.

96. Sayyah M, Rashidi MR, Delazar A, et al. Effect of peppermint water on prevention of nipple cracks in lactating primiparous women: a randomized controlled trial. *Int Breastfeed J.* 2007;2(7):1-18.

97. Melli MS, Rashidi MR, Nokhoodchi A, et al. A randomized trial of peppermint gel, lanolin ointment, and placebo gel to prevent nipple crack in primiparous breastfeeding women. *Med Sci Monit.* 2007;13(9):CR406-CR411.

98. Jeengar MK, Kumar PS, Thummuri D, et al. Review on emu products for use as complementary and alternative medicine. *Nutrition.* 2015;31(1):21-27.

99. Zanardo V, Giarrizzo D, Maiolo L, Straface G. Efficacy of topical application of emu oil on areola skin barrier in breastfeeding women. *J Evid Based Complementary Altern Med.* 2016;21(1):10-13.

100. Newman J, Pittman T. *Dr. Jack Newman's Guide to Breastfeeding.* 3rd ed. London, England: Pinter and Martin; 2014.

101. Ray L. A list of skin care ingredients that shouldn't be used while breastfeeding. Livestrong website. https://www.livestrong.com /article/76800-list-skin-care-ingredients-shouldnt/. Published June 13, 2017. Accessed October 15, 2017.
102. Dhivya S, Padma VV, Santhini E. Wound dressings: a review. *BioMedicine*. 2015;5(4):22.
103. Stout E, McKessor A. Glycerin-based hydrogel for infection control. *Adv Wound Care*. 2012;1(1):48-51.
104. La Leche League International. How do I heal sore nipples? La Leche League International website. www.llli.org. Published 2011. Accessed October 16, 2017.

Additional Resources

Genna CW. *Selecting and Using Breastfeeding Tools*. Amarillo, TX: Hale Publishing; 2009.

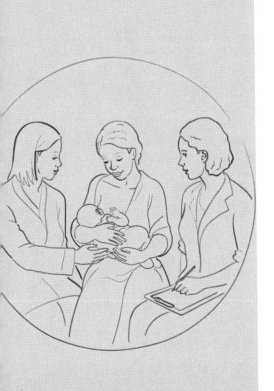

SECTION III

Professional

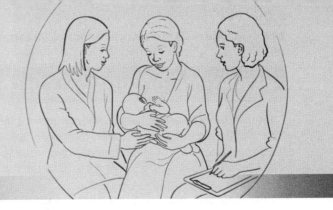

CHAPTER 25

Professional Standards for Lactation Care Providers

Elizabeth C. Brooks
Elizabeth K. Stehel

OBJECTIVES

- Identify major practice-guiding documents that define mandatory and best practice (or model) expectations of professional practice for International Board Certified Lactation Consultants (IBCLCs).
- Discuss elements of the major practice-guiding and ethics-related documents as they relate to lactation consultant practice for IBCLCs.
- Describe practice-guiding authority for members of other healthcare professions that may care for families who are breastfeeding or using human milk.
- Recognize situations that require IBCLCs to assess professional behaviors in light of the major practice-guiding documents.
- Describe when and how to report violations of the International Board of Lactation Consultant Examiners (IBLCE) Code of Professional Conduct for IBCLCs.

DEFINITIONS OF COMMONLY USED TERMS

Advisory Opinion An opinion published by the IBLCE describing the organization's position about expected and acceptable professional behaviors.

Clinical Competencies for the Practice of International Board Certified Lactation Consultants (IBCLCs) An IBLCE document that identifies mandatory skills expanding each of the broader six duty and clinical areas defined in the IBLCE *Scope of Practice for International Board Certified Lactation Consultant (IBCLC) Certificants*.

Code of Professional Conduct for IBCLCs An IBLCE document that describes the IBCLC profession's mandatory ethical code of conduct and outlines the professional behaviors expected of IBCLCs.

Documentation Guidelines An IBLCE document that provides basic suggestions for clinical record keeping.

(continues)

DEFINITIONS OF COMMONLY USED TERMS

International Board of Lactation Consultant Examiners (IBLCE) An international certification board for the lactation consultant profession; formed in 1985.

***International Code of Marketing of Breast-milk Substitutes* (WHO Code)** An international health policy framework for breastfeeding promotion adopted by the World Health Assembly, the decision-making body of the World Health Organization (WHO), in 1981.

International Lactation Consultant Association (ILCA) A voluntary international professional association for lactation consultants.

Scope of Practice for International Board Certified Lactation Consultant (IBCLC) Certificants An IBLCE document that describes mandatory clinical, educational, professional, and advocacy activities in which a certified IBCLC may engage.

Standards of Practice for International Board Certified Lactation Consultants (IBCLCs) An ILCA document that serves as a compendium of best professional practices in which IBCLCs should engage.

Any use of the term *mother*, *maternal*, or *breastfeeding* is not meant to exclude transgender or nonbinary parents who may be breastfeeding or providing human milk to their infant.

▶ Overview

Lactation support has been provided ever since humans began living together in communities. For centuries, breastfeeding (and the companion activities of cross- or shared feeding, or collection and use of human milk) was the only means to feed and nurture offspring. Humans showed other humans how to breastfeed. With the overall decline in breastfeeding rates in the 20th and 21st centuries, there was a similar decline in the ability of family members, friends, and neighbors to help a new parent navigate challenges to successfully breastfeed. But the need for help—including skilled lactation care—was always there. The modern-day rise in chronic disease rates (in parents) and improved survival rates for infants born extremely early or at extremely low weights have increased the need for skilled clinical lactation care. Many families today need more than parent-to-parent advice and support. As families fell away from breastfeeding (that is, fewer family members or friends had much lactation experience), organizations of breastfeeding support volunteers and healthcare professionals began to fill the gap in care at the lay level and the skilled clinical level.

Although a family can now tap into many options for help, the choices can be confusing and overwhelming for new parents who just want answers to common quandaries (e.g., "Why do my nipples hurt, and why does my milk supply seem low?"). There are different levels of education, training, and clinical experience required for similarly named lactation care providers.[1] Trusted, licensed healthcare providers (physicians, nurses, midwives, dietitians, etc.) may not have received any specific training or education in breastfeeding and lactation, either in school or on the job. Thus, many caregivers who legitimately can help with lactation may come to the field with anywhere from a few hours to many years of preparation.

This chapter will explore the professional practice-guiding documents for IBCLCs and key elements from practice-guiding documents of other professions or organizations for breastfeeding and human lactation support. The chapter will also review major concepts and offer practice-based examples for IBCLCs and other healthcare providers who commonly provide some lactation care.

I. The Need for Professional Support to Breastfeed

A. Most families will not need the specialized clinical care that an IBCLC or breastfeeding medicine specialist can provide.

1. Most families will be well-served by someone with training in basic lactation physiology and management and counseling skills, just as, historically, they would have received kind and accurate advice from friends, neighbors, and family members, all of whom had breastfed their own children.

2. In an ideal world, every family would be able to easily access the right level of care for their lactation issue, the visit would be covered by their health insurance, and the person offering care would be paid for providing sensitive counseling and clinical care.

3. There are many kinds of breastfeeding and lactation supporters (volunteer and paid) who are eager to help new families. There are also many primary healthcare providers who have made an effort to learn more about breastfeeding and lactation because their formal education rarely requires it.
4. The homework of discerning who is the right lactation care provider often falls to the new parent.

B. Whether the person offering lactation care is a volunteer or paid healthcare provider, each will have official parameters for professionalism.
   1. Typically, parameters for professionalism include the following:
      a. An ethical or professional code of conduct that defines ethics requirements.
      b. A scope of practice or a clinical competencies description that defines the specific areas in which the person is trained to offer skilled help.
      c. Laws and regulations covering workplace setting behaviors (ranging from broad-reaching laws of national, provincial, or state governments to policies and procedures that are applicable to only one workplace).
   2. Many IBCLCs acquire certification after obtaining licensure or registration as another kind of healthcare provider (doctor, nurse, midwife, dietitian, etc.) and thus have guidance from within those professions. IBCLCs with multiple roles may have overlapping, but different, ethical and legal responsibilities.
   3. Most healthcare professions have guideposts to impart the best professional practices.
      a. Some elements of clinical care and professional judgment are mandatory.
      b. Some professional behaviors are considered discretionary, best practices, or model behaviors.

II. IBCLC Practice Documents

A. Mandatory practice-guiding documents outline the professional behaviors that all IBCLCs must follow. All IBLCE documents may be viewed and downloaded at www.iblce.org.
   1. IBLCE *Code of Professional Conduct for IBCLCs* (referred to as the Code of Professional Conduct).[2]
   2. IBLCE *Disciplinary Procedures for the Code of Professional Conduct for IBCLCs for the International Board of Lactation Consultant Examiners* (referred to as Disciplinary Procedures).[3]
   3. IBLCE *Scope of Practice for International Board Certified Lactation Consultant (IBCLC) Certificants* (referred to as Scope of Practice).[4]
   4. IBLCE *Clinical Competencies for the Practice of International Board Certified Lactation Consultants (IBCLCs).*[5]
   5. IBLCE *Documentation Guidelines.*[6]
   6. *International Code of Marketing of Breast-milk Substitutes* (WHO Code) and subsequent relevant World Health Assembly resolutions.[7,8] (See Chapter 29, *Initiatives to Protect, Promote, and Support Breastfeeding.*)
      a. The WHO Code is an international health policy framework for breastfeeding promotion adopted by the World Health Assembly, the decision-making body of the World Health Organization (WHO), in 1981.
      b. The WHO Code is a mandatory document if it has been enacted into law by the country where the IBCLC practices, or if the IBCLC works in a facility officially designated by WHO/UNICEF as a Baby-friendly Hospital.
      c. Otherwise, the WHO Code is considered a discretionary, best practices, or model document, and any IBCLC and healthcare worker can choose to follow the WHO Code as though it were required by law.
   7. Workplace policies and procedures specific to the place of employment.
      a. Lactation care, advocacy, and education are provided in various work settings, such as hospitals, birth centers, physician or midwifery practices, clinics, public health agencies, educational institutions, companies, policy-setting nongovernmental agencies, and private practice.
      b. Generally, a workplace-established policy or procedure is a mandatory practice-guiding document for healthcare providers employed within that work setting. It is a condition of employment to follow the employer's policies and procedures.

    c.   When conflicts arise between the employer's policy and the profession's practice-guiding documents, the employer's policy must be respected as the greater authority until and unless it is changed to better encompass the clinical role of IBCLCs and other lactation care providers.

B.   Discretionary, best practices, or model practice-guiding documents outline those professional behaviors for IBCLCs (i.e., IBCLCs should endeavor to follow them but will not be sanctioned for failure to do so).

    1.   ILCA *Standards of Practice for International Board Certified Lactation Consultants (IBCLCs)* (referred to as Standards of Practice).[9]

    2.   ILCA *Position Paper on the Role and Impact of the IBCLC*.[10]

    3.   Three Advisory Opinions from the IBLCE: Frenulotomy[11]; Professionalism in the Social Media Age[12]; and Assessment, Diagnosis, and Referral.[13]

    4.   The WHO Code[7,8] is discretionary unless legally required.

        a.   Even if WHO Code elements have not been enacted into law by a country, respecting its tenets as though the Code were the law is a discretionary, best practice, or model action that any supporter of the WHO Code may choose to take.

        b.   The nonbinding introduction to the IBLCE Code of Professional Conduct encourages IBCLCs to respect and support the WHO Code, even though the Code of Professional Conduct cannot require them to do so.[14]

III. Certification Authority of IBLCE

A.   IBLCE is an international certification board for the lactation consultant profession, formed in 1985. Its role is to administer the IBCLC certification exam, award the IBCLC credential to those who pass the exam, and protect the public health, safety, and welfare through discipline procedures for IBCLCs.[3]

B.   An IBCLC is the only internationally certified healthcare provider with clinical expertise in breastfeeding and human lactation, which is required as a part of certification.

    1.   An IBCLC earns the credential by successful completion of lactation-specific education, substantial clinical practice, and the certification exam administered by the IBLCE.[15]

    2.   The IBLCE has sole international authority to offer the IBCLC certification examination and confer the IBCLC credential. Accreditation is awarded by an independent organization, the National Commission for Certifying Agencies (NCCA).[16]

        a.   The NCCA operates under the umbrella of the Institute for Credentialing Excellence (ICE).[17] The IBLCE is solely a certification testing authority and does not provide any of the education that is required to meet exam requirements.

        b.   "NCCA Standards were developed to help ensure the health, welfare, and safety of the public. They highlight the essential elements of a high-quality program."[17(para 2)]

    3.   The IBLCE certification process includes education, clinical training, and examination. It is meant to measure the skill of practitioners who will use expertise in their clinical, advocacy, and educational duties.

        a.   There are many kinds of lactation caregivers, including healthcare providers and lay breastfeeding supporters, who have obtained additional education and clinical experience in the areas of breastfeeding and human lactation.

        b.   IBCLC candidates use a variety of educational offerings to satisfy their educational requirements, including accredited academic lactation programs, elective college courses, and short-term courses of study. The requirements for each training type vary significantly.[1] (See Chapter 30, *Lactation Education for Health Professionals*.)

IV. The IBLCE Code of Professional Conduct for IBCLCs

A.   Ethics is a body of philosophy designed to guide decision making and behaviors, based on morals and legal principles, to achieve a good, right, or just objective.

    1.   There must be a disciplinary process in place at the certifying authority to ensure that the health, welfare, and safety of the public is protected against healthcare providers who do not practice using the requisite professional skills.[16]

    2.   The IBLCE Disciplinary Procedures fulfill this requirement.[3]

B.	The IBLCE Code of Professional Conduct serves as the IBCLC's mandatory ethical code of conduct; it outlines the professional behaviors expected of IBCLCs. Refer to the IBLCE website (www.iblce.org) to see the most current version of the Code of Professional Conduct, which is periodically reviewed and updated by the IBLCE according to best practices.

C.	The prematter to the Code of Professional Conduct states the IBLCE's position on several points.

1.	The IBLCE encourages IBCLCs to support the WHO Code.[2]

a.	IBCLCs are considered health workers under the WHO Code.

b.	It is important for IBCLCs to understand the principles of the WHO Code, which predates the profession of lactation consultation. (See Chapter 29, *Initiatives to Protect, Promote, and Support Breastfeeding*.)

2.	The IBLCE embraces two United Nations Conventions (or position statements) about human rights standards. They provide authority for protecting a child's right to good health and a woman's right to appropriate health care and nutrition during pregnancy and lactation. Promoting and protecting breastfeeding are seen as integral to optimal infant and young child feeding (the child's human right) provided by the parent (the parent's human right).[18,19]

3.	The IBLCE embraces the Council of Medical Specialty Societies "Code for Interactions With Companies," which is a model voluntary code to guide professional healthcare societies in programs, policies, and advocacy positions to avoid commercial influences from pharmaceutical and medical device manufacturers.[20]

D.	The Code of Professional Conduct is a mandatory practice-guiding document describing the IBCLC's authority and responsibilities.

1.	The Code of Professional Conduct is the authoritative document from the IBLCE that describes the minimum standards that IBCLCs must meet in their professional practice.

2.	The expectation is that IBCLCs will follow these guidelines in the conduct of their duties. The Code of Professional Conduct is the standard against which complaints of misconduct will be evaluated.

3.	The Code of Professional Conduct states that IBCLCs consent, when obtaining certification, to any future adjudication of complaints against them under the disciplinary process, timetable, and procedures established and enforced by the IBLCE.

CLINICAL TIP

Although the Code of Professional Conduct describes minimum standards that IBCLCs must meet in their professional practice, IBCLCs and other healthcare professionals are encouraged to practice in a manner that sets a higher bar of ethical conduct (for example, abiding by the health worker elements of the WHO Code, regardless of its legislative status in the IBCLC's country).

E.	Every IBCLC is required to practice in accordance with the principles of the Code of Professional Conduct.

1.	Principle 1 requires IBCLCs to "provide services that protect, promote and support breastfeeding."[2(p2)]

a.	This principle embraces the concept of family-centered and culturally sensitive care. Social, cultural, religious, political, familial, and personal beliefs about breastfeeding vary widely. IBCLCs should provide information and support in a manner that is respectful of the personal and cultural beliefs of the family to help them meet their infant feeding goals.

b.	In partnership with the family, IBCLCs strive to understand these goals and needs and provide the most up-to-date information and evidence-informed care in a compassionate and caring manner. This helps the family make informed decisions about their care.

c.	Caution is to be exercised when a perceived conflict exists (e.g., a hospital or a private-practice IBCLC has the potential for financial gain from equipment rental or sales).

i.	The family should recognize that the recommendation to use equipment is based on their clinical need, not on the lactation caregiver's financial interests.

ii.	When consulting with a family about the use of any commercial product (e.g., a medical device, such as a breast pump, or equipment for supplemental feedings), information should be unbiased and tailored to the family's clinical needs.

2. Principle 2 requires IBCLCs to "act with due diligence."[2(p2)]
    a. This principle discusses the IBLCE Scope of Practice,[4] which describes the boundaries within which IBCLCs may practice.
        i. The aim of the Scope of Practice is to protect the public by ensuring safe, competent, and evidence-informed care.
        ii. The Scope of Practice defines the areas in which IBCLCs are educated and have clinical skills, as authorized by IBCLC certification.
        iii. Also helpful in describing the range and boundaries of IBCLC expertise is the ILCA *Position Paper on the Role and Impact of the IBCLC*.[10] This document substantiates the assertion that IBCLCs play an integral role in the health care of a family as an advocate, clinical expert, collaborator, educator, facilitator, investigator, policy consultant, professional, and promoter. It can be an effective advocacy tool to explain and support the need for IBCLC-specific care within a healthcare system.
    b. This principle stresses the collaborative nature of the role of IBCLCs.
        i. IBCLCs must work with other members of the healthcare team in taking care of the family so that lactation care can be aligned with and included in the overall care plan (a notion underscored by the IBLCE's Advisory Opinion on Assessment, Diagnosis, and Referral).[13]
        ii. IBCLCs do not practice medicine nor diagnose, but they do assess, document, and refer for diagnosis.
    c. IBCLCs should take responsibility for their personal behavior and clinical practice, regardless of practice setting; obey laws governing practice by IBCLCs or similar allied healthcare providers; and adhere to the rules and policies in place at the work setting.
    d. IBCLCs are specifically required to respect intellectual property rights, which is a vast area of law governing copyrights, trademarks, service marks, and patents. The implication is that intellectual property law infringement is a de facto violation of the IBLCE Code of Professional Conduct.
        i. Permission must be obtained to use any copyright-protected material.
        ii. Seeking permission to use another person's copyright-protected materials can be as simple as sending an email to the originator describing the material that is sought for reuse and the conditions under which it will be shown and credited.
        iii. IBCLCs should receive permission before using the material and retain proof of the permission sought and granted to defend any challenge to its use.
        iv. IBCLCs who prepare scholarly works (position papers, book chapters, or articles for publication in a professional journal or text) may cite sources in a bibliography, without prior permission, under the traditional conventions of academic and professional writing. When giving educational presentations that discuss another's work, the original author should be credited.
    e. IBCLCs must obey all applicable laws for the workplace and geopolitical setting where they practice.
3. Principle 3 requires IBCLCs to "preserve the confidentiality of clients."[2(p2)]
    a. IBCLCs may not reveal information about a family or a lactation consultation unless the client permits it, it is required as part of a court or legal proceeding, or when imminent harm is suspected.
    b. Of particular note is the high standard for the use of any images. Prior written consent must be obtained from the parent before any images are obtained, for any use whatsoever, of the parent or child.
    c. Prior permission is not required from the client for IBCLCs to discuss the case anonymously with colleagues who are not part of the healthcare team. However, it is good practice to ask as a matter of respect because the client has placed trust in the lactation caregiver. IBCLCs must be cognizant to avoid using bits of information that may unwittingly identify the parent.
    d. Particular care should be taken to avoid the use of client identification clues when sharing case studies on websites or at conferences. IBCLCs must not share details that have even a remote chance of specifically identifying the parent and child, unless the parent has first consented. It is best practice for IBCLCs to receive permission to discuss the case in such a forum, even if the family is not to be identified.

4. Principle 4 requires IBCLCs to "report accurately and completely to other members of the health-care team."[2(p3)]

   a. This principle describes the IBCLC's responsibility to share information about the lactation consultation with other members of the family's healthcare team.

      i. Receiving permission from the parent to share health concerns with the primary health-care provider is a precondition of care.

      ii. In certain rare circumstances, the parent may have legitimate reasons to not have their identifying information sent to a healthcare provider. For example, if the parent and children are at risk and under protection from domestic abuse or threats, the parent will not want the home address and phone number included in a report to the pediatrician if the child's other parent can access the pediatric file. IBCLCs should speak to the healthcare provider by phone or in person to describe the lactation assessment and care plan. IBCLCs should also describe the reasons for the verbal report in the parent's lactation chart.

   b. This principle recognizes that IBCLCs, as caregivers in the earliest days after birth, may identify early warning signs of possible health or personal safety complications.

      i. When the health and safety of either the parent, baby, or a coworker is at risk or appears to be at risk, IBCLCs should inform the involved parties and, if appropriate, supervisors and authorities.

      ii. IBCLCs have a responsibility for the safety of parents and children and to the profession of lactation consulting. IBCLCs who are practicing under conditions in which health, safety, or professional decision making are compromised or at risk cannot provide competent, ethical care.

      iii. When other IBCLCs become aware of or suspect such professional liabilities in a colleague, they should consider addressing their concerns with the colleague in question. They should also share these concerns with the lactation consultant's supervisor or administrator to trigger appropriate remedial and mitigating measures.

      iv. In many countries, IBCLCs are legally required to report any suspicion of child abuse to the appropriate authorities. Although there is no mandatory requirement to report a suspicion of domestic partner violence, IBCLCs should be aware of and provide information about available resources to safely assist the client.

5. Principle 5 requires IBCLCs to "exercise independent judgment and avoid conflicts of interest."[2(p3)]

   a. Full and advance disclosure of relationships that constitute real or perceived conflicts of interest, coupled with a consent to consult, is important to maintain public trust in an IBCLC's professional practice.

   b. Generally speaking, a conflict of interest arises when an IBCLC appears to be more concerned about their own professional or financial interests than those of the client. Fully disclosing any relationship with any commercial entity is important to maintain professional integrity.

   c. When clinically indicated, IBCLCs can, and should, talk about the use of breastfeeding equipment and supplies with a parent. The brand names, prices, advantages, and disadvantages must all be discussed so the family can make a fully informed decision about the care plan that will work best for them, given their circumstances. IBCLCs should be certain the parent is aware that the discussion about products is a necessary element in devising the care plan and is not because the IBCLC has any financial interest in the outcome of the consultation.

   d. A conflict of interest does not prevent a consultation from occurring. A conflict of interest can be negated by full disclosure of the IBCLC's interests before the consultation begins and with the family's consent to proceed.

   e. IBCLCs who teach in a program that awards IBLCE-approved continuing education recognition points must avoid any affiliation with commercial entities when preparing, delivering, or being compensated for teaching. An IBLCE policy warns that such an affiliation may deny or void the continuing education recognition point award and that it violates elements of the IBLCE Code of Professional Conduct pertaining to conflicts of interest.[21]

6. Principle 6 requires IBCLCs to "maintain personal integrity."[2(p4)]
   a. IBCLCs must be just and honest in their professional practice.
   b. IBCLCs must treat all families fairly and equitably, harboring no ill will or prejudice based on the characteristics or circumstances of the client.
   c. IBCLCs who are impaired by addiction or substance abuse could render compromised care, placing the public in danger. Such an IBCLC should withdraw from practice until the addiction or abuse has been addressed with an effective treatment and recovery program. When the IBCLC is meeting all recovery program requirements, they can resume practice.
   d. If an IBCLC already has an established professional relationship and cannot put aside personal bias for whatever reason, a referral to another lactation provider must occur, and client files must be forwarded. If a professional relationship has not yet commenced, it is not obligatory, but it is helpful, to share resources for finding other lactation caregivers with the family.

7. Principle 7 requires IBCLCs to "uphold the professional standards expected of an IBCLC."[2(p4)]
   a. Every IBCLC is expected to use professional behaviors that conform to those described in the Code of Professional Conduct.
   b. Any advertising or marketing of IBCLC services must accurately and honestly describe what a lactation consultation involves: how fees, payment, or reimbursement are handled; the IBCLC's obligation to share concerns with other healthcare providers; the protection of private health information; the parent's role in devising and implementing a care plan; and how follow-up is arranged.
   c. A family expecting to be seen by an IBCLC must be seen by an IBCLC, not another kind of lactation care provider. Only those who are currently certified by the IBLCE as an IBCLC may use that acronym and title.
   d. It is impossible for IBCLCs to guarantee a particular breastfeeding outcome.
      i. IBCLCs can provide evidence-based information and support and deliver professional services in a responsive, efficient, and ethical manner.
      ii. IBCLCs should strive to help every client achieve the breastfeeding goal and the best possible health outcome.
   e. IBCLCs may work with or supervise other lactation care providers. Indeed, parent-to-parent counselors are the backbone of most community-based breastfeeding support programs around the world.
      i. The client must always have a clear understanding of the limitations in the clinical care that a non-IBCLC can provide.
      ii. IBCLCs may serve as mentors and help train and educate those who are fulfilling requirements to become an IBCLC. As time progresses, those students operate with diminishing direct supervision. These clinical training arrangements are an acceptable and ethical means to educate trainees. The family should always be informed that part of their consultation is being spent with a student, with oversight provided by the responsible IBCLC.
      iii. The use of terms such as *IBCLC candidate* or *student IBCLC* are potentially misleading to the public. The student is advised to use a generic descriptor, such as *student lactation consultant* or *lactation trainee*.

8. Principle 8 requires IBCLCs to "comply with the IBLCE Disciplinary Procedures."[2(p4)]
   a. This principle governs the disciplinary procedures of the IBLCE Ethics and Discipline Committee that are intended to enforce the Code of Professional Conduct and to protect the health, safety, and welfare of the public.
   b. The process and procedures for handling complaints are detailed in the IBLCE Disciplinary Procedures.[3]
   c. IBCLCs may be disciplined under the auspices of other licenses or certifications they carry, which is an automatic violation of the IBLCE Code of Professional Conduct. IBCLCs should evaluate their practice and behavior to ensure that they provide professional and ethical practice, protect the public, and minimize the risk of violations of the Code of Professional Conduct and subsequent disciplinary complaints. For details about how to report a violation of the Code of Professional Conduct, refer to the IBLCE website (www.iblce.org).

F.   IBLCE Advisory Opinions describe the organization's positions about expected and acceptable professional behaviors.

   1.   IBLCE has issued three Advisory Opinions:
      a.   Frenulotomy.[11]
      b.   Professionalism in the Social Media Age.[12]
      c.   Assessment, Diagnosis, and Referral.[13]
   2.   The other way to learn how the IBLCE evaluates IBCLC behaviors is by reviewing published public sanctions after an Ethics and Discipline Committee case has been adjudicated.

V. The IBLCE Scope of Practice for IBCLC Certificants

A.   A scope of practice is a defined list of skill areas in which a practitioner may engage.

B.   The IBLCE Scope of Practice describes clinical, educational, professional, and advocacy activities in which a certified IBCLC may engage. Refer to the IBLCE website (www.iblce.org) for the most current version of the Scope of Practice, which is periodically reviewed and updated by the IBLCE.

CLINICAL TIP

The IBLCE Scope of Practice clearly defines the IBCLC's role as a member of the healthcare team. The Scope of Practice for IBCLCs who have additional training (e.g., speech pathology, midwifery, doctor of medicine, registered dietitian, registered nurse) might encompass a wider range of clinical competencies. Those who hold more than one credential must be clear as to which clinical role they are assuming when consulting with a breastfeeding parent. Scopes of practice are meant to describe and define all practices in which the practitioner is allowed to engage. They are not intended to list forbidden practices.

C.   The Scope of Practice describes activities in which IBCLCs can competently engage. IBCLCs who are challenged to substantiate why their professional behaviors are within the IBLCE Scope of Practice will need to demonstrate how their actions and practice were fairly contained within the clinical, educational, advocacy, and professional activities described by the Scope of Practice.

D.   The Scope of Practice lists six major duties for which IBCLCs have specialized skill and training to practice with competent and evidence-based care to protect the public.

   1.   IBCLC certificants have the duty to uphold the standards of the IBCLC profession.
      a.   This duty requires IBCLCs to practice under ethical and professional guidelines described by the IBLCE Code of Professional Conduct, while competently providing the clinical care and education enumerated in the IBLCE clinical competencies, IBLCE detailed content outline,[22] and within the legal framework of the practice setting and geopolitical setting.
         i.   The legal framework encompasses laws, regulations, and institutional policies in the IBCLC's work setting.
         ii.   IBCLCs must follow the rules of the place where they work. Despite international certification demonstrating that IBCLCs are educated and trained in the same lactation-related subjects, they work in vastly different settings.
         iii. Policies and procedures for IBCLCs can differ in hospitals that are across the street from one another. This does not prevent IBCLCs from seeking to change policies by educating their peers and superiors if current policies are no longer supported by evidence-based and best practices.
      b.   IBCLCs must stay up to date on emerging and evolving clinical practice based on new research.
   2.   IBCLC certificants have the duty to protect, promote, and support breastfeeding.
      a.   Breastfeeding advocacy encompasses preconception to weaning and applies to everyone from parents to the community at large.
         i.   It includes providing education at all ages in the school system, from elementary to postgraduate.
         ii.   It involves preventive health care, from infancy until weaning.
      b.   IBCLCs should educate families and colleagues and seek substantive policy changes.

    c.   IBCLCs who offer holistic care are concerned about the whole person, including medical, biological, and social factors, not just treatment of symptoms.

    d.   Evidence-based practice will guide how IBCLCs provide their expertise.

3.   IBCLC certificants have the duty to provide competent services for parents and families.

    a.   This duty defines the boundaries (or scope) within which IBCLC clinical expertise rests.

    b.   A comprehensive assessment of the parent and child, and an assessment of an entire feeding and sometimes multiple feedings at the breast, will be needed for IBCLCs to identify issues that may require a care plan.

    c.   A thorough lactation assessment may identify a situation requiring a referral for a definitive diagnosis or a medication. IBCLCs are not authorized to make a diagnosis or instruct a parent on which medications should be used.

        i.   Families are entitled to evidence-based information about the impact on lactation of complementary therapies, drugs, alcohol, and tobacco.

        ii.   IBCLCs can tell parents how lactation may be impacted if various substances are ingested and how complementary therapies may be part of a lactation care plan.

    d.   This duty requires a lactation care plan to be developed in consultation with the parent, using teaching principles of family-centered care.

        i.   IBCLCs have a duty to help parents successfully meet their infant feeding goals. This is different from simply helping the parent breastfeed.

        ii.   Not all parents breastfeed, and not all families provide human milk the same way. A family may include adoptive parents, same-sex parents, grandparents raising their grandchildren, or parents who have had surgeries that curtail lactation. All are entitled to learn how to induce lactation, maximize milk production, obtain safe donor human milk, and use special feeding devices to assist them (including the benefits and risks associated with the devices).

4.   IBCLC certificants have the duty to report truthfully and fully to the parent's or infant's primary healthcare provider and to the healthcare system.

    a.   IBCLCs should chart or prepare reports accurately and as close in time to the consultation as possible.

    b.   The mandatory IBLCE *Documentation Guidelines*[6] offer basic suggestions for clinical record keeping.

5.   IBCLC certificants have the duty to preserve client confidence.

    a.   It is the duty of all IBCLCs to preserve the privacy of the client. This is a common requirement for any practitioner in any healthcare profession.

    b.   Use the client's name only when in confidential discussions with other healthcare providers; discuss the case anonymously with others who may offer clinical insight but are not in the circle of care.

    c.   Take care not to allow client files to be seen or copied.

    d.   Be aware of privacy laws and regulations for the geopolitical setting (such as the U.S. Health Insurance Portability and Accountability Act [HIPAA] requirement to provide a notice of privacy practices[23]), in addition to this Scope of Practice mandate.

    e.   Although social media platforms are a great way to share general information of interest, they are nonsecure, nonprivate platforms that are inappropriate for any kind of specific clinical discussion of a case, even if the family has agreed to let the situation be discussed.

        i.   Not even parental permission can remove the privacy requirements IBCLCs must meet (such as electronic security standards for HIPAA in the United States, described under the Health Information Technology for Economic and Clinical Health [HITECH] Act).[24]

        ii.   Telemedicine platforms differ; they are often encrypted, secure, and intended for one-to-one communication.

        iii.   Using public social media or cloud-based electronic systems for specific clinical discussions presents privacy risks and is fraught with the possibility for misunderstanding, given the two-dimensional nature of communication. For additional guidance, see the IBLCE Advisory Opinion on Professionalism in the Social Media Age.[12]

6.   IBCLC certificants have the duty to act with reasonable diligence.

    a.   *Reasonable diligence* is a significant phrase in the eyes of the law. It admonishes IBCLCs to exhibit professional excellence in the exercise of any activity described under all duties in the IBLCE Scope of Practice.

b.   This includes the duty to uphold the standards of the profession; the duty to promote, protect, and support breastfeeding; the duty to provide competent services; the duty to report truthfully and fully; and the duty to preserve client confidence.

VI. IBLCE Clinical Competencies for IBCLC Practice

A.   The IBLCE clinical competencies are patterned after, and expand upon, each of the six duties described in the IBLCE Scope of Practice.

   1.   Customarily, a clinical competency statement simply describes the skills for which a healthcare practitioner has particular training and expertise.

   2.   The IBLCE clinical competencies detail the clinical, educational, and advocacy practices that a healthcare practitioner might be called upon to use, given the particular needs of the family being served.

B.   The language of the clinical competencies identifies skills (described as *duties*) that expand each of the broader six duty and clinical areas defined in the IBLCE Scope of Practice.

   1.   IBCLCs do not have a duty to cover each of these clinical areas at each consultation. The clinical competencies simply describe, in great detail, all of the topics about which an IBCLC has some expertise.

   2.   IBCLCs might discuss some of these competencies if teaching and clinical topics are relevant in a lactation consultation. Other elements might be covered in advocacy and education venues where the IBCLC is sharing knowledge and expertise, for example.

VII. ILCA Standards of Practice for IBCLCs

A.   The ILCA was formed in 1985 as a voluntary international professional membership association.

   1.   Open to anyone who supports and promotes breastfeeding, the ILCA membership primarily includes IBCLCs who care for breastfeeding families.

   2.   The ILCA offers continuing education and professional development opportunities; promotes IBCLCs and the profession to the public; engages in international policy making as a nongovernmental organization, with recognized status at the WHO; and publishes the *Journal of Human Lactation*, a peer-reviewed scientific journal.[25]

B.   The ILCA Standards of Practice[9] serves as a compendium of best professional practices in which IBCLCs should engage. Failure to do so, however, brings no sanctions.

C.   The Standards of Practice offers a guideline of tasks and skills that IBCLCs "should be able to perform in the course of fulfilling the duties of the profession."[9(p1)] The four major standards are described here. Refer to the ILCA website (www.ilca.org) for the most current version of this important practice-guiding document, which is periodically reviewed and updated.

   1.   Standard 1, Professional Responsibilities, says "the IBCLC has a responsibility to maintain professional conduct and to practice in an ethical manner, accountable for professional actions and legal responsibilities."[9(p2)]

      a.   Many of the model behaviors described as IBCLC professional responsibilities echo those described in the IBLCE Code of Professional Conduct and Scope of Practice.

      b.   The discretionary, best practices, or model professional activities should encompass and mirror the mandatory behaviors.

      c.   The ILCA Standards of Practice outline expected practices clearly, succinctly, and with an active voice, indicating what to do and what actions to refrain from.

   2.   Standard 2, Legal Considerations, says "the IBCLC is obligated to practice within the laws of the geopolitical region and setting in which the IBCLC works . . . [and] must practice with consideration for rights of privacy and with respect for matters of a confidential nature."[9(p2)]

      a.   IBCLCs who follow the laws of their land and the rules of their workplace operate to the highest professional standard.

      b.   Workplace rules and procedures may vary, sometimes widely, within the same region. IBCLCs may worry that they are practicing at risk of liability if their clinical approach (dictated by their facility's policies and procedures) differs from facilities nearby.

      c.   IBCLCs may always seek to change policies within a facility if newer research suggests a revision in policy. Because IBCLCs are obligated to practice evidence-informed care, they should attempt to make changes, but the responsibility to effectuate change does not rest solely with IBCLCs.

  3. Standard 3, Clinical Practice, says "IBCLC practice focuses on providing clinical lactation care and management."[9(p3)]

      a.   "This is best accomplished by promoting optimal health through collaboration and problem-solving with the patient/client and other members of the health care team."[9(p3)]

      b.   For IBCLCs, the best clinical practice is accomplished when the parent and the entire healthcare team collaborate on a plan of care.

         i.   As a practical matter, IBCLCs will construct the care plan with the family's assistance then, if the situation warrants, share the plan with the primary healthcare providers to keep them apprised of the IBCLC's interventions.

        ii.   A lactation consultation ideally involves a comprehensive assessment, plan development, realistic implementation elements, and an opportunity for evaluation and revision of the foregoing. The importance of ongoing communication cannot be overemphasized.

  4. Standard 4, Breastfeeding Education and Counseling, says that "breastfeeding education and counseling are integral parts of the care provided by the IBCLC."[9(p4)]

      a.   The education of families and healthcare providers is a large part of the IBCLC's role.

      b.   Effective teaching allows for informed decision making by the client. Involving family members in discussing care that accounts for their personal needs and special considerations will make it feasible for them to follow the care plan.

      c.   Education is the cornerstone of advocacy efforts to change administrative or public health policies that involve breastfeeding and lactation.

VIII. Practice Guidance for Lactation Care from Other Professional Organizations

  A. Guidance for breastfeeding and lactation care comes from many sources beyond the IBLCE and ILCA.

  B. Other healthcare providers, parent–peer supporters, public health policy advocates, and organizations establish baselines of professional care for breastfeeding families.

    1. United States Breastfeeding Committee's core competencies:

      a.   The United States Breastfeeding Committee (USBC) is a U.S. governmental, nonprofit, cross-disciplinary advocacy organization for breastfeeding promotion and protection.

      b.   The USBC identified core competencies for basic breastfeeding and lactation care that any healthcare provider—regardless of specialty or practice area—should be able to meet.

      c.   The competencies were developed to "provide health professionals with a guideline and framework to integrate evidence-based breastfeeding knowledge, skills, and attitudes into their standard health care delivery practices."[26(p2)] The core competencies are available online at no charge.

    2. Academy of Breastfeeding Medicine's (ABM) protocols and position papers:

      a.   The ABM is a worldwide organization of physicians who are dedicated to the promotion, protection, and support of breastfeeding and human lactation.

      b.   The ABM has several position statements on breastfeeding advocacy matters and scores of evidence-based best practice clinical protocols for offering care on various lactation-related matters.

      c.   All of these resources are available free online for public access and are offered in several languages.[27]

    3. U.S. Surgeon General's call to action to support breastfeeding:

      a.   The Surgeon General is the leading public health authority for the United States.

      b.   The advocacy statement urges "support of family members, communities, clinicians, health care systems, and employers . . . to make breastfeeding become the easy choice, the default choice."[28(p37)]

    4. American Academy of Pediatrics (AAP):

      a.   The AAP, officially a U.S.-based professional organization, has worldwide esteem, and pediatricians from all over the globe favorably cite AAP policies to guide their practice.

      b.   The AAP policy on breastfeeding and the use of human milk[29] provides core endorsement for breastfeeding as a public health imperative.

5. American College of Obstetricians and Gynecologists (ACOG):
   a. The ACOG enjoys international esteem, and their website (www.acog.org) offers several web-based resources available to the public.
   b. A tool kit, clinical guidelines, and protocols are offered for healthcare providers.
   c. Materials also link families in need to breastfeeding resources.[30]
6. Emergency Nutrition Network (ENN):
   a. The ENN is an interagency international group that provides training and guidance for relief workers caring for families in natural or manmade disasters.
   b. Its operational guidance on infant feeding in emergencies (OG-IFE) version 3.0 offers strong policy guidance to help families with young children fleeing disasters and to avoid practices that could disrupt lactation (such as distribution of formula and feeding supplies in a manner that disrupts breastfeeding).[31]
7. These are just a few of the numerous examples that healthcare providers from many disciplines might find.
   a. There are similar organizations throughout the world offering guidance within their profession for ethical and clinical care for breastfeeding and families who use human milk.
   b. It is incumbent upon any healthcare provider who is licensed or certified beyond IBCLC to be familiar with the obligations and guidance offered by their profession.

▶ Key Points from This Chapter

A. There are many kinds of breastfeeding and lactation supporters (volunteer and paid) who are eager to help new families.
B. There are primary healthcare providers who have made an effort to learn more about breastfeeding and lactation because their formal education rarely requires it.
C. Although many IBCLCs practice under the authority of that credential alone, others have earned the IBCLC credential in addition to a preexisting healthcare professional license or registration.
D. When offering support to families, the practitioner must be cognizant of the obligations mandated by ethical codes of professional conduct, scopes of practice, and workplace rules.
E. The lactation practitioner should endeavor to follow the best practices described in discretionary model practice-guiding documents.

🔍 CASE STUDY

Cate is 10 days postpartum, having delivered baby Mari at the local birth center. Cate and Mari have been home for 7 days, and Cate's mother calls the postpartum care team at the birth center with questions about Mari's feeding patterns. Cate and her mother bring Mari to the center to meet with you. Cate's mother is carrying Mari, and Cate appears exhausted, with large circles under her eyes. At the beginning of the session Cate barely participates in the conversation, and her mother is outspoken and appears to be solicitous of Cate's needs. Cate's mother asks questions about how often Mari should eat and how many wet and dirty diapers are expected. You ask if Mari is receiving only breastmilk, and Cate's mother confirms that all feeds are at the breast. Cate is still not interactive and sits slumped in a chair. When she is questioned directly, Cate mumbles or her mother answers. You ask to talk with Cate alone, and her mother takes Mari for a short walk. With further questioning, Cate says she is scared to hold her baby and is not sleeping well because of worry about acting impulsively and harming Mari. Cate mumbles that her mother cannot keep Mari safe from the bad people who are after them, then she starts crying and quits responding. When her mother and Mari return a few minutes later, Cate is staring into space and unresponsive.

Questions
1. What is your impression of Cate's mental status at the visit?
2. What follow-up is appropriate regarding Cate's situation?

References

1. Massachusetts Breastfeeding Coalition. The landscape of breastfeeding support. Massachusetts Breastfeeding Coalition website. https://massbreastfeeding.org/landscape/. Published March 30, 2014. Accessed October 10, 2017.

2. International Board of Lactation Consultant Examiners. Code of professional conduct for IBCLCs. International Board of Lactation Consultant Examiners website. https://iblce.org/wp-content/uploads/2017/05/code-of-professional-conduct.pdf. Published September 2015. Accessed September 26, 2017.

3. International Board of Lactation Consultant Examiners. Disciplinary procedures for the code of professional conduct for IBCLCs for the International Board of Lactation Consultant Examiners (IBLCE). International Board of Lactation Consultant Examiners website. https://iblce.org/wp-content/uploads/2017/05/disciplinary-procedures.pdf. Updated November 3, 2016. Accessed October 10, 2017.

4. International Board of Lactation Consultant Examiners. Scope of practice for International Board Certified Lactation Consultant (IBCLC) certificants. International Board of Lactation Consultant Examiners website. https://iblce.org/wp-content/uploads/2017/05/scope-of-practice.pdf. Published September 15, 2012. Accessed October 10, 2017.

5. International Board of Lactation Consultant Examiners. Clinical competencies for the practice of International Board Certified Lactation Consultants (IBCLCs). International Board of Lactation Consultant Examiners website. https://iblce.org/wp-content/uploads/2017/05/clinical-competencies.pdf. Published September 15, 2012. Accessed October 10, 2017.

6. International Board of Lactation Consultant Examiners. IBLCE documentation guidelines. International Board of Lactation Consultant Examiners website. https://iblce.org/wp-content/uploads/2017/05/documentation-guidelines.pdf. Published February 28, 2012. Accessed October 10, 2017.

7. World Health Organization. International code of marketing of breast-milk substitutes. World Health Organization website. http://www.who.int/nutrition/publications/code_english.pdf. Published 1981. Accessed October 10, 2017.

8. International Baby Food Action Network. The full code. International Baby Food Action Network website. http://ibfan.org/the-full-code. Accessed October 10, 2017.

9. International Lactation Consultant Association. Standards of practice for international board certified lactation consultants. International Lactation Consultant Association website. https://higherlogicdownload.s3.amazonaws.com/ILCA/e3ee2b6e-c389-43de-83ea-f32482f20da5/UploadedImages/Learning/Resources/Standards%20of%20Practice%20for%20International%20Board%20Certified%20Lactation%20Consultants%20(newlogo).pdf. Revised December 2013. Accessed October 10, 2017.

10. International Lactation Consultant Association. Position paper on the role and impact of the IBCLC. International Lactation Consultant Association website. https://higherlogicdownload.s3.amazonaws.com/ILCA/e3ee2b6e-c389-43de-83ea-f32482f20da5/UploadedImages/WHY%20IBCLC/Role%20of%20IBCLC/Role%20%20Impact%20of%20the%20IBCLC.pdf. Published June 2011. Accessed October 10, 2017.

11. International Board of Lactation Consultant Examiners. Advisory opinion—frenulotomy. International Board of Lactation Consultant Examiners website. https://iblce.org/wp-content/uploads/2017/05/advisory-opinion-frenulotomy-english.pdf. Published February 2013. Accessed October 10, 2017.

12. International Board of Lactation Consultant Examiners. Advisory opinion: professionalism in the social media age. International Board of Lactation Consultant Examiners website. https://iblce.org/wp-content/uploads/2017/11/Advisory-Opinion-Social-Media-Professionalism.pdf. Published September 2015. Accessed October 10, 2017.

13. International Board of Lactation Consultant Examiners. Advisory opinion: assessment, diagnosis, and referral. International Board of Lactation Consultant Examiners website. https://iblce.org/wp-content/uploads/2017/05/advisory-opinion-assessment-diagnosis-referral-english.pdf. Published March 22, 2017. Accessed October 10, 2017.

14. International Board of Lactation Consultant Examiners. Frequently asked questions (FAQs) regarding the code of professional conduct for IBCLCs. International Board of Lactation Consultant Examiners website. https://iblce.org/wp-content/uploads/2017/05/code-of-professional-conduct-faqs.pdf. Published March 2013. Accessed October 10, 2017.

15. International Board of Lactation Consultant Examiners. Step 1: prepare for IBCLC certification. International Board of Lactation Consultant Examiners website. https://iblce.org/certify/eligibility-criteria/. Accessed October 10, 2017.

16. Institute for Credentialing Excellence. NCCA accreditation process and resources (table: NCCA certification accreditation: self-assessment checklist). Institute for Credentialing Excellence website. http://www.credentialingexcellence.org/p/cm/ld/fid=87. Accessed October 10, 2017.

17. Institute for Credentialing Excellence. NCCA accreditation. Institute for Credentialing Excellence website. http://www.credentialingexcellence.org/p/cm/ld/fid=86. Published 2017. Accessed October 10, 2017.

18. United Nations. Convention on the elimination of all forms of discrimination against women (article 12). United Nations website. http://www.un.org/womenwatch/daw/cedaw/. Published 1979. Accessed October 10, 2017.

19. United Nations. Convention on the rights of the child. United Nations website. http://www.ohchr.org/EN/ProfessionalInterest/Pages/CRC.aspx. Published November 20, 1989. Accessed October 10, 2017.

20. Council of Medical Specialty Societies. Code for interactions with companies. Council of Medical Specialty Societies website. https://cmss.org/wp-content/uploads/2016/02/CMSS-Code-for-Interactions-with-Companies-Approved-Revised-Version-4.13.15-with-Annotations.pdf. Published April 2015. Accessed September 26, 2017.

21. International Board of Lactation Consultant Examiners. Minimising commercial influence on education policy. International Board of Lactation Consultant Examiners website. https://iblce.org/wp-content/uploads/2017/05/minimising-commercial-influence-on-education-policy.pdf. Published May 1, 2017. Accessed October 10, 2017.

22. International Board of Lactation Consultant Examiners. International Board Certified Lactation Consultant (IBCLC) detailed content outline. International Board of Lactation Consultant Examiners website. https://iblce.org/wp-content/uploads/2017/05/ibclc-detailed-content-outline-for-2016-for-publication.pdf. Published 2014. Updated January 2016. Accessed October 10, 2017.

23. U.S. Department of Health and Human Services. Notice of privacy practices for protected health information. U.S. Department of Health and Human Services website. https://www.hhs.gov/hipaa/for-professionals/privacy/guidance/privacy-practices-for-protected-health-information/index.html. Updated July 26, 2013. Accessed October 10, 2017.

24. U.S. Congress. Omnibus final rule, including Health Information Technology for Economic and Clinical Health Act (HITECH). 78 Fed. Reg. 5566. Government Publishing Office website. https://www.gpo.gov/fdsys/pkg/FR-2013-01-25/pdf/2013-01073.pdf. Published January 25, 2013. Accessed October 10, 2017.

25. International Lactation Consultant Association. About ILCA. International Lactation Consultant Association website. http://www.ilca.org/about/values-vision-mission. Published 2017. Accessed October 10, 2017.

26. United States Breastfeeding Committee. Core competencies in breastfeeding care and services for all health professionals. United States Breastfeeding Committee website. http://www.usbreastfeeding.org/core-competencies. Published 2010. Accessed October 10, 2017.

27. Academy of Breastfeeding Medicine. Resources. Academy of Breastfeeding Medicine website. http://www.bfmed.org/resources. Accessed January 15, 2018.

28. U.S. Surgeon General. The Surgeon General's call to action to support breastfeeding. U.S. Department of Health and Human Services website. https://www.surgeongeneral.gov/library/calls/breastfeeding/index.html. Published 2011. Accessed October 10, 2017.

29. American Academy of Pediatrics. Breastfeeding and the use of human milk. American Academy of Pediatrics website. http://pediatrics.aappublications.org/content/129/3/e827.full#content-block. Published March 2012. Accessed October 10, 2017.

30. American Congress of Obstetricians and Gynecologists. Breastfeeding. American Congress of Obstetricians and Gynecologists website. https://www.acog.org/About-ACOG/ACOG-Departments/Breastfeeding. Accessed October 10, 2017.

31. Emergency Nutrition Network. Operational guidance on infant feeding in emergencies (OG-IFE) version 3.0. Emergency Nutrition Network website. http://www.ennonline.net/operationalguidance-v3-2017. Published October 2017. Accessed October 10, 2017.

32. Association of Women's Health, Obstetric and Neonatal Nurses. Breastfeeding. Journal of Obstetric, Gynecologic and Neonatal Nursing website. http://www.jognn.org/article/S0884-2175(15)31769-X/pdf. Published November 2014. Accessed October 10, 2017.

33. Academy of Nutrition and Dietetics. Practice paper: promoting and supporting breastfeeding. EatRightPRO website. www.eatrightpro.org/resource/practice/position-and-practice-papers/practice-papers/practice-paper-promoting-and-supporting-breastfeeding. Published March 2015. Accessed January 15, 2018.

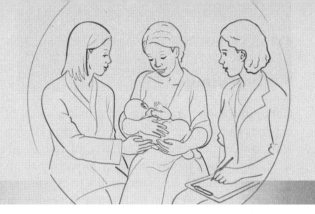

CHAPTER 26
Counseling and Communication

Laurie K. Scherer
Angela Love-Zaranka

OBJECTIVES

- Use effective counseling techniques for supporting families.
- Identify sources of breastfeeding support for the family.
- Apply the counseling process to real-life situations.
- Modify communication based on family composition, language differences, culture, and specific situations such as bereavement.
- Identify different learning styles and limitations in communication abilities.
- Respect patient privacy in real-life patient encounters.
- Describe the responsibility to report child abuse.
- Communicate effectively with other healthcare providers to support the family in attaining their breastfeeding goals.

DEFINITIONS OF COMMONLY USED TERMS

active listening A communication technique in which the listener attends to the speaker and reflects back understanding of the content and the meaning of the speaker's statements.

motivational interviewing A counseling technique designed to meet clients at their point of willingness to change and to support clients in incremental steps toward a goal.

rapport A close and harmonious relationship in which people or groups seek to understand each other's feelings or ideas and work to communicate well.

shared decision making An approach to working collaboratively in a medical setting that gives agency to the individual patient or family along with important medical information from the healthcare team.

vicarious trauma The emotional impact of witnessing the pain, fear, or terrors that trauma causes in clients and families. Vicarious trauma may lead to burnout, or helper fatigue.

Any use of the term *mother*, *maternal*, or *breastfeeding* is not meant to exclude transgender or nonbinary parents who may be breastfeeding or providing human milk to their infant.

▶ Overview

Communication depends on the provider's state of mind and approach to the counseling situation as much as it depends on having good clinical knowledge. Utilizing effective communication and counseling skills builds rapport with families, allowing them to feel comfortable and able to receive new information. A respectful relationship builds trust, improves a family's capacity to participate in their care, and allows them to adopt behaviors to reach their goals. A lactation consultant's ability to explain, listen, and empathize can have a profound effect on self-efficacy. Effective communication results in positive interactions with colleagues to provide support services to a family and increases positive interactions during unexpected events.

I. Counseling Basics

A. Lactation consultants must understand the basic goals of counseling.
    1. Helping families successfully breastfeed requires the consultant to have knowledge about breast-feeding and clinical skills and to have good communication skills.
    2. The first contact with a family can set the tone for the entire helping relationship.
    3. Utilizing effective communication skills begins with active listening, which includes the following:
        a. Attending to communication by facing the family and utilizing appropriate eye contact.
        b. Responding appropriately by using rephrasing and questions.
    4. To be effective, clinical information needs to be shared with the family to allow:
        a. The family to understand the information.
        b. The family to utilize the information to make the best decisions for them.
    5. Attend to nonverbal communication to obtain more cues about the mental status and capabilities of family members.[1] (See Chapter 18, *Maternal Mental Health and Breastfeeding*.)
        a. The types of nonverbal communication include the following:
            i. Gestures.
            ii. Posture.
            iii. Body movements.
            iv. Eye contact and movement.
            v. Tone of voice.
            vi. Facial expression.
        b. Certain forms of nonverbal communication may have different meanings to members of different cultures.
B. Skills to facilitate communication include the following:
    1. Maintain appropriate eye contact to encourage sharing.
    2. Attend to nonverbal communication.
    3. Notice which family members answer questions.
    4. Observe communication patterns to gain insight into the roles and influences within the family.
    5. Notice language comprehension differences that might affect communication.
    6. Watch for indications of understanding, such as head nods and appropriate responses.[1]
    7. If there is no clear indication that the family understands, ask for feedback.
    8. Listen for specific words the family uses to refer to body parts or relationships and use the same ter-minology, if appropriate, while offering technical and scientific terms that will help the family com-municate effectively with medical personnel.
    9. To build respect and rapport, provide the family with full attention and allow them time to formulate full responses.[1]
    10. If communication problems result from language differences, utilize interpretive services.
        a. Professional interpreters will provide services without adding or subtracting information to ensure concise communication.
        b. Using a family member as an interpreter is not recommended because the family member may not relay exactly what is being said and may not know technical terms.

C. Lactation consultants should assess the composition of the family.
   1. Each family situation is different, and approaching a family without assumptions allows for respectful communication.
   2. Never assume genders or relationships based on outward appearance.
   3. Ask about pronouns and use them to effectively build rapport, especially when a client's appearance or situation is not typical.
   4. Often biological information will be included in medical charts or records before you meet the family, but if relationships and connections of the people who are present are not known, they will have to be assessed.
   5. Traditionally the mother is the biological parent of the child, and she experienced a pregnancy and birth resulting in the new family member; but be careful not to assume biological connections.
   6. The biological mother of the child may identify as a male and be providing milk through a supplemental breastfeeding aid, usually referred to as chest feeding, if breast tissue is absent.
   7. Families may include a single parent, two or more parents in a committed relationship, or other combinations.
   8. It is important to identify the main emotional support people for the breastfeeding dyad and include them in your planning.
   9. When working with a family, observe how each family member interacts and relates to the other family members.
D. Understand different belief systems that may affect parenting and feeding choices.[2]
   1. Avoid assuming that a family fits in a clearly defined category.
   2. Cultural humility is imperative. (See Chapter 28, *Cultural Humility*.)
   3. A working knowledge about different religions and cultural experiences is a starting point to begin asking sensitive and respectful questions about how a particular family operates and observing how the family members interact and speak.
E. Lactation consultants must utilize effective counseling skills.
   1. The technical information being conveyed is only part of the interaction.
   2. The lactation consultant offers information, and the listeners need to hear and understand the information.
   3. A relationship between the provider and family should include mutual respect for information to be effectively shared, understood, and utilized.
   4. The shared decision-making model used in medical settings since the 1980s provides a respectful framework for working with people who are making healthcare decisions.[3]
      a. Shared decision making starts with offering choices and information to the client and allowing time for reactions and questions.
      b. A mental stepping back must occur to allow space for the parent and family to consider the new information and process uncertainties.
      c. Describe options, harms, and benefits, and then support the family in making their own decision.
      d. Engage in dialogue to assess their understanding of the options.
      e. Help the family make a decision by focusing on their personal preferences and continuing to check for understanding.
      f. Reviewing the options and decisions can help the family move toward closure and feel comfortable with their decision.
      g. If decision making can be deferred, let the family know they have time to think and process the information.
      h. If the situation is emergent, offer information quickly and continue to respect the family's right to make a decision that is best for them.[3]
      i. Work with the expectation that the family makes the decisions, and provide care within that context.

CLINICAL TIP

Using unconditional positive regard requires the lactation consultant to deeply and genuinely care for the client. Although the consultant does not have to approve of every behavior exhibited by the client, the client is accepted and supported in that moment. Research indicates that prizing, accepting, and valuing the client in a nonpossessive way leads to greater chances for successful outcomes in counseling.[4]

II. Effective Counseling Sessions

A. Lactation consultants should understand the counseling setting.
1. Consider using space creatively and utilizing doors and curtains to create an atmosphere that allows the new family to relax.
2. A meeting held in a private office may provide a space that feels comfortable and safe for discussing concerns and observing adult–baby interactions.
3. Assessments in a hospital room may require more attention to creating an emotionally safe and comfortable environment.[5]
4. Environmental factors may affect communication and cause disruptions in understanding.
5. Move furniture to facilitate ease of communication and to include all family members and professionals.
6. Consider the breastfeeding parent's level of modesty and comfort with being exposed or touched.
7. Ensure comfort by creating privacy and explaining the necessity of physical exams.
8. When the physical organization of the room feels comfortable, proceed with the session.
B. Begin the assessment with the following factors in mind:
1. Always begin interactions by introducing yourself and your function in the care of the family.
2. Include an introduction of the professionals in the room and the purpose of the visit.
3. Clearly state the names the family members should use to address professionals, such as, "Hi, I'm Tonya, the lactation consultant" or "Hello, I'm Dr. Anderson."
4. Ask about relationships and responsibilities within the family or group, and include all people in the room when you speak.
5. Directly ask what names family members use and their preferred pronouns.
6. Use the preferred names and pronouns when addressing the family members to show respect and build rapport.
7. Avoid calling family members *mom, baby, dad,* and *family member* because these terms may contribute to making clients feel disrespected and disempowered.
8. When talking to clients, pay attention to responses that indicate differences in comprehension or ability to communicate.
9. Be sensitive about labeling differences as problems or disabilities.
10. It may be common to hear people referred to by their condition or disability, especially within a medical setting, but make it a practice to use names and correct pronouns at all times to maintain the humanity and dignity of the clients.
11. Showing people respect will help them feel at ease during a time of immense life change.[6]
12. Clearly explain the purpose of the visit to the clients, especially in a hospital setting where there are many different care providers.
13. Ask everyone at the visit if it is OK to proceed.
14. Provide an overview of how the session will progress.
15. Inform the clients of any limits to confidentiality, and explain who will have access to the notes taken at the visit.
16. Explain the payment terms clearly, if applicable, including how any third-party billing and reimbursement will occur.
17. If the assessment will include touching, obtain permission before you touch an adult or a child.
    a. Ask for the parent's permission before touching their child to communicate that the parent is the person who is responsible for caring for the child and to encourage acquisition of the parental role.
    b. Explain the measures used to ensure safety, such as hand washing or wearing gloves.
18. Narrate the actions and observations made so that everyone in the room understands what is happening and learns more about infant behavior and breastfeeding.
C. Ascertain the breastfeeding goals.
1. Part of the responsibility of working with new families is to normalize breastfeeding and help adults understand their new baby's requirements for care.
2. Lactation consultants may have personal experiences with breastfeeding and individual beliefs about what is best for baby.

CLINICAL TIP

Know the legal requirements for reporting suspected abuse. Mandated reporting may include reporting suspected child abuse, domestic violence, elder abuse, sexual abuse, or other abuses as defined by local law. The requirements may depend on the place of practice, such as private practice, hospital, or clinic, and may differ markedly in different regions or countries. It is the clinician's responsibility to understand the reporting mandate and to explain the reporting process to the family. Seek consultation with a trusted colleague or supervisor to ensure you are fully aware of your responsibilities in cases of suspected abuse. Always include a written report of your observations and consultations, and place a copy of the report in the client's record or chart.

3. As a professional, it is imperative to keep opinions and personal experiences separate from professional support.
4. Observing new families during an assessment allows the consultant to notice indications that the family might be confused or have concerns.
5. Offer everyone the opportunity to raise questions, and let them know their concerns are important, even if they are based on misinformation.
6. Adapt to cultural beliefs rather than dismissing them as irrelevant.[7]
7. If adults believe they are being addressed in a condescending way, they may be openly hostile and more likely to discount the provided information.
8. Look for clues to differences in learning styles.
    a. Auditory and verbal learners can listen to explanations and conversations, then utilize the information.
    b. Visual learners need to see behaviors demonstrated and like to have written notes or diagrams for reference.
    c. Kinesthetic learners obtain new information best by performing behaviors with guidance or even moving their bodies while listening.
    d. Encourage clients to take notes, imitate your actions, ask questions, or contact you later with questions.
    e. Identifying a particular learning style is less important than offering information in different forms and checking for comprehension and acquisition of knowledge.[4]

D. Misunderstandings may occur because a clinician is unaware of differing intellectual abilities.
    1. When a parent or family member appears to be argumentative or unsupportive, consider asking clarifying questions, and be curious about why the communication is challenging.
    2. Change the wording you use and slow down your speech when sharing information, and allow time for the listener to process what was heard.
    3. Continued difficulties may require asking the family for suggestions or resources.
    4. Community social service resources may be helpful, if they are available in your locality.

E. A client may have experienced trauma associated with pregnancy, birth, medical procedures, or interactions with other healthcare professionals, which can manifest as a lack of engagement in conversation, hostility, or unusual responses.[5]

F. Consider that the mood and responses of the client may be related to personal factors, and adjust the communication to focus on acceptance and support.
    1. Hormonal changes, exhaustion, and mental health concerns can impact the ability of a parent to adequately engage in self-care and the baby's care.
    2. When communication is impaired due to trauma or other factors particular to the client, it may be best to stop the session and refer the client to other professionals for counseling or treatment. Continue to provide breastfeeding support as appropriate.[5]

G. After sharing information and listening carefully to the family members, a general idea of the family's breastfeeding expectations will emerge.
    1. Start with understanding the parents' goals, and provide objective information to help them achieve their goals.
    2. Use positive words and encouragement.

3. If there is a conflict between the family's breastfeeding goals and the medical recommendations, address the difference clearly and offer options to the family.
   a. Another medical professional might have told a lactating parent to pump their breasts to feed a baby who is experiencing challenges, but the parent might not want to pump.
   b. The lactation consultant can explain why it is important to provide the parent's milk and listen carefully to the parent's concerns and worries and assure the family that they will make the final decision.
4. Education combined with acknowledgement of the family's responsibility for making the final choice increases rapport between the consultant and the family and allows the relationship to continue.
5. Maintaining the relationship allows for continued education and might change decisions that affect breastfeeding.

CLINICAL TIP

Basic counseling skills can be remembered by using the acronym LOVE[8]:
- **L:** Listen.
- **O:** Ask Open-ended questions.
- **V:** Validate the client's concerns.
- **E:** Educate, targeting client-specific concerns.

III. Counseling Skills for Challenging Situations

A. Parents' behaviors may not support their stated goals.
   1. A parent may state a goal to exclusively breastfeed but is breastfeeding the baby only every 4 hours, indicating a gap between the stated goal and the behavior.
   2. Motivational interviewing can clarify the difference between the end goals and the behaviors that do not support attaining the goals.[9]
      a. Motivational interviewing skills are used when the healthcare provider notices a gap and then uses positive, supportive counseling skills to help the client move toward the stated goal.
      b. The steps of motivational interviewing include asking about the client's goals, listening to the explanation, asking questions to fully understand, and then sharing clinical information.
      c. A client may not be ready to completely change behaviors but may agree to adopt smaller behavioral changes that move in the direction of the goal.
         i. It is important for the lactation consultant to indicate that the baby needs to be fed. If the parent is not willing to engage in behaviors that allow for complete breastfeeding, other feeding options must be considered.
         ii. Defining success for a particular parent may include helping redefine the goal and using combined feeds or a supplemental feeding system.
B. Parents may be unable to meet the stated goals due to health or situational factors.
   1. A family may face a difficult or unexpected situation that complicates infant feeding.
   2. One family member might not support breastfeeding, creating enough pressure that the parents choose not to breastfeed to maintain their relationship with that family member.
   3. Parents facing infant health problems may need to reassess their feeding options.
   4. The lactating parent's health may affect feeding choices.
   5. Helping a family to accept a different reality than expected requires supportive counseling and recognition that grief may be involved in changing the goals.
   6. Sharing specific technical information is important so the family will understand the options.
   7. Recognize that each family member might react in a different way or grieve a loss differently.
   8. Continue respectful communication and offer options, with empathy, to provide the best support for the family.
   9. Some families find immense comfort in donating expressed milk when they experience an infant loss; others want to stop lactation as quickly as possible.[10,11] See "Lactation Support for the Bereaved

Mother" article for more information and a toolkit about bereavement situations.[11] (See Chapter 23, *Breastfeeding and Infant Birth Injury, Congenital Anomalies, and Illness.*)

    10. Listen, offer support, and accept the decisions of the lactating parent and family.

C. Certain problems require a referral to psychological care.

    1. When a parent's behavior seems concerning or the parent expresses emotional struggling, it is important to provide a referral for appropriate help.

    2. Knowing the common signs of postpartum depression can help a lactation consultant recognize depression before parenting is impaired and to help the parent find psychological support while continuing to breastfeed (see **BOX 26-1**).

    3. Ask about previous experience with depression or a family history that may increase the likelihood of depression.

    4. Refer to counseling and psychiatric care if needed.

    5. Normalize seeking help for depression, and educate the family about the availability of medications for depression that are compatible with breastfeeding.[12]

    6. Postpartum depression is recognized as a mental health disorder experienced after birth. There are other mental health disorders that can occur in the postpartum period and require referral and treatment.

    7. Although a lactation consultant does not need to be familiar with all diagnoses, it is imperative that problems be recognized and appropriate referrals be made.

    8. Recognize that symptoms of stress may be present and need to be treated.

        a. Acute stress disorder is diagnosed within 1 month of experiencing a traumatic event.

        b. Posttraumatic stress disorder is diagnosed if symptoms persist for more than 1 month and include the following[13]:

            i. A perceived traumatic event was experienced.

            ii. History of childhood or previous adult trauma or abuse.

            iii. Feelings of hopelessness, intense fear, or horror.

            iv. Subjective sense of numbing or absence of emotional response.

            v. Lack of memory of traumatic event.

            vi. Reexperiencing parts of a traumatic event.

            vii. Hypervigilance.

            viii. Exaggerated startle response.

            ix. Irritability.

            x. Sleep problems unrelated to infant care.

            xi. Poor concentration.

            xii. Symptoms of trauma overlap with symptoms of depression and other mental health diagnoses.

        c. The recognition of troubling symptoms is more important than a specific diagnosis.

        d. Refer the patient to a competent trauma therapist and medical care if trauma symptoms are present.

        e. Family members may react to the same experience with different symptoms based on their coping skills, resilience, and history of trauma.

        f. Inform the family that treatments compatible with breastfeeding are available.[13]

BOX 26-1 Symptoms of Postpartum Depression

The symptoms of postpartum depression include the following[13]:

- Depressed or dysphoric mood.
- Anhedonia (inability to experience pleasure in normally pleasurable activities).
- Sleep difficulties unrelated to infant care.
- Fatigue; be aware of the assumption that all new parents are exhausted.
- Concentration difficulties.
- Hopelessness.
- Marked changes in appetite.
- Increased anger, hostility, and thoughts of death.
- Anxiety.

    D.   Lactation consultants must handle their personal emotions in difficult situations.

        1. Lactation care professionals are expected to keep their opinions and personal experiences from affecting their work with a family.

        2. Unexpected events may trigger a stress response in the consultant or remind the consultant of personal trauma.

        3. If the lactation consultant's emotional state is affecting the situation, it is important for the consultant to recognize what is happening and take steps for self-care.

        4. Notice the reaction and work to calm the physiological arousal by stepping away, taking deep breaths, and returning to a grounded state before interacting with the family.

        5. In some situations it may be best to find another professional to work with the family.

        6. Self-care can prevent vicarious traumatization, which manifests as extreme exhaustion and loss of hopefulness in helping others.[5]

IV. Communicating with Professionals

    A.   Lactation consultants are part of a healthcare team that supports new families, and they need to communicate with other providers.

    B.   Communication among healthcare providers allows for all professionals interacting with the parents to know what has occurred in other patient encounters.

    C.   In a hospital or clinic, everyone working with the family might have access to central charts that include descriptions of various interactions and the provided education and support.

    D.   In other settings, the lactation consultant may write a formal letter to a medical provider or make a phone call to share concerns.

    E.   Communication provides the opportunity to educate other professionals about the role of the lactation consultant and to share information about basic breastfeeding management.

        1. Use appropriate titles when addressing other professionals and clearly state your title.

        2. Clearly communicate when and where family interactions occurred and state your concerns in a concise manner.

        3. Outline the recommendations you made to the family.

        4. Include contact information so other professionals can ask questions.

        5. Record contacts with other healthcare providers.

    F.   When communication with other professionals takes place in an emergency situation, be concise and clear. Use words that describe behavior, and refrain from diagnosing the client or using overly emotional language.

    G.   Keep communications short and include only the necessary information, then trust the other professionals to do their jobs.

    H.   If another professional prescribes a treatment that interrupts breastfeeding or is counter to the family's goals, continuing respectful communication with the professional and providing support for the family can help empower the family and educate the professional about lactation.

    I.   Maintaining a respectful, ongoing relationship with other professionals creates acceptance of different roles and opportunities for continued growth and education.

▶ Key Points from This Chapter

    A.   Effective communication begins with respect and unconditional positive regard for the client; it includes attention to both verbal and nonverbal information.

    B.   Beneficial counseling sessions begin with creating a safe and welcoming physical space, include respect for gender identity and family structure, and always include an attitude of cultural humility.

    C.   Shared decision making provides a framework that incorporates evidence-informed treatment with the client's abilities, preferences, and values.

    D.   Active listening, LOVE counseling, and motivational interviewing are practical counseling tools that can be utilized to help families meet their breastfeeding goals.

🔍 *CASE STUDY 1*

A new mother, Ana, arrives for a breastfeeding help session. Her first baby, Ben, is 6 weeks old. Ana appears tired but is dressed appropriately and is responsive to questions. Ana holds Ben and interacts appropriately with him. Ana says her main concern is that she does not have enough milk. She brought bottles of artificial baby milk with her to the appointment.

Talking with Ana during the initial discussion produces the following facts: Ben was born vaginally at 40 weeks with no identified health problems. Ana is healing from the birth and did not have significant tearing or an episiotomy. Breastfeeding was encouraged right after birth, and Ben was held skin to skin for the first few hours of life. He was then taken for a bath and a newborn physical exam.

Ana says that since they have been home she has been tired, and Ben seems to want to breastfeed all the time. Ana is struggling with tending to herself, making her meals, getting rest, and feeding Ben. She has family members who live with her, and sometimes they will hold Ben if she needs to sleep. Ana is certain she does not have enough milk because of the frequency of Ben's feedings. Ana's mother helped in the early days of Ben's life and introduced bottles of artificial baby milk so Ana could sleep longer.

Questions

How would you approach this helping session so Ana is most likely to be successful in meeting her breastfeeding goals?

1. Utilize the LOVE counseling framework to form rapport, ascertain Ana's goals, and make a plan that works for the family:
   - L: Listen.
   - O: Ask open-ended questions.
   - V: Validate the client's concerns.
   - E: Educate, targeting client-specific concerns.

   The first goal is to understand Ana's desires for breastfeeding. Asking her directly could feel confrontational, so the best first step is to listen. When appropriate, ask open-ended questions that elicit information about Ana's experiences during Ben's birth and the breastfeeding relationship so far. For example, "How do you feel the breastfeeding is going?" Listen for cues that she is overly exhausted or not feeling supported by her family and friends. Note any misunderstandings about how breastfeeding works or behaviors that do not support successful breastfeeding. If Ana says she is supplementing with artificial baby milk, note the information for later and validate her feelings.

   It can be difficult to refrain from quickly correcting misinformation when a parent or family members says something incorrect about breastfeeding. However, if you continue to listen and validate their feelings, you will help them feel comfortable and begin to form rapport.

   After you have validated the client's feelings, you can gently begin to offer education and help set appropriate goals. Utilize wording that reflects the way the client talks. Check often for indications the client understands what is said. Make a plan and review it with the client. Document the plan so the client can refer to the steps at home.

2. If there is a discrepancy between the parent's stated goals and behaviors, employ motivational interviewing. Gather information to assess the parent's readiness to change, and help the parent identify behaviors to move toward the stated goals.

🔍 *CASE STUDY 2*

Cate delivered her baby, Mari, at the local birth center 10 days ago. Cate's mother called the birth center with questions about Mari's feeding patterns, and the birth center referred Cate and her mother to a lactation consultant. Cate and her mother met with the lactation consultant, along with baby Mari. Cate's mother arrived, carrying Mari, and Cate appeared exhausted and had large dark circles under her eyes.

At the beginning of the session, Cate barely replies to the conversation, while her mother is outspoken and appears to be solicitous of Cate's needs. Cate's mother asks questions about how often Mari should eat and how many wet and dirty diapers she should expect. The lactation consultant asks questions and learns that Mari is receiving only Cate's milk, and Cate's mother confirms that all feedings are at the breast. Cate is still not participating in the conversation and is sitting slumped in the chair. When the lactation consultant questions Cate directly, she mumbles or her mother

(continues)

CASE STUDY 2 *(continued)*

answers. The lactation consultant asks if she can talk to Cate alone, and Cate's mother takes Mari for a short walk. When her mother is gone, Cate says she is scared to hold her baby and is not sleeping because she is worried that she will act impulsively and hurt Mari. Cate mumbles that her mother is better for Mari than she is, then she stops responding and starts to cry. When her mother and Mari return a few minutes later, Cate is staring into space and is unresponsive.

Questions

1. What is your impression of Cate's mental status at the visit?

   There are indications that Cate may be exhausted, depressed, or experiencing some other mental health symptoms. Lactation consultants should take note when working with a client who is unresponsive or makes statements about possibly harming the baby. Even with concerns about Cate's well-being, the first response is to utilize basic counseling skills to elicit more information while continuing to offer empathy.

   Employ the LOVE counseling techniques:

   - L: Listen to the mother. Continue to listen to Cate's mother while including Cate with eye contact and encouraging her to participate.
   - O: Ask open-ended questions. Be curious about what is happening with this family. Continue to stay engaged and watch for nonverbal cues. By responding without alarm, the family will feel more comfortable sharing any mental health history or current concerns.
   - V: Validate the client's concerns. In this case, both Cate and her mother need validation and understanding. Point out what they are doing well and praise them for ensuring that Mari is receiving all feedings at the breast. Cate's mother is an integral part of the breastfeeding relationship because it appears she is providing care for both Mari and Cate.
   - E: Educate, targeting client specific concerns. Suggest some resources or referrals that can provide a formal assessment of Cate's mental health and provide treatment if necessary. By maintaining a calm tone and conveying empathy, the lactation consultant can ensure that Cate and her mother feel supported and not just passed off to another provider. If there is any indication that Cate is a threat to herself or Mari, an immediate call to security or emergency services is necessary. The best course of action is to keep Cate and her family in the office while planning for further care. Continue to talk with Cate and her mother in a respectful and honest manner to help normalize the referral. Maintaining a calm demeanor will help reduce Cate's and her mother's fears.

2. What do you need to do to support the breastfeeding relationship?

   Cate should be referred to a mental health professional who can provide an adequate assessment and treatment options. Protecting the breastfeeding relationship is paramount, but Cate's mental health requires an intervention. Ideally, treatment can be obtained that benefits Cate and allows her to continue breastfeeding Mari. Cate's doctors can choose medications, if needed. The lactation consultant can provide information about how medications are transferred through the milk and how they may impact Cate's milk production. If Cate's treatment requires her to be separated from Mari, it would be appropriate to provide education to Cate and her mother about maintaining Cate's milk production and alternative feeding methods to ensure adequate nutrition for Mari. Document the session and referral information, and offer to communicate with other healthcare providers as needed to support the family.

References

1. Corey G. Adlerian therapy. In: *Theory and Practice of Counseling and Psychotherapy*. 9th ed. Belmont, CA: Brooks/Cole; 2012:101-135.
2. Lauwers J. Special counseling circumstances. In: *Counseling the Nursing Mother: A Lactation Consultant's Guide*. 6th ed. Burlington, MA: Jones & Bartlett Learning; 2016:475-495.
3. Elwyn G, Frosch D, Thomson R, et al. Shared decision making: a model for clinical practice. *J Gen Intern Med.* 2012;10:1361-1367.
4. Lauwers J. Empowering women to breastfeed. In: *Counseling the Nursing Mother: A Lactation Consultant's Guide*. 6th ed. Burlington, MA: Jones & Bartlett Learning; 2016:69-92.
5. Van der Kolk B. *The Body Keeps the Score: Brain, Mind, and Body in the Healing of Trauma*. New York, NY: Viking; 2014.
6. Institute for Healthcare Communication. Impact of communication in healthcare. Institute for Healthcare Communication website. http://healthcarecomm.org/about-us/impact-of-communication-in-healthcare/. Published July 2011. Accessed February 2018.
7. National Institute for Children's Health Quality. Cultural sensitivity for better breastfeeding outcomes. NICHQ website. https://www.nichq.org/insight/cultural-sensitivity-better-breastfeeding-outcomes. Accessed February 2018.
8. Taylor E. LOVE counseling. Paper presented at: Virginia Collaborative Learning Session; May 2016; Richmond, VA.

9. Rollnick S, Miller WR, Butler CC. *Motivational Interviewing in Health Care: Helping Patients Change Behavior.* New York, NY: Guilford Press; 2008.

10. Wellborn JM. The experience of expressing and donating breast milk following a perinatal loss. *J Hum Lactation.* 2012;28:506-510. doi:10.1177/0890334412455459.

11. Wellborn J. Jones F, ed. Lactation support for the bereaved mother. Human Milk Banking Association of North America. 2012. Available at https://www.hmbana.org/publications.12.

12. Hale T, Rowe H. Commonly used antidepressants—suitability in lactation. In: *Medications and Mothers' Milk.* 17th ed. New York, NY: Springer Publishing; 2017:1030.

13. American Psychiatric Association. *Diagnostic and Statistical Manual of Mental Disorders.* 5th ed. Washington, DC: American Psychiatric Association; 2013.

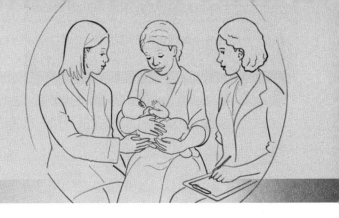

CHAPTER 27

Problem Solving and Documentation

Angela Love-Zaranka

Laurie K. Scherer

OBJECTIVES

- Summarize the content that is expected in a lactation health record.
- Describe the key elements of a breastfeeding history.
- Identify events that may occur during pregnancy, labor, and birth and that may affect breastfeeding.
- Evaluate potential and existing factors that may impact a parent's breastfeeding goals.
- Organize observations and clinical assessments to analyze the current situation, apply problem solving, calculate clinical algorithms, and utilize critical thinking skills.
- Develop a plan of care that incorporates adult learning principles.

DEFINITIONS OF COMMONLY USED TERMS

Bristol Breastfeeding Assessment Tool (BBAT)[1] An assessment tool used to measure breastfeeding proficiency in clinical practice and research.

Bristol Tongue Attachment Tool (BTAT)[2] An assessment tool used to assist with tongue-tie identification. A visual and digital assessment of an infant's tongue function.

critical thinking Process of purposeful self-regulatory judgment that gives reasoned consideration to evidence, contexts, conceptualizations, methods, and criteria.

Hazelbaker Assessment Tool for Lingual Frenulum Function (HATLFF)[3] An assessment tool used to assist with tongue-tie identification. A visual and digital assessment of an infant's tongue function.

Infant BreastFeeding Assessment Tool (IBFAT)[4-6] A validated assessment tool used to evaluate the effectiveness of early breastfeeding.

intrapartum Occurring during labor and delivery.

(continues)

DEFINITIONS OF COMMONLY USED TERMS *(continued)*

Latch, Audible swallowing, Type of nipple, Comfort, maternal Help (LATCH).[4,5,7] A validated assessment tool used to evaluate the effectiveness of early breastfeeding.

Preterm Infant Breastfeeding Behavior Scale (PIBBS).[8,9] An assessment tool used to evaluate preterm infants' breastfeeding behaviors.

problem-oriented medical record.[10] A type of record keeping in a problem-solving system. Information includes a defined database of information, a problem list, a plan of action for each problem, and progress notes on each problem.

Any use of the term *mother*, *maternal*, or *breastfeeding* is not meant to exclude transgender or nonbinary parents who may be breastfeeding or providing human milk to their infant.

▶ Overview

A comprehensive medical history and clinical evaluation is an integral part of lactation care. The documentation of relevant lactation history, observations, and assessments is necessary to understand the comprehensive picture of the breastfeeding dyad and each breastfeeding relationship. The synthesis of information with critical thinking and analytical skills will assist the lactation consultant and other healthcare providers to develop an appropriate, evidence-informed plan of care. Respectful communication skills will aid in constructive dialogue with the family to implement techniques and processes to help them meet their breastfeeding goals. Lactation consultants are a part of a multidisciplinary team. Appropriate communication with other healthcare professionals regarding distinct observations, assessments, and the lactation care plan is necessary to ensure preservation of the parent's breastfeeding goals.

I. Stages of Skill Acquisition and Critical Thinking

A. As the depth of lactation evidence, knowledge, and clinical skills grows, an increased level of expertise is necessary. The role of the International Board Certified Lactation Consultant (IBCLC) is based on an advanced practice model.

B. The Dreyfus and Dreyfus Five Stages of Skill Acquisition[11-14] describes a five-stage model of the mental activities involved in directed skill acquisition.

1. Novice:
   a. Follows specific rules or protocols to learn.
   b. Has minimal or no context or situational experience.
   c. Applies protocols or rules to all situations.
   d. "Just tell me what to do and I'll do it."

2. Advanced beginner:
   a. Achieved after considerable experience.
   b. Follows more sophisticated rules that are situational.
   c. Begins to recognize meaningful elements and situational components.
   d. Develops principles, based on experience, to guide actions.

3. Competent:
   a. Achieved after more experience, usually 2 to 3 years.
   b. Possesses a sense of importance and is able to establish priorities based on levels of importance.
   c. Able to cope with and manage many contingencies.
   d. Uses a hierarchal procedure for decision making.
   e. Conscious and deliberate planning helps achieve efficiency and organization.
   f. Accepts responsibility for choices.

4. Proficient:
   a. Uses intuition based on past experiences.
   b. Intuition is "the product of deep situational involvement and recognition of similarity."[12(p18)]
   c. Gains a deep understanding of the entire situation and provides a holistic approach to problem solving.

     d.   Perceives which attributes and aspects in a current situation are important.

     e.   Intuitive-based cognition is coupled with detached decision making.

   5. Expert:

     a.   Knowledge becomes tacit, with loss of awareness of intuition and decision making.

     b.   Sees, but sometimes does not recognize that he or she sees.

     c.   Performs fluidly without reflecting on every behavior.

     d.   Reflects and considers alternatives when presented with time and critical outcomes.

     e.   Engages in critical reflection of his or her own assumptions, thereby enhancing performance.

C. Benner's application of this model to the nursing profession[13,14] can be applied to the lactation consultant profession as well.

   1. Students move from reliance on abstract principles learned in their didactic education to concrete experiences as paradigms.

   2. Through their clinical training, they are able to distinguish between a compilation of equally relevant bits of information and pieces of information that are germane to an individual parent–baby dyad.

   3. Creating a care plan employs problem solving and critical thinking skills that demonstrate the student is moving from novice to competent practitioner.

   4. The lactation consultant is considered a competent practitioner of skilled lactation care. Continued support of the breastfeeding couplet further deepens and strengthens the foundation of knowledge for the lactation consultant to assist families in a variety of situations.

D. The utilization of critical thinking and analytical skills will assist the practitioner to define solutions and guide the family toward an optimal care plan.

   1. Critical thinking is the process used to make a judgment about what to believe and what to do about the symptoms the patient is presenting for evaluation and treatment.[15]

   2. Core critical thinking skills include the following[16]:

     a.   Analysis.

     b.   Interpretation.

     c.   Inference.

     d.   Explanation.

     e.   Evaluation.

     f.   Self-correction or self-regulation.

II. Key Elements in a Lactation Health Record

A. A lactation history includes medical conditions that could impact lactogenesis I, lactogenesis II, and lactogenesis III (galactopoiesis).

B. The previous breastfeeding history for a multiparous woman may provide insight to assess the current situation. Guiding the inquiries of the mother and a review of previous medical documentation will aid in compiling objective and subjective information for a comprehensive history.

C. Significant events or diagnoses are provided in the following list, which is not all inclusive. An asterisk refers to a clinical practice that is best suited for an IBCLC.[17] Breastfeeding and lactation care may be provided by a variety of lactation support providers. This chapter assumes that all professionals who provide breastfeeding care will operate within their scope of practice.

   1. Prepregnancy:

     a.   Hormonal imbalance* (e.g., polycystic ovarian syndrome, hyperprolactinemia, hyperandrogenism).

     b.   Autoimmune disorders* (e.g., Type 1 diabetes, thyroiditis, Graves disease, Hashimoto thyroiditis, systemic lupus erythematosus).

     c.   Endocrine disorders* (e.g., hypothalamic amenorrhea, hyperprolactinemia).

     d.   Childhood cancer, specifically involving radiation to pituitary or hypothalamus.*

     e.   Psychiatric (e.g., diagnosed conditions, previous trauma).

     f.   Surgery* (e.g., breast augmentation or reduction, weight loss surgery).

     g.   Previous lactation history:

        i.   Parity.

        ii.   Acute or chronic* nipple trauma.

        iii.   Acute or recurrent* mastitis.

        iv.   Acute or chronic* bacterial or fungal infections.

        v.   Milk production* (overabundant or insufficient).

        vi.   Duration and reason for weaning.

        vii.   Parent's perception of previous breastfeeding experience.

2.   Pregnancy (obstetric complications)*:

    a.   Hypertension.

    b.   Gestational diabetes.

    c.   Multiples.

    d.   Surgery during pregnancy.

3.   Intrapartum (labor):

    a.   Duration of labor.

    b.   Induction or spontaneous labor.

    c.   Labor medications.

4.   Intrapartum (delivery method):

    a.   Vaginal delivery:

        i.   Infant presentation (breech, occiput anterior, or occiput posterior).*

        ii.   Episiotomy or tear.

        iii.   Instrument assisted (e.g., vacuum, forceps).

    b.   Vaginal delivery after cesarean.

    c.   Cesarean section.*

    d.   Instrument-assisted delivery (e.g., vacuum, forceps).

5.   Intrapartum complications:

    a.   Maternal complications*:

        i.   Placental (e.g., abruption, previa).

        ii.   Preeclampsia.

        iii.   Hemorrhage.

        iv.   Excessive IV fluid intake.

        v.   Chorioamnionitis.

    b.   Infant complications*:

        i.   Gestational age (e.g., preterm, late preterm).

        ii.   Small for gestational age or large for gestational age.

        iii.   Transient tachypnea of the newborn or respiratory distress.

        iv.   Meconium aspiration.

        v.   Hypoglycemia.

        vi.   Sepsis (rule out).

6.   Postpartum:

    a.   Timing of first feeding.

    b.   Hospital practices to support optimal breastfeeding (rooming in, skin-to-skin care, supplementation only when medically necessary).

    c.   Maternal acute complications*:

        i.   Postpartum hemorrhage.

        ii.   Chorioamnionitis.

        iii.   Retained products of conception.

        iv.   Postpartum preeclampsia.

    d.   Common infant complications:

        i.   Late preterm gestation.

        ii.   Physiologic hyperbilirubinemia.

        iii.   Hypoglycemia.

        iv.   Oral/motor dysfunction (e.g., ankyloglossia).

        v.   Precipitous weight loss in newborn.

        vi.   Newborn birth trauma.

7.   Uncommon or persistent complications*:

    a.   Continued weight loss after day 5.

    b.   Failure to regain birth weight by 2 to 3 weeks of age.

      c.   Pathologic hyperbilirubinemia.

      d.   Colic.

8.   Significant infant disorders, illnesses, and chronic conditions*:

      a.   Born at less than 37 weeks' gestation.

      b.   Metabolic disorders (phenylketonuria, galactosemia).

      c.   Congenital heart defect.

      d.   Cleft palate, lip, or both.

      e.   Hypotonia.

      f.   Genetic syndromes (e.g., Down syndrome, Pierre Robin syndrome).

      g.   Oral, abdominal, or chest surgeries.

9.   Assessment of the current situation:

      a.   Frequency of feeding.

      b.   Duration of feedings.

      c.   Hand expression and pumping:

         i.   Type.

         ii.   Frequency.

         iii.   Amount extracted.

      d.   Supplementation:

         i.   Expressed breastmilk, pasteurized donor human milk, or breastmilk substitutes.

         ii.   Mode of delivery.

      e.   Maternal physical exam:

         i.   Scarring, specifically on the torso.*

         ii.   Overall physique.

         iii.   Age.*

         iv.   Breasts.

         v.   Speech or communication barriers.*

         vi.   Cognitive deficits.*

         vii.   Other aids to help mother communicate or care for the baby.

         viii.   Demeanor.

      f.   Infant physical exam:

         i.   Respiration.

         ii.   Neurologic.*

         iii.   Behavior.

         iv.   Extremities, specifically movement.

         v.   Skin.

         vi.   Head, eyes, ears, neck, throat (HEENT).*

         vii.   Oral assessment.

         viii.   Digital suck examination.*

      g.   Breastfeeding session:

         i.   Position of the baby at the breast.

         ii.   Latch.

         iii.   Nutritive versus nonnutritive sucking.

         iv.   Signs of milk transfer (e.g., swallowing, breast changes, and satiety).

III. Documentation

A.   Documentation provides a written record of assessments, recommendations, plans of care, and evaluations of treatments utilized.

B.   Charting is an integral part of providing safe, quality care and is a reflection of the standard of care provided.

    1.   It can help practitioners monitor what has been done, what has been effective, and how to move toward positive outcomes.

    2.   It provides other healthcare providers with valuable and unique information on the parent, the baby, and the dynamic of the dyad.

    3.   It may include consent to assess, treat, and provide information to others.

C. In many countries documentation is a legal record and may serve as evidence in an ethics dispute or court of law.
1. Meaningful information can supplement the practitioner's memory of crucial events.
2. A review of the documentation can help the practitioner self-reflect and improve critical thinking, which is important for professional development and continuous improvement of clinical skills.

D. Documentation should include the following assessments:
1. Medical history of parent and baby.
2. Birth.
3. Postpartum.
4. Parent.
5. Baby.

E. Documentation should include the following elements of the encounter:
1. Evidence of parental consent for care, based on country, state, province, or locality rules and regulations with regard to privacy, disclosure of information, and consent for medical care. (See Chapter 25, *Professional Standards for Lactation Care Providers*.)
   a. Written consent, signed and dated by the parent, to:
      i. Touch the parent and baby (or babies).
      ii. Obtain medical information and disclose it to other healthcare professionals.
      iii. Obtain medication information and disclose it to third-party payers (in the United States).
   b. Verbal consent immediately prior to touching the parent or baby.
2. History.
3. Presenting problem.
4. Parental goals.
5. Assessments.
6. Care plan and recommendations.
7. Evaluation of care.

F. Documentation should include a written report to other healthcare professionals (as appropriate by jurisdiction).
1. The report should be clear, concise, factual, and objective.
2. Elements of the report include the following:
   a. Patient identifiers.
   b. Major findings.
   c. Recommendations.
   d. Plans for follow-up care.
3. Urgent situations, especially in an outpatient setting, may require immediate and direct communication with other healthcare providers or the primary healthcare provider who is ultimately responsible for the patient. These situations include the following:
   a. Retained placenta.
   b. Hyperbilirubinemia.
   c. Persistent inadequate infant weight gain.
   d. Suspected abuse.

G. Maintain documentation of all contacts, assessments, feeding plans, recommendations, and evaluations of care; and retain records for the time specified by the local jurisdiction.

H. There are two types of charting methods[18]:
1. Narrative charting uses a diary or story format. It includes documentation of the time of assessment, care, and information provided. This type of charting is utilized less frequently in favor of flow sheets and clinical care plans.
2. Problem-oriented medical records[10] utilize subjective, objective, assessment, and plan (SOAP) notes (see **BOX 27-1**):
   a. Subjective: Information from the parents, including when the problem started, symptoms, and descriptions of symptoms (e.g., nipple pain with initial latch, not confident in milk production).
   b. Objective: Observations that can be measured (e.g., baby's skin color, weight, or output; parent's pain score; and number of feedings per day).
   c. Assessment: Bring the objective information together to make an assessment of the current situation.

BOX 27-1 Example of a SOAP Note for a Breastfeeding Encounter

Subjective

Parent's information:

1. Concerns about milk production ("baby always seems hungry, especially at night," or unable to hand express "much" after feeding).
2. Nipple pain with initial latch ("baby slurps onto the breast").

Objective

Information from medical record, including history and lactation consultant observations:

1. First pregnancy and first live birth (G1P1).
2. Vaginal delivery.
3. 38 weeks' gestation.
4. Baby 82 hours old at time of visit.
5. Breastfed 10 times in previous 24 hours.
6. Reported output is four voids and four stools; previous stool was green.
7. Weight loss of 5 percent since birth.
8. Amount expressed after feeding is 15 mL.
9. Latch, Audible swallowing, Type of nipple, Comfort, maternal Help (LATCH) score is 8 (L = 1, A = 2, T = 2, C = 1, H = 2).
10. Cradle hold used for feeding.

Assessment

Lactation consultant's assessment of the situation:

1. Nipple pain caused by ineffective position and latch technique, resulting in shallow latch.
2. Milk production appropriate considering age of baby, infant output, and amount of milk extracted via hand expression.

Plan

Parent's goals and steps needed to achieve goal; for example, pain-free and exclusive breastfeeding:

1. Cross-cradle hold with asymmetric latch.
2. Education about normal newborn feeding patterns and circadian rhythms.
3. Objective standards to know if baby is getting enough (e.g., track intake and output over a 24-hour period).
4. Plan for follow-up with lactation support or pediatric provider.

      d.   Plan: Specific steps to meet the parent's goals:
            i.   Interventions: Measures recommended to achieve expected outcome.
           ii.   Evaluation of care: Analysis of the effectiveness of the plan and interventions.
          iii.   Time frame for follow-up with lactation consultant or primary care provider.

IV. Problem-Solving Steps

   A.   Problem solving involves organizing observations and clinical assessments to analyze the current situation, applying problem-solving and critical thinking skills and clinical algorithms, and incorporating adult learning principles in formulating a plan of care.

   B.   Identify the key issues.
      1.   Collect maternal information:
         a.   Relevant medical history.
         b.   Breast assessment.
         c.   Expression of milk:
            i.   Hand or mechanical.
           ii.   Frequency.
          iii.   Amount extracted.

    2.   Collect infant information:
        a.   Relevant medical history.
        b.   General condition of the baby.
        c.   Infant oral assessment using the appropriate tool as needed; for example, Hazelbaker Assessment Tool for Lingual Frenulum Function (HATLFF),[3] Bristol Tongue Attachment Tool (BTAT),[2] or lingual frenulum protocol from Martinelli et al.[19]
    3.   Assess the current situation:
        a.   Observe a breastfeeding session.
        b.   Document the observation with an assessment tool[20]; for example, LATCH,[4,5,7] Infant Breast-Feeding Assessment Tool (IBFAT),[4-6] Bristol Breastfeeding Assessment Tool (BBAT),[1] or Preterm Infant Breastfeeding Behavior Scale (PIBBS).[8,9]
        c.   Digitally assess the infant suck as appropriate.
    4.   Note any clinical concerns or problems.

C.   Understand everyone's interests.
    1.   Assess the parent's understanding and goals through reflections and open-ended questions; clarify as necessary.
    2.   Assess the parent's support network; discuss the pressures, expectations, and understanding of baby feeding behavior by engaging both the parent and supporters who are present.
    3.   Assess the parent's ability to communicate effectively, follow directions, and willingness to learn and use new information.

D.   Discuss possible solutions or options utilizing a shared decision-making process.[21-23] (See Chapter 26, *Counseling and Communication.*)
    1.   Share information to support possible solutions.
    2.   Ask the parent and supporters for ideas, respectfully considering the family's viewpoint.
    3.   Consider every possible solution, accepting the family's ideas.
    4.   Generate a list of possible solutions that are acceptable to the parent and family.

E.   Evaluate the options.
    1.   Share objective information about possible options that can be implemented, clarifying any risks.
    2.   Provide evidence-informed information to parents regarding the use of techniques and devices.
    3.   Reframe any unrealistic plans by being positive and adding education to help the parent understand the effectiveness of each option.
    4.   Provide appropriate education as needed, taking into account the parent's ability to comprehend.
    5.   Utilize motivational interviewing to encourage the parent to consider possible behavioral changes to meet agreed-upon goals. (See Chapter 26, *Counseling and Communication.*)

CLINICAL TIP

"To arrive at a judgment about what to believe and what to do, a clinician should consider the unique character of the symptoms (evidence) in view of the patient's current health and life circumstances (context), using the knowledge and skills acquired over the course of their health sciences training and practice (methods, conceptualizations), anticipate the likely effects of a chosen treatment action (consideration of evidence and criteria), and finally monitor the eventual consequences of delivered care (evidence and criteria)."[15(p2)]

F.   Select and document an agreement to an option or options.
    1.   Select the best options for the family and obtain their agreement of the final choices.
    2.   Provide a written plan with clearly defined behaviors in language the parent and supporters can understand.

G.   Agree on contingencies, monitoring, and evaluation.
    1.   Clarify that the family can follow the agreed-upon plan.
    2.   Provide appropriate anticipatory guidance.
    3.   Provide follow-up information and set a time frame for follow-up.

4. List clear measurements for the parent to assess progress (e.g., ounces of milk fed, time at breast, audible swallows heard, time expressing milk, skin-to-skin time, and wet and dirty diapers).
5. List symptoms and behaviors that require immediate intervention, and provide phone numbers of medical care providers and emergency contacts.

V. Essential Characteristics of a Plan of Care

A. Feed the baby and provide supplementation as necessary.
　　1. Use the appropriate amount of supplement for adequate weight gain.[24]
　　2. Choose the feeding method that interferes the least with direct breastfeeding; consider safety, efficiency, effectiveness, and the parent's ability to replicate the method.[25] (See Chapter 24, *Breastfeeding Devices and Topical Treatments*.)
　　3. The supplementation choices, in order of priority, are as follows:
　　　　a. Parent's own expressed milk.
　　　　b. Pasteurized donor milk.
　　　　c. Human milk substitute.
B. Support milk production, including one of the following types of milk expression as needed:
　　1. Hand expression.
　　2. Multiuser pump.
　　3. Single-user pump.
C. Address all elements of the problem.
D. Consider other factors that will lead to meeting the parent's goals.
　　1. Focus on the breast for feedings.
　　　　a. Provide any supplements at the breast.
　　　　b. Supplement with the baby resting on the breast.
　　　　c. Use nipple shields as necessary.
　　2. Keep the frustration level low.
　　　　a. Reinforce that only positive things happen at the breast.
　　　　b. Encourage skin-to-skin care.
　　　　c. Reinforce positive bonding with baby.
　　3. Make sure all of the parent's questions are answered.
E. Evaluate the parents' understanding of all provided information and education and assess their ability to accept and integrate the information.
　　1. Ask the parents to verbalize their understanding in their own words.
　　2. Ask for a return demonstration, or teach back, of techniques.
　　3. Measure behavioral change.
　　　　a. Reinforce accurate responses.
　　　　b. If the parents' response indicates a lack of understanding, do the following:
　　　　　　i. Clarify the information.
　　　　　　ii. Reassess the parents' comprehension and modify the teaching technique.
　　4. Document the parents' verbalized understanding and note any inconsistency between their verbalized understanding and their body language. (See Chapter 26, *Counseling and Communication*, for a discussion of motivational interviewing.)
F. Provide a written care plan.
　　1. Ensure that the parents and family are comfortable with the care plan and that it addresses the parents' goals.
　　2. Use operational words and positive language.
　　3. Identify the agreed-upon interventions.
　　4. Indicate specified criteria for follow-up.
　　　　a. Time frame.
　　　　b. Parents and baby reaching certain targets.
　　　　c. Criteria for unexpected or urgent issues, including contact information.

▶ **Key Points from This Chapter**

A. Know the components of a comprehensive history and how the history may affect current concerns.

B. Perform a thorough assessment of the current problem.

C. Communicate effectively with other care providers and document the contact.

D. Follow logical steps during an assessment to identify problems and generate solutions while considering family input.

E. Share the risks and benefits of generated solutions through shared decision making, and provide information and follow-up plans to the family.

F. Provide a written care plan that clearly states agreed-upon goals, behaviors to reach those goals, and indications of any problem that requires intervention.

🔍 *CASE STUDY*

Tonya requested a consultation for her 3-week-old baby, Michael. She complained of nipple pain and expressed concern that Michael is not "getting enough." Michael was born vaginally at 39 weeks' gestation. There is no other relevant medical history for Tonya or Michael. Tonya reports that she had no nipple pain during the first 7 days postpartum, but she noticed increasing pain after the first 7 to 10 days. Tonya believes that Michael is not getting enough because of his short feedings at the breast and repeatedly coming off the breast during feedings. Michael is exclusively breastfeeding, and he was fed nine times in the previous 24 hours. His output every 24 hours has been six to eight heavy, wet diapers and two to three yellow stools.

Assessment

The lactation consultant assessed Michael, and the findings were unremarkable. The oral assessment revealed that Michael can open his mouth symmetrically, and he lifts his tongue to his palate and lateralizes bilaterally. His lingual frenulum was not obviously visualized, but the lactation consultant found it to be elastic upon manipulation. Michael's labial frenulum is attached high on the alveolar ridge, is pliable, and does not blanch when his lip is lifted to the philtrum.

The lactation consultant also assessed Tonya's breasts and found that they are symmetrical and slightly engorged, and areolar edema is present. Tonya is using the cradle position and leaning over Michael when she feeds him. Michael initially has difficulty grasping the nipple. Midway through a feeding, he coughs, chokes, reattaches, then clamps down on the breast. Tonya complains of nipple pain when this happens.

Feeding Adjustments

The lactation consultant teaches Tonya how to use reverse pressure softening and a hand expression technique to soften the breasts and reduce areolar edema. The consultant discussed and demonstrated the laid back breastfeeding position, also known as a semireclined position, and she placed Michael parallel to or just above the level of the nipple and areola. Michael was able to latch more easily and to remain latched without coming off the breast. The feeding was complete in 7 minutes. Tonya noticed that her breasts were slightly softer after the feeding, but one breast was a bit fuller and slightly uncomfortable. The lactation consultant noted that Michael displayed contented behaviors; she pointed them out to Tonya, who could see that Michael was no longer demonstrating hunger cues. Tonya said that Michael appeared to be satiated and content.

Care Plan

The lactation consultant provided written instructions for reverse pressure softening, hand expression prior to feeding, and laid back breastfeeding. Tonya was able to provide a return demonstration of these techniques. The consultant provided information about milk production and sufficiency, including how to know if Michael is getting enough (i.e., Michael's weight gain and behavior, instead of time at the breast). The lactation consultant discussed the overproduction of milk and overactive milk ejection reflex with Tonya, along with how to manage breast discomfort between feedings and how to mitigate excessive milk production if it continues to be problematic.

Questions

1. What is the cause of Tonya's nipple pain?
2. What lets you know that Michael is getting enough milk?
3. How do you conclude that Tonya's nipple pain was caused by Michael's biting?

4. What aspects of the care plan include anticipatory guidance?
5. What is the subjective information in the case study?
6. What is the objective information in the case study?
7. What lets you know that Tonya understands the information you provided?

References

1. Ingram J, Johnson D, Copeland M, Churchill C, Taylor H. The development of a new breastfeeding assessment tool and the relationship with breastfeeding self-efficacy. *Midwifery*. 2015;31:132-137. doi:10.1016/j.midw.2014.07.001.
2. Ingram J, Johnson D, Copeland M, Churchill C, Taylor H, Emond A. The development of a tongue assessment tool to assist with tongue-tie identification. *Arch Dis Child Fetal Neonatal Ed*. 2015;100(4):F344-F349. doi:10.1136/archdischild-2014-307503.
3. Hazelbaker A. *Tongue Tie Morphogenesis, Impact, Assessment and Treatment*. Columbus, OH: Aidan and Eva Press; 2010.
4. Altuntas N, Turkyilmaz C, Yildiz H, et al. Validity and reliability of the infant breastfeeding assessment tool, the Mother Baby Assessment Tool, and the LATCH scoring system. *Breastfeed Med*. 2014;9:191-195. doi:10.1089/bfm.2014.0018.
5. Chapman D, Doughty K, Mullin E, Perez-Escamilla R. Reliability of lactation assessment tools applied to overweight and obese women. *J Hum Lactation*. 2015;32(2):269-276. doi:10.1177/0890334415597903.
6. Matthews MK. Developing an instrument to assess infant breastfeeding behaviour in the early neonatal period. *Midwifery*. 1988;4:154-165.
7. Jensen D, Wallace S, Kelsay P. LATCH: a breastfeeding charting system and documentation tool. *J Obstet Gynecol Neonatal Nurs*. 1994;23:27-32.
8. Radzyminski S. Neurobehavioral functioning and breastfeeding behavior in the newborn. *JOGNN*. 2005;34:335-341.
9. Nyqvist KH, Sjoden, P-O, Ewald U. The development of preterm infants' breastfeeding behavior. *Early Hum Dev*. 1999;55:247-264.
10. Simons S, Cillessen F, Hazelzet J. Determinants of a successful problem list to support the implementation of the problem-oriented medical record according to recent literature. *BMC Med Inform Decis Mak*. 2016;16(1):1. doi:10.1186/s12911-016-0341-0.
11. Dreyfus SE, Dreyfus HO. *A Five-Stage Model of the Mental Activities Involved in Directed Skill Acquisition*. Berkeley, CA: University of California; 1980.
12. Dreyfus H, Dreyfus S. *Mind over Machine: The Power of Human Intuition and Expertise in the Era of the Computer*. New York, NY: Free Press; 1986.
13. Benner P. *From Novice to Expert: Excellence and Power in Clinical Practice*. Menlo Park, CA: Addison Wesley; 1984.
14. Benner P. Using the Dreyfus model of skill acquisition to describe and interpret skill acquisition and clinical judgment in nursing practice and education. *Bull Sci Technol Soc*. 2004;24(3):188-199.
15. Facione N, Facione P. *Critical Thinking and Clinical Reasoning in the Health Sciences: An International Multidisciplinary Teaching Anthology*. Millbrae, CA: California Academic Press; 2008.
16. Facione P. *Critical Thinking: What Is It and Why It Counts*. Millbrae, CA: California Academic Press; 2015.
17. Mannel R. Defining lactation acuity to improve patient safety outcomes. *J Hum Lactation*. 2011;27(2):163-170. doi:10.1177/0890334410397198.
18. Brooks E, Genna CW, Mannel R. The lactation consultant: roles and responsibilities. In: Wambach K, Riordan J, eds. *Breastfeeding and Human Lactation*. 5th ed. Burlington, MA: Jones & Bartlett Learning; 2016:3-40.
19. Martinelli L, Marchesan I, Berretin-Felix G. Lingual frenulum protocol with scores for infants. *Int J Orofacial Myology*. 2012;38:104-112.
20. Sartorio BT, Coca KP, Marcacine KO, Abuchaim, ESV, Abrão ACFV. Breastfeeding assessment instruments and their use in clinical practice. *Rev Gaúcha Enferm*. 2017;38(1):e64675. doi:10.1590/1983-1447.2017.01.64675.
21. Opel D. A push for progress with shared decision-making in pediatrics. *Pediatrics*. 2017:e20162526. doi:10.1542/peds.2016-2526.
22. Barry MJ, Edgman-Levitan S. Shared decision making: the pinnacle of patient-centered care. *N Eng J Med*. 2012;366:780-781.
23. Fried T. Shared decision making—finding the sweet spot. *N Engl J Med*. 2016;374:104-106.
24. Kellams A, Harrel C, Omage S, Gregory C, Rosen-Carole C, Academy of Breastfeeding Medicine. ABM clinical protocol #3: supplementary feedings in the healthy term breastfed neonate. *Breastfeed Med*. 2017;12:188-198. doi:10.1089/bfm.2017.29038.ajk.
25. Wilson-Clay B, Hoover K. Infant states and infant assessment. In: *The Breastfeeding Atlas*. 6th ed. Manchaca, TX: LactNews Press; 2017:7-16.

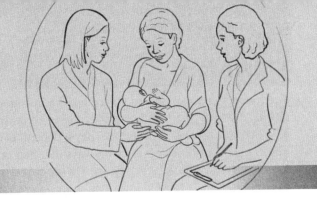

CHAPTER 28

Cultural Humility

Nekisha L. Killings

DEFINITIONS OF COMMONLY USED TERMS

cultural humility The delicate application of cultural knowledge and information in a way that allows for the client's lived experiences to supersede what the clinician believes to be true about members of that culture based on the clinician's own studies or previous interactions.[1]

dominant culture In a societal structure with multiple cultures, the culture that controls the conceptual maps and encompasses the most power, and is thereby able to impose its values and norms on subcultures or vulnerable populations.[2]

equipoise Balance of power or interest.[3]

humility Interpersonal and intrapersonal modesty exhibited by respect, empathy, openness, and a sense of self as not higher in relation to others; integrity of belief, behavior, and motivation.[4]

implicit bias Inherent prejudices and attitudes that unconsciously impact one's decision making.[5]

institutional bias Discriminatory practices that go beyond individual-level prejudice and occur at the institutional level through biased policies or practices as seen most blatantly in outcomes across entire groups.[6]

Latinx A gender-neutral term used to describe a person of Latin American origin or descent.

vulnerable population In a societal structure with multiple people groups, the population that is underrepresented and has less presence, power, and influence than another group.[7]

Any use of the term *mother*, *maternal*, or *breastfeeding* is not meant to exclude transgender or nonbinary parents who may be breastfeeding or providing human milk to their infant.

▶ Overview

The concept of cultural competence in the clinician–client relationship is a cornerstone of establishing rapport and, ultimately, trust. If a healthcare provider is unaware of the cultural norms, language, ethnotheories, and customs of the communities they support, they will be ill equipped to meet the most basic needs of breastfeeding families. The clinician can easily misstep in ways that halt or stall communication in the consultation. Perhaps even more important than cultural competence in a support setting is the practice of cultural humility—the delicate application of cultural knowledge and information in a way that allows for the client's lived experiences to supersede what the clinician believes to be true about members of that culture based on the clinician's previous trainings or interactions. Unlike cultural competence, which is finite in scope, cultural humility involves ongoing lifelong learning from the community that is being supported. It involves shifting the power balance in the interaction between a clinician and a client and, often, also dismantling bias at an organizational level.

I. Cultural Humility and Its Relationship to Cultural Competency

A.   Cultural humility is a multilayered concept that involves a broad perception of the terms culture and humility.

   1.   Culture is defined as knowledge, values, beliefs, and norms shared among a group—shared meaning.[2]

   2.   Cultural humility is a concept that dates back to the landmark work of Melanie Tervalon and Jann Murray-Garcia in their research of physician education outcomes in multicultural education.[1] It is defined as having a relational attitude that focuses on others instead of oneself.[8] It removes what one thinks they know to be true about a group and replaces it with a constant readiness to learn from the client they are relating to in the moment.

   3.   To be most effective, one must approach interpersonal encounters with those from a different culture with respect and humility toward an individual culture's background or experience.[8]

   4.   Cultural humility shifts the power balance in the relational experience between a clinician and a client to allow the client's needs and values to guide the recommendations by the provider. This is especially important when there is an added layer of structural or historical oppression compounding the imbalance.[9]

   5.   Common factors that are influential in a power differential are race, religion, language, physical ability, socioeconomic status, age, education, sexuality, and gender identity. Often several of these components are present, and they combine to affect the interaction between a client and a clinician.

   6.   Equipoise is present when the power imbalance between a clinician and a client is removed.[3]

   7.   A broad and generous application of humility on the part of the power holder helps to reduce and potentially eliminate obstacles to communication and trust building.

   8.   Constant self-evaluation is key to maintaining cultural humility and to applying it appropriately.

B.   Cultural humility is a distinctly different approach from cultural competence, which can be harmful if inappropriately applied.

   1.   The false or inadequate application of cultural competency can easily shift to cultural hubris, which is the opposite of cultural humility.

   2.   Cultural hubris is pride based on limited knowledge and contextual insight of cultures other than one's own. It is characterized by a reluctance to become a continuous and humble learner about other cultures' languages, norms, and nuances, making it impossible to incorporate those new learnings into the care relationship.

   3.   Cultural competence is finite in scope, whereas cultural humility involves continually learning from the community that is being supported. Consistently interacting with families from underrepresented populations provides more opportunities for exposure to nuances and norms within the culture.

   4.   Although the cultural competence model is a similar and somewhat related model to the patient-centered care model, neither fully captures the continual learning and relational component of cultural humility, which is the key distinctive quality.[10]

C.   Bridging cultural competence and cultural humility is the key to providing optimal care.

   1.   Cultural competence and cultural humility rely on each other and both are necessary for culturally adequate and appropriate care.

2. Cultural competence alone provides a narrow, limited perspective on a community and disallows potential for growth into a trusting and productive relationship. It is often limited to knowledge and awareness of primarily race and ethnicity information about the client, and it ignores other more nuanced differences, such as attitudes and ethnotheories that are prominent within any given culture.

3. Cultural competence has been criticized for centering the dominant culture as the norm and stereotyping anyone who is not a member of the dominant culture.[11]

4. Cultural humility cannot exist without acquiring some level of knowledge and competence of the community that is being supported. Coupled, the two provide didactic and experiential knowledge of a community, alongside context for a fuller understanding of how nuanced individual and community needs are.

5. The added layer of humbly listening and receiving information from the population that is being served is the bridge from competence to humility.

II. Cultural Humility and Power

A. Power dynamics and the biases associated with them are inherent in encounters between a clinician and a client.

B. Power is at play even when the care provider is from the same culture, speaks the same language, identifies as the same gender, and lives in the same community as the client seeking support.

C. These factors often compound the baseline power differential that already exists due to a perceived social hierarchy in which care providers are ranked higher than care seekers.

D. It is the responsibility of the care provider to seek and achieve equipoise through the practice of cultural humility to promote a client-centered approach to care.

III. Bias

A. Implicit bias involves inherent prejudices and attitudes that unconsciously impact one's decision making.

1. Implicit bias at the institutional or organizational level is common and undermines individual or intraorganizational attempts at equipoise.

2. Institutional bias is exhibited by discriminatory practices that go beyond individual-level prejudice and occurs at the institutional level through biased policies or practices as seen most blatantly in outcomes across entire groups.

B. Confronting and dismantling bias should be the ongoing goal of individuals and organizations in order to provide appropriate care to all clients in a community.

1. Dismantling bias at institutional levels is a massive undertaking and often involves replacement of people, policies, and practices that sustain oppressive disparities among the client base. Organizations must work simultaneously to provide excellent care and address gaps in the quality of care received by vulnerable populations.[12]

2. Institutions that are responsible for the training and preparation of healthcare and lactation care providers have an obligation to provide culturally appropriate and sensitive information that relates to a wide swath of underrepresented groups.[13]

   a. Cultural competence should be accompanied by a focus on listening and counseling skills specifically related to groups that are prevalent in the local community and that are different from the care provider's own culture, language, and race.

   b. Clinical instructors, mentors, and preceptors would benefit from training in relational skills that provide insights into perceiving the education of students and mentees as an opportunity to learn about building trust and open communication with other cultures. (See Chapter 26, *Counseling and Communication*, for more information about counseling skills.)

   c. Perpetual learning as a vital component of the cultural humility approach can be reinforced by course offerings in lactation and other healthcare provider training.

3. Opportunities to assess and confront one's own biases and to do the work necessary to eliminate them should be made available for the novice and experienced provider alike, and continuously over the course of a career.

C. Implicit bias has a direct impact upon cultural humility and must be addressed and dismantled to create a respectful and empathic care environment.

1. Authentic cultural humility cannot exist where implicit biases negatively impact the perceptions of the caregiver toward the community being served.[5]

2. Implicit bias refers to inherent prejudices and attitudes that unconsciously impact one's decision making. Because implicit bias is not something a person is consciously aware of, it often goes unaddressed and unresolved.

3. Implicit association tests expose hidden biases that affect interactions and attitudes. They are available through various organizations; Harvard University's Project Implicit is the most commonly used tool for assessing implicit cognition.[14] An implicit association test can be used to identify particular biases that are present as an initial step in a process to address and eliminate impediments to the practice of cultural humility in the clinician–client relationship.

4. Inherent biases toward or against populations can greatly impact the quality of care families receive from healthcare providers.[15] A 2007 study of racial implicit bias in physicians uncovered a direct correlation between the level of care provided and the perceptions of the patients. Biases against black patients and toward white patients impacted care. The study exposed a prevailing perception that black patients are less cooperative. The greater the bias, the less likely the physicians were to treat black patients with thrombolysis.[16]

5. Multiple studies have shown a notable difference in the level of breastfeeding information shared with expectant parents by healthcare providers and nutrition counselors in the U.S. Special Supplemental Nutrition Program for Women, Infants, and Children (WIC) program. One study revealed that being African American was associated with less likelihood of receiving breastfeeding information and a greater likelihood of receiving bottle feeding information from a nutrition counselor.[17] A literature review reported a trend among African American populations wherein the quality of human milk feeding information shared by healthcare providers was either inadequate or inaccurate.[18]

D. Recent studies have uncovered some ways in which implicit bias can be addressed and dismantled with focused attention and intention.

1. Recognizing one's hidden biases is only the first step in addressing them. Working to dismantle and eliminate bias are the necessary next and final steps in better serving a vulnerable population.

2. One method of reducing implicit bias among healthcare professionals was addressed in a 2012 study of habit-breaking strategies to address implicit bias specifically related to race.[19] There was a sustained reduction in implicit bias among psychology students after 12 weeks. The focused intervention program involved stereotype replacement, counterstereotypic imaging, individuation, perspective taking, and increasing opportunities for contact. Individuals and organizations should consider applying this five-pronged approach to identifying and addressing implicit bias in lactation care.

a. Stereotype replacement is recognizing personally held stereotypes, acknowledging them, then reflecting on them. This reflection is followed by deliberate consideration of how such a stereotype could be avoided in the future by replacing one's original response with an unbiased one.

b. Counterstereotypic imaging is a mental exercise to intentionally recall individuals who are of the stereotyped group yet do not exhibit the stereotypic behaviors. This process deposits positive images of members of the stereotyped group into one's conscience.

c. Individuation involves seeking and attaining information about real subjects of the stereotyped group. This helps to see members of the group as individuals and not only as group members.

d. Perspective taking involves adopting a first-person perspective of a stereotyped group member. This process creates psychological closeness to the group and reduces snap judgments based on assumptions.

e. Increasing opportunities for contact is simply creating and taking advantage of opportunities for exposure to the group to personally get to know members.

3. Another study on group-based reflection to identify personal implicit biases shows promise as a tool to eliminate bias when it is exposed in a group-reflection setting.[20]

a. In this study, small groups of six to eight 3rd year medical students engaged in reflection discussions after being exposed to a provocative trigger (implicit association tests).

b. The facilitated discussions led to discovery of personal biases and discussions of ways to dismantle bias to ensure that equitable care is provided in the hospital setting.

IV. Cultural Humility and Race, Gender Identity, and Sexuality

A. At present, race, gender identity, and sexuality are some of the most sensitive issues to tread due to global political and cultural shifts.

B. As healthcare professionals, lactation support persons are required to provide equitable quality care for families of any race, gender identity, or sexuality, regardless of whether they differ from the care provider.

C. Providers may find themselves serving families they have had little to no experience supporting in the past. These families are in dire need of support due to multiple factors related to long-standing systemic or structural discrimination.

D. Lactation care providers who are personally challenged by providing care to families that differ greatly from their own experiences or belief systems still have an obligation to provide equitable and quality care. Ethics codes for most lactation care providers specify this point, and the consequences for refusing to adhere to said codes are clear. For example, the *Code of Professional Conduct for IBCLCs*, in section 6.3 under Principle 6: Maintain Personal Integrity, states that every International Board Certified Lactation Consultant (IBCLC) shall "treat all clients equitably without regard to ability/disability, gender identity, sexual orientation, sex, ethnicity, race, national origin, political persuasion, marital status, geographic location, religion, socioeconomic status, age, within the legal framework of the respective geo-political region or setting."[21(p4)] Please see your certification's code of ethics for more information.

E. A referral to a colleague is appropriate when a provider is still learning and does not yet consider him- or herself competent to serve certain groups. However, this should be considered a temporary option while the care provider works to build both competence and humility to serve all families in the community.

V. Interdisciplinary Applications of Cultural Humility

A. Considering cooperative teams wherein lactation care providers are integral members, it is imperative that cultural humility is a priority for all team members.

B. System-wide trainings in bias and equity would benefit all providers in a care setting. All trainings are not equal, however. Special care should be taken to identify training that works both to identify challenges within a particular organization and to dismantle any contributors to those challenges.

　　1. Sources of solid organization or team-wide equity training include Harvard University's Project Implicit and Race Forward (formerly The Center for Social Inclusion). Lactation support organizations would be well served by affiliating with their local and state breastfeeding coalitions. Among other benefits, this relationship provides direct access to tremendous equity training and education resources from the United States Breastfeeding Committee.

　　2. Anyone who frequently interacts with breastfeeding families has a personal responsibility to pursue continuing education and opportunities for exposure to groups that are considered underserved or most vulnerable in the community. In cases of private practice or community providers who only occasionally interact with other members of a family's care team, the onus is on the provider to gain as much knowledge and garner as much trust as possible to become recognized as a community ally who can provide care in a safe environment.

　　3. Although there is no appropriate prescriptive approach to supporting entire demographic groups in the clinician–client interaction, there are some key practices for clinicians that support a culturally humble approach to care, honors all individuals, and works to dismantle the power imbalances at play in the breastfeeding consultation. Consider the following tools in the care setting:

　　　　a. At the start of the interaction, ask the client how they would prefer that you address them. The response might include preferred pronouns, official titles, formal titles, or nicknames. The goal is to best relate to the client in the way they prefer. Practice using their preferred title throughout the interaction.

　　　　b. After the initial introduction, consider sitting at eye level with the client for the duration of the consult, but position yourself at a comfortable enough distance to not invade their personal space.

　　　　c. Meet clients where they are. Ask open-ended questions about their experiences and symptoms. Listen intently without interrupting. Do not judge them. Believe them.

    d.   Explain to the client that breastfeeding is most often successful when the breastfeeding parent has a support system. Support systems may include partners, friends, relatives, support groups, any combination of these, or something entirely different. If appropriate, ask the client questions such as "do you have a support system?" or "what does a support system look like for you?" If appropriate, consider asking the client if they would like their support person to be included in the consultation. Welcome the support person so they can receive the same advice and guidance as the breastfeeding parent. Having multiple listeners helps to reinforce the information at home.

    e.   Remember that although you are the clinical expert, the parent is the expert of their experiences. Offer to partner with them in the creation of the care plan. Frequently ask a question such as "what does that look like for you?" Allow the client to relate the details of the care plan back to you in their own words. For example, if you recommend that the parent breastfeeds on demand over the next 7 days, asking what that looks like for the parent might reveal that the parent needs education about hunger cues, or perhaps the parent is planning to sleep upright in a recliner holding the baby at the breast for days on end. Whatever the response, follow up with clarifying information using respectful language and tone.

    f.   If you need to touch the client, ask for permission first and explain the technique you are practicing as you do it. Encourage the parent to attempt it on their own so they are empowered and equipped to perform the same task at home.

    g.   If language is a barrier, either provide a translator or welcome a support person who can help relate information between you and the parent.

▶ Key Points from This Chapter

    A.   Humility is respect in action.
    B.   Cultural humility is another-centric approach to care.
    C.   Cultural humility involves continual learning from the community being served.
    D.   Cultural humility is not cultural competence, but it can work alongside cultural competence to enhance the patient–provider experience.
    E.   Cultural competence without cultural humility can lead to cultural hubris.

The following case studies are examples of real interactions between healthcare providers and clients that show ways in which a cultural humility approach might have improved the care experience and relational outcomes.

🔎 CASE STUDY 1

A black mother and college professor shared a personal account in which a resident actively negated the patient's lived experience and failed to acknowledge that symptoms may present differently in people with dark skin.

Experience: "Through all three of my children's pregnancies I have been prone to dehydration and low blood pressure. I have become accustomed to identifying the symptoms (which don't correspond to the symptoms that white people show when dehydrated). When I was pregnant with the last, I went to the doctor's office, and told him that I was dehydrated. The resident insisted that I was wrong and that I wasn't pale (I don't get pale), my eyes weren't sunken, and my skin wasn't crepey (soft, fragile, and paper thin). This resident totally dismissed me, and told me to go home, and that my symptoms (faintness, extreme nausea, extreme headache) were just common pregnancy symptoms. I reminded him that I know my body, and my own pregnancy symptoms, as I was on my third baby. I told him in my professor tone to consult with his attending, and to order a urine specific gravity test. He did, and shamefacedly reported within a few minutes that I would need two bags of IV fluid."

Application: A resident practicing cultural humility might have been open to learning from a darker-skinned patient about how dehydration presents differently across ethnicities. Asking questions about the patient's past experience and identifying key signs that led to the diagnosis in prior pregnancies would have honored the patient's experience and provided an opportunity for open communication and education.

🔍 CASE STUDY 2

The following account from Germany shows institutional bias.

Experience: "When you check into some German hospitals or do pre-op paperwork, they ask for your religion, and the options are Catholic or Protestant, in essence asking, 'What type of Christian are you?' This ignores the non-Christian and atheist patients in the community served."

Application: The use of forms and policies that ignore swaths of the population or assume homogeneity creates a sentiment that the facility does not see or understand the groups that are not included. This issue could be corrected by providing many more options or adding open-ended questions for patients to self-identify according to their preferences.

🔍 CASE STUDY 3

The following account from a lactation student who was shadowing an IBCLC shows how problematic cultural competence is without cultural humility.

Experience: "When I was orienting to inpatient, I shadowed the hospital staff IBCLC, a white woman. We saw a Latinx family. Mom, who was very self-conscious about her English (which was fluent), asked the exact same questions as every white mom we had seen. 'How do I know if I'm making enough milk for my baby?'' How do I know if he's getting enough?' In what was one of the most horrific moments of my career, I had to stand by silently (because I was 'learning' from this woman) while the white IBCLC shouted at this mom 'In your culture, you're taught that mom's milk isn't enough, but that's not true.'"

Application: This provider could have treated the patient with much more dignity and respect, not making stereotypic or possibly insulting general statements. Listening to this patient's concerns and treating her as an individual with valid concerns would have gone much further in fostering mutual trust and respect.

🔍 CASE STUDY 4

The following account describes a conversation between a physician and a mother of black children, which included insensitive language.

Experience: "My daughter was being evaluated for precocious puberty and the pediatric endocrinologist told me that African American girls mature faster than 'normal' girls."

Application: To suggest that some girls are normal implies that others are abnormal. Word choice is of utmost importance in ensuring that patients feel valued, respected, and understood. Positive, appropriate, and sensitive language fosters an environment in which the provider can learn from the patient.

🔍 CASE STUDY 5

In the following account a young woman describes an awkward conversation with her obstetrician, who appeared to be uncomfortable counseling patients in same-sex relationships.

Experience: "I got a lecture from my gynecologist when I said I was sexually active and not using birth control. I explained I'd been having sex with my female partner of 10 years with no pregnancies so far."

Application: Taking the time to listen to and engage with this patient about her specific situation would have led to an understanding of her lived experiences. Avoiding stating information that might be appropriate for heterosexual patients would have circumvented this exchange and would have created an environment of mutual respect.

References

1. Tervalon M, Murray-Garcia J. Cultural humility versus cultural competence: a critical distinction in defining physician training outcomes in multicultural education. *J Health Care Poor Underserved*. 1998;9(2):117-125.
2. Young P, Adler SA, Shadiow LK. *Representation: Cultural Representations and Signifying Practices in Cultural Foundations of Education*. Columbus, OH: Pearson; 2006.

3. Elwyn G, Edwards A, Kinnersley P, Grol R. Shared decision making and the concept of equipoise: the competences of involving patients in healthcare choices. *Br J Gen Pract.* 2000;50(460):892-899.

4. Davis DE, Worthington EL Jr, Hook JN. Humility: review of measurement strategies and conceptualization as personality judgment. *J Posit Psychol.* 2010;5(4):243-252.

5. Greenwald AG, Banaji MR. Implicit social cognition: attitudes, self-esteem, and stereotypes. *Psychol Rev.* 1995;102:4-27.

6. Henry PJ. Institutional bias. In: Dovidio JF, Hewstone M, Glick P, Esses VM, eds. *The Sage Handbook of Prejudice, Stereotyping and Discrimination.* London, UK: SAGE Publishing Ltd; 2010:426-440.

7. Vulnerable populations: who are they? *Am J Manag Care.* 2006;12(suppl):S348-S352.

8. Hook JN, Davis DE, Owen J, Worthington EL Jr, Utsey SO. Cultural humility: measuring openness to culturally diverse clients. *J Couns Psychol.* 2013;60(3):353-366. doi:10.1037/a0032595.

9. Gallardo ME. *Developing Cultural Humility: Embracing Race, Privilege and Power.* Los Angeles, CA: Sage; 2013.

10. Saha S, Beach MC, Cooper LA. Patient centeredness, cultural competence and healthcare quality. *J Natl Med Assoc.* 2008;100(11):1275-1285.

11. Yeager KA, Bauer-Wu S. Cultural humility: essential foundation for clinical researchers. *Appl Nurs Res.* 2013;26(4):251-256.

12. Griffith DM, Mason M, Yonas M, Eng E, Jeffries V, Plihcik S, Parks B. Dismantling institutional racism: theory and action. *Am J Community Psychol.* 2007;39(3-4):381-392.

13. U.S. Department of Health and Human Services. The national CLAS standards. U.S. Department of Health and Human Services Office of Minority Health website. https://minorityhealth.hhs.gov/omh/browse.aspx?lvl=2&lvlid=53. Accessed March 11, 2018.

14. Project Implicit. Project Implicit social attitudes, Project Implicit mental health, Project Implicit featured task. Harvard University website. https://implicit.harvard.edu/implicit/. Published 2011. Accessed February 21, 2017.

15. FitzGerald C, Hurst S. Implicit bias in healthcare professionals: a systematic review. *BMC Med Ethics.* 2017;18(1):19.

16. Green AR, Carney DR, Pallin DJ, et al. Implicit bias among physicians and its prediction of thrombolysis decisions for black and white patients. *J Gen Intern Med.* 2007;22(9):1231-1238.

17. Beal AC, Kuhlthau K, Perrin JM. Breastfeeding advice given to African American and white women by physicians and WIC counselors. *Public Health Rep.* 2003;118(4):368-376.

18. DeVane-Johnson S, Woods-Giscombé C, Thoyre S, Fogel C, Williams R. Integrative literature review of factors related to breastfeeding in African American women: evidence for a potential paradigm shift. *J Hum Lactation.* 2017;33(2):435-447.

19. Devine PG, Forscher PS, Austin AJ, Cox WT. Long-term reduction in implicit race bias: a prejudice habit-breaking intervention. *J Exp Soc Psychol.* 2012;48(6):1267-1278.

20. Teal CR, Shada RE, Gill AC, et al. When best intentions aren't enough: helping medical students develop strategies for managing bias about patients. *J Gen Intern Med.* 2010;25(2):115-118.

21. International Board of Lactation Consultant Examiners. Code of professional conduct for IBCLCs. International Board of Lactation Consultant Examiners website. https://iblce.org/wp-content/uploads/2017/05/code-of-professional-conduct.pdf. Published September 2015. Accessed September 26, 2017.

Additional Resources

Publications

2014 Lactation Summit Design Team. *Summary Report of the 2014 Lactation Summit: Addressing Inequities within the Lactation Profession.* Morrisville, NC: ILCA; 2014. https://higherlogicdownload.s3.amazonaws.com/ILCA/e3ee2b6e-c389-43de-83ea-f32482f20da5/UploadedImages/Values%20Images/Summary%20Report_2014LactationSummit-FINAL(1).pdf.

Chapman EN, Kaatz A, Carnes M. Physicians and implicit bias: how doctors may unwittingly perpetuate health care disparities. *J Gen Intern Med.* 2013;28(11):1504-1510.

Foronda C, Baptiste DL, Reinholdt MM, Ousman K. Cultural humility: a concept analysis. *J Transcult Nurs.* 2016;27(3):210-217.

Good Mojab C. An American IBCLC's observations on breastfeeding in Iran. *J Hum Lactation.* 2008;24(1):13.

Good Mojab C. Ethics, culture, and lactation: essential concepts and principles for lactation specialists. 2017 International Lactation Consultant Association Conference: knowledge, diversity, equity. *J Hum Lactation.* 2017;33(3):614-634.

Good Mojab C. Pandora's box is already open: answering the ongoing call to dismantle institutional oppression in the field of breastfeeding. *J Hum Lactation.* 2015;31(1):32-35. http://www.lifecirclecc.com/yahoo_site_admin/assets/docs/PandorasBoxGoodMojab2015.pdf.

Good Mojab C, Healy E. Undoing institutional racism in perinatal support organizations: first steps for eliminating racial inequity in breastfeeding support. In: Smith PH, Labbok M, eds. *It Takes a Village: The Role of the Greater Community in Inspiring and Empowering Women to Breastfeed.* Amarillo, TX: Praeclarus Press; 2015:72-78.

Johnson RL, Saha S, Arbelaez JJ, Beach MC, Cooper LA. Racial and ethnic differences in patient perceptions of bias and cultural competence in health care. *J Gen Intern Med.* 2004;19(2):101-110.

Schuldberg J, Fox NS, Jones CA, et al. Same, same—but different: the development of cultural humility through an international volunteer experience. *Int J Humanit Soc Sci.* 2012;2(17):17-30.

Websites

Race Forward. https://www.raceforward.org.
United States Breastfeeding Committee. http://www.usbreastfeeding.org.

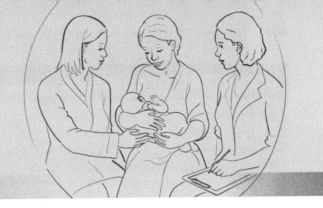

CHAPTER 29

Initiatives to Protect, Promote, and Support Breastfeeding

Suzanne Hetzel Campbell
Joan Younger Meek
Tina Revai

OBJECTIVES

- Describe current evidence-based initiatives that promote and support breastfeeding.
- Recognize the determinants of breastfeeding success and advocate for breastfeeding families in all areas, including environments that are not supportive of breastfeeding.
- Define the role of healthcare professionals in compliance with the World Health Organization's (WHO) *International Code of Marketing of Breast-milk Substitutes* (WHO Code).
- Provide examples of the lactation consultant's role as a change agent in the protection, promotion, and support of breastfeeding at individual, community, political, and global levels.
- Articulate the key elements of a Baby-friendly hospital, according to the Baby-friendly Hospital Initiative (BFHI).
- Describe some of the barriers and facilitators to implementing a Baby-friendly neonatal intensive care unit (NICU) according to Baby-friendly Hospital Initiative for Neonatal Wards (Neo-BFHI) protocols.
- Describe global successes and challenges to implementing the Ten Steps to Successful Breastfeeding (BFHI).
- Identify evidence-based breastfeeding protocols.
- Describe Baby-friendly policies and practices at multiple levels, including hospital, clinical practice, and community.

DEFINITIONS OF COMMONLY USED TERMS

Baby-friendly Hospital Initiative (BFHI) Global initiative led by UNICEF and WHO to protect, promote, and support breastfeeding.

change agent A catalyst for change; one who leads change or one who facilitates change.[1]

cultural humility As defined by the First Nations Health Authority, "Cultural humility is a process of self-reflection to understand personal and systemic biases and to develop and maintain respectful processes and relationships based on mutual trust... [this] involves humbly acknowledging oneself as a learner when it comes to understanding another's experience."[2(para 6)]

cultural safety A call for healthcare providers to respond to the colonizing histories and experiences of indigenous people,[3] an approach used (with some critique) for a diverse range of groups that are underserved in the healthcare system.[4]

health equity The state in which everyone has the opportunity to attain their highest level of health.[5]

health promotion Advocating for and the process of enabling people to increase their control over their health and improve their health.[6]

public health The science and art of preventing disease, prolonging life, and promoting health through the organized efforts of society.[7]

social determinants of health The economic and social conditions that shape the health of individuals, communities, and jurisdictions as a whole.[8,9]

socioecological model A framework for understanding the complex interplay among individual, relationship, community, and societal factors that influence health.[10] An approach that focuses on both population-level and individual-level determinants of health and interventions; recognizes that health is determined by influences at multiple levels (e.g., public policy, community, institutional, interpersonal, and intrapersonal factors).[11]

UNICEF Global agency that protects and promotes the rights of every child in 190 countries and regions.

World Health Assembly The forum through which the WHO is governed by its 194 member states.

World Health Organization (WHO) Global agency composed of the health ministers from its member states; considered the world's foremost policy-setting body for health.

Any use of the term *mother*, *maternal*, or *breastfeeding* is not meant to exclude transgender or nonbinary parents who may be breastfeeding or providing human milk to their infant.

▶ Overview

The awareness of breastfeeding as an important public health initiative to ensure healthy outcomes for mothers and infants has driven improvement in the systems that support breastfeeding, both globally and in individual countries worldwide. The health impact pyramid is a way to conceptualize the lactation consultant's role in the promotion and protection of breastfeeding. The pyramid takes into consideration socioeconomic factors; changing contexts for health decision making; long-lasting protective interventions, including clinical, counseling, and education interventions; and concrete support of families by all healthcare practitioners.[12]

There is a considerable opportunity for change in formal health systems in which many lactation consultants are positioned, in that healthcare systems have a commitment to provide evidence-based care. However, the full protection, promotion, and support of breastfeeding consists of integrated efforts not only within formal health systems, but at all levels of society. With this broader goal in mind, the lactation consultant understands that the fundamental commitment to act is not only at the level of the clinical encounter; it also includes the context that enables true breastfeeding choice. When lactation care is conceptualized beyond the clinical encounter, it becomes clear that "the success or failure of breastfeeding [is] not solely the responsibility of the woman. Her ability to breastfeed is very much shaped by the support and the environment in which she lives. There is a broader responsibility of governments and society to support women through policies and programs in the community."[13,14(para.5)]

Additionally, health promotion work recognizes that social justice is a prerequisite to health.[6] Therefore, breastfeeding is necessarily a health issue with equity considerations.[15] Accordingly, the lactation consultant works in partnership with populations that bear the burden of suboptimal breastfeeding rates to identify challenges and find accessible and acceptable evidence-informed solutions.

This chapter will review evidence, relevant policy, and potential strategies that will guide the lactation consultant toward action that protects, promotes, and supports breastfeeding at all levels of the healthcare system, and indeed throughout society, so the option to breastfeed becomes a truly empowered and realistic choice for every parent.

I. Lactation Consultant as Change Agent at the Individual Level

A. Globally, there is broad support in recognizing the importance of protecting, promoting, and supporting breastfeeding.

B. It is in the point-of-care interaction with soon-to-be parents, families, and other health professionals where most direct-care lactation consultants have multiple opportunities to make a difference as change agents.

C. This starts with one parent and child at a time, and one healthcare professional at a time.

D. Taking a person-centered public health approach to the clinical encounter sensitizes the lactation consultant to the determinants of health that may affect the dyad's situation.

II. Determinants of Breastfeeding and Opportunities for Change

A. Knowing the determinants of breastfeeding as a health behavior and ensuring that clinical practice is evidence informed and culturally safe (see **FIGURE 29-1**) will guide the lactation consultant to be responsive and respectful at the level of the clinical encounter, while holding a view that is broader than that of individual responsibility for breastfeeding outcomes.

B. Access to social resources: Evidence shows that the general pattern across most populations is that supportive social connections for breastfeeding parents correlate to higher breastfeeding rates.

1. Breastfeeding parents who live with a partner are significantly more likely to breastfeed.[16,17]

2. In the United States, the availability of a family member who can help care for the baby is significantly associated with exclusive breastfeeding lasting 4 months or longer.[18]

C. Access to material resources: In developed countries, the data shows a general trend where low income and education are associated with suboptimal breastfeeding rates. In low- and middle-income countries, the highest income quintile and people with higher education have an increased risk of suboptimal breastfeeding rates.

1. An analysis of 44 countries with the highest rate of maternal and child mortality showed that when rates of breastfeeding were broken into four income quintiles, the poorest and richest quintiles were least likely to initiate breastfeeding. The richest quintile was the least likely to practice exclusive breastfeeding.[19]

2. Canadian data showed that women with a household income of $100,000 CAD or more had a 2.11 odds ratio for exclusive breastfeeding, and multivariate analysis showed that years of education was a significant predictor of 6-month exclusive breastfeeding.[16]

3. Spanish data showed temporal trends of education as a factor in duration of breastfeeding. Women with a secondary education or higher had lower rates of breastfeeding until 1980; thereafter the rates were significantly higher.[20]

4. Australian data showed that women who did not complete high school were four times more likely to wean earlier, compared to those with a university education.[21]

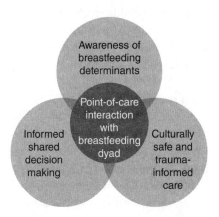

FIGURE 29-1 Point-of-care interaction with breastfeeding dyad.

5. Cambodian data showed a gap in healthcare professionals' knowledge and practice to support families to exclusively breastfeed, especially in the areas of latch, milk production, and feeding frequency. The conclusion was that the message, on its own, to exclusively breastfeed was not sufficient for success.[22]

D. Self-efficacy: The parent's confidence in the ability to breastfeed is positively correlated with breastfeeding rates.[21,23,24] A 2017 meta-analysis of educational and supportive interventions to increase breastfeeding self-efficacy demonstrated effectiveness, and mothers in the intervention groups were 1.56 and 1.66 times more likely to be breastfeeding at 1 and 2 months postpartum.[23]

E. Experience of trauma: Global estimates indicate that about 1 in 3 women have experienced either physical or sexual violence at some point in their life.[25] The rate of birth trauma is estimated at 21.4 percent in the Netherlands[26] to 34 percent in the United States.[27]

1. Women with a history of childhood sexual abuse may be more likely to initiate breastfeeding than their counterparts with no history of abuse.[28]

2. For women who have experienced birth trauma, breastfeeding can either facilitate healing or compound the experience of trauma.[29]

3. A strategy to implement trauma-informed practice—a universal precaution approach—assumes that all service users may be survivors of trauma.[30]

F. Smoking: A consistent trend is that smoking is inversely related to both initiation and duration of breastfeeding.[16,17,21,31]

G. Obesity: Obesity is associated with a risk for delay in lactogenesis (odds ratio 1.02–1.10), and parents who are obese are more likely than parents with a normal body mass index to never attempt breastfeeding.[32]

H. Specific populations: Populations or groups of individuals who have been historically stigmatized and marginalized within a given society may have a tendency toward suboptimal breastfeeding rates.

1. Regardless of whether lactation consultants hold direct membership in these groups, they have an obligation to go beyond advocating at the level of direct care based on their knowledge of inequitable access or quality of care.

2. Lactation consultants have a mandate to work toward healthcare system transformation that sees the population in question as part of a more equitable healthcare system redesign. Although there is research noting that disparities are often associated with membership in or identification with groups that are marginalized due to economic status, skin color, nationality, employment, religion, age, gender, or sexual orientation, it is beyond the scope of this section to cover the complexities of why this occurs and interventions that address this issue. (See Chapter 28, *Cultural Humility*, for more extensive research and suggested strategies.)

3. Research indicates promising practices for racialized and other groups:

   a. Racialized groups[33,34]:

      i. A systematic review about psychosocial interventions for enhancing breastfeeding rates among African American women found a need for an integrative approach because of the complex and interrelated barriers experienced across the layers of the social–ecological system.[35]

      ii. Similarly, exclusive breastfeeding rates that traditionally fell short of Healthy People 2010 goals in a low-income, predominantly Latina community, were found to improve with well-structured, intensive breastfeeding support and community-based peer counseling.[36,37]

      iii. An ecological perspective of breastfeeding in an indigenous community found patterns related to influences among the indigenous and mainstream cultures, barriers that were communication related, and socioeconomic and support issues that defined a need for more culturally relevant programs.[38]

   b. Other groups:

      i. Individuals from diverse communities, including lesbian, gay, bisexual, transgender, queer, questioning, and intersex, face significant barriers in accessing health care that is appropriate for meeting their parenting and breastfeeding goals. Lactation consultants need to be aware of the unique needs of nontraditional families and use the approaches described throughout this text to provide culturally sensitive care that takes into consideration the traditions and context of diverse cultures.[39]

      ii. Adolescent or young mothers: An education and support intervention was found to be effective for adolescent mothers between 15 and 18 years of age,[40] and a scale to measure instrumental, informational, and emotional appraisal support for adolescent mothers has been developed.[41] A systematic review of intervention studies supporting breastfeeding in adolescent mothers found the interventions to be resource intensive and lacking in theoretical foundations, with an aim at increasing duration and exclusivity. It was suggested that involving mothers and partners of young mothers was more likely to improve outcomes.[42]

      iii.   Mothers with disabilities: There are potential pregnancy complications for women with disabilities.[43] A national study in the United Kingdom found that improvement in communication for more individualized care, including support for infant feeding, was warranted.[44]

I.   Consider the following strategies for change:
1. Utilize proportionate universal approaches rather than targeted programs that may contribute to stigma.[45]
2. Increase control over defining breastfeeding issues, setting priorities, and designing interventions.
3. Increase diversity within the healthcare profession both broadly and, specifically, in lactation care.[46]
4. Utilize patient-oriented research, especially that which evaluates the experience of care.

III. Using a Socioecological Approach to Identify Opportunities for Change

A.   Implementing evidence-based practice and advocating for change within the healthcare system and beyond is seldom done by a single lactation consultant. Efforts require partnering with others and implementing multiple strategies.

B.   An important framework for conceptualizing health beyond the individual is the social–ecological model of care[10] (**FIGURE 29-2**). An ecological approach is a theory-based understanding of the multifaceted and interactive effects of personal and environmental factors that determine health behaviors and that, importantly, identify opportunities for leveraging change.

IV. Lactation Consultant as Change Agent at the Family Level

A.   Recognize the influence of the fathers.
1. The father's attitude is more influential than that of healthcare professionals.[47]
2. Mothers whose partners receive information about overcoming breastfeeding challenges have greater breastfeeding rates than mothers whose partners do not receive that information.[48]

B.   Recognize the influence of grandmothers.
1. In a systematic review, most studies showed a significant positive impact on breastfeeding when grandmothers had their own breastfeeding experience or were positively inclined toward breastfeeding.[49]
2. Although grandmothers exert influence, if they are not supportive they may undermine a mother's efforts to exclusively breastfeed.[50]
3. A systematic review indicated that lactation programs seeking to influence exclusive breastfeeding should include grandmothers in their interventions as valuable potential influencers.[51]

C.   Strategies for influencing families include the following:
1. Breastfeeding advice, support, and education should include the family and partner and be responsive to their needs and concerns.
2. Incorporate patient-oriented research and outcomes that matter to patients and how they experience their care.

V. Lactation Consultant as Change Agent at the Community Level

A.   Access to community resources (e.g., peer support groups), knowledgeable healthcare providers, and skilled specialist help, especially when delivered in the home, is particularly effective.[52-56]

B.   Strategies for change include Baby-friendly initiatives for the community, community engagement and development, and group processes (facilitators and barriers).[57,58]
1. Community building for breastfeeding promotion includes support of new parents.

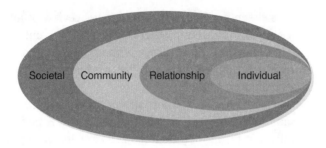

FIGURE 29-2 Social–ecological model of care.

Reproduced from Centers for Disease Control and Prevention (CDC). The social-ecological model: a framework for prevention. CDC website. https://www.cdc .gov/violenceprevention/overview/social-ecologicalmodel.html. Updated March 25, 2015. Accessed October 21, 2017.[10]

2. Home- and family-based interventions are particularly effective at improving exclusive breastfeeding (risk ratio 1.48), continued breastfeeding (risk ratio 1.26), any breastfeeding (risk ratio 1.16), and early initiation of breastfeeding (risk ratio 1.74).[13]
3. Work to implement health policies for support programs following the Baby-friendly initiative.[59,60]
4. Incorporate multidisciplinary team-led programs.
5. Involve parents and families in designing, promoting, and evaluating support programs.
6. Partner with community-based organizations for support.

VI. Lactation Consultant as Change Agent at the Organizational Level

A. The BFHI, developed by the WHO and UNICEF in 1991, is an organizational certification process that ensures the implementation of specific evidence-based hospital practices to promote exclusive breastfeeding; that is, the infant receives only breastmilk—no other food or drink, not even water.[61]
1. To be designated as Baby-friendly, hospitals must implement the Ten Steps to Successful Breastfeeding (**BOX 29-1**).[62]
2. Maternity care facilities designated as Baby-friendly must not accept free infant formula, bottles, or nipples or teats.
3. Implementation of the evidence-based Ten Steps to Successful Breastfeeding has been shown to improve breastfeeding outcomes.[63,64] In a meta-analysis of the elements of BFHI, the provision of individual breastfeeding counseling and group education, immediate breastfeeding support at delivery, and skilled lactation management were specific interventions that increased exclusive

---

BOX 29-1 Ten Steps to Successful Breastfeeding (Revised 2018)

Critical Management Procedures
1a. Comply fully with the *International Code of Marketing of Breast-milk Substitutes* and relevant World Health Assembly resolutions.
1b. Have a written infant feeding policy that is routinely communicated to staff and parents.
1c. Establish ongoing monitoring and data-management systems.
2. Ensure that staff have sufficient knowledge, competence, and skills to support breastfeeding.

Key Clinical Practices
3. Discuss the importance and management of breastfeeding with pregnant women and their families.
4. Facilitate immediate and uninterrupted skin-to-skin contact and support mothers to initiate breastfeeding as soon as possible after birth.
5. Support mothers to initiate and maintain breastfeeding and manage common difficulties.
6. Do not provide breastfed newborns any food or fluids other than breastmilk, unless medically indicated.
7. Enable mothers and their infants to remain together and to practice rooming-in 24 hours a day.
8. Support mothers to recognize and respond to their infants' cues for feeding.
9. Counsel mothers on the use and risks of feeding bottles, teats, and pacifiers.
10. Coordinate discharge so that parents and their infants have timely access to ongoing support and care.

Reproduced from World Health Organization. Baby-friendly Hospital Initiative. WHO website. http://www.who.int/nutrition/bfhi/ten-steps/en/. Accessed April 14, 2018.[62]

breastfeeding by 49 percent (95 percent confidence interval 33–68) and any breastfeeding by 66 percent (95 percent confidence interval 34–107).[13]

    4.   According to a 2017 WHO report,[65] although the majority of countries have established a national BFHI program, only 10 percent of births worldwide occur in facilities that have been designated or redesignated as Baby-friendly within the prior 5 years.

B.   The Neo-BFHI Core document was published in 2015.[66,67] The aim was to modify and adapt the Ten Steps to Successful Breastfeeding to protect, promote, and support breastfeeding in the NICU setting. (See Chapter 14, *Breastfeeding and the Preterm Infant*.)

    1.   Three guiding principles were developed[68]:

       a.   Staff attitudes toward the mother must focus on the individual mother and her situation.

       b.   The facility must provide family-centered care, supported by the environment.

       c.   The health care system must ensure continuity of care from pregnancy to after the infant's discharge.

    2.   Research supports the importance of peer counselors in supporting breastfeeding in this vulnerable population.[68]

C.   Change within health systems is challenging.

    1.   Research demonstrates that it takes approximately 17 years for evidence-based-practice to reach the bedside.[69]

    2.   Countries throughout the world experience facilitators and barriers to effecting BFHI and Neo-BFHI.

       a.   Facilities in Austria found that a complex interplay of factors is required to become a Baby-friendly hospital, especially during implementation.

          i.   Hospitals seeking BFHI certification may benefit from distinct and intensive investments in planning and preparation before putting the steps into practice.

          ii.   Staff members, parents, and families require extensive information and the continuous participation of healthcare professionals.

          iii.   Allowing room for debate and a staggered step implementation, depending on the context, is paramount.

          iv.   Adjusting activities or expanding them during the BFHI certification process lead to sustainable implementation.[70]

       b.   Hospitals in Canada identified the following barriers and facilitators in expanding BFHI to the NICU:

          i.   The barriers included infant health status, parent and infant separation, workloads and patterns of staffing, gaps in staff knowledge and skills, and lack of continuity in breastfeeding support.

          ii.   The facilitators included breastfeeding education and champions, and interprofessional collaboration. BFHI was recognized as a facilitator of family-centered care, and the recommendations included promoting it as such, developing champions in the NICU, and increasing access to lactation consultants for parents and staff members.[57]

       c.   Hospitals in Spain identified barriers and challenges through a national survey, and a new national strategy to promote BFHI was implemented with promising results.

          i.   The recognition of threats highlighted the healthcare professionals' fear of change[71] and the need to counteract noncompliance with the WHO Code regarding marketing of breastmilk substitutes.

          ii.   The recognized strengths included the enthusiasm of generous volunteers and the power of an increasing number of parents who recognize their right to support in attaining their breastfeeding goals.[72-74]

       d.   Health professionals in Brazil perceived the following barriers to Neo-BFHI implementation[75]:

          i.   Limited infrastructure to support 24-hour parental presence, overcrowded units, and insufficient staff.

          ii.   Lack of protocols.

          iii.   Lack of education for clinical staff on preterm breastfeeding and resistance to change.

          iv.   Inadequate interdisciplinary communication.

          v.   Cultural and socioeconomic challenges of families (i.e., social determinants of health).

e. In contrast, the perceived facilitators in Brazil included the following[75]:
    i. BFHI implemented at all sites.
    ii. National law permitting parental access to infants 24/7.
    iii. Multidisciplinary teams to assist with families' needs.
    iv. Training in BFHI policies.
    v. Support of human milk bank staff.

D. Continuity of care requires the lactation consultant to work collaboratively with the healthcare team:
    1. Develop professionally mediated or peer support programs.[37,76,77]
    2. Provide interactive group education during the prenatal phase, which was shown to be effective in increasing breastfeeding initiation and duration.[78]
    3. Provide information to healthcare providers when patients are referred. Establish practice and referral opportunities with physicians, midwives, nurses, pharmacists, and other healthcare providers.[79]
    4. Provide ongoing support that is evidence based at the point of care.
    5. Provide breastfeeding education and training for fellow healthcare providers in the system and community.

E. Evidence demonstrates that supportive birthing practices and facility organizational structure increase breastfeeding.
    1. A BFHI facility provides more supportive birthing practices.[58]
    2. Midwife attendant, doula, peer counselor, and International Board Certified Lactation Consultant (IBCLC) combinations are important as support systems, especially for adolescent new parents.[42,80]
    3. The elements of policy and practice that support breastfeeding include the following:
        a. Skin-to-skin care.[81]
        b. Rooming in.[82]
        c. Adequate breastfeeding education for staff members.[83]
        d. Access to skilled help.[54]
        e. Teleconferencing of hospital lactation consultants with low-income women at community centers.[84]
        f. Breastfeeding support in community pharmacies.[58,83-87]

F. A summary of a BFHI global perspective and safety issues includes the following:
    1. Evidence shows that the more BFHI steps that are in place, the more likely women are to breastfeed.
        a. Among women who intended to breastfeed for more than 2 months, 30 percent of those who experienced no supportive maternity practices had stopped breastfeeding before 6 weeks; however, only 3 percent of those who experienced six of the BFHI steps had stopped breastfeeding by 6 weeks.[64]
        b. Interventions as simple as minimizing mother–infant separation can have significant implications.[88-90]
    2. Baby-friendly implementation occurs within the context of breastfeeding, sleep, and safety.
        a. Although critical components of BFHI include skin-to-skin contact in the immediate postpartum period, exclusive breastfeeding, and continuous rooming in, an increase in both neonatal falls and sudden unexpected postnatal collapse have been reported with skin-to-skin care.
        b. Sudden unexpected postnatal collapse is seen more commonly in the following situations:
            i. Neonates with infection, concern for infection, any signs of distress, congenital heart defects, prematurity, metabolic defects, and anemia.
            ii. Neonates that have been placed in the prone position.
            iii. Lack of consistent supervision in the immediate postpartum period while infants are experiencing skin-to-skin contact.[91]
            iv. Mothers who are primiparous, exhausted, sedated, have infections, and are alone.
        c. Mothers and newborns with the above risk factors should have continuous clinical supervision in the immediate postpartum period, with the infant's face visualized and the head uncovered, according to the American Academy of Pediatrics.[92] Bedside nurses should be trained to provide this continuous supervision and assessment with minimal interference to skin-to-skin contact or breastfeeding.

      d.   Globally, there are a variety of opinions related to sleep and breastfeeding, and this continues to be an area of clinical controversy.

         i.   The American Academy of Pediatrics Task Force on Sudden Infant Death Syndrome recommends breastfeeding to decrease the risk of sudden infant death syndrome.[93] The task force advocates room sharing and discourages bed sharing. It suggests that infants should sleep in the supine position on a separate sleep surface with no loose bedding.

        ii.   Caregivers should avoid the use of tobacco, alcohol, and illicit drugs.

      iii.   Pacifiers are recommended to reduce the risk of sudden infant death syndrome; however, in breastfed infants, pacifiers should be introduced only after breastfeeding has been established.[94]

      e.   Public health messaging in some jurisdictions has moved beyond a "just say no" approach, particularly when research has demonstrated that many breastfeeding mothers will continue to sleep with their infant, at least some of the time, even in areas where this has been discouraged.[95-97]

         i.   In the United Kingdom and British Columbia, Canada, public health resources have been developed that support the clinician in a person- and situation-centered shared decision-making conversation with families.[98,99]

        ii.   Infant solitary sleep recommendations are not particularly effective at stopping mothers and infants from sharing sleep, and when breastfeeding mothers practice solitary sleeping arrangements it is strongly associated with less breastfeeding on all dimensions, including frequency,[100] exclusivity, and duration.[97,101]

      iii.   A mother's decision to sleep with the infant, in the absence of additional risk factors, seems like a reasonable option[102] for nighttime parenting and maintenance of breastfeeding. The development of decision-making tools to support more tailored advice is a promising approach for lactation consultant practice.

      iv.   Parents who choose to sleep with their infants should be advised to avoid alcohol, tobacco, and medication, and they should sleep on a firm surface without excessive bedding. Older children and pets should not share the bed. Sleeping with infants in chairs and on sofas is not recommended.[98,99]

VII. Lactation Consultant as Change Agent at the Workplace Level and in the Sociocultural Context

  A.   Government guidelines and public policies that are conducive to breastfeeding include the following:

    1.   The right to breastfeed in public.[103]

    2.   Economic policies that support workers' rights for paid maternity and paternity leave and breastfeeding breaks.[104-106] (See Chapter 11, *Breastfeeding and Employment*.)

    3.   Breastfeeding in public is normalized when mothers see other mothers breastfeeding without discrimination and with full community support.[8,9] Social mobilization and integrated mass media increased timely initiation by 86 percent (95 percent confidence interval 33–159) and exclusive breastfeeding by 20 percent (95 percent confidence interval 3–39).[13]

  B.   Strategies for creating a social movement through social marketing include the following:

    1.   "Breastfeeding is the biological norm for infant feeding, and is also a social construct. As such, its rates and practices are determined by the same social determinants that shape health inequalities and inequities."[127(p3)]

    2.   When breastfeeding is protected, promoted, and supported equitably at all levels of the healthcare system and throughout society, the option to breastfeed becomes a fully enabled choice for all parents.

    3.   A scaling up of breastfeeding promotion programs in low- and middle-income countries has been suggested as the breastfeeding gear model, which takes into consideration public health, public policy, and the ramifications in the social support of breastfeeding families.[107,108]

    4.   Devoting attention to the AIDED framework and breastfeeding gear model[108] can lead to scaling up of efforts and overall promotion of breastfeeding as the gold standard and cultural norm. The AIDED framework addresses the following:

      a.   Assess the landscape (baseline needs).

      b.   Innovate to fit user receptivity (media, BFHI, Baby-friendly promotion).

     c.   Develop support.

     d.   Engage user groups (individual approach, dispel myths).

     e.   Devolve efforts for spreading innovation.

    5.   A total of 22 enabling factors and 15 barriers are mapped and used to build the breastfeeding gear model.[108,109]

VIII. Lactation Consultant as Change Agent at the National and Global Levels

    A.   The WHO approved the *International Code of Marketing of Breast-milk Substitutes* in 1981 to limit the marketing of artificial breastmilk substitutes.

        1.   The *International Code of Marketing of Breast-milk Substitutes* is known as the WHO Code.[110,111]

        2.   The WHO Code prohibits the following:

            a.   Advertising of formula directly to consumers.

            b.   Distributing free formula to consumers.

            c.   Promotion by formula companies in healthcare facilities.

            d.   Healthcare workers accepting personal samples of infant formula or other gifts.

            e.   Idealizing artificial feeding in pictures or in the marketing of artificial feeding devices.

        3.   The WHO Code may be adapted in individual countries as appropriate. Formula manufacturers are expected to comply, even when an individual country does not choose to enact the code and enforce sanctions.

            a.   Evidence supports the efficacy of enacting the WHO Code into national law.

            b.   In 1992 India created strong legislation and a monitoring system for implementing the WHO Code, and the country has significantly higher breastfeeding rates and lower national formula sales despite a higher birth rate, compared to China, where there is weak support for the WHO Code.[112]

        4.   The International Baby Food Action Network (IBFAN) campaigns for the enactment of the WHO Code and works to protect infant health and mothers' rights by vigilance to ensure that the marketing of baby food does not have a negative impact on child or parental health.[113] IBFAN's seven principles are as follows:

            1.   Infants and young children everywhere have the right to the highest attainable standard of health.

            2.   Families, and in particular women and children, have the right to access adequate and nutritious food and sufficient and affordable water.

            3.   Women have the right to breastfeed and to make informed decisions about infant and young child feeding.

            4.   Women have the right to full support to breastfeed for two years or more and to exclusively breastfeed for the first six months.

            5.   All people have the right to access quality health care services and information free of commercial influence.

            6.   Health workers and consumers have the right to be protected from commercial influence which may distort their judgement and decisions.

            7.   People have the right to advocate for change which protects, promotes, and supports basic health, in international solidarity.[114]

        5.   The *Code of Professional Conduct for IBCLCs* states that "a crucial part of an IBCLC's duty to protect mothers and children is adherence to the principles and aim of the *International Code of Marketing of Breast-milk Substitutes* and subsequent relevant World Health Assembly's resolutions."[115(p1)] Product information provided to healthcare workers should be factual and scientific.

    B.   In 1990 the WHO and UNICEF developed the *Innocenti Declaration on the Protection, Promotion and Support of Breastfeeding* in support of maternal and child health.[116]

        1.   Four primary goals were to be met by 1995:

            a.   Appoint "a national breastfeeding coordinator [and establish] a multisectoral national breastfeeding committee composed of representatives from relevant government departments, non-governmental organizations, and health professional associations;"[116(p2)]

      b. Ensure "that every facility providing maternity services fully practices all ten of the *Ten Steps to Successful Breastfeeding*"; [116(p2)]

      c. Enact "the International Code of Marketing of Breast-milk Substitutes and subsequent relevant World Health Assembly resolutions in their entirety; and," [116(p2)]

      d. Enact "legislation protecting the breastfeeding rights of working women and establish means for its enforcement." [116(p2)]

   2. In 2005, 15 years after the *Innocenti Declaration*, a call was issued to governments, civil society, and donors to implement the targets of the declaration and the targets established in 2003 within the Global Strategy for Infant and Young Child Feeding[117] to ensure that every child has a right to adequate nutrition.

C. The Global Strategy for Infant and Young Child Feeding addressed the importance of appropriate infant and young child feeding as a cornerstone for childhood development, acknowledging that 30 percent of children younger than age 5 years have stunted growth as a result of poor feeding and repeated infections.[118] The strategy called for the following actions:

- All governments should develop and implement a comprehensive policy on infant and young child feeding, in the context of national policies for nutrition, child and reproductive health, and poverty reduction.
- All mothers should have access to skilled support to initiate and sustain exclusive breastfeeding for 6 months and ensure the timely introduction of adequate and safe complementary foods with continued breastfeeding up to two years or beyond.
- Health workers should be empowered to provide effective feeding counselling, and their services be extended in the community by trained lay or peer counsellors.
- Governments should review progress in national implementation of the *International Code of Marketing of Breastmilk Substitutes* and consider new legislation or additional measures as needed to protect families from adverse commercial influences.
- Governments should enact imaginative legislation protecting the breastfeeding rights of working women and establishing means for its enforcement in accordance with international labour standards.[118(para 4)]

D. *Protection, Promotion and Support of Breastfeeding in Europe: A Blueprint for Action* was published in 2004 as a project cofunded by the Directorate General for Health and Consumer Protection of the European Commission.[119] The blueprint established the protection, promotion, and support of breastfeeding as a public health priority throughout Europe. The blueprint's six priority areas included the following[119]:

   1. Policy and planning to implement the Global Strategy for Infant and Young Child Feeding.

   2. Information, education, and communication to reestablish a breastfeeding culture and enact the WHO Code.

   3. Evidence-based training for all healthcare workers, especially those in frontline maternity and childcare areas (training should not be influenced by manufacturers of infant formula).

   4. Protection, promotion, and support of breastfeeding to enable all parents to exclusively breastfeed their infant for 6 months and to continue thereafter.

   5. Monitoring of breastfeeding initiation, exclusivity, and duration rates through standardized methods.

   6. Research marketing practices under the scope of the WHO Code, comprehensive maternity protection legislation, different communication strategies, and ethical guidelines ensuring freedom from commercial interests and disclosure of conflicts of interest.

E. The Academy of Breastfeeding Medicine (ABM), founded in 1994, is a worldwide organization of physicians dedicated to the protection, promotion, and support of breastfeeding and human lactation.[120]

   1. The ABM provides physician education directly through annual international conferences and calls upon medical training institutions to incorporate breastfeeding into medical training for all physicians during medical school, residency training, and beyond.[121]

   2. The ABM publishes evidence-based, peer-reviewed clinical protocols translated into multiple languages to guide clinical practice. Lactation consultants should be aware of these resources and incorporate the guidance into their clinical practice and policy development.[122]

F. In 2011, the U.S. Surgeon General issued a Call to Action to Support Breastfeeding.[123] The initiative called for the enactment of 20 action steps involving families, friends, communities, clinicians, healthcare leaders, employers, and policy makers to help support parents who choose to breastfeed and to eliminate barriers that parents may face in achieving their breastfeeding goals. One step includes ensuring access to services provided by IBCLCs.

G. In 2010, a nonprofit agency called 1,000 Days was founded to address the period of time from a woman's pregnancy through the child's second birthday.[124]

    1. The 1,000 Days initiative is supported by the U.S. Government, the Government of Ireland, the Bill & Melinda Gates Foundation, InterAction, and the Global Alliance for Improved Nutrition.

    2. The 1,000 Days initiative works to improve nutrition for the most vulnerable populations in some of the poorest parts of the world. The organization believes that exclusive breastfeeding is a cornerstone of child survival and child health, providing essential, irreplaceable nutrition for a child's growth and development.

H. In 2016, *The Lancet's* breastfeeding series provided statistics regarding breastfeeding and its impact on health and global economic development.[125] The findings suggest the importance of scaling up breastfeeding promotion and support of exclusive breastfeeding.[126]

    1. Globally, only 37 percent of infants are exclusively breastfed during the first 6 months of life, according to the WHO.

    2. Improving breastfeeding practices could save more than 820,000 lives per year, with 87 percent of the preventable deaths occurring in infants aged 6 months or younger.

    3. The estimated costs associated with not breastfeeding amount to $300 billion per year.[13]

I. The Pontifical Academy of Sciences held a working group on breastfeeding, science, and society in 1995 at the Vatican.[127] Specific addresses by Catholic pontiffs that addressed breastfeeding included the following:

    1. Pope Pius XII urged Catholic mothers to nourish their children themselves.[127]

    2. Pope John Paul II said that "mothers need time, information, and support" and that "no one can substitute for the mother in this natural activity."[127(para 8)]

    3. Pope Francis called upon mothers to engage in breastfeeding publically during church services, including infant baptismal, indicated that crying hungry infants during long ceremonies should be nursed without fear. It is all normal![128]

J. A systematic review of the BFHI impact on child health found that adherence to the BFHI Ten Steps to Successful Breastfeeding has a positive impact on short-term, medium-term, and long-term breastfeeding outcomes.

    1. A dose–response exposure to the Ten Steps to Successful Breastfeeding demonstrates an increased likelihood of improved breastfeeding outcomes (early breastfeeding initiation, exclusive breastfeeding at hospital discharge, any breastfeeding, and exclusive breastfeeding duration).

    2. Community support through implementation of Step 10 of the Ten Steps appears to be essential for sustaining the positive breastfeeding impacts of BFHI in the longer term.[129]

    3. The evidence base for BFHI is robust. When used in combination with other interventions, the largest effects on breastfeeding outcomes are achieved.[13,62]

K. Key issues related to large-scale and sustainable breastfeeding promotion on a global level include the following:

    1. Maternity and parental leave. (See Chapter 11, *Breastfeeding and Employment*.)

    2. Workplace legislation.

    3. Enforcement of the WHO Code.

    4. Training of administrators, healthcare professionals, and paraprofessionals.

    5. Improvements in medical and nursing school curricula.

▶ Key Points from This Chapter

A. Lactation consultants have the opportunity to act as change agents at many levels—individual, organizational, community, and globally—to help in breastfeeding initiation, promotion, protection, and support.

B. Global policies such as BFHI, Neo-BFHI, and the WHO Code provide the political insight to promote and support breastfeeding, and individuals in the community (including healthcare workers) can use these policies to guide community action.

C. Investment in breastfeeding, the initiation, support, promotion, and protection of breastfeeding families has the potential to affect world health, economics, and the future health of our global citizens.

References

1. Naccarella L, Butterworth I, Moore T. Transforming health professionals into population health change agents. *J Public Health Res.* 2016;5(1):21-26.
2. First Nations Health Authority. Cultural humility. FHNA website. http://www.fnha.ca/wellness/cultural-humility. Accessed August 14, 2017.
3. Ramsden I. Towards cultural safety. In: Wepa D, ed. *Cultural Safety in Aotearoa New Zealand.* 2nd ed. Melbourne, Australia: Cambridge University Press; 2015:5-25.
4. Browne AJ, Varcoe C, Smye V, Reimer-Kirkham S, Lynam MJ, Wong S. Cultural safety and the challenges of translating critically oriented knowledge in practice. *Nurs Philos.* 2009;10:167-179.
5. American Public Health Association. Health equity. APHA website. https://www.apha.org/topics-and-issues/health-equity. Accessed August 14, 2017.
6. World Health Organization. The Ottawa charter for health promotion. WHO website. http://www.who.int/healthpromotion/conferences /previous/ottawa/en/. Published November 21, 1986. Accessed October 2, 2017.
7. Acheson D. *Public Health in England: The Report of the Committee of Inquiry into the Future Development of the Public Health Function.* London, England: HMSO; 1988.
8. Rapheal D. *Social Determinants of Health.* 3rd ed. Toronto, Canada: Canadian Scholars' Press; 2016.
9. Raphael D. Social determinants of health: present status, unanswered questions, and future directions. *Int J Health Serv.* 2006;36(4):651-677.
10. Centers for Disease Control and Prevention (CDC). The social-ecological model: a framework for prevention. CDC website. https:// www.cdc.gov/violenceprevention/overview/social-ecologicalmodel.html. Updated March 25, 2015. Accessed October 21, 2017.
11. McLeroy KR, Bibeau D, Steckler A, Glanz K. An ecological perspective on health promotion programs. *Health Educ Q.* 1988;15(4):351-377.
12. Frieden TR. A framework for public health action: the health impact pyramid. *Am J Public Health.* 2010;100(4):590-595.
13. Rollins NC, Bhandari N, Hajeebhoy N, et al. Why invest, and what it will take to improve breastfeeding practices? *Lancet.* 2016;387(10017):491-504.
14. Hodal K. Breastfeeding could prevent 800,000 child deaths, Lancet says. *The Guardian.* January 28, 2016. https://www.theguardian.com /global-development/2016/jan/28/breastfeeding-could-prevent-800000-child-deaths-lancet-says. Accessed February 9, 2018.
15. Griswold MK. Reframing the context of the breastfeeding narrative: a critical opportunity for health equity through evidence-based advocacy. *J Hum Lactation.* 2017;33(2):415-418.
16. Al-Sahab B, Lanes A, Feldman M, Tamim H. Prevalence and predictors of 6-month exclusive breastfeeding among Canadian women: a national survey. *BMC Pediatrics.* 2010;10(1):20.
17. McInnes RJ, Love JG, Stone DH. Independent predictors of breastfeeding intention in a disadvantaged population of pregnant women. *BMC Public Health.* 2001;1:10.
18. Pitonyak JS, Jessop AB, Pontiggia L, Crivelli-Kovach A. Life course factors associated with initiation and continuation of exclusive breastfeeding. *Matern Child Health J.* 2016;20(2):240-249.
19. Mason F, Rawe K, Wright S. *Superfood for Babies: How Overcoming Barriers to Breastfeeding Will Save Children's Lives.* London, England: Save the Children Fund; 2013. https://www.savethechildren.org.uk/content/dam/global/reports/health-and-nutrition/superfood -for-babies-UK-version.pdf. Accessed April 7, 2018.
20. Colodro-Conde L, Sanchez-Romera JF, Tornero-Gomez MJ, Perez-Riquelme F, Polo-Tomas M, Ordonana JR. Relationship between level of education and breastfeeding duration depends on social context: breastfeeding trends over a 40-year period in Spain. *J Hum Lactation.* 2011;27(3):272-278.
21. Baghurst P, Pincombe J, Peat B, Henderson A, Reddin E, Antoniou G. Breast feeding self-efficacy and other determinants of the duration of breast feeding in a cohort of first-time mothers in Adelaide, Australia. *Midwifery.* 2007;23(4):382-391.
22. Bazzano AN, Oberhelman RA, Storck Potts K, Taub L, Var C. What health service support do families need for optimal breastfeeding? An in-depth exploration of young infant feeding practices in Cambodia. *Int J Womens Health.* 2015;7:249-257.
23. Brockway M, Benzies K, Hayden KA. Interventions to improve breastfeeding self-efficacy and resultant breastfeeding rates: a systematic review and meta-analysis. *J Hum Lactation.* 2017;33(3):486-499.
24. Wilhelm SL, Rodehorst TK, Stepans MB, Hertzog M, Berens C. Influence of intention and self-efficacy levels on duration of breastfeeding for midwest rural mothers. *Appl Nurs Res.* 2008;21(3):123-133.
25. World Health Organization. Violence against women: intimate partner and sexual violence against women fact sheet. WHO website. http://www.who.int/mediacentre/factsheets/fs239/en/. Updated November 2017. Accessed February 9, 2018.
26. Olde E, van Der Hart O, Kieber RJ, Van Son MM, Wijnen HA, Pop VM. Peritraumatic dissociation and emotions as predictors of PTSD symptoms following childbirth. *J Trauma Dissociation.* 2005;6(3):125-142.
27. Soet JE, Brack GA, DiIorio C. Prevalence and predictors of women's experience of psychological trauma during childbirth. *Birth.* 2003;30(1):36-46.
28. Kendall-Tackett KA. Violence against women and the perinatal period: the impact of lifetime violence and abuse on pregnancy, postpartum, and breastfeeding. *Trauma Violence Abuse.* 2007;8(3):344-353.
29. Beck CT, Watson S. Impact of birth trauma on breast-feeding: a tale of two pathways. *Nurs Res.* 2008;57(4):228-236.
30. *Trauma-Informed Practice Guide.* British Columbia; 2013. http://bccewh.bc.ca/wp-content/uploads/2012/05/2013_TIP-Guide.pdf. Accessed October 3, 2017.
31. Liu J, Rosenberg KD, Sandova AP. Breastfeeding duration and perinatal cigarette smoking in a population-based cohort. *Am J Public Health.* 2006;96(2):309-314.
32. Lepe M, Bacardi Gascón M, Castañeda-González LM, Pérez Morales ME, Jiménez Cruz A. Effect of maternal obesity on lactation: systematic review. *Nutr Hosp.* 2011;26(6):1266-1269.
33. Jones KM, Power ML, Queenan JT, Schulkin J. Racial and ethnic disparities in breastfeeding. *Breastfeed Med.* 2015;10(4):186-196.

34. Miller J, Garran AM. Racism in the United States: implications for helping professions. In: Miller J, Garran AM, eds. *Racism in the United States: Implications for Helping Professions.* Belmont, CA: Thomason Brooks/Cole; 2008:13-33.

35. Johnson A, Kirk R, Rosenblum KL, Muzik M. Enhancing breastfeeding rates among African American women: a systematic review of current psychosocial interventions. *Breastfeed Med.* 2015;10(1):45-62.

36. Anderson AK, Damio G, Young S, Chapman DJ, Pérez-Escamilla R. A randomized trial assessing the efficacy of peer counseling on exclusive breastfeeding in a predominantly Latina low-income community. *Arch Pediatr Adolesc Med.* 2005;159(9):836-841.

37. Chapman DJ, Damio G, Young S, Pérez-Escamilla R. Effectiveness of breastfeeding peer counseling in a low-income, predominantly Latina population: a randomized controlled trial. *Arch Pediatr Adolesc Med.* 2004;158(9):897-902.

38. Dodgson JE, Duckett L, Garwick A, Graham BL. An ecological perspective of breastfeeding in an indigenous community. *J Nurs Scholarsh.* 2002;34(3):235-241.

39. Farrow A. Lactation support and the LGBTQI community. *J Hum Lactation.* 2015;31(1):26-28.

40. Wambach KA, Aaronson L, Breedlove G, Domian EW, Rojjanasrirat W, Yeh H-W. A randomized controlled trial of breastfeeding support and education for adolescent mothers. *West J Nurs Res.* 2011;33(4):486-505.

41. Grassley JS, Spencer BS, Bryson D. The development and psychometric testing of the supportive needs of adolescents breastfeeding scale. *J Adv Nurs.* 2013;69(3):708-716.

42. Sipsma HL, Jones KL, Cole-Lewis H. Breastfeeding among adolescent mothers: a systematic review of interventions from high-income countries. *J Hum Lactation.* 2015;31(2):221-229.

43. Mitra M, Clements KM, Zhang J, Iezzoni LI, Smeltzer SC, Long-Bellil LM. Maternal characteristics, pregnancy complications, and adverse birth outcomes among women with disabilities. *Med Care.* 2015;53(12):1027-1032.

44. Redshaw M, Malouf R, Gao H, Gray R. Women with disability: the experience of maternity care during pregnancy, labour and birth and the postnatal period. *BMC Pregnancy Childbirth.* 2013;13:174. http://europepmc.org/abstract/MED/24034425. Published September 13, 2013. Accessed November 2017.

45. Carey G, Crammond B, De Leeuw E. Towards health equity: a framework for the application of proportionate universalism. *Int J Equity Health.* 2015;14(1):81.

46. Griswold MK. "You are not alone": toward equity in breastfeeding and skilled lactation care: president's address given at the 2016 meeting of the International Lactation Consultant Association. *J Hum Lactation.* 2016;32(4):596-600.

47. Rempel LA, Rempel JK. The breastfeeding team: the role of involved fathers in the breastfeeding family. *J Hum Lactation.* 2011;27(2):115-121.

48. Pisacane A, Continisio GI, Aldinucci M, D'Amora S, Continisio P. A controlled trial of the father's role in breastfeeding promotion. *Pediatrics.* 2005;116(4):e494.

49. Yazgan H, Yazgan Z, Keleş E, Gebeşçe A. The effect of family members on breastfeeding practices among Turkish mothers. *Breastfeed Med.* 2013;8(2):232.

50. Bernie K. The factors influencing young mothers' infant feeding decisions: the view of health professionals and voluntary workers on the role of the baby's maternal grandmother. *Breastfeed Med.* 2014;9(3):161-165.

51. Negin J, Coffman J, Vizintin P, Raynes-Greenow C. The influence of grandmothers on breastfeeding rates: a systematic review. *BMC Pregnancy Childbirth.* 2016;16(1):91.

52. Castrucci BC, Hoover KL, Lim S, Maus KC. A comparison of breastfeeding rates in an urban birth cohort among women delivering infants at hospitals that employ and do not employ lactation consultants. *J Public Health Manag Pract.* 2006;12(6):578-585.

53. U.S. Preventive Services Task Force. Final recommendation statement. Breastfeeding: primary care interventions. U.S. Preventive Services Task Force website. https://www.uspreventiveservicestaskforce.org/Page/Document/RecommendationStatementFinal/breastfeeding-primary-care-interventions. Published October 2016. Accessed August 13, 2017.

54. McFadden A, Gavine A, Renfrew MJ, et al. Support for healthy breastfeeding mothers with healthy term babies. *Cochrane Database Syst Rev.* 2017;2:CD001141. doi:10.1002/14651858.CD001141.pub5.

55. Anderson AK, Damio G, Young S, Chapman DJ, Pérez-Escamilla R. A randomized trial assessing the efficacy of peer counseling on exclusive breastfeeding in a predominantly Latina low-income community. *Arch Pediatr Adolesc Med.* 2005;59(9):836-841.

56. Morrow AL, Guerrero ML, Shults J, et al. Efficacy of home-based peer counselling to promote exclusive breastfeeding: a randomised controlled trial. *Lancet.* 1999;353(9160):1226-1231.

57. Benoit B, Semenic S. Barriers and facilitators to implementing the Baby-Friendly Hospital Initiative in neonatal intensive care units. *J Obstet Gynecol Neonatal Nurs.* 2014;43(5):614-624.

58. Semenic S, Childerhose JE, Lauziere J, Groleau D. Barriers, facilitators, and recommendations related to implementing the Baby-Friendly Initiative (BFI): an integrative review. *J Hum Lactation.* 2012;28(3):317-334.

59. MacEnroe T. The Baby-Friendly Hospital Initiative. *Breastfeed Med.* 2010;5(5):247-248.

60. Breastfeeding Committee for Canada. *The Baby-Friendly Initiative (BFI) in Canada.* Drayton Valley, Canada: Breastfeeding Committee for Canada; 2012. http://breastfeedingcanada.ca/documents/BFI_Status_report_2012_FINAL.pdf. Accessed November 26, 2016.

61. World Health Organization. Exclusive breastfeeding. WHO website. http://www.who.int/nutrition/topics/exclusive_breastfeeding/en/. Accessed January 8, 2018.

62. World Health Organization. Baby-friendly Hospital Initiative. WHO website. http://www.who.int/nutrition/bfhi/ten-steps/en/. Accessed April 14, 2018.

63. Grummer-Strawn LM, Shealy KR, Perrine CG, et al. Maternity care practices that support breastfeeding: CDC efforts to encourage quality improvment. *J Womens Health.* 2013;22(2):107-112.

64. DiGirolamo AM, Grummer-Strawn LM, Fein SB. Effect of maternity-care practices on breastfeeding. *Pediatrics.* 2008;122(suppl 2):S43-S49.

65. World Health Organization. *National Implementation of the Baby-friendly Hospital Initiative, 2017.* Geneva, Switzerland: World Health Organization; 2017.

66. International Lactation Consultant Association. The Neo-BFHI: The Baby-Friendly Hospital Initiative for neonatal wards. ILCA website. http://www.ilca.org/main/learning/resources/neo-bfhi. Accessed December 7, 2016.

References 473

67. Nyqvist KH, Maastrup R, Hansen MN, et al. Neo-BFHI: The Baby-Friendly Hospital Initiative for Neonatal Wards. Core Document with Recommended Standards and Criteria. Nordic and Quebec Working Group; 2015.

67. Nyqvist KH, Maastrup R, Hansen MN, et al. *Neo-BFHI: The Baby-Friendly Hospital Initiative for Neonatal Wards. Core Document with Recommended Standards and Criteria.* Nordic and Quebec Working Group; 2015. http://www.ilca.org/i4a/pages/index.cfm?pageid=4214.

68. Merewood A, Chamberlain LB, Cook JT, Philipp BL, Malone K, Bauchner H. The effect of peer counselors on breastfeeding rates in the neonatal intensive care unit: results of a randomized controlled trial. *Arch Pediatr Adolesc Med.* 2006;160(7):681-685.

69. Morris ZS, Wooding S, Grant J. The answer is 17 years, what is the question: understanding time lags in translational research. *J R Soc Med.* 2011;104(12):510-520.

70. Wieczorek CC, Schmied H, Dorner TE, Dür W. The bumpy road to implementing the Baby-Friendly Hospital Initiative in Austria: a qualitative study. *Int Breastfeed J.* 2015;10(1):3.

71. Reddin E, Pincombe J, Darbyshire P. Passive resistance: early experiences of midwifery students/graduates and the Baby Friendly Health Initiative 10 steps to successful breastfeeding. *Women Birth.* 2007;20(2):71-76.

72. Alonso Diaz C, Utrera-Torres M, Alba-Romero C, Flores-Anton B, Escuder-Vieco D, Pallas-Alonso C. PS-270 breastfeeding support in Spanish Nicus and the Baby-friendly Hospital Initiative: a national survey. *Arch Dis Child.* 2014;99(suppl 2):A210.

73. Alonso-Diaz C, Utrera-Torres I, de Alba-Romero C, Flores-Anton B, Lora-Pablos D, Pallas-Alonso CR. Breastfeeding support in Spanish neonatal intensive care units and the Baby-Friendly Hospital Initiative. *J Hum Lactation.* 2016;32(4):613-626.

74. Hernández-Aguilar MT, Lasarte-Velillas JJ, Martín-Calama J, et al. The Baby-Friendly Initiative in Spain: a challenging pathway. *J Hum Lactation.* 2014;30(3):276-282.

75. Balaminut T, Scochi CGS, Leite AM, et al. *Prevalence of Breastfeeding in Premature at Discharge and Home in Brazilian's Baby Friendly Hospital Initiative.* 2nd Annual Neo-BFHI Conference; Uppsala, Sweden; 2015.

76. Vari PM, Camburn J, Henly SJ. Professionally mediated peer support and early breastfeeding success. *J Perinat Educ.* 2000;9(1):22-30.

77. Schafer E, Vogel MK, Viegas S, Hausafus C. Volunteer peer counselors increase breastfeeding duration among rural low-income women. *Birth.* 1998;25(2):101-106.

78. Hannula L, Kaunonen M, Tarkka M. A systematic review of professional support interventions for breastfeeding. *J Clin Nurs.* 2008;17(9):1132-1143.

79. Witt AM, Smith S, Mason MJ, Flocke SA. Integrating routine lactation consultant support into a pediatric practice. *Breastfeed Med.* 2012;7(1):38-42.

80. Nommsen-Rivers LA, Mastergeorge AM, Hansen RL, Cullum AS, Dewey KG. Doula care, early breastfeeding outcomes, and breastfeeding status at 6 weeks postpartum among low-income primiparae. *J Obstet Gynecol Neonatal Nurs.* 2009;38(2):157-173.

81. Blomqvist YT, Frölund L, Rubertsson C, Nyqvist KH. Provision of kangaroo mother care: supportive factors and barriers perceived by parents. *Scand J Caring Sci.* 2013;27(2):345-353.

82. Yamauchi Y, Yamanouchi I. The relationship between rooming-in/not rooming-in and breastfeeding variables. *Breastfeed Rev.* 1992;2(5):238-241.

83. Tender JAF, Cuzzi S, Kind T, Simmens SJ, Blatt B, Greenberg L. Educating pediatric residents about breastfeeding. *J Hum Lactation.* 2014;30(4):458-465.

84. Friesen CA, Hormuth LJ, Petersen D, Babbitt T. Using videoconferencing technology to provide breastfeeding support to low-income women: connecting hospital-based lactation consultants with clients receiving care at a community health center. *J Hum Lactation.* 2015;31(4):595-599.

85. Cox A. Breastfeeding promotion and support in the Colorado region of Kaiser Permanente. *Breastfeed Med.* 2010;5(5):259-259.

86. Tiedje LB, Schiffman R, Omar M, et al. An ecological approach to breastfeeding. *Am J Maternal Child Nurs.* 2002;27(3):154-161.

87. Lenell A, Friesen C, Hormuth L. Breastfeeding support in a community pharmacy. *J Hum Lactation.* 2015;31(4):577-581.

88. Anderson GC. Risk in mother-infant separation postbirth. *J Nurs Scholarsh.* 1989;21(4):196-199.

89. Bystrova K, Ivanova V, Edhborg M, et al. Early contact versus separation: effects on mother–infant interaction one year later. *Birth.* 2009;36(2):97-109.

90. Crenshaw J. Care practices that promote normal birth #6: no separation of mother and baby with unlimited opportunity for breastfeeding . . . including commentary by Klaus PH, and Klaus MH. *J Perinat Educ.* 2004;13:35-41.

91. Herlenius E, Kuhn P. Sudden unexpected postnatal collapse of newborn infants: a review of cases, definitions, risks, and preventive measures. *Transl Stroke Res.* 2013;4:236-247.

92. Feldman-Winter L, Goldsmith JP. Safe sleep and skin-to-skin care in the neonatal period for healthy term infants. *Pediatrics.* 2016;138(3):e1-e11.

93. Thompson JMD, Tanabe K, Moon RY, et al. Duration of breastfeeding and risk of SIDS: an individual participant data meta-analysis. *Pediatrics.* 2017;140(5). doi:10.1542/peds.2017-1324.

94. Task Force on Sudden Infant Death Syndrome. SIDS and other sleep-related infant deaths: updated 2016 recommendations for a safe infant sleeping environment. *Pediatrics.* 2016;138:e1-e11.

95. Lahr MB, Rosenberg KD, Lapidus JA. Maternal-infant bedsharing: risk factors for bedsharing in a population-based survey of new mothers and implications for SIDS risk reduction. *Maternal Child Health J.* 2007;11(3):277-286.

96. Ateah CA, Hamelin KJ. Maternal bedsharing practices, experiences, and awareness of risks. *J Obstet Gynecol Neonatal Nurs.* 2008;37(3):274-281.

97. Ball HL, Howel D, Bryant A, Best E, Russell C, Ward-Platt M. Bed-sharing by breastfeeding mothers: who bed-shares and what is the relationship with breastfeeding duration? *Acta Paediatr.* 2016;105(6):628-634.

98. The Lullaby Trust. Co-sleeping with your baby. The Lullaby Trust website. https://www.lullabytrust.org.uk/safer-sleep-advice/co-sleeping/. Accessed November 3, 2017.

99. Perinatal Services BC. Safe infant sleep: a practice support tool for healthcare professionals. http://www.perinatalservicesbc.ca/Documents/Resources/HealthPromotion/Sleep/SaferSleepTool.pdf. Accessed April 16, 2018.

100. McKenna JJ, Mosko SS, Richard CA. Bedsharing promotes breastfeeding. *Pediatrics.* 1997;100(2):214.

101. Santos IS, Mota DM, Matijasevich A, Barros AJD, Barros FCF. Bed-sharing at 3 months and breast-feeding at 1 year in southern Brazil. *J Pediatr.* 2009;155(4-4):505-509.

102. Blair PS. Bed-sharing and breastfeeding: the importance of giving the correct advice. *Acta Paediatr.* 2016;105(6):570-571.

103. Azulay Chertok IR, Hoover ML. Breastfeeding legislation in states with relatively low breastfeeding rates compared to breastfeeding legislation of other states. *J Nurs Law.* 2009;13(2):45-53.

104. Heymann J, Raub A, Earle A. Breastfeeding policy: a globally comparative analysis. *Bull World Health Organ.* 2013;91:398-406.

105. Carothers C, Hare I. The business case for breastfeeding. *Breastfeed Med.* 2010;5(5):229-231.

106. Ortiz J, McGillan K, Kelly P. Duration of breast milk expression among working mothers enrolled in an employer-sponsored lactation program. *Pediatr Nurs.* 2006;30(2):111.

107. Pérez-Escamilla R, Hall Moran V. Scaling up breastfeeding programmes in a complex adaptive world. *Maternal Child Nutr.* 2016;12(3):375-380.

108. Pérez-Escamilla R, Chapman D. BF protection, promotion, and support in US: a time to nudge, a time to measure. *J Hum Lactation.* 2012;28(2):118-121.

109. Perez-Escamilla R, Curry L, Minhas D, Taylor L, Bradley E. Scaling up of breastfeeding programs in low- and middle-income countries: the "breastfeeding gear" model. *Adv Nutr.* 2012;3(6):790-800. https://www.ncbi.nlm.nih.gov/pmc/articles/PMC3648703/. Published November 6, 2012. Accessed February 8, 2018.

110. World Health Organization. *International Code of Marketing of Breas-tmilk Substitutes.* Geneva, Switzerland: World Health Organization; 1981. http://www.who.int/nutrition/publications/infantfeeding/9241541601/en/. Accessed March 9, 2017.

111. Gray H. A quick guide to the International (WHO) Code. *Leader Today.* January 12, 2017. http://leadertoday.breastfeedingtoday-llli .org/a-quick-guide-to-the-who-code/. Accessed October 2, 2017.

112. Piwoz EG, Huffman SL. The impact of marketing of breast-milk substitutes on WHO-recommended breastfeeding practices. *Food Nutr Bull.* 2015;36(4):373-386.

113. International Baby Food Action Network. About IBFAN. IBFAN website. http://ibfan.org/about-ibfan. Accessed August 11, 2017.

114. International Baby Food Action Network. Seven principles. IBFAN website. http://ibfan.org/seven-principles. Accessed February 8, 2018.

115. International Board of Lactation Consultant Examiners. *Code of Professional Conduct for IBCLCs.* IBLCE website. https://iblce.org /resources/professional-standards/. Updated September 2015. Accessed April 17, 2018.

116. World Health Organization, UNICEF. *Innocenti Declaration on the Protection, Promotion and Support of Breastfeeding.* Florence, Italy: UNICEF; 1991. http://www.who.int/elena/titles/breastfeeding_care_facilities/en/. Accessed April 17, 2018.

117. UNICEF. Innocenti declaration 2005 on infant and young child feeding. UNICEF website. https://www.unicef-irc.org/publications/435/. Published 2007. Accessed August 11, 2017.

118. World Health Organization. Global strategy for infant and young child feeding. WHO website. http://www.who.int/nutrition/topics /global_strategy_iycf/en/. Accessed August 11, 2017.

119. EU Project on Promotion of Breastfeeding in Europe. *Protection, Promotion and Support of Breastfeeding in Europe: A Blueprint for Action.* European Commission website. http://ec.europa.eu/health/ph_projects/2002/promotion/fp_promotion_2002_frep_18_en.pdf. Published 2004. Accessed August 11, 2017.

120. Academy of Breastfeeding Medicine. About ABM. ABM website. http://www.bfmed.org. Accessed August 14, 2017.

121. Academy of Breastfeeding Medicine. Educational objectives and skills for the physician with respect to breastfeeding. *Breastfeed Med.* 2011;6(2):99-105.

122. Academy of Breastfeeding Medicine. Resources. http://www.bfmed.org/resources. Accessed August 14, 2017.

123. U.S. Department of Health and Human Services. The Surgeon General's call to action to support breastfeeding. U.S. Surgeon General website. https://www.surgeongeneral.gov/library/calls/breastfeeding/index.html. Updated August 12, 2014. Accessed August 15, 2017.

124. 1,000 Days. 1,000 Days principles. 1,000 Days website. https://thousanddays.org/about/1000days-principles/. Accessed August 15, 2017.

125. Victora CG, Bahl R, Barros AJD, et al. Breastfeeding in the 21st century: epidemiology, mechanisms, and lifelong effect. *Lancet.* 2016;387(10017):475-490.

126. Bhandari N, Iqbal Kabir AKM, Adbus Salam M. Mainstreaming nutrition into maternal and child health programmes: scaling up of exclusive breast-feeding. *Maternal Child Nutr.* 2008;4(1):5-23.

127. Breastfeeding Promotion Network of India, Maharashtra. Pope John Paul II on breastfeeding. BreastfeedingIndia website. http://www .breastfeedingindia.com/articles/articles_pope.html. Accessed November 18, 2017.

128. Hersher R. Pope Frances reiterates support for public breast-feeding. NPR website. https://www.npr.org/sections/thetwo-way /2017/01/09/508927895/pope-francis-reiterates-support-for-public-breastfeeding. Published January 9, 2017. Accessed January 9, 2018.

129. Pérez-Escamilla R, Martinez JL, Segura-Pérez S. Impact of the Baby-friendly Hospital Initiative on breastfeeding and child health outcomes: a systematic review. *Maternal Child Nutr.* 2016;12(3):402-417.

Additional Resources

Email Addresses

UNICEF Adviser, Infant Feeding. smhossain@unicef.org.

World Health Organization, Department of Child and Adolescent Health and Development. cah@who.int.

World Health Organization, Department of Nutrition for Health and Development. nutrition@who.int.

Publication

Public Health Agency of Canada. *Protecting, Promoting and Supporting Breastfeeding: A Practical Workbook for Community-Based Programs.* 2nd ed. Ottawa, Canada: Public Health Agency of Canada; 2014. https://www.canada.ca/content/dam/phac-aspc/migration/phac-aspc/hp-ps/dca-dea/publications/pdf/ppsb-ppsam-eng.pdf.

Websites

Academy of Breastfeeding Medicine. www.bfmed.org.
Innocenti +15. www.innocenti15.net.
International Baby Food Action Network. www.ibfan.org.
International Lactation Consultant Association. www.ilca.org.
La Leche League International. www.lalecheleague.org.
Wellstart International. www.wellstart.org.
World Alliance for Breastfeeding Action. http://waba.org.my/.

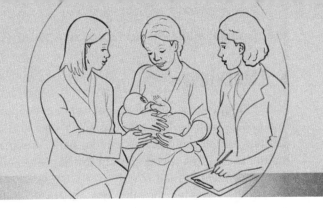

CHAPTER 30

Lactation Education for Health Professionals

Alisa Sanders
Debi Ferrarello
Andrea Bulera Judge

OBJECTIVES

- Apply appropriate educational methods to teach healthcare professionals.
- Design a sample breastfeeding training for various healthcare professionals.
- Identify key breastfeeding competencies for healthcare professionals.

DEFINITIONS OF COMMONLY USED TERMS

clinical instructor A skilled practitioner who provides guidance and education to students and trainees within a formal, structured program; responsible for connecting previous didactic training to real-life applications in clinical settings.

IBCLC® International Board Certified Lactation Consultant®.

mentor A person who teaches or gives help and advice to a less-experienced person.[1]

preceptor In health care, a skilled practitioner or faculty member who supervises students in a clinical setting to allow practical experience with patients.

Any use of the term *mother, maternal,* or *breastfeeding* is not meant to exclude transgender or nonbinary parents who may be breastfeeding or providing human milk to their infant.

▶ Overview

A core competency in professional lactation support is to provide evidence-informed education and information to families, aspiring lactation consultants, and other healthcare professionals. Lactation consultants, physicians, dietitians, nurses, and other members of the breastfeeding parent's healthcare team provide clinical care and information to families. It is important for all professionals to have adequate clinical and didactic lactation education that is pertinent to their role.

An effective educator will assess student attributes and needs and craft training sessions that are appropriate for the students' level of education, interest, role, and need. Trainings that are interactive and multimodal will be more effective than lectures alone. Quality programs include role play, simulations, videos, interviews, guest speakers, and group work.

Experienced lactation consultants often provide informal clinical instruction to healthcare students, professionals, and aspiring lactation professionals. Such teaching allows a single practitioner to impact large numbers of families through growth of the lactation consultant profession and education of other healthcare providers. The still-young lactation consultant profession depends on increasing access to quality, formal clinical training opportunities simultaneously through an effective interdisciplinary approach to lactation care with appropriate education of the healthcare team.

I. General Principles of Adult Education

Adult education denotes ongoing learning processes, formal or otherwise. Adult learners develop their abilities, enrich their knowledge, and improve their technical or professional qualifications to meet their own needs and those of society.[2,3] The theories of adult learning are as follows:

  A. Andragogy, the art and science of helping adults learn, captures general characteristics of adult learners and offers guidelines for planning instruction for learners who tend to be self-directed and independent.[4]

  B. Reflective practice, or knowing in action, links theory to practice.[5]

  C. Brain-based learning refers to teaching methods, lesson designs, and programs that are based on the latest scientific research about how the brain learns. It includes such factors as cognitive development—how students learn differently as they age, grow, and mature socially, emotionally, and cognitively.[6-8]

  D. Connectivism is a learning theory for the digital age. It posits that knowledge has a decreasing half-life, and the need for continuous updates is imperative in a digital society.[9]

  E. A digital age learning matrix is an evaluation tool for the application of digital technology in learning.[10]

II. Types of Learning Styles

The three primary learning styles are visual, auditory, and kinesthetic. Information retention improves when all these learning styles are used.

  A. Visual learners learn by looking, seeing, viewing, and watching.
    1. They pay attention to the face, body, and language of an instructor to fully understand the concepts of the lesson.
    2. They usually sit toward the front of the classroom or near the teacher to avoid distraction.
    3. They tend to think of pictures and learn best from visual displays.
    4. They take detailed notes to absorb information.

  B. Auditory learners learn by listening, hearing, and speaking.
    1. They learn best through lecture, discussion, and brainstorming.
    2. Written material has little meaning until it is spoken.
    3. Reading out loud or listening to audio versions of lessons facilitates learning.

  C. Kinesthetic learners learn by moving or a hands-on approach.
    1. They learn best through activities and hands-on practice.
    2. They have trouble sitting for long periods of time.

III. Education for Aspiring Lactation Professionals

Multiple educational opportunities combine lactation education and clinical experience in different ways. Ultimately it is up to the learner or the clinical instructor to make sure the minimum competencies are met and the combination of knowledge and experience is well rounded.

A.   LEAARC provides recognition for didactic education.

   1.   The Lactation Education Accreditation and Approval Review Committee (LEAARC) establishes standards for lactation education programs, ensuring courses are taught by appropriate faculty, are free from bias, meet minimum curriculum requirements, and are in compliance with the World Health Organization's (WHO) *International Code of Marketing of Breast-milk Substitutes*, commonly referred to as the WHO Code.[11]

   2.   LEAARC provides three forms of recognition for lactation education.

      a.   Recognition of breastfeeding courses designed for breastfeeding counselors and educators.

      b.   Approval of courses designed to provide 90 hours of instruction in lactation management.

      c.   Recommendation for accreditation by the Commission on Accreditation of Allied Health Education Programs (CAAHEP) for academic programs; programs accredited by CAAHEP are recognized by the International Board of Lactation Consultant Examiners (IBLCE) as satisfying Pathway 2 criteria for exam eligibility.

   3.   The LEAARC curriculum identifies essential competencies needed for a comprehensive lactation education program. (See the *Additional Resources* section later in this chapter.)

B.   Clinical instruction requires qualified and skilled clinical instructors and mentors.

   1.   The requirements for clinical instructors and mentors are as follows:

      a.   Clinical instructors who train IBCLC candidates must be IBCLCs.

      b.   Several years of experience in a variety of clinical settings is preferred.

   2.   Being a clinical instructor or mentor offers many rewards.

      a.   Professional growth as teaching skills are developed.

      b.   Knowledge base is continually renewed and updated.

      c.   Potential for increased income.

      d.   Increased access to lactation care for families.

      e.   Increased community outreach, which improves awareness of lactation care.

   3.   The challenges of being a clinical instructor or mentor are as follows:

      a.   Time constraints.

      b.   Potential for conflict in personality or work style.

   4.   The responsibilities of a formal clinical instructor or mentor are as follows:

      a.   Structure clinical opportunities.

      b.   Monitor student and intern progress.

      c.   Establish time lines for skills acquisition.

      d.   Create opportunities to obtain skills in varied settings (e.g., hospital, outpatient clinic, public health offices, private practice), which allow students to practice the skills learned in didactic education.

      e.   Provide regular, specific feedback to guide the intern throughout the program.

   5.   A memorandum of understanding should be developed, and it should include the following:

      a.   Outline the responsibilities, costs, and time line of the clinical instruction relationship. (See the *Additional Resources* section later in this chapter.)

      b.   A formal, written understanding is particularly important if instruction takes place outside an academic setting where those elements would already be established.

C.   Clinical evaluations include the following elements:

   1.   Ensure that students demonstrate the necessary skills and competencies:

      a.   Student has completed or is concurrently completing a 90-hour course in lactation management if pursuing IBCLC certification.

      b.   Student demonstrates proficiency in the clinical competencies identified by the profession

      c.   Evaluation tools track progress and improve communication regarding strengths and weaknesses. (See the *Additional Resources* section later in this chapter.)

    d. Critical thinking skills are developed through assignments and clinical practice:
        i. Students learn to think through complex problems.
        ii. Students consider clinical information and the social ecological framework as it applies to decision making.
    e. Self-reflection activities encourage the practice of continual self-assessment to foster continued learning throughout the students' careers.
  2. Solicit feedback from students at the end of the internship, asking for a candid evaluation and suggestions for improvement.[12]

IV. Becoming an IBCLC

A. The IBLCE sets the standards for exam eligibility and is responsible for certifying IBCLCs.
B. The IBLCE is not prescriptive as to how aspiring IBCLCs are to gain didactic education and clinical experience.
  1. There are three pathways for exam eligibility:
    a. Pathway 1 applicants may learn clinical skills in lactation as part of their work as a healthcare professional or volunteer breastfeeding counselor.
    b. Pathway 2 and Pathway 3 applicants are required to have supervised clinical experiences. Various models are available.
  2. All three pathways share a combination of the following:[13,14]
    a. Background health science education in specific subjects outlined by the IBLCE.
    b. Ninety hours of education in human lactation and breastfeeding:
        i. Pathways 1 and 3 can include education from various sources; it is the student's responsibility to ensure that education hours are well-rounded and comprehensive.
        ii. Pathway 2 programs, which must be accredited by CAAHEP, ensure a comprehensive didactic curriculum.
C. The three pathways vary in the clinical practice experience required for certification.[13,14]
  1. Pathway 1 requires 1,000 hours working with breastfeeding families through paid or volunteer work in the past 5 years.
  2. Pathway 2 clinical experience, coordinated with didactic instruction in a CAAHEP accredited program, requires clinical hours directly supervised by IBCLCs and completion of all core competencies in the LEAARC curriculum.
  3. Pathway 3 requires 500 hours directly supervised by IBCLCs while following a preapproved Pathway 3 Plan.[14]
  4. All pathway candidates should meet the current clinical competencies as defined by the IBLCE.[15]
D. Examples of formal clinical programs for IBCLC candidates are as follows:
  1. Clinical experience through an accredited Pathway 2 program:
    a. Clinical experience is available to direct-entry students. Prospective students may find current Pathway 2 programs on the CAAHEP website (www.caahep.org).
    b. Students complete all didactic courses and clinical instruction through supervised practice.
    c. The program integrates didactic instruction with clinical experiences at hospitals, community centers, public health clinics, outpatient clinics, and in other community programs.
    d. The program covers the full spectrum of the breastfeeding continuum.
  2. Clinical programs that accommodate Pathway 3 are as follows (see the *Additional Resources* section later in this chapter):
    a. Community-based programs:
        i. The student must have completed all required didactic training prior to clinical skills mentoring.
        ii. The student is responsible for obtaining liability insurance and current immunizations, and is responsible for developing a proposed schedule of availability.
        iii. The mentor and the student meet and develop a routine schedule to obtain the needed hours.
        iv. The student may obtain experience in hospitals, community centers, public health clinics, outpatient clinics, and other community programs.

          v.   Some internships charge no fee for clinical mentoring and arrange with the student to provide an agreed-upon number of hours of service after becoming an IBCLC.

    b.   Educator-based programs:

        i.   The student must have completed all required didactic training prior to clinical skills mentoring.

        ii.   Interns are placed at participating area hospitals and outpatient facilities.

        iii.   The program director establishes affiliation agreements with hospitals outside the immediate area where students find placements.

        iv.   The program prescreens potential interns for health clearance; training in patient privacy compliance, occupational safety, and infection control; liability insurance; personal health insurance; background check and drug screening; and preapproval from the IBLCE.

        v.   The program requires reports and evaluations of the student's activities.

    c.   Academic medical center programs:

        i.   Interns spend 6 months full time gaining clinical experience.

        ii.   Experiences are available in teaching hospitals, children's hospitals, outpatient lactation clinics, Baby-friendly Hospitals in the community, local milk banks, and other community settings.

E.   The IBLCE requires recertification every 5 years.[16]

    1.   At 5 years, Continuing Education Recognition Points (CERPs) can be used to recertify.

        a.   The IBCLC must obtain 75 CERPs in the 5-year period.

        b.   CERPs can be obtained by attending or presenting formal classes and lectures, staff or peer education, learning new lactation-related skills, and mentoring.

    2.   IBCLCs have the option to recertify by exam at 5 years instead of through CERPs.

    3.   Recertification by exam is required at least every 10 years.

F.   Membership and participation are encouraged in local, state, national, and international organizations dedicated to promoting lactation support and fostering continuing education.

V. Lactation Education for Healthcare Professionals

A.   The objectives for lactation management education are as follows:[17]

    1.   Level I: Awareness:

        a.   Target group: Medical, nursing, dental, and allied health students (preservice education).

        b.   Example objectives:

            i.   Discuss, in general terms, findings from the basic and social sciences of lactation.

            ii.   Describe the general benefits of breastfeeding for the infant and basic methods of support.

    2.   Level II: Generalist:

        a.   Target group: Pediatricians, obstetricians, family medicine physicians, and advanced practice nurses.

        b.   Example objectives:

            i.   Apply the findings from the basic and social sciences to breastfeeding and lactation issues.

            ii.   Describe the unique properties of human milk for human infants.

            iii.   Describe the advantages of preterm milk for preterm infants.

    3.   Level III: Specialist:

        a.   Target group: Advanced or independent study, fellowships.

        b.   Example objectives:

            i.   Critique the findings from the basic and social sciences and evaluate their applicability to clinical management issues.

            ii.   Discuss in detail the components of human milk and their functions.

            iii.   Describe in detail the suitability of preterm human milk for preterm infants.

            iv.   Demonstrate the ability to provide basic breastfeeding support for breastfeeding dyads, including facilitating latch and positioning.

B. Education for nurses working in perinatal and postpartum settings includes the following:
   1. In most settings, IBCLCs work with patients in a consultative role, whereas nurses have 24/7 responsibility for patient care. Nurses must have the training and education needed to provide basic breastfeeding management and to identify patients who need the level of care provided by the IBCLC.
   2. The Baby-friendly Hospital Initiative requires that all nurses working in perinatal and postpartum settings have a minimum of 20 hours of education, including 5 hours of skills competency demonstration.[18]
   3. The didactic portion of nurse education may be delivered by computer-based modules or instructor-led courses.

C. The education considerations for physicians and other clinicians include the following:
   1. Provider education and support of breastfeeding are critical to parents seeking information from clinicians.
   2. Physicians need the education necessary to promote, protect, and support breastfeeding in their roles.
   3. Almost all physicians will care for breastfeeding families at some point in their practice.
      a. They need a basic understanding of the physiology of lactation.
      b. They need an appreciation for the importance of breastfeeding to the health of the parent and child.
   4. The knowledge required by obstetricians, family physicians, and pediatricians is more extensive than that required of radiologists, internists, and anesthesiologists, yet all professionals must have the information and skills needed to provide appropriate support, instruction, and referrals to their breastfeeding patients.
   5. The Academy of Breastfeeding Medicine Clinical Protocol #19 guides physicians who provide prenatal and perinatal education and support.[19]
   6. The Baby-friendly Hospital Initiative requires that physicians and clinicians who care for parents in the prenatal and perinatal period, and who care for breastfeeding dyads during the postpartum period, have a minimum of 3 hours of breastfeeding education that is pertinent to their role.[18]
      a. Physician education can be provided by online modules, conferences and webinars, or instructor-led trainings.
      b. See **BOX 30-1** for Baby-friendly USA requirements.
   7. Obstetricians, midwives, and family physicians play an important role in breastfeeding promotion, initial counseling, and management.
   8. Pediatricians play an important role in breastfeeding management and counseling.
   9. Pediatricians, obstetricians, midwives, and family physicians need to understand anatomy and physiology related to breastfeeding, including long-term health impact and risks associated with not breastfeeding.
   10. Pediatricians and family physicians should be well versed in basic breastfeeding management through toddlerhood, including normal infant behavior, feeding patterns, common problems, and developmental changes.
   11. Providers should cultivate a network of fellow clinicians, including IBCLCs, otolaryngologists, and physical and speech therapists, for collaboration and referrals to foster optimal patient care.
   12. Physicians providing direct care to breastfeeding families are encouraged to spend time in a mentoring relationship with IBCLCs to develop the clinical skills required to provide counsel and support to new parents.
   13. The American Academy of Pediatrics provides a curriculum for breastfeeding education for resident physicians.[20]

D. Other healthcare providers also benefit from lactation education.
   1. Dietitians are uniquely positioned to understand the importance of the initial nutrition of lactation. Clinical experience in lactation during training is vital.
   2. Dentists, speech therapists, and other providers may encounter breastfeeding patients with particular challenges. They benefit from lactation training pertinent to their role (see **BOX 30-2**).

BOX 30-1 Baby-friendly USA Breastfeeding Education Requirements for Healthcare Providers

Training for Healthcare Providers

The Baby-friendly Hospital Initiative requires that healthcare providers, such as physicians, advanced practice nurses, nurse midwives, and physician assistants working in labor and delivery, maternity, and nursery and newborn care should have a minimum of 3 hours of breastfeeding management education that is pertinent to their role.

All healthcare providers must demonstrate an understanding of the benefit of exclusive breastfeeding, physiology of lactation, how their specific field of practice impacts lactation, and how to learn about safe medications for use during lactation.

It is expected that healthcare providers will know how, when, and to whom they should make a referral for breastfeeding support beyond their level of expertise.

Baby-friendly facilities should determine the amount and content of training required for staff members in other units and in other roles according to their anticipated workplace exposure to breastfeeding parents and infants.

Training for Other Healthcare Professionals

Training for staff members working outside a maternity unit will be developed by each facility, based on job description and workplace exposure to breastfeeding couplets. Examples of training for staff members outside a maternity unit include, but are not limited to, the following:

- Pharmacist: Importance of exclusive breastfeeding, medications acceptable for breastfeeding
- Social worker, discharge planner: Importance of exclusive breastfeeding, community resources that support breastfeeding
- Anesthesiologist: Importance of exclusive breastfeeding, importance of immediate skin-to-skin contact
- Radiology: Importance of exclusive breastfeeding, where to find out about safe medications for use during lactation, where to find appropriate information on use of radioisotopes during lactation
- Dietary: Importance of exclusive breastfeeding, practices that support breastfeeding
- Housekeeping staff: Importance of exclusive breastfeeding, practices that support breastfeeding, the facility's philosophy on infant nutrition, who to call when help is needed

Modified from Baby-friendly USA. *Guidelines and Evaluation Criteria for Facilities Seeking Baby-friendly Designation*. Rev 2016. Albany, NY: Baby-friendly USA; 2016. https://www.babyfriendlyusa .org/get-started/the-guidelines-evaluation-criteria. Accessed September 5, 2017.[18]

BOX 30-2 Interdisciplinary Considerations in Lactation Training

Interdisciplinary Application

- Lactation education must be tailored to the needs of each learner.
- Customized patient-centered care may require referral to speech therapists, otolaryngologists, registered dietitians, physicians, nurses, IBCLCs, and other healthcare professionals.
- All members of the team lend particular expertise to foster breastfeeding success.

CLINICAL TIP

Comments from students about the most helpful parts of an internship:

"Allowing us to advance at our own pace and not pushing us into uncomfortable situations. Asking the 'correct' questions when counseling moms."

"Observing the different 'teaching' styles of many IBCLCs. Letting our own personalities and 'teaching' styles shine through with moms and class."

Comments from a mentor:

"Solid lists of competencies helped keep us on track but it was hard. We couldn't cover all the topics. Lunch reviews of topics, 15–20 minutes left time to discuss and just socialize."

▶ Key Points from This Chapter

   A. Education should be based on the principles of adult learning.
   B. Training content should be shaped by the roles and learning needs of the learners.
   C. Mentoring provides a learning opportunity for both mentors and mentees.
   D. Mentoring aspiring lactation professionals is a key to sustainability of the profession.

References

1. Mentor. Merriam-Webster website. http://www.merriam-webster.com/dictionary/mentor. Accessed September 15, 2017.
2. Adult education. Encyclopedia Britannica website. https://www.britannica.com/topic/adult-education. Accessed September 15, 2017.
3. Palis AG, Quiros PA. Adult learning principles and presentation pearls. *Middle East Afr J Ophthalmol.* 2014;21(2):114-122.
4. Knowles MS. *Andragogy in Action: Applying Modern Principles of Adult Learning.* San Francisco, CA: Jossey Bass; 1984.
5. Schon, DA. *Reflective Practitioner: How Professionals Think in Action.* New York, NY: Basic Books; 2000.
6. Jensen E. Brain-based learning—a reality check. *Educational Leadership.* 2000;57(7):76-79.
7. Blakemore SJ, Frith U. *The Learning Brain: Lessons for Education.* Malden, MA: Blackwell Publishing; 2005.
8. Abbott SE. Hidden curriculum. In: Abbott S, ed. *The Glossary of Education Reform.* http://edglossary.org/hidden-curriculum. Accessed November 7, 2017.
9. Siemens G. Connectivism: a learning theory for the digital age. *International Journal of Instructional Technology and Distance Learning.* 2005;2(1):3-10.
10. Starkey L. Evaluating learning century: a digital age learning matrix. *Technol Pedagogy Educ.* 2011;20(1):19-39.
11. World Health Organization. *International Code of Marketing of Breast-milk Substitutes.* Geneva, Switzerland: World Health Organization; 1981. http://apps.who.int/iris/bitstream/10665/40382/1/9241541601.pdf. Accessed September 2, 2017.
12. MindTools. Kirkpatrick's four-level training evaluation model: analyzing training effectiveness. Mind Tools website. https://www.mindtools.com/pages/article/kirkpatrick.htm. Accessed September 5, 2017.
13. International Board of Lactation Consultant Examiners. Pathways. http://iblce.org/certify/pathways/. Accessed September 5, 2017.
14. International Board of Lactation Consultant Examiners. *Pathway 3 Plan Guide.* Fairfax, VA: International Board of Lactation Consultant Examiners; 2017. https://iblce.org/wp-content/uploads/2017/05/pathway-3-plan-guide.pdf. Accessed September 2, 2017.
15. International Board of Lactation Consultant Examiners. *Clinical Competencies for the Practice of International Board Certified Lactation Consultants (IBCLCs).* Fairfax, VA: International Board of Lactation Consultant Examiners; 2012. https://iblce.org/wp-content/uploads/2017/05/clinical-competencies.pdf. Accessed September 5, 2017.
16. International Board of Lactation Consultant Examiners. *Recertification Guide.* Fairfax, VA: International Board of Lactation Consultant Examiners; 2015. https://iblce.org/wp-content/uploads/2017/09/recertification-guide-english.pdf. Accessed September 5, 2017.
17. Wellstart International. *Lactation Management Self-Study Modules Level I.* 4th ed. Shelburne, VT: Wellstart International; 2014. http://www.wellstart.org/Self-Study-Module.pdf. Accessed September 15, 2017.
18. Baby-friendly USA. *Guidelines and Evaluation Criteria for Facilities Seeking Baby-friendly Designation.* Rev 2016. Albany, NY: Baby-friendly USA; 2016. https://www.babyfriendlyusa.org/get-started/the-guidelines-evaluation-criteria. Accessed September 5, 2017.
19. Rosen-Carole C, Hartman S, Academy of Breastfeeding Medicine. ABM clinical protocol #19: breastfeeding promotion in the prenatal setting, revision 2015. *Breastfeeding Med.* 2015;10(10):451-457. http://www.bfmed.org/Media/Files/Protocols/Protocol%2019%20Prenatal%20Setting%202015%20English%20Version.pdf. Accessed September 15, 2017.
20. American Academy of Pediatrics. Breastfeeding: welcome to the breastfeeding residency curriculum. https://www.aap.org/en-us/advocacy-and-policy/aap-health-initiatives/Breastfeeding/Pages/Residency-Curriculum.aspx. Accessed September 5, 2017.

Additional Resources
Publications

Allen TD, Eby LT. *The Blackwell Handbook of Mentoring: A Multiple Perspectives Approach.* Malden, MA: Blackwell Publishing; 2007.
Altman D. *Mentoring Our Future Clinics in Human Lactation.* Amarillo, TX; Praeclarus Press; 2010.
International Lactation Consultant Association. *Clinical Instruction in Lactation: Teaching the Next Generation.* Amarillo, TX: Praeclarus Press; 2012.
Ragins BR. Diversity and workplace mentoring relationships: a review and positive social capital approach. In: Allen TD, Eby LT, eds. *The Blackwell Handbook of Mentoring: A Multiple Perspectives Approach.* Oxford, UK: 2007. doi: 10.1111/b.9781405133739.2007.00017.x.
Wellstart International. *Lactation Management Self-Study Modules Level I.* 4th ed. Shelburne, VT: Wellstart International; 2014. http://www.wellstart.org/Self-Study-Module.pdf.

World Health Organization, UNICEF, Wellstart International. *Baby-friendly Hospital Initiative. Revised Updated and Expanded for Integrated Care. Section 3: Breastfeeding Promotion and Support in a Baby-friendly Hospital. A 20-Hour Course for Maternity Staff*. Geneva Switzerland: World Health Organization; 2009. http://www.unicef.org/french/nutrition/files/BFHI_2009_s3.1and2.pdf.

Websites

Lactation Education Accreditation and Approval Review Committee. Curriculum; memorandum of understanding; resource guide for clinical internships; criteria for course recognition or approval; standards for accreditation; directories of recognized breastfeeding courses; approved lactation courses; courses accredited by CAAHEP; and clinical opportunities. www.leaarc.org.

United States Breastfeeding Committee. Core competencies in breastfeeding care and services for all health professionals. http://www.usbreastfeeding.org/core-competencies.

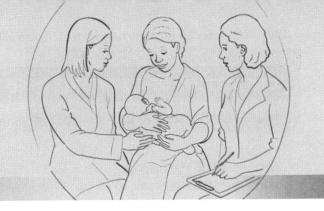

CHAPTER 31

Expression and Use of Human Milk

Frances Jones
Gillian Weaver

OBJECTIVES

- Describe key concepts and strategies for supporting human milk expression.
- Explain how milk and equipment should be safely handled.
- Describe the length of appropriate milk storage times at room temperature, in the refrigerator, and in the freezer.
- Describe the testing and processing of milk for donation and sharing.
- Explain how donors are safely recruited and screened by milk banks.
- List how milk should be transported.
- Outline the differences between human milk banking and other forms of milk sharing.

DEFINITIONS OF COMMONLY USED TERMS

donor human milk (DHM) Milk expressed by a parent and provided freely to a human milk bank to be fed to another parent's child. Also called donor breastmilk.

engorgement Condition in which the breasts are overly full of fluid and are hard and usually painful.

European Milk Bank Association (EMBA) The European Milk Bank Association was founded in 2010 and is based in Milan, Italy. It provides oversight and education to more than 200 nonprofit milk banks located in 28 European countries.

hands-on pumping A technique suggested to increase milk production when using a pump.

human milk bank An establishment that collects human milk from screened donors. The milk is pasteurized, tested, and distributed to infants with a medical need for human milk, mainly in hospitals.

(continues)

DEFINITIONS OF COMMONLY USED TERMS   *(continued)*

Human Milk Banking Association of North America (HMBANA) Organization founded in 1985 that provides oversight and education to nonprofit member milk banks and developing human milk banks in North America.

lactogenesis II The onset of copious milk production after the birth of a baby.

milk processing company A commercial, for-profit human milk company that provides financial or other incentives to parents and sells human milk and other products.

milk sharing The exchange of human milk among parents or other individuals seeking human milk. The milk is freely shared or paid for.

oral immune therapy Placing drops of colostrum inside the baby's cheek every 2 hours, or less frequently, while the baby is not able to feed orally.

pasteurized donor human milk (PDHM) Donor milk that has been heat treated using the Holder pasteurization process.

pump dependent Using a breast pump to establish milk production, or pumping exclusively to feed milk to a baby who is not directly breastfeeding.

Any use of the term *mother, maternal,* or *breastfeeding* is not meant to exclude transgender or nonbinary parents who may be breastfeeding or providing human milk to their infant.

▶ Overview

Parents should be supported to breastfeed or provide their own milk for their babies whenever possible. In North America, the emphasis in the 21st century seems to have moved for many parents from direct breastfeeding to providing the product—human milk—no matter where the source of the milk. Education about feeding options is important so parents and their families can make informed, supported decisions.

Direct breastfeeding provides optimal outcomes and is only rarely contraindicated. When breastfeeding is not possible, milk expression allows parents to feed expressed milk to their baby. Ideally, information about milk expression begins prenatally, particularly in high-risk cases, such as when a preterm infant is expected. All parents should receive information about establishing and maintaining milk production, and storage and handling of milk. In the absence of the breastfeeding parent's milk, the World Health Organization (WHO) recommends donor milk from a human milk bank.[1] The American Academy of Pediatrics (AAP) and the European Society for Pediatric Gastroenterology, Hepatology and Nutrition (ESPGHAN) also recommend donor milk from a milk bank for preterm infants whose parents have insufficient milk.[2,3] Few countries have complete equity of access to donor milk. With the increase in information from the internet and misinformation about milk sharing and milk donation, evidence-based information is needed.

I. Reasons for Milk Expression

A. Milk production works on supply and demand. Although milk is made on an ongoing basis, frequent expression results in better milk production and maintenance of milk production.[4] Unrelieved engorgement is painful and is believed to negatively affect milk production at a cellular level through pressure and negative feedback factors in the milk.[5]

B. Milk expression is needed if a baby is unable to effectively breastfeed or if a parent is separated from the baby, such as with a neonatal intensive care unit (NICU) admission.

C. Milk expression may be chosen due to concern about adequate milk production, return to work, embarrassment, reluctance to engage in direct breastfeeding, or other cultural reasons.[6]

D. Expressing milk to feed to a baby by bottle is an increasingly common practice in North America, with employment being a common reason for the practice.[7,8] Evidence indicates that infant weight gain may be associated not only with the type of milk consumed, but also the mode of delivery, with increased weight gain being associated with bottle feeding.[9] In addition, bottle feeding expressed milk may not provide the same health benefits as breastfeeding, such as reducing the risk of otitis media.[10]

II. Validity of Information about Establishing and Maintaining Milk Production

Lactation consultants should caution parents about using the internet as a source of information.

    A.   Many parents use the internet to access information about milk expression and breast pumps.

    B.   Much of the information on the internet is not evidence based, and it is inconsistent and incomplete.

    C.   Companies selling breastfeeding equipment may present milk expression as a convenient option[11] that is equivalent to breastfeeding.[12]

        1.   Breast pumps can be expensive and, if not used properly, can result in bruising or nipple trauma.

        2.   Milk expression is time consuming and requires additional work due to the cleaning of pump parts and storage and handling of milk.

        3.   The amount of milk expressed does not always correlate with actual milk production because some parents find it difficult to express milk, and breast pumps do not completely drain the breasts.[13]

    D.   Evidence-based antenatal and postpartum education for parents and their partners encourages support for breastfeeding, appropriate expression of milk when needed, and, when the parent is returning to work, the use of lactation rooms and milk expression breaks to increase the rates of breastfeeding and provision of expressed milk.[14]

III. Strategies to Help Establish and Maintain Milk Production

    A.   Milk may be removed through hand expression or use of breast pump.

        1.   Methods of expression include hand expression, electric hospital multiuser pumps, and pumps designed to be used by one individual (electric or hand pumps). If the parent is considering using a secondhand pump, either through purchase or loan, it is important that the manufacturer's instructions be checked regarding the pump's suitability or the parent may increase contamination in the milk by using an unsuitable pump. Websites such as KellyMom.com provide good basic information. (See *Additional Resources* later in this chapter.)

        2.   Low-cost techniques that may result in greater volumes of milk include early hand expression initiation when the baby is not able to breastfeed effectively, listening to relaxing music, massaging the breasts before and during pumping, and warming the breasts prior to and during pumping.[15]

        3.   The decision regarding the expression method depends on whether the parent is establishing and maintaining milk production with pumping or expressing extra milk with a baby who breastfeeds effectively.

            a.   For an extremely preterm baby, a good quality electric pump is important.

            b.   For a healthy term infant requiring only occasional milk expression (e.g., a return to full-time or part-time work), hand expression or a hand pump may be sufficient.

            c.   Some pump-dependent parents find that renting a hospital-grade pump works well because they can pump both breasts simultaneously and purchase a greater range of breast flange sizes. The motor is also more durable over time, compared to personal pumps.

            d.   In addition to effectiveness, the ease of use, portability, noise level, and cost are important factors when choosing a pump.

            e.   Pumps with a compression component, versus those that work with suction only, are more effective at removing milk.[16]

            f.   Cultural factors are another consideration, including the availability of parental leave, resources, attitudes toward breasts and equipment, and support for breastfeeding.

    B.   It is useful for every breastfeeding parent to learn how to express milk by hand.

        1.   Milk can be expressed without special equipment.

        2.   Hand expression is particularly useful in the first 24 hours when there is a very small volume of viscous colostrum.[17,18] The drops obtained through hand expression can be collected and given to the infant rather than losing them in the pumping equipment.

        3.   Early hand expression has been shown to increase breastfeeding rates by 25 percent at 2 months, compared to pumping.[19]

4. Teach parents the mechanics of hand expression.
   a. Gently massage the breast in circles toward the areola.
   b. Place a clean collection container beneath the nipple.
   c. Place the thumb and second finger on opposite sides of the breast, about 3 cm (1.5 inches) back from the nipple.
   d. Leaning forward over the container, gently press the thumb and finger back toward the chest wall without pulling or sliding along the skin.
   e. Compress the breast, then release the pressure. Repeat the process several times.
   f. Reposition the hand and repeat the compressions, moving around the breast to compress all the milk ducts.

5. Traditional Russian practices combine hand expression and breast massage for milk removal, engorgement, plugged ducts, and mastitis.[20] The technique can be viewed in an online video.[21]

C. The use of an effective electric breast pump will protect milk production when the breastfeeding dyad is separated.

1. In the first few days, milk production progresses from a few drops to a few ounces per feed. By 4 days postpartum, parents who depend on a pump should be producing 500 mL or more per day.[22] Those with lower volumes are at risk for inadequate milk volumes by 6 weeks.
   a. Delayed initiation of milk expression results in decreased milk volumes and may increase the time to lactogenesis II. Delayed initiation is also associated with inadequate breastfeeding duration in the preterm population.[23,24]
   b. Expression should start ideally within an hour of birth[25] and definitely by 6 hours postpartum.[26,27]
   c. Expression of milk as soon as possible after birth for babies admitted to the NICU supports the availability of oral immune therapy for preterm and critically ill babies.[28]

2. Pump selection should be based on objective factors including reason for use, comfort, ease of use, effectiveness, and cost.[15,29]

3. The most suitable method of expression depends on the individual parent and baby and the reason for expressing milk.[15]
   a. Milk expression should mimic the pattern of a healthy breastfed baby. Research indicates that eight or more expressions per day support adequate milk production.[23,30]
   b. A recent review demonstrated that using an effective electric pump, either alone or in combination with hand expression, provides greater milk volumes when replacing, rather than augmenting, breastfeeding.[29]
   c. The use of an electric double pump saves time, although some parents may prefer sequential pumping with a single pump. The amount of milk pumped in the early weeks has been shown to be greater with double pumping and when using a pump that is comfortable.[31]
   d. Research indicates that using techniques like hands-on pumping—combining hand expression, breast massage, and compression and electric pumping—results in higher milk volumes[13] and milk with higher caloric value.[32]

4. Pumping guidelines:
   a. The manufacturers' instructions provide guidance on appropriate use and cleaning of pumps and their parts. Use the following cleaning procedure for pump parts that come in contact with milk:
      i. Take them apart.
      ii. Rinse them in lukewarm water after use to remove milk solids.
      iii. Wash them in hot soapy water with liquid dish soap in a clean pan reserved for this purpose.
      iv. Rinse them well in hot water.
      v. Dry them with a clean paper towel or shake them to remove extra moisture, then air dry them on a clean towel.
      vi. Store them in a covered clean container when they are dry.
      vii. Wash and dry the bowl or pan used for washing the pump parts.
   b. Pump parts should be disinfected once a day by boiling for 5 minutes after cleaning if the pumping is for an ill or preterm infant.[33]
   c. To promote success when expression is needed, instruct the parent on mechanics, beginning with good hand washing technique.[34] There are a number of online videos to assist.
      i. Assemble the clean pump parts and center the breast shields over the nipples.

ii. Lean forward to encourage milk to flow into the collection container.

iii. Turn on the pump with the suction at the lowest setting, and gradually increase the suction according to comfort.

iv. With a double pump, pump for about 10 minutes or until the milk stops spraying and the breasts are soft. With a single pump, pump for about 5 minutes per breast and switch back and forth until the breasts are soft and milk is no longer flowing easily. Expressing for a couple of minutes after milk stops flowing is often suggested for increasing milk production.

v. Warming the breast flanges has been shown to improve the efficiency of milk removal.[35]

vi. Keeping a milk diary can be useful in monitoring milk production and knowing when to seek help if production falters. A daily review by hospital staff provides timely support and encouragement for milk expression in the NICU.[36]

CLINICAL TIP

Except in rare situations, all parents need ongoing and skilled support to breastfeed or express milk to meet their breastfeeding goals. In the absence of the parent's own milk, pasteurized donor milk from a recognized milk bank is the next best option, especially for high-risk and ill babies. In many NICUs, the use of pasteurized donor milk is the standard of care when the parent's milk is unavailable or insufficient.

IV. Storage and Handling of Milk

A. Education about careful technique and using clean hands and equipment result in milk with less contamination, which is desirable for milk storage.[37]

B. The following factors should be considered with regard to storage time:

1. The storage of human milk, whether at room temperature for short periods or for longer times in a refrigerator or freezer, has an impact on its composition.[38,39]

2. Ideally, expressed milk should be placed in a refrigerator or freezer immediately after expression, particularly if expressing for a preterm or ill infant.[40]

3. Milk that is collected cleanly can safely be left for up to 6 hours at the bedside on the postpartum unit if there is no refrigerator available.

4. Milk with higher contamination or in a unit with a higher ambient temperature (warmer than 27°C) should be stored for a shorter time out of the refrigerator (i.e., 3 to 4 hours or less).[41-43]

5. Milk should be stored at 4°C in a refrigerator[44] and at −18 to −20°C in a freezer.[45] See **TABLE 31-1** for human milk storage guidelines.[46,47]

6. Milk that is stored in a refrigerator or freezer should be placed away from the door because of temperature fluctuations. Placing it in an additional storage container with a lid will ensure that other foods or liquids do not contaminate the milk.

C. Use the following guidelines when choosing a storage container:

1. Any clean food-grade container with a lid is appropriate for term, preterm, healthy, or ill infants.[46]

2. Milk storage bags are convenient for milk storage at home but may be expensive.

3. Each expression in the NICU should be placed in a new container because when a container is opened there is an increased chance of contamination. For a healthy baby at home, milk can be layered. Chill the first expression and add additional milk after it has been chilled for a period of about 12 hours and then freeze as each addition increases the chance of greater bacterial contamination.[48]

4. Leave about 0.5 inch at the top of the storage container to allow for expansion as the milk freezes.

D. Refer to the following guidelines for labeling and storage of milk:

1. Carefully label all stored milk with the date it was expressed. For hospital storage, note the date, patient name, and other information as needed.

2. Package the milk in serving sizes when possible to minimize waste, decrease the chance of contamination, and reduce the loss of nutrients if the unused milk were poured into another container.

TABLE 31-1 Guidelines for Storage of Human Milk		
Any storage of human milk outside the breast can negatively impact the milk components. For ill and preterm babies, the shorter the length of storage, the better. For healthy babies at home, particularly if they are being breastfed and receive stored milk only occasionally, longer storage is not a problem. Milk should be expressed and stored under the cleanest conditions possible.		
Temperature by Location	**Parent's Own Expressed Milk**	**Pasteurized Donor Human Milk**
Room temperature	≤ 4 hours Ideally, refrigerate immediately	≤ 4 hours
Refrigerator: Between 2°C and 4°C	2–8 days 48–72 hours for NICU babies Previously frozen and thawed: 12–24 hours	24–48 hours after thawed Do not refreeze previously frozen milk
Freezer: Between –18°C and –20°C	3–12 months	3–12 months 12 months from the time of expression

Data from Human Milk Banking Association of North America. *2011 Best Practice for Expressing, Storage and Handling Human Milk in Hospitals, Homes, and Child Care Settings.* Fort Worth, TX: Human Milk Banking Association of North America; 2011[46]; British Dietetic Association. *Guidelines for the Preparation and Handling of Expressed and Donor Breast Milk and Special Feeds for Infants and Children in Neonatal and Paediatric Health Care Settings.* Birmingham, UK: British Dietetic Association; 2016.[47]

E. When stored milk is ready to be used, consider the following guidelines:
1. In the hospital, milk can be defrosted in a milk warmer or refrigerator, or it can be thawed in its container in warm water (keep the lid out of the water to avoid contamination). Defrosting in the refrigerator results in less fat loss, compared to using warm water.[49]
2. Milk for full-term infants does not need to be warmed.[50]
3. For ill or preterm babies, bringing milk to body temperature is thought to be appropriate, although the optimal temperature has been shown to vary and further research is needed.[51]
4. Do not microwave milk because this cooks some milk properties and may result in hot spots, which can burn the baby.[52]

V. Transporting Human Milk

A. The length of time milk will remain frozen is affected by the following:
1. How much milk is in each container; partially filled bottles defrost easier than totally filled containers.
2. How many bottles are being transported together.
3. Length of time from freezer to freezer.
4. How the chilled or frozen milk is packed.
5. Temperatures the shipping container is exposed to.
B. The following are guidelines for short trips of less than 4 hours in a temperate climate:
1. Chilled or frozen milk can be packed in a clean plastic bag and placed in a thermal lunch kit with frozen gel packs added for travel to the hospital if the trip from refrigerator to refrigerator, or freezer to freezer, is less than 4 hours.
2. The gel packs need to be frozen solid to keep the milk chilled, and any extra air in the thermal lunch kit should be removed with clean towels or clean newspaper.
3. Larger amounts of milk that cannot fit into a thermal lunch kit can be packed in a regular hard-sided picnic cooler (see the next section).

C. The following are guidelines for trips of 4 to about 20 hours in a temperate climate:
    1. Line a hard-sided picnic cooler with a clean plastic bag, place frozen gel packs on the bottom and sides, and pack the frozen milk containers (in clean plastic bags that can be zipped) solidly together in the middle of the cooler.
    2. Place frozen gel packs on top of the milk and tie the bag shut to remove all extra air.
    3. Remove any extra air in the cooler with clean paper or towels. Seal the lid with packing tape if needed.
    4. Pack the milk for transport just prior to leaving so the milk will remain in the freezer as long as possible. Place it in a freezer upon arrival at the destination after checking that the milk is still frozen.
D. Dry ice may be needed for longer trips or trips in very hot weather. Call a shipping company or check online for instructions on handling dry ice.
E. For air travel, check with the airline because regulations change. Check the appropriate websites before traveling to confirm the current information. The U.S. Transportation Security Administration website[53] currently lists the following guidelines for carrying on human milk:
    1. Ice packs, freezer packs, frozen gel packs, and other accessories required to chill milk are permitted.
    2. Separate the milk from other liquids and aerosols, which are limited to 3.4 ounces or 100 milliliters. Human milk is not restricted to a quart-size bag.
    3. Notify the screening officer that the bag contains human milk.
    4. Tell the officer to not open the container. Other methods of testing can be used if needed. Be aware that the U.S. Food and Drug Administration says there are no known adverse effects from eating food, drinking beverages, or using medicine that was screened with X-rays.

CLINICAL TIP

Evidence indicates that after human milk is expressed, any storage method impacts the composition and effectiveness of the milk. Storage and handling may also impact contamination. There is a lack of independent evidence regarding contamination based on different types of breast pumps that are currently on the market. In addition, research on the effect of handling and fortification of human milk in clinical areas, such as at the bedside in the NICU, is needed.

VI. Sharing of Human Milk

A. The demand for human milk for infants whose parents are unable to, or choose not to, breastfeed has expanded significantly in recent years, although data about the extent of human milk sharing is lacking.[54]
B. Parents wish to provide the best for their babies, and the acknowledged health disadvantages for infants and young children who are not fed with human milk[55] has led to increasing demands by parents and caregivers for donor milk.[2,54,56,57]
C. Milk may be shared with or sought from established nonprofit human milk banks, from commercial human milk enterprises, or via milk sharing and milk selling.[58]
    1. Milk that is donated to a nonprofit human milk bank is provided to preterm and sick infants who have the greatest medical need and some banks provide milk to community recipients.[59]
    2. Milk can be sold on internet sites or to companies that source human milk on behalf of for-profit companies.[60]
D. Milk is sometimes shared among parents.
    1. The sharing of milk among parents has existed throughout human history.[61]
    2. In the 20th century, sharing began to occur among relatives and friends in undocumented numbers.[60]
    3. In the 21st century, groups and individuals began sharing milk via online milk sharing groups.
        a. Parents who do not know each other connect online, and some of these connections have resulted in friendships.
        b. The safety risk of using milk from a relative, friend, or stranger is unknown because every situation involves many unmeasurable factors.

c. Milk is affected by the health and lifestyle of the donor, the cleanliness of the environment where the milk is expressed, the type of storage container, the storage conditions, milk handling, the shipping conditions, and the handling, storage, and preparation by the receiver.

d. In a home environment, it is not possible to screen donors and milk to the same standards as screening by a milk bank. The family decides if the risks of possible contamination, transmission of disease, presence of drugs, or presence of other fluids are acceptable.

e. Ideally, all parents should receive adequate support, including maternity leave, so they can breastfeed their own children and reduce the need for milk sharing.[59,62]

VII. History of Sharing Human Milk

A. Throughout history, sharing human milk through direct breastfeeding (wet nursing) or providing expressed milk to another parent's infant made it possible for babies to survive despite the parent's death, ill health, or lactation insufficiency, or because of separation for a variety of reasons.[61] There is no historical data regarding any harm these children experienced from milk sharing. In the absence of their parent's own milk, they faced certain death without wet nursing.

B. Wet nursing was commonplace until the 20th century. It was largely an altruistic act for a relative, friend, or community member, and it could be a source of income for both individuals and those who worked for bureaus of wet nurses.

1. Worldwide, wet nursing remains the means by which many babies receive human milk, although it became far less common in the 20th century with the widespread availability of infant formula based on cow's milk.

2. The successful use of a wet nurse requires the infant to be physically mature and healthy enough to fully obtain their nutritional requirements while directly breastfeeding. This is not possible for most preterm infants and ill babies, especially those with compromised breathing.

C. With improvements in neonatal medicine and the ability to keep increasingly lower-gestational-aged infants alive, the need for a way to feed these babies was key to their survival. Artificial feedings could be avoided only with expressed milk. As a result, parents were recruited to express their milk, and various feeding implements were developed to allow at-risk infants to be fed without aspirating.

D. Milk banking has a long history throughout the world.

1. The location of the first formal milk bank is generally attributed to Vienna in modern-day Austria.[63] It was established in 1909, and the European Milk Bank Association (EMBA) celebrated the centenary anniversary with its 2009 conference in Vienna.[64]

2. It is very likely that similar operations were concurrently operational in Switzerland and other European countries.

3. The centenary anniversary of the first such North American establishment, located at the Tufts Medical Center's Floating Hospital for Children in Boston, was celebrated at the Human Milk Banking Association of North America (HMBANA) International conference in Boston in 2010.

4. The terms *breast milk dairy* and *milk bureau* were initially used prior to the use of the term *milk bank*, which came into being in the mid-20th century.[65]

5. Parents received small payments for the milk they provided; they are still financially reimbursed to cover their expenses in some northern European countries, including Norway and Germany.

6. Other parents' milk was instrumental in the successful feeding of many infants, with the most famous being the identical Dionne quintuplets born in Canada in 1934 and the St. Neots quads born in the United Kingdom in 1935.

a. Frozen milk for the Dionne quintuplets was shipped by train from southern Ontario and Quebec to the small village of Corbeil in northern Ontario.[66]

b. Milk for the St. Neots quads traveled 100 miles by plane from London. The first milk bank in the United Kingdom was established as a direct result of the successful feeding of the St. Neots quads.[67]

7. The fortunes of milk banks waxed and waned globally according to infant feeding preferences and national and local circumstances.

a. Globally the numbers dropped significantly in the 1980s following the development of specialist preterm infant formula and the discovery that HIV can be transmitted through breastmilk.[68]

b. A 1980s feeding trial conducted in the United Kingdom showed that preterm babies gained weight more rapidly when fed with preterm formula, compared to donor milk.[69] This led to the further demise of milk banks. It is noteworthy that the donor milk used was so-called drip milk, which is lower in fat and energy than milk that has been expressed according to current milk bank requirements.

VIII. Milk Banking Today

A. There is renewed confidence in the safety of donor milk.
1. Following the closure of milk banks globally, it was later confirmed that heat treating human milk at greater than 56°C for 30 minutes inactivates HIV.[70] This led to renewed confidence in the safety of human milk bank operations.
   a. Holder pasteurization at 62.5°C for 30 minutes followed by rapid cooling has been widely adopted due to the known inactivation of pathogenic bacteria and viruses combined with the preservation of much of the anti-infective components in the milk.[71]
   b. Further results from the research cautioned that preterm babies who are fed with formula rather than human milk showed significantly increased rates of necrotizing enterocolitis, a disease with a high mortality rate and severe associated morbidities.[72] A systematic review published in 2014 confirmed this, adding that the data suggests that feeding with formula significantly increases the risk of feeding intolerance in preterm and low birth weight infants.[73]
   c. Subsequently, standardized heat treatments for donor milk were incorporated into most milk bank guidelines. The use of pasteurized donor milk began to increase, and new milk banks began to be established.
2. Globally, most milk banks can trace the milk from donor to recipient. Milk is provided to recipients anonymously, the same as blood, organs, and tissues.
3. Some milk banks screen and process milk for a parent's own baby; this is the norm in France, Belgium, and some parts of South America. Most other countries avoid heat processing milk for the parent's own baby to maintain maximum benefits for the child.
4. Human milk is now included in the ISBT 128 global standard[74] coding guidelines, with codes applied to different types and stages of human milk (e.g., colostrum, raw milk, and heat-treated milk). The process employs bar code tracking, which aids the traceability of milk through milk banking processes.
B. Human milk banks are operated as follows:
1. PATH, an organization based in Seattle, Washington, is active in more than 70 countries and leads the way in providing global support for the development of safe and sustainable human milk banking operations.[75]
2. The operation of human milk banks differs widely from country to country, and sometimes within a single country. The differences include the following:
   a. Reimbursement or payment for milk versus free donations.
   b. Milk testing regimens both before and after heat treatment.
   c. Standardized and novel heat treatments versus raw milk.
   d. Donor serological screening.
   e. Widely varying time limits both for the length of time after giving birth that a donor can continue donating, and for acceptance of frozen stored milk before and after heat treatment.
3. National guidelines are available in many, but not all, locations. They are freely available online from the United Kingdom, France, Italy, Norway, Sweden, and Switzerland. The EMBA website provides further details,[65] and the HMBANA guidelines can be purchased online.
4. National guidelines provide recommendations for every stage in the milk banking process:
   a. Donor recruitment.
   b. Donor screening, including serology testing.
   c. Storage, handling, and transportation of raw milk.
   d. Storage of donor milk in the milk bank.
   e. Microbiological testing of milk prior to and after heat treatment.
   f. Heat treatment, including time and temperature parameters.
   g. Milk tracking to ensure traceability throughout the process.
   h. Storage and distribution, including transportation from the milk bank.

C.   Milk donors are carefully screened.
    1.   Milk donors generally fall into three main groups:
        a.   Ongoing donors express milk at home, usually once per day, and freeze it in containers supplied by the milk bank. It is transported to the milk bank after a sufficient quantity has been collected.
        b.   One-time donors donate frozen milk they stored prior to recruitment. These donors may continue to express and donate their milk.
        c.   Bereaved parents are asked to consider donating their stored milk to a human milk bank. Donating milk has been shown to be beneficial to their grieving. Some bereaved parents continue to express, store, and donate milk for several weeks or months.[76]
    2.   Donor selection criteria differ among, and sometimes within, countries.
        a.   Not all lactating parents are able to donate their milk. Selection is mainly based on health criteria obtained through questionnaires about risk reduction.
        b.   Lactating parents are not usually able to donate their milk if they meet the following criteria:
            i.   Smoke or use nicotine substitutes, including e-cigarettes.
            ii.   Drink more than a specified number of units of alcohol daily (some guidelines recommend no alcohol).
            iii.   Use recreational or street drugs.
            iv.   Have recently received a blood transfusion or blood products or tissues.
            v.   Use certain medications.
            vi.   Have undergone certain diagnostic tests or therapeutic treatments.
            vii.   Have recently been exposed to certain infections through travel or contact (e.g., Ebola virus, Zika virus, West Nile virus, and tuberculosis).
        c.   If prospective donors are not deferred as a result of initial screening, further screening is usually required, including serology tests. They should be provided with evidence of their blood test results. Different national recommendations include screening for some or all of the following:
            i.   HIV-1 and HIV-2.
            ii.   Human T lymphotropic viruses I and II.
            iii.   Hepatitis B.
            iv.   Hepatitis C.
            v.   Syphilis.
         d.   Further tests may be requested depending on the location of the milk bank or the donor, the operational regimes, and the traveling history of the donor.
        e.   The presence of cold sores, infectious illnesses such as varicella within the family, and influenza will usually lead to temporary deferment. Short courses of medications and some treatments may require only temporary deferment.
D.   Milk bank requirements ensure safe collection, storage, handling, and processing of the milk.
    1.   Donors receive information (verbal and written) from the milk bank outlining the bank's expectations and requirements.
        a.   This process facilitates safe collection, storage, and handling of expressed milk, including cleaning and disinfecting equipment.
        b.   The storage of donor milk should adhere to the following guidelines:
            i.   Optimal storage of human milk for donation requires that it be fast frozen in a −20°C freezer as soon as possible following expression; however, most milk banks also accept refrigerated storage. The length of refrigerated storage time varies.
            ii.   Milk banks require that daily temperature records be kept of all refrigerators and freezers used to store the milk at any milk storage depot or facility and in the milk bank itself. Some milk banks require this with refrigerators and freezers in the donor's home.
            iii.   Milk bank freezers should have continuous monitoring and be fitted with audible and visible alarms. They should preferably be connected to security systems to prevent milk being lost in the event of a power failure.
        c.   To ensure optimal milk quality, the milk should be protected from light and temperature increases during transport. Additional transportation considerations include the following:
            i.   Distances traveled and ambient temperature conditions.

      ii.   The use of dry ice or refrigerated vehicles.

      iii. The use of easy-to-clean, insulated transport containers.

      iv. Temperature monitoring throughout transportation or on arrival at the destination (this is recommended for both raw donor milk arriving at the milk bank and pasteurized donor milk arriving at the recipient hospital).

2. Safety and quality checks of donor human milk include the following:

    a. Globally, recommendations related to quality and safety checks for donated milk vary. Most define microbiological cultures for some, if not all, milk. Cultures may be performed on the milk prior to heat treatments, after pasteurization, or at both times.

    b. Current HMBANA guidelines do not require routine prepasteurization culturing, although many banks do perform this step. Culturing and acceptance criteria are included if the milk is to be fed raw, although the use of raw milk from HMBANA banks is extremely rare.[77]

    c. Raw milk may be an option for particular patients, as determined by a physician. The microbiological limits for raw milk are as follows:

      i.   Less than or equal to 10^4 cfu/mL of normal skin flora (e.g., coagulase negative staphylococci, diphtheroids, *Staphylococcus epidermidis*, or *Streptococcus viridans*).

      ii. The presence of any pathogens is unacceptable.

    d. Guideline 93 published by the National Institute for Health and Care Excellence (NICE) in the United Kingdom recommends that all milk be tested prior to heat treatment.[71] The microbiological limits for acceptance of the milk are as follows:

      i.   Total viable count (TVC) less than 10^5 cfu/mL.

      ii. Coagulase positive staphylococci less than $< 10^4$ cfu/mL.

      iii. Enterobacteriaceae less than 10^4 cfu/mL.

    e. Other published guidelines, such as those from Australia,[78] recommend that all milk be tested prior to heat treatment. The acceptance criteria include a TVC of less than 10^5 cfu/mL, but milk should not be used if any pathogens are detected.

    f. If the tested milk fails the acceptance criteria, the donor should be taught how to minimize contamination during collection and handling of the milk. The guidance should include how to decontaminate and sterilize the equipment as well as personal and hand hygiene.

3. Donor milk is heat treated according to the following procedures:

    a. Holder pasteurization is the most widely recommended temperature and time combination. This process heats the milk to 62.5°C and maintains this temperature for 30 minutes. This is followed by rapid cooling to prevent unnecessary exposure to high temperatures, which reduces most of the active immunological, and some of the nutritional, components in the milk.

    b. Holder pasteurization is currently accepted as the most practical and cost-effective method for preserving anti-infective components while simultaneously inactivating harmful bacteria and viruses.

    c. Alternative methods that are used widely in the food industry are being investigated and developed for use in human milk banks. They include high-pressure pasteurization; high temperature, short time treatments; and microwave and other forms of radiation.[79]

4. Considerations for quality and safety testing of pasteurized donor human milk include the following:

    a. Cooled pasteurized donor milk is transferred to a holding refrigerator or freezer while awaiting postpasteurization test results prior to being cleared as ready to dispense. Samples of pasteurized donor milk should show no growth to demonstrate efficacy of the heat treatment.

    b. The guidelines vary as follows:

      i.   Testing a sample from every batch (HMBANA).

      ii. Testing once every 10 batches (NICE) or more frequently if indicated.

      iii. Testing less frequently.

IX. Use of Raw versus Pasteurized Donor Milk

A. Before the 1980s, the use of raw donor milk (i.e., without any heat treatment) was more prevalent, especially if it showed low levels of bacterial contamination on testing. Raw milk is still used in some places.

   1. In Norway, most donor milk in hospital NICUs is used raw.

BOX 31-1   Suggested Uses of Pasteurized Donor Human Milk

The use of pasteurized donor human milk (PDHM) in NICUs varies in criteria, such as weight restrictions, use in maternity areas for medical issues such as hypoglycemia to support exclusive breastfeeding, and use for outpatients who have a medical need (with a physician's prescription). When quantities are limited, the PDHM is distributed based on medical priority (both maternal and infant factors), with the tiniest and sickest infants having top priority. Additional requests are referred to another milk bank. Generally, priority criteria for the use of PDHM are as follows:

1. Preterm infants.
2. Infants younger than 12 months with medical conditions that are likely to respond to donor human milk therapy.
3. Individuals older than 12 months with medical conditions that are likely to respond to donor human milk therapy.
4. Clinical use in well-designed studies through research contracts.
5. Individuals older than 12 months with chronic conditions that require small amounts.
6. Individuals older than 12 months with chronic conditions that require large amounts.
7. Infants with no specific medical conditions who require short-term use.
8. Laboratory research milk that is not suitable for human consumption.

PDHM may be provided for the following conditions:

1. Preterm infants and infants whose parents have insufficient milk.
2. Children with certain medical conditions (e.g., cardiac, kidney, and gastrointestinal problems). Children with a chylothorax may receive low-fat milk.
3. Children with an allergy to formula that results in bleeding from the bowel or anaphylactic shock.
4. Children who do not thrive without human milk and whose parents are unable to provide sufficient milk.

Data from Human Milk Banking Association of North America. *Guidelines for the Establishment and Operation of a Donor Human Milk Bank*. Fort Worth, TX: Human Milk Banking Association of North America; 2015.[77]

---

2. In some NICUs in Germany, raw donor milk is provided to very preterm or sick infants.[80] Donor milk from mothers who are positive for cytomegalovirus or whose milk fails the criteria for raw feeding, will be pasteurized and fed to higher-gestation and lower-risk neonates.
3. Milk banks in Norway and Germany undertake additional donor screening, including for cytomegalovirus, which is inactivated by pasteurization but only partially inactivated by freezing.
B. The clinical uses of pasteurized donor milk include the following:
1. In line with recommendations from the WHO, AAP, and ESPGHAN, pasteurized donor milk is mainly fed to preterm infants in the hospital when the baby's parent is unable to provide any or enough milk.[2,3,56] (See **BOX 31-1**.)
2. The parent's milk is the preferred food for all babies, especially those born with immature or compromised immune and digestive systems. The availability of pasteurized donor milk should not undermine lactation support for the baby's parent or be used instead of the parent's milk (except in rare and clinically justified circumstances).
3. Randomized controlled trials have not been undertaken for most clinical uses of pasteurized donor milk. However, a growing body of evidence demonstrates the potential short-, medium-, and long-term disadvantages of feeding artificial formula to infants.[81]
4. To reduce infant mortality, support for human milk banking through resource and policy development needs to be integrated into newborn care, particularly for ill and high-risk newborns.[82]

X. Nonprofit Milk Banks

A. Globally, there are an estimated 560 nonprofit human milk banks.
B. The largest milk banking system in the world is in Brazil. In the 1980s, the country's Ministry of Health supported the development of milk banks as a strategy to improve child health by avoiding the use of formula. In 2016 there were 210 milk banks and more than 100 milk depots.
1. The milk banks are a large part of breastfeeding support centers. Together with kangaroo care, they help ensure that all preterm infants receive human milk.
2. Expressed human milk is screened and processed mostly within the milk banks, and any surplus milk is automatically donated for babies in need.

3. The Brazilian model of milk banking has been widely used in other South and Central American countries.[83] This model differs from milk banking in North America and the majority of centers globally.
   a. Prepasteurization milk testing includes Dornic acidity tests rather than bacteriological screening, which is used in other global centers.
   b. Dornic acidity is an indirect measurement of bacterial content in milk because bacteria ferment lactose into lactic acid. A Dornic acidity test is a simple and economical way to identify milk that is suitable for pasteurization.[84]
4. The Brazilian model is followed by the milk bank in Cabo Verde, a former Portuguese colony off the coast of Africa. In Africa, there is interest at a national level in developing milk banks in a growing number of countries, including Kenya and Ethiopia. In South Africa, thriving national groups have supported the widespread development of milk banks.[85]
5. In Europe, there are 224 established and 16 planned milk banks in 28 countries,[64] including several new milk banks in Russia, Poland, and Lithuania. The continent includes some of the longest-operating milk banks in the world, dating back to the early years of the 20th century. The numbers of banks per country and per 1,000 people vary widely. There are currently at least 20 milk banks in Germany, 36 in France, 37 in Italy, and 16 in the United Kingdom.[64]
6. In North America, 27 HMBANA-accredited human milk banks operate, and 5 more milk banks are under development. The oldest two (one in the United States and one in Canada) have operated continuously since 1974. Since 2000, the amount of milk distributed by HMBANA banks has grown yearly. In 2017, the HMBANA milk banks distributed over 6 million ounces (over 170,000 liters) of pasteurized donor milk.
7. In recent years, India has seen a rapid increase in the number of milk banks. The oldest milk bank dates to the late 1980s and was the only one for many years. Now there are more than 45 milk banks, and more are planned.
8. Vietnam recently opened its first milk bank in Da Nang. There are milk banks in Southeast Asia, Taiwan, the Philippines, and Thailand. The numbers of milk banks are growing in China and Japan as well.
9. Australia has five milk banks, with others planned. New Zealand is exploring how to use the milk bank in Christchurch as a regional hub for the South Island that can work alongside a similar facility for the North Island.

XI. For-Profit Milk Processing Companies

A. The 21st century has seen the development of commercial companies that generally provide payment to donors for their milk.
   1. Their products include frozen heat-treated human milk, frozen human milk fortifier (derived from human milk and used to increase the nutritional content of the parent's own milk or donor human milk for preterm infants), and ultra-heat-treated human milk stored at ambient temperatures.[59]
   2. With the increased buying and selling of human milk and human milk products, the word *donor* seems inappropriate in most commercial contexts. Globally recognized terminology for purchased human milk has not yet been adopted.
   3. In 2017 in India, the term *milk bank* was replaced by the term *lactation management center* to refer to nonprofit milk banks. The change recognizes that the focus is on supporting parents to breastfeed their own infants, and pasteurized donor milk is available when the parent's own milk is insufficient or unavailable.
   4. Large-scale commercial human milk processing companies are a 21st-century phenomenon.
      a. Currently, few are in operation globally.
      b. There are several in the United States, one in Europe, and one being developed in India.
      c. The selling of human milk and human milk products seems to be on the rise, including from overseas sources. This raises a number of concerns, not the least of which is the potential for exploitation of parents and babies.[58]

B.   There are major concerns within the nonprofit human milk banking sector that the commercialization of human milk reduces the availability of donated milk. In the face of rising demands from hospitals for pasteurized donor milk, commercialization could create shortages.

    1.   In 2011, the U.S. Department of Health and Human Services released *The Surgeon General's Call to Action to Support Breastfeeding*, which includes an action to "identify and address obstacles to greater availability of safe banked donor milk for fragile infants."[86 (p49)] This action recognizes the need for a national strategy to address the issues of providing banked milk particularly to the vulnerable infant population.

    2.   A recently published policy statement from the AAP notes an increase in the use of pasteurized donor milk for high-risk infants (categorized as weighing less than 1,500 g or with severe intestinal disorders).[57]

        a.   The statement endorses the use of pasteurized donor milk, which it concludes is safe when the milk is from an established human milk bank that screens donors and uses appropriate measures to collect, store, and pasteurize the milk.

        b.   The statement notes the importance of the development of public policy to increase access to pasteurized donor milk. The AAP does not recommend the use of nonpasteurized donor milk and other forms of direct, internet-based, or informal milk sharing because of the risks of bacterial and viral contamination and the possibility of exposure to medications, drugs, or herbs in human milk.

▶ Key Points from This Chapter

A.   Direct breastfeeding between a parent and baby provides optimal outcomes and is only rarely contraindicated.

B.   All methods of storage outside the breast negatively affect the components in human milk.

C.   If an infant is separated from the parent, milk expression, ideally by 1 hour postpartum and definitely before 6 hours postpartum, is imperative for the provision of oral immune therapy and establishing milk production.

D.   Good hand washing, appropriate storage containers, clean pump parts, and appropriate storage temperatures are key to safe milk storage.

E.   In the absence of the parent's milk, the alternative recommended by the WHO is pasteurized donor milk from a human milk bank.

F.   Families need evidence-based recommended feeding options to make informed decisions.

G.   Nonprofit milk banking is expanding globally to meet the needs of infants, particularly ill and preterm infants.

🔍 *CASE STUDY 1*

Jennifer was expecting her third baby. Her pregnancy went well, and she went into labor at 37 weeks. After 14 hours of labor something went dreadfully wrong, and her daughter was stillborn. Jennifer's nurse on the postpartum unit reviewed the options for Jennifer's milk. The nurse explained that Jennifer could express milk to provide comfort as needed and let her milk gradually dry up, or she could express milk and donate it to the milk bank. Jennifer decided on the second option and began regular expression. The nurse notified the milk bank, and Jennifer received a call from the milk bank at about 2 weeks postpartum. Jennifer explained that she did not yet know why her baby died but that donating milk was a meaningful way to honor her baby daughter. She said, "Something good will come from something terrible. I will be helping lots of other babies through my daughter's gift and that, in a small way, helps." Jennifer donated milk for 3 months. She lived near the milk bank and dropped off her donations in person. On her last donation she said, "I am ready to let go. This is my last donation." Jennifer had already sought information about weaning off the breast pump. She received a note from the milk bank thanking her for her special donation.

Questions

1.   What can the milk bank do to ensure all staff immediately recognize that Jennifer is a bereaved donor and take this into account when discussing her milk donation?

2.   How would practical support for Jennifer throughout her donation period differ from support given to donors with a living child?

🔍 CASE STUDY 2

Randeep's baby, Aarush, was born at 27 weeks and went immediately to the NICU with respiratory distress. Randeep began hand expressing within an hour of delivery, and her scant drops of milk were sent to the NICU for Aarush. Randeep received ongoing support to express milk at regular intervals. After 48 hours, she was discharged, and her husband accompanied her to their home, which was 2 hours away. All of the couple's relatives live in India. Randeep came to the hospital every day to be with her baby; she often traveled by bus because she did not have a car. At home, she tried to regularly express her milk. She spent many hours holding Aarush directly against her skin, but her milk production began to decrease and eventually did not meet her baby's needs. Aarush received pasteurized donor milk in the NICU in addition to Randeep's expressed milk. The primary nurse checked with Randeep daily regarding her milk expression and gave her some tips on what might help. Randeep connected with a friend who began driving her to and from the hospital. Gradually, her milk production began to increase. At 37 corrected weeks, Aarush was discharged and almost completely on Randeep's milk with about 2 ounces per day of pasteurized donor milk. Randeep indicated that she knew mother's milk is best, and this information was reinforced by the staff. In addition, the fact that the hospital provided donor milk rather than formula conveyed to her how important human milk is for Aarush, especially her own milk.

Questions

1. What would you explore as the causes of Randeep's difficulty with sufficient milk production?
2. What would you introduce to routine hospital care to make it easier for parents in Randeep's situation to provide enough of their own milk?
3. How did the availability of donor milk affect Randeep's motivation to breastfeed?

References

1. World Health Organization. Donor human milk for low-birth-weight infants. World Health Organization website. http://www.who.int/elena/titles/donormilk_infants/en/. Accessed November 16, 2017.
2. American Academy of Pediatrics. Breastfeeding and the use of human milk. *Pediatrics*. 2012;129(3):e827-e841. http://pediatrics.aappublications.org/content/pediatrics/129/3/e827.full.pdf. Published February 27, 2012. Accessed November 16, 2017.
3. ESPGHAN Committee on Nutrition, Arslanoglu S, Corpelein W, et al. Donor human milk for preterm infants: current evidence and research directions. *J Pediatr Gastroenterol Nutr*. 2013;57(4):535-542.
4. Flaherman VJ, Lee HC. "Breastfeeding" by feeding expressed mother's milk. *Pediatr Clin North Am*. 2013;60(1):227-246.
5. Weaver SR, Hernandez LL. Autocrine-paracrine regulation of the mammary gland. *J Dairy Sci*. 2016;99(1):842-853.
6. Johns HM, Forester DA, Amir LH, McLachlan HL. Prevalence and outcomes of breast milk expressing in women with healthy term infants: a systematic review. *BMC Pregnancy Childbirth*. 2013;13:212. doi:10.1186/1471-2393-13-212.
7. Labiner-Wolfe J, Fein SB, Shealy KR, Wang C. Prevalence of breast milk expression and associated factors. *Pediatrics*. 2008;122(suppl 2):S63-S68.
8. Geraghty S, Davidson B, Tabangin M, Morrow A. Predictors of breastmilk expression by 1 month postpartum and influence on breastmilk feeding duration. *Breastfeed Med*. 2012;7(2):112-117.
9. Li RL, Magadia J, Fein SB, Grummer-Strawn LM. Risk of bottle-feeding for rapid weight gain during the first year of life. *Arch Pediatr Adolesc Med*. 2012;166(5):431-436. doi:10.1001/archpediatrics.2011.1665.
10. Boone KM, Geraghty SR, Keim SA. Feeding at the breast and expressed milk feeding: associations with otitis media and diarrhea in infants. *J Pediatr*. 2016;174:118-125.
11. McInnes RJ, Arbuckle A, Hoddinott P. How UK internet websites portray breast milk expression and breast pumps: a qualitative study of content. *BMC Pregnancy Childbirth*. 2015;2(15):81.
12. Sheehan A, Bowcher WL. Messages to new mothers: an analysis of breast pump advertisements. *Matern Child Nutr*. 2017;13(2). doi:10.1111/mcn.12313.
13. Morton J, Hall JY, Wong RJ, Thairu L, Benitz WE, Rhine WD. Combining hand techniques with electric pumping increases milk production in mothers of preterm infants. *J Perinatol*. 2009;29(11)757-764.
14. Tsai SY. Influence of partner support on an employed mother's intention to breastfeed after returning to work. *Breastfeed Med*. 2014;9(4):222-230.
15. Becker GE, Smith HA, Cooney F. Methods of milk expression for lactating women. *Cochrane Database Syst Rev*. 2015;27(2):CD006170. doi:10.1002/14651858.CD006170.pub4.
16. Alekseev NP, Ilvin VI. The mechanics of breast pumping: compression stimuli increased milk ejection. *Breastfeed Med*. 2016;11:370-375.
17. Santoro W, Martinez FE, Ricco RG, Jorge SM. Colostrum ingested during the first day of life by exclusively breastfed healthy newborn infants. *J Pediatr*. 2010;156(1):29-32.
18. Ohyama M, Watabe H, Hayasaka Y. Manual expression and electric breast pumping in the first 48 h after delivery. *Pediatr Int*. 2010;52(1):39-43.
19. Flaherman VJ, Gay B, Scott C, Avins A, Lee KA, Newman TB. Randomised trial comparing hand expression with breast pumping for mothers of term newborns feeding poorly. *Arch Dis Child Fetal Neonatal*. 2012;97(1). doi:10.1136/adc.2010.209213.

20. Bolman M, Saju L, Oganesyan K, Kondrashova T, Witt AM. Recapturing the art of therapeutic breast massage during breastfeeding. *J Hum Lact.* 2013;29(3):328-831.

21. Bolman W. The basics of breast massage and hand expression [Video]. http://bfmedneo.com/resources/videos/. Published 2013. Accessed February 1, 2018.

22. Hill PD, Aldag JC. Milk volume on day 4 and income predictive of lactation adequacy at 6 weeks of mothers of nonnursing preterm infants. *J Perinat Neonatal Nurs.* 2005;19(3):273-282.

23. Hill PD, Aldag JC, Chatterson RT, Zinaman M. Primary and secondary mediators' influence on milk output in lactating mothers of preterm and term infants. *J Hum Lactation.* 2005;21(2):138-150.

24. Maastrup R, Hansen BM, Kronborg H, et al. Factors associated with exclusive breastfeeding of preterm infants: results from a prospective national cohort study. *PLOS One.* 2014;9(2):e89077. doi:10.1371/journal.pone.0089077.

25. Parker LA, Sullivan S, Kruger C, Muellier M. Association of timing of initiation of breastmilk expression on milk volume and timing of lactogenesis stage II among mothers of very low-birth-weight infants. *Breastfeed Med.* 2015;10(2):84-91.

26. Furman L, Minichin N, Hack M. Correlates of lactation in mothers of very low birth weight infants. *Pediatrics.* 2002;109(4):e57.

27. Parker LA, Sullivan S, Kruger C, et al. Effect of early milk expression on milk volume and timing of lactogenesis stage II among mothers of very low birth weight infants: a pilot study. *J Perinatal.* 2013;32:H205-H209.

28. Pletsch D, Ulrich C, Angelini M, Fernandes G, Lee DS. Mothers' "liquid gold": a quality improvement initiative to support early colostrum delivery via oral immune therapy (OIT) to premature and critically ill newborns. *Nurs Leadersh.* 2013;26(spec no 2013):34-42.

29. Meier P, Patel A, Hoban R, Engstrom J. Which breast pump for which mother: an evidenced based approach to individualizing breast pump technology. *J Perinatol.* 2016;36(7):493-499.

30. Hill PD, Aldag JC, Chatterton RT Jr. Breastfeeding experience and milk weight in lactating mothers pumping for preterm infants. *Birth.* 1999;26(4):233-238.

31. Fewtrell MS, Kennedy K, Ahluwalia JS, Nicholl R, Lucas A, Burton P. Predictors of expressed breast milk volume in mothers expressing milk for their preterm infant [published online ahead of print March 2, 2016]. *Arch Dis Child Fetal Neonatal Ed.* doi:10.1136/archdischild-2015-308321.

32. Morton J, Wong RJ, Hall JY, et al. Combining hand techniques with electric pumping increases the caloric content of milk in mothers of preterm infants. *J Perinatol.* 2012;32(10):791-796.

33. Smith SL, Serke L. Case report of sepsis in neonates fed expressed mother's milk [published online ahead of print July 30, 2016]. *J Obstet Gynecol Neonatal Nurs.* doi:10.1016/j.jogn.2016.05.006.

34. Qi Y, Zhang Y, Fein S, Wang C, Lovo-Berrios N. Maternal and breast pump factors associated with breast pump problems and injuries. *J Hum Lactation.* 2014;30(1):62-72.

35. Kent JC, Geddes DT, Hepworth AR, Hartmann PE. Effect of warm breast shields on breast milk pumping. *J Hum Lactation.* 2011;27(4):331-338.

36. Wu B, Zheng J, Zhou M, et al. Improvement of expressed breast milk in mothers of preterm infants recording breast milk pumping dairies in a neonatal unit in China. *PLOS One.* 2015;10(12):e0144123. doi:10.1371/journal.pone.0144123.e.

37. Karimi M, Eslami Z, Moradi J, Ahmadi J, Baghianimoghadam B. The effect of educational intervention on decreasing mothers' expressed breast milk bacterial contamination whose infants are admitted to neonatal intensive care unit. *J Res Health Sci.* 2012;29;13(1):43-47.

38. Chang YC, Chen CH, Lin MC. The macronutrients in human milk change after storage in various containers. *Pediatr Neonatol.* 2012;53(3):205-209.

39. Hanna N, Ahmed K, Anwar M, Petrova A, Hiatt M, Hegyi T. Effect of storage on breast milk antioxidant activity. *Arch Dis Child Fetal Neonatal Ed.* 2004;89(6):F518-F520.

40. Government of Canada. Safe food storage. Government of Canada website. http://healthycanadians.gc.ca/eating-nutrition/healthy-eating-saine-alimentation/safety-salubrite/tips-conseils/storage-entreposage-eng.php. Updated November 14, 2014. Accessed November 16, 2017.

41. Eteng MU, Ebong PE, Eyong EU, et al. Storage beyond three hours at ambient temperature alters the biochemical and nutritional qualities of breastmilk. *Afr J Reprod Health.* 2001;5:130-134.

42. Hamosh M, Ellis LA, Pollock DR, Henderson TR, Hamosh P. Breastfeeding and the working mother: effect of time and temperature of short- term storage on proteolysis, lipolysis, and bacterial growth in milk. *Pediatrics.* 1996;97:492-498.

43. Igumbor EO, Mukura RD, Makandiramba B, et al. Storage of breast milk: effect of temperature and storage duration on microbial growth. *Centr Afr J Med.* 2000;46:247-251.

44. Pardou A, Serruys E, Mascart-Lemone F, Dramaix M, Vis HL. Human milk banking: influence of storage processes and of bacterial contamination on some milk constituents. *Biol Neonate.* 1994;65(5):302-309.

45. Silvestre D, López MC, March L, Plaza A, Martínez-Costa C. Bactericidal activity of human milk: stability during storage. *Br J Biomed Sci.* 2006;63(2):59-62.

46. Human Milk Banking Association of North America. *2011 Best Practice for Expressing, Storage and Handling Human Milk in Hospitals, Homes, and Child Care Settings.* Fort Worth, TX: Human Milk Banking Association of North America; 2011.

47. British Dietetic Association. *Guidelines for the Preparation and Handling of Expressed and Donor Breast Milk and Special Feeds for Infants and Children in Neonatal and Paediatric Health Care Settings.* Birmingham, UK: British Dietetic Association; 2016.

48. Eglash A, Liliana S, The Academy of Breastfeeding Medicine. ABM clinical protocol #8: human milk storage information for home use for full-term infants, revised 2017. *Breastfeed Med.* 5(3):127-30.

49. Thatrimontrichai A, Janijindamai W, Puwanant M. Fat loss in thawed breast milk: composition between refrigerator and warm water. *Indian Pediatr.* 2012;49(11):877-880.

50. Thomas E. Warming feeds is unnecessary and hazardous. *BMJ.* 2000;15;320(7241):1078.

51. Dumm M, Hamms M, Sutton J, Ryan-Wenger N. NICU breast milk warming practices and the physiological effects of breast milk feeding temperatures on preterm infants. *Adv Neonatal Care.* 2013;13(4):279-287. doi:10.1097/ANC.0b013e31829d8c3a.

52. Sando WC, Gallaher KJ, Rodgers BM. Risk factors for microwave scald injuries in infants. *J Pediatr.* 1984;105(6):864-867.

53. Transportation Security Administration. Traveling with children. Department of Homeland Security website. https://www.tsa.gov/travel/special-procedures/traveling-children. Accessed January 25, 2017.

54. Palmquist AE, Doehler K. Contextualizing online human milk sharing: structural factors and lactation disparity among middle income women in the U.S. *Soc Sci Med.* 2014;122:140-147. doi:10.1016/j.socscimed.2014.10.036.

55. Stuebe A. The risks of not breastfeeding for mothers and infants. *Rev Obstet Gynecol.* 2009;2(4): 222-231.

56. American Academy of Pediatrics Committee on Fetus and Newborn. Donor human milk for the high-risk infant: preparation, safety, and usage options in the United States. *Pediatrics.* 2017;139(1):e20163440. doi:10.1542/peds.2016-3440.

57. Palmquist AE, Doehler K. Human milk sharing practices in the US. *Matern Child Nutr.* 2016;12(2):278-290.

58. Buia C. The booming market for breast milk. *Newsweek.* May 23, 2015. http://www.newsweek.com/2015/06/05/booming-market-breast-milk-335151.html. Accessed January 24, 2017.

59. Jones F. Milk sharing: how it undermines breastfeeding. *Breastfeed Rev.* 2013;21(3):21-25.

60. Keim SA, McNamara KA, Dillon CE, et al. Breastmilk sharing: awareness and participation among women in the Moms2Moms study. *Breastfeed Med.* 2014;9:398-406.

61. Stevens EE, Patrick TE, Pickler R. A history of infant feeding. *J Perinat Educ.* 2009;18(2):32-39.

62. Perinatal Services BC. *Informal (Peer-to-Peer) Milk Sharing: The Use of Unpasteurized Donor Human Milk.* Vancouver, Canada: Perinatal Services BC; 2016. http://www.perinatalservicesbc.ca/Documents/Guidelines-Standards/HealthPromotion/InformalMilkSharing_PracticeResource.pdf. Accessed November 16, 2017.

63. Titmuss RM, Oakey A, Ashton J, eds. *The Gift Relationship: From Human Blood to Social Policy.* London, UK: LSE Books; 1997.

64. European Milk Bank Association. About EMBA. European Milk Bank Association website. www.europeanmilkbanking.com. Accessed January 25, 2017.

65. Swanson K. *Banking on the Body.* Cambridge, MA: Harvard University Press; 2014.

66. Berton P. Dionne quintuplets. The Canadian Encyclopedia website. http://www.thecanadianencyclopedia.ca/en/article/dionne-quintuplets/. Accessed January 23, 2017.

67. Williams AS. *Women and Childbirth in the Twentieth Century: A History of the National Birthday Trust Fund.* Stroud, Gloucestershire: Alan Sutton Publishing; 1997.

68. Department of Health and Social Security. HIV infection, breastfeeding and human milk banking. London HMSO 1989 (PL/MO(89)4 and PL/MO(89)3, June 1989).

69. Lucas A, Gore SM, Cole TJ, et al. Multicentre trial on feeding low birthweight infants: effects of diet on early growth. *Arch Dis Child.* 1984;59:722-730.

70. Orloff SL, Wallingford J, McDougall JS. Inactivation of human immunodeficiency virus type I in human milk: effects of intrinsic factors in human milk and pasteurisation. *J Hum Lactation.* 1993;9:13-17.

71. National Institute for Health and Care Excellence. Donor milk banks: service operation. NICE website. https://www.nice.org.uk/guidance/cg93. Published February 2010. Accessed November 16, 2017.

72. Lucas A, Cole TJ. Breast milk and neonatal necrotizing enterocolitis. *Lancet.* 1990;336:1519-1523.

73. Quigley M, McGuire W. Formula versus donor breast milk for feeding preterm or low birth weight infants. *Cochrane Database Syst Rev.* 2014;4:CD002971. doi:10.1002/14651858.CD002971.

74. ICCBBA. ISBT 128—the global information standard for medical products of human origin. ICCBBA website. http://www.iccbba.org. Accessed November 16, 2017.

75. PATH. Strengthening human milk banking: a global implementation framework, version 1.1. PATH website. http://www.path.org/publications/detail.php?i=2433. Published December 2013. Accessed November 16, 2017.

76. Welborn JM. The experience of expressing and donating breastmilk following a perinatal loss. *J Hum Lactation.* 2012;28(4):506-510. doi:10.1177/0890334412455459.

77. Human Milk Banking Association of North America. *Guidelines for the Establishment and Operation of a Donor Human Milk Bank.* Fort Worth, TX: Human Milk Banking Association of North America; 2015.

78. Hartmann BT, Pang AD, Keil AD, Hartmann PE, Simmer K. Best practice guidelines for the operation of a donor human milk bank in an Australian NICU. *Early Hum Dev.* 2007;83(10):667-673.

79. Peila C, Emmerik NE, Giribaldi M, et al. Human milk processing: a systematic review of innovative techniques to the ensure safety and quality of donor milk. *J Pediatr Gastroenterol Nutr.* 2017;64(3):353-361.

80. Kühn T. *Use of Breast Milk for Feeding Preterm Infants.* Bremen, Germany: UNI-MED; 2016.

81. Victora CG, Bahl R, Franca GV, et al. Breastfeeding in the 21st century: epidemiology, mechanisms, and lifelong effect. *Lancet.* 2016;387(10017):475-490.

82. DeMarchis A, Israel-Ballard K, Mansen KA, Engmann C. Establishing an integrated human milk banking approach to strengthen newborn care. *J Perinatol.* 2017;37(5):469-474.

83. UNICEF. Breast milk banks are a sound investment in the health of Brazil's premature babies. UNICEF website. https://www.unicef.org/infobycountry/brazil_70944.html. Updated November 15, 2013. Accessed January 23, 2017.

84. Vázquez-Román S, Garcia-Lara NR, Escuder-Vieco D, Chaves-Sánchez F, De la Cruz-Bertolo J, Rosa Pallas-Alonso C. Determination of Dornic acidity as a method to select donor milk in a milk bank. *Breastfeed Med.* 2013;8(1):99-104.

85. Human Milk Banking Association of South Africa. HMBASA. HMBASA website. www.hmbasa.org.za/. Accessed January 23 2017.

86. U.S. Department of Health and Human Services. *The Surgeon General's Call to Action to Support Breastfeeding.* Washington, DC: U.S. Department of Health and Human Services, Office of the Surgeon General; 2011. https://www.surgeongeneral.gov/library/calls/breastfeeding/calltoactiontosupportbreastfeeding.pdf. Accessed November 16, 2017.

Additional Resources

Policy

The Global Breastfeeding Collective. Ensuring equitable access to human milk for all infants. https://www.path.org/publications/files/MNCHN
_EquitableAccesstoHumanMilk_PolicyBrief.pdf. Published November 2017. Accessed January 29, 2018.

The Global Breastfeeding Collective (UNICEF, WHO, & PATH) released a policy brief in late 2017 outlining global actions needed to support
breastfeeding and the provision of donor milk as needed.

Information about Breast Pumps

KellyMom.com. What should I know about buying a new or used breastpump? http://kellymom.com/bf/pumpingmoms/pumping
/buying-a-used-or-new-pump/.

Videos about Hand Expression

Stanford Medicine. Hand expression of breastmilk. https://med.stanford.edu/newborns/professional-education/breastfeeding/hand
-expressing-milk.html.

Healthy Families BC. A video on hand expressing breastmilk. https://www.healthyfamiliesbc.ca/home/articles/video-hand-expressing
-breastmilk.

Milk Bank Development

PATH. A workshop for developing a hazard analysis critical control points plan for your human milk bank. https://www.path.org
/publications/detail.php?i=2679.

Other Websites

Human Milk Banking Association of North America. https://www.hmbana.org.

European Milk Bank Association. http://europeanmilkbanking.com.

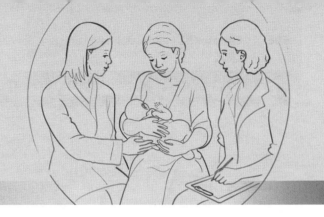

CHAPTER 32

Interdisciplinary Lactation Services

Rebecca Mannel

Suzanne Hetzel Campbell

Elizabeth K. Stehel

OBJECTIVES

- Outline the variety of disciplines involved in lactation services and care.
- Describe the current perspective of interdisciplinary lactation services.
- Define interdisciplinary health care.
- Illustrate the role of lactation consultants as they collaborate and partner with other healthcare professionals, patients, and families for the provision of lactation services at multiple levels.
- Provide examples of the lactation consultant's role as a change agent in working collaboratively with the rest of the healthcare team to provide coordinated services to families.
- Review Baby-friendly infant feeding policy tenets using the principles of interdisciplinary care.
- Apply effective interdisciplinary care to a real-life situation given case studies and examples.
- Demonstrate leadership and cultural awareness when communicating within an organization and when representing an organization to others.

DEFINITIONS OF COMMONLY USED TERMS

acuity As related to patients in health care, a prioritization based on how critical, or acute, their presenting symptoms are related to the severity of illness and the amount of care required.[1]

collaboration The process of working together toward a common end by various participants. Whereas compromise is a passive process of conceding something to find middle ground, collaboration is an active process that involves creating something to grow or achieving mutual gain.[2]

interdisciplinary health care "When multiple health workers from different professional backgrounds work together with patients, families, carers, and communities to deliver the highest quality of care."[3(p7)]

(continues)

DEFINITIONS OF COMMONLY USED TERMS *(continued)*

interprofessional practice When healthcare workers from various backgrounds learn about, with, and from each other to negotiate a plan of care that best meets patient, family, and community health and wellness needs while respecting individual choice and decision making. Relies on interprofessional education, interprofessional learning, interprofessional collaboration, and interprofessional teamwork.[4]

lactation acuity A measure of the severity of breastfeeding or lactation complications and the intensity of lactation care that a breastfeeding couplet requires.[5]

patient-centered care Design of patient care wherein institutional resources and personnel are organized around patients rather than specialized departments.[6,7] The U.S. Institute of Medicine (IOM) defines patient-centered care as "providing care that is respectful of, and responsive to, individual patient preferences, needs and values, and ensuring that patient values guide all clinical decisions."[8(p3)]

postnatal A term that clarifies confusion between postpartum (lactating parent only) and neonatal (baby only). Refers to all issues pertaining to the lactating parent and baby dyad from birth to 6 weeks (42 days).[3]

Any use of the term *mother*, *maternal*, or *breastfeeding* is not meant to exclude transgender or nonbinary parents who may be breastfeeding or providing human milk to their infant.

▶ Overview

The important role that healthcare professionals play in providing accurate information to families regarding the feeding and care of their children has been shown to affect the intention, initiation, and successful meeting of parents' goals related to infant feeding. This is especially true with vulnerable populations, such as adolescents, indigenous families, and infants in neonatal intensive care.[9-13] Yet research provides conflicting evidence of the benefit of healthcare professionals in roles such as advocate, informer (risk versus benefit), and supporter.[14,15] Given the opportunities for providing lactation support from a variety of professionals, this chapter provides information about the benefits and challenges of interdisciplinary lactation services and provides suggestions for education in basic breastfeeding support and interprofessional teamwork. Geddes encourages us to "discard the stereotype, strengthen the science, and experience success" by letting go of our own prejudices and labels of "researchers as closeted and unapproachable old men, midwives as pushy, lactation consultants as overly zealous, and doctors as detached."[16(p122)] She provides examples of groups who have pushed aside stereotypical assumptions to work together toward a common goal, such as New Zealand's approach to implementing the Baby-friendly Hospital Initiative. Although the focus was on obtaining research rigor, with methodologies and measurements of outcomes, and appreciating the roles played by various parties—from researcher, to clinician, to statistician, to patient—the concept is similar to finding ways to come together as healthcare professionals to support parents in their breastfeeding goals. Almost 50 percent of the world's gross national income is lost ($302 billion annually) as a result of not breastfeeding.[17] It is imperative to come together as healthcare professionals to support what the global vice president of the World Bank stated about breastfeeding: "Just in sheer, raw bottom-line economic terms, [breastfeeding is] the single most effective investment a country can make in any sector for any reason!"[18(p386)]

I. Interdisciplinary Health Care

A. Interdisciplinary or interprofessional health care is a fairly recent concept in delivering healthcare services. The major movements began with the following events:
   1. In 2003 with the IOM's *Health Professions Education: A Bridge to Quality*.[19]
   2. In 2010 with the release of a report in *The Lancet*, "Health Professionals for a New Century: Transforming Education to Strengthen Health Systems in an Interdependent World."[20]
B. Traditional healthcare settings for most of the 20th century typically employed a hierarchical system. The clinician focused on treating the disease and relying mostly on their own knowledge and skills to make decisions about the management of a particular patient's care, with little focus on the patient's perspective.

C. A transition occurred in health care, by early innovators, beginning with a focus on the patient called patient-centered care by the early innovators.
    1. It evolved to focus on the important roles of all members on the healthcare team.
    2. The explosion of knowledge in medicine and health care has led to increased specialization and recognition that one clinician cannot be the expert in all areas.
    3. The emerging concept of interdisciplinary care encourages collaboration among various healthcare disciplines or professions to capitalize on the larger body of knowledge and skills.
D. As the input of all members on the healthcare team has become more valued, the notion of the patient's role as a critical member of the healthcare team has become better understood, and efforts to incorporate patient voices and perspectives is happening in the broader community.[4]
E. For interprofessional care to impact patients' health and healthcare outcomes, concepts of interprofessional practice need to be embedded in healthcare practitioner education across disciplines and incorporated in practice through continuing education and learning on the job.[4]

II. Interdisciplinary Education

A. There is a need to realign the education of healthcare professionals and interprofessional practice in the workforce.
    1. A model that can allow for the development of a professional identity and also provide ample opportunities for interprofessional education and collaborative care is needed.[4]
    2. "Multidisciplinary staff training may increase knowledge and can increase initiation rates and duration of breastfeeding, although evidence is limited. Lack of staff training is an important barrier to implementation of effective interventions."[11(piii)]
B. Over the last half century the interest in interprofessional education has grown among healthcare disciplines.
    1. Since 2000 a renewed interest has occurred due to concerns about quality, cost, access, and safety in health care.
    2. The focus of interprofessional education is on outcomes, including the impact and importance of interprofessional collaboration in care delivery improvements, such as patient and staff satisfaction, safety, quality, cost containment, and value.[4]
C. Improvements in learning must be made, and the link among "patient, population and system outcomes"[4(p18)] must be emphasized.
    1. Updates to interprofessional competencies identify a triple aim to improve the patient experience, the health of populations, and healthcare costs.[21,22] See the *Additional Resources* section.
    2. "Although there is a widespread and growing belief that interprofessional education may improve interprofessional collaboration, promote team-based health care delivery, and enhance personal and population health, definitive evidence linking interprofessional education to desirable intermediate and final outcomes does not yet exist."[4(p25)]
D. The importance of interprofessional education for better healthcare outcomes is well recognized; however, a Cochrane Review that looked specifically at interprofessional education found that the heterogeneity and methodological limitations of the studies identified for meta-analysis require caution when interpreting the results.[23] Although an array of positive effects were identified for interprofessional education, the small sample sizes and lack of control groups made it hard to conclude that interprofessional education positively impacted client or patient healthcare outcomes or professional practice.

III. Institute of Medicine: Measuring the Impact

A. The IOM asserts there is a "moral imperative to work together to combat a specific disease (e.g., cancer diagnosis and treatment) or public health crisis (e.g., Ebola and Zika epidemics) but also increasingly in Western countries, is driven by concerns about the overall health of the population, the quality and safety of health care, and health care costs."[4(p29)]
B. Other industries, including the military and the airline industry, have incorporated interprofessional education and team-based collaboration better than the healthcare industry. The reasons for this are unclear; possibly there is better alignment between education and practice (see **FIGURE 32-1**).

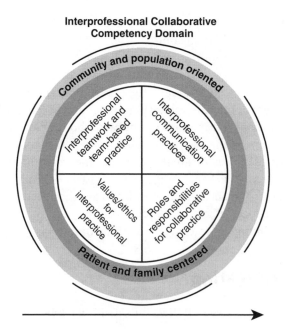

FIGURE 32-1 Interprofessional collaboration competency domain.

C.   Many questions remain, including what the IOM means when it refers to "treatment and dose" and when and how much interprofessional education and practice is most effective.[4] In an effectiveness review, interprofessional education was shown to "nurture collaborative knowledge, skills and attitudes" and it was observed that "more limited but growing evidence [exists] that interprofessional education can help enhance collaborative practice and improve patient care."[4(p161)]

IV.   Examples of Interdisciplinary Collaboration

A.   Successful examples of interdisciplinary collaboration in health care include the management of diabetes and cancer. Relying on the expertise of various disciplines improves the overall management and quality of care in these complex diseases.[24-29]

B.   People with diabetes may receive care from several healthcare professionals.

1.   They may have had screenings by a nurse, a diagnosis by a physician, counseling on nutritional choices by a dietitian, and education about managing their disease by a diabetes educator.

2.   Diabetic patients with complications might receive care from a physical therapist to help manage neuropathies, care from an ophthalmologist to treat glaucoma, or care from an endocrinologist to manage kidney function.

3.   All these providers need to have knowledge about diabetes as it relates to their field of expertise. Further, they need to be in communication with each other to have a complete picture of the patient's current health.

C.   A cancer patient may receive an initial screening from a primary care provider and receive a referral to an oncologist for further work-up.

1.   Cancer patients may be sent to numerous healthcare providers to confirm a diagnosis. They will likely have multiple visits at healthcare centers to obtain blood tests, radiology scans, or X-rays.

2.   They may have surgery performed by a surgical oncologist, chemotherapy prescribed by a medical oncologist and administered by a nurse, radiation therapy given by a radiation oncologist, nutrition therapy managed by a dietitian, and help with transportation or family lodging from a social worker.

3.   All healthcare team members have an important role in caring for the patient. When the team members work interprofessionally, they must understand and value the role of each team member and the necessity for communication and collaboration.

V. Interdisciplinary Teams

A. Building a collaborative, interdisciplinary team requires trust, open communication, respect, and an understanding that every team member has positive intent.[30]
   1. Building trust with an interprofessional team starts with institutional leadership demonstrating trust in each member of the team and valuing their knowledge and expertise.
      a. Regular, positive communication helps maintain trust.
      b. Demonstrating humility by listening and learning from each other is a key component in building trust.
   2. Open communication in an interdisciplinary team requires team members to speak the same language.
      a. Members work to help the team understand the language of their particular specialty.
      b. Members of different disciplines are open to learning and valuing differing insights.
      c. Questions are allowed and encouraged to promote clarity and understanding for open communication to exist.
   3. Respect for each team member and valuing the knowledge and skills they bring to the table are crucial.
      a. No one team member possesses all the needed knowledge or expertise.
      b. There is strength in examining issues from different perspectives.
   4. Strong interdisciplinary teams assume that each team member wants to provide quality care and improve patient outcomes.[31]
      a. When unexpected outcomes occur, the team avoids placing blame.
      b. The team evaluates what happened and what can be done differently in the future to achieve a better outcome.
B. Team decision making involving a breastfeeding dyad includes several considerations. When exploring a particular course of action or recommendation, ask these questions:
   1. What is the family's current breastfeeding goal?
   2. What is the potential impact on the breastfeeding duration?
   3. What is the impact on the parent?
   4. Can the parent follow through with the recommended plan?
   5. What is the impact on the baby?
   6. What resources are available to support this course of action?

VI. Interdisciplinary Care for Lactation

A. Lactation is a prime example of the need for interdisciplinary care. Optimal care involves all family members, including the lactating parent, the infant or child, and the support persons surrounding them.
B. Obstetric providers coordinate pregnancy care and may refer parents to prenatal breastfeeding education taught by a breastfeeding educator or a nurse trained in basic breastfeeding counseling.
C. At the time of birth, the baby is delivered by a midwife or physician and is placed in skin-to-skin contact with the parent for the initial feeding. The baby–birth parent dyad is assessed and monitored by a nurse during the first 1 to 2 hours postpartum. That same nurse or a skilled lactation support provider will assist with the first breastfeeding.
D. Pediatric and obstetric providers need to consider the dyadic nature of breastfeeding when caring for the infant and birth parent. Treatments and interventions for the lactating parent could affect the baby, and vice versa.
E. The baby might develop respiratory distress requiring neonatal intensive care managed by the neonatal–pediatric provider. In this case, the breastfeeding couplet has a higher acuity that requires care from a certified lactation consultant.
F. At the time of hospital discharge, the lactating parent and the baby will need a referral to community support to sustain breastfeeding. This may include the following:
   1. Direct referral to a certified lactation consultant for continued management of any breastfeeding complications.
   2. Referral to a community support group where peer support is beneficial.

G. A 2015 research article highlighted the importance of continuing education to support expanding clinicians' roles in breastfeeding support.[32] An online continuing education tutorial for physicians and nurses was created to contribute to Healthy People 2020 Maternal, Infant, and Child Health objectives in the United States to support facilities pursuing Baby-friendly Hospital Initiative designation.[32]

VII. Patient-Centered Care

A. Patient-centered care is another important development in health care that can improve the quality of interdisciplinary care.

B. Patient-centered care involves including the patients' needs, values, and perceptions in decisions made about their care.[33]

1. Paternalism in health care is no longer an acceptable standard of care.
   a. A renewed focus on partnership between the healthcare team and the patient is evolving.
   b. This more personalized care model is much more patient centered.

2. Childbirth and lactation are good examples of the benefit of patient-centered care.
   a. Historically, the traditional maternity care model involved separating the dyad.
   b. After delivering the baby, designated nurses cared for the baby in a nursery, and postpartum nurses cared for the mother in a postpartum room. Contact between the mother and the baby was rigidly scheduled.
   c. This model evolved due to prevailing views at the time that mothers needed rest to recover and that newborns were initially best cared for in incubators to maintain their temperature and protect them from infection.
   d. Hospitals were constructed around this model, so some outdated practices have continued due to the physical layout. All care revolved around the routines of the hospital staff and clinicians.
   e. Fathers or other support people were often not encouraged to visit, and sometimes they were not allowed to be present during the birth.
   f. Research demonstrates the stress that mother–infant separation places on the newborn infant.[34]

3. A patient-centered or family-centered model involves identifying the parents' goals for childbirth and infant feeding and including key support prenatally, such as the partner, a female relative, or a doula.
   a. Leading up to and at the birth of the baby, the support team is present, and the dyad remains together unless one or both experience medical complications.
   b. The remainder of the hospital birth stay involves the nursing and lactation staff caring for the dyad as a couplet, and obstetric and pediatric team members performing routine exams in the patient's room.
   c. All care revolves around the needs of the dyad.

VIII. Interprofessional Education and Patient-Centered Care

A. Lactation care can be provided in many settings and may be needed over the course of months or years, starting during pregnancy and continuing through weaning.

1. A parent who has several children and breastfeeds each child for 1 to 2 years, as recommended internationally, can easily require lactation care that spans 10 to 20 years, depending on birth spacing.
2. Lactation care typically occurs in both the hospital and the community.
3. Lactation care is best started with early education about breast development in the elementary school system, including education that breasts develop to make milk to feed babies. The conversation can continue during the teenage years with education about fertility and ways to plan the timing of childbirth.
4. Every professional discipline that provides care for breastfeeding children and lactating parents needs education about lactation physiology and basic lactation support.[9,35-37]

B. Breastfeeding education and lactation support are provided in hospitals and birthing centers.
    1. Basic breastfeeding education can be provided in obstetrical triage units where expecting families are monitored for possible hospital admission.
    2. Lactation consultants and healthcare providers furnish education and support on antepartum care units where women with high-risk pregnancies are admitted and may stay until birth. These high-risk patients may have difficulty with breastfeeding, and early lactation support and education will help anticipate challenges and allow for early intervention to promote breastfeeding success.
    3. Labor and delivery nurses and obstetric providers initiate skin-to-skin contact and breastfeeding initiation at birth.
    4. Nurses and lactation consultants on postpartum units regularly assess breastfeeding until discharge.
    5. Neonatologists, neonatal nurse practitioners, nurses, lactation consultants, speech pathologists, and occupational therapists provide breastfeeding support in neonatal intensive care units (or special-care nurseries) where preterm and critically ill infants are admitted and all lactation care is high acuity.
    6. Lactation support providers, including lactation consultants, registered dietitians, occupational therapists, and speech pathologists, provide lactation support and consultation in pediatric general and intensive care units where breastfeeding babies may be readmitted due to other health issues (e.g., abnormality on the newborn screening) or breastfeeding complications (e.g., significant jaundice or weight loss).
    7. Lactation support providers furnish lactation consultations in emergency departments where a breastfeeding dyad may be evaluated, either related to a breastfeeding complication (e.g., mastitis) or a health issue that may impact breastfeeding (e.g., infant illness leading to poor feeding).
    8. Lactation support providers also provide lactation consultations in other general or intensive care adult hospital units where a breastfeeding parent may be admitted for routine surgery (e.g., cholecystectomy) or medical complications (e.g., cardiomyopathy).
C. Breastfeeding education and lactation support are provided in community lactation care settings.
    1. Lactation support caregivers provide lactation care and consultation in private homes where families may receive care. These caregivers can include public health nurses, community health workers, peer support counselors (such as La Leche League Leaders), or breastfeeding peer counselors and community-based certified lactation consultants.
    2. Lactation support caregivers provide lactation care and consultation in clinics where families may receive prenatal and postpartum care or where the baby is receiving regular well-baby checkups. Ideally these clinics will have staff members trained in basic breastfeeding management and either employ a certified lactation consultant or collaborate with community-based certified lactation consultants to provide skilled care for higher-acuity situations.
    3. Lactation support caregivers provide lactation care and consultation in local health departments that may provide some postnatal care or well-baby checkups, including scheduled childhood immunizations.
        a. In the United States, the parent and baby may be enrolled in the Department of Health and Human Services Special Supplemental Nutrition Program for Women, Infants, and Children (WIC).
        b. Breastfeeding mothers enrolled in WIC receive prenatal breastfeeding information, supplemental food packages throughout the first year of breastfeeding, and access to breast pumps and other supplies needed to sustain breastfeeding.
        c. Breastfeeding infants enrolled in WIC receive age-appropriate supplemental food packages to complement breastfeeding past 6 months of age and regular nutritional checkups.
        d. Health departments and WIC clinics employ or collaborate with community-based certified lactation consultants (e.g., IBCLCs).
    4. Dental offices may have providers trained in evaluating and treating ankyloglossia (tongue-tie), which can interfere with the infant's ability to latch effectively at the breast.
    5. Community support groups, such as La Leche League, Australian Breastfeeding Association, Baby Café, and others, provide lactation care and peer support. These groups typically utilize some type of trained lay counselor to facilitate the groups and identify situations requiring referral for higher-acuity lactation or medical care. The value of the groups is the peer support received from others who are breastfeeding.

6.   Doulas, or birth companions, are usually nonmedically educated individuals trained to provide help and support before, during, and after birth. As with some home visiting staff members, doulas establish a relationship during pregnancy that continues for some time after the baby's birth. Doulas also attend the birth in the hospital or birthing center.

D.   Special social situations may require additional lactation support and care.

1.   Incarcerated lactating women requiring community-based admission to a facility for treatment of conditions such as drug dependency need access to breastfeeding support.

a.   Employees of these facilities can work with the community to create a breastfeeding plan in the same fashion as a plan for prenatal care of pregnant individuals in the facility.

b.   In some situations, the dyad is separated, and the plan might need to include accommodations for milk expression and storage. (See Chapter 31, *Expression and Use of Human Milk*.)

2.   Homeless parents might need infant feeding and other assistance as they struggle to find a safe place for themselves and their infants.

3.   Breastfeeding children and their parents might experience extended separation, such as during work time for flight attendants, during deployments for military personnel, or due to parental separation such as divorce.

E.   The interdisciplinary team of healthcare providers and support personnel for breastfeeding families is extensive.

1.   Specialists on the healthcare team who provide care to breastfeeding families can include some or all of the following providers (alphabetical and not inclusive):

a.   Chiropractors

b.   Dentists

c.   Dietitians

d.   Lactation consultants (e.g., IBCLCs)[38]

e.   Midwives

f.   Nurses, including advanced practice nurses

g.   Occupational therapists

h.   Pharmacists[39-40]

i.   Physical therapists or physiotherapists

j.   Physician assistants

k.   Physicians

l.   Social workers

m.   Speech–language pathologists[41]

2.   Lactation support providers include the following:

a.   Breastfeeding counselors

b.   Breastfeeding educators

c.   Breastfeeding peer counselors

d.   Certified lactation counselors

e.   Community health workers

3.   Public health staff members, such as the state or regional breastfeeding coordinator, may be part of the team.

4.   Other critical members of the team include administrative leaders in both inpatient and outpatient settings. Although they do not provide direct patient care, they are responsible for creating, or allowing the creation of, programs that support evidence-based lactation care.

F.   Hospital and community collaboration provides continuity of lactation care.

1.   Providers working in hospitals or clinics rely on relationships with community resources to help address social and clinical needs of parents and newborns.

2.   Establishing those connections and networks can be a challenge for busy providers and clinical staff members.

3.   Some healthcare systems provide home visits by trained staff members (e.g., midwives, nurses, and community health workers) for several weeks after a baby is born.

4.   In other systems, parents must actively seek follow-up appointments or other support for themselves and their newborn. Having a list of local contacts to facilitate the recommended parental and newborn follow-up is vital.

5. The World Health Organization (WHO) defines best practice in postnatal care as follows[42]:
    a. Provide postnatal care in the first 24 hours for every birth:
        i. Delay facility discharge for at least 24 hours.
        ii. In the case of home births, visit the breastfeeding dyad within the first 24 hours.
    b. Provide four postnatal visits:
        i. On the first day (within 24 hours of birth).
        ii. On day 3 (48 to 72 hours after birth).
        iii. Between days 7 and 14 after birth.
        iv. At 6 weeks after birth.
    c. Offer home visits by midwives, other skilled providers, or well-trained and supervised clinical health workers.
    d. Use chlorhexidine for umbilical cord care after home deliveries in settings with high newborn mortality.
    e. Reemphasize and support elements of quality postnatal care for birth parents and newborns, including identification of issues and referrals.
6. The WHO guidelines[42] may be applied differently, depending on the resources available in a given country. Identifying issues related to breastfeeding for parents and their newborns is a key aspect of the WHO's guidelines.
    a. Staff members who provide postnatal care need to be trained in basic breastfeeding management and provide referrals to a certified lactation consultant (e.g., IBCLC) when they identify higher-acuity lactation issues.[5,43]
    b. Breastfeeding parents need referral to community support for managing breastfeeding after they return to work.[43]
    c. Breastfeeding must be promoted and supported, particularly during emergencies such as natural disasters, civil unrest, and in refugee camps.[44]
        i. Donations of human milk substitutes (e.g., formula) must be avoided.
        ii. When needed, human milk substitutes (e.g., formula) must be placed under the control of appropriate health agencies for monitoring of need, expiration dates, and access to safe water supplies.
7. Local public health departments and regional breastfeeding coalitions are good sources of information about resources.
    a. Local La Leche League groups, which are available in 89 countries, are knowledgeable about quality resources.
    b. Regional or national lactation consultant groups and national breastfeeding committees can help find local resources.
    c. The International Board of Lactation Consultant Examiners (IBLCE) maintains an online registry of currently certified IBCLCs in more than 100 countries. An IBCLC's current certification status can be verified by entering his or her name.
    d. For more information on this topic, see the websites listed in the *Additional Resources* section.

IX. Policy Development Resources for Interdisciplinary Lactation Care

A. The Baby-friendly Hospital Initiative[45] is a good example of a project requiring interdisciplinary lactation care.
    1. This initiative is a concrete example of the importance of interprofessional care because the designation cannot typically be earned without a multidisciplinary team working on the project. It involves too many aspects of parental and infant care for one person to have sufficient power to successfully mandate and incorporate all requirements into clinical care. (See Chapter 29, *Initiatives to Protect, Promote, and Support Breastfeeding*, for details about the Baby-friendly Hospital Initiative.)
    2. A fundamental tenet of the Baby-Friendly USA guidelines is that "the health care delivery environment should be neither restrictive nor punitive and should facilitate informed health care decisions on the part of the mother and her family."[46(p8)] Applying this tenet involves the effort of every member of the healthcare team.

3. Step 2 of the *Ten Steps to Successful Breastfeeding* (the evidence-based foundation for Baby-friendly Hospital Initiative practices) requires sufficient education of every hospital professional that provides care to breastfeeding families.[45] Baby-friendly USA guidelines include the following directives:

    a. Maternal and newborn nursing staff members who provide the bulk of care to breastfeeding couplets are required to have 20 hours of education and training in basic breastfeeding management.[46]

    b. Healthcare providers with privileges in labor, delivery, maternity, and newborn care need to have at least 3 hours of breastfeeding education pertinent to their role.[46]

    c. Healthcare providers and staff members in other hospital units need training pertinent to their role and possible workplace exposure to breastfeeding couplets.[46] Pharmacists, for example, need to understand the importance of exclusive breastfeeding and medication safety during lactation.[39]

B. Published data on the experience in Canada with implementing the Baby friendly Hospital Initiative for neonatal units (Neo-BFHI) for neonatal care reveals why an interdisciplinary team is critical.

    1. Barriers included concern about infant health, parent–infant separation, staff workload, lack of continuity in breastfeeding support, and inadequate staff knowledge and skills.[47]

    2. Getting staff buy-in and identifying perceived barriers and facilitators enhances the ability for interprofessional communication and team support of the family, especially for more vulnerable patients and their families.

C. Hospital breastfeeding policies can emphasize the interdisciplinary team approach in caring for breastfeeding families.

    1. The Academy of Breastfeeding Medicine has a model hospital policy available for free download from its website (www.bfmed.org).

    2. The policy introduction might include statements related to infant feeding from various national and international professional associations (e.g., American Academy of Pediatrics, American College of Obstetricians and Gynecologists, and Academy of Breastfeeding Medicine), national governmental organizations (e.g., Centers for Disease Control and Prevention and European Union), and international nongovernmental organizations (e.g., WHO and UNICEF).

    3. The institutional commitment to a system-wide multidisciplinary approach is often stated in policies to clarify the institutional and professional commitment to encouraging breastfeeding while also respecting parental choice.

    4. The expectation within institutions is that the role of the various disciplines that interact directly or indirectly with either the breastfeeding parent or infant will be outlined. Expectations describe in detail the barriers practitioners are responsible for removing and their active support in providing patient-centered care according to the *Ten Steps to Successful Breastfeeding*.

    5. The interdisciplinary team coming to an agreement on a work flow that incorporates the *Ten Steps to Successful Breastfeeding* requires creating policies and working through specific issues, such as the contraindications to breastfeeding. An interdisciplinary team approach to crafting and reworking the work flow for their given context will lead to better buy-in and more successful implementation of the *Ten Steps to Successful Breastfeeding* in the facility.

    6. Monitoring adherence after policy implementation requires the ongoing efforts of many interdisciplinary team members and will be supported by incorporating evaluation and quality improvement measures as well as ongoing education and professional development.

    7. Although it appears these steps might typically take place in the hospital or at the local health authority, it is possible to have a regional or national policy to support families in a Baby-friendly way that is then translated by all healthcare staff members, from prenatal to intrapartum to postpartum care. Examples include the Baby-friendly Initiative in Canada[48] and the BFHI in the United Kingdom.[49]

    8. Providing consistent and sufficient education about breastfeeding to all staff members can be a challenge, but is necessary to overcome mixed messages to the family.[50,51] Scripting can be a useful way to ensure a consistent message for families from staff members representing various disciplines (e.g., physicians and lactation) and among staff members within a discipline (e.g., day and night shift nurses).

X. The Lactation Consultant as a Key Partner

A. Certified lactation consultants (e.g., IBCLCs) play a major role as key partners who can teach healthcare providers and work collaboratively with the healthcare team, community, and patients to support and advocate for interprofessional lactation services.

B. The IBCLC scope of practice supports the role of IBCLCs as members of an interdisciplinary healthcare team. (See Chapter 25, *Professional Standards for Lactation Care Providers.*)

   1. Lactation consultants are advocates for evidence-based breastfeeding care and policies. By maintaining an up-to-date practice with evidence-informed and evidence-based care guidelines, they can provide education, references, and support to interdisciplinary partners, parents, and the community.

   2. Communication with healthcare professionals includes the following:

      a. Provide teaching, professional development education opportunities, and in situ learning opportunities in units, clinics, institutions, and the community.

      b. Establish practice and referral opportunities with other providers.[52]

   3. Lactation consultants can work to implement support programs.

      a. Multidisciplinary team-led programs that address the context and population needs of their community.

      b. Community-based support systems that integrate multiple disciplines, patients, and governments.

      c. Partnerships with existing groups, such as parent support and peer support programs, breastfeeding support, local classes, and practitioners.

▶ Key Points from This Chapter

A. Identify the healthcare professionals and disciplines available in a community that can improve the care of breastfeeding families.

B. Develop processes to ensure interdisciplinary collaboration and communication.

C. Interprofessional education is critical to the provision of quality lactation care.

D. Patient-centered care involves the family in decisions about the care of the breastfeeding dyad.

E. Patient-centered care acknowledges the parent's goals for childbirth and breastfeeding.

F. Lactation care must occur in and be incorporated into many settings, including the community, hospital, and outpatient facility, to make the needed support available for the breastfeeding dyad.

🔍 CASE STUDY 1

Baby Noah was born at term and is exclusively breastfed. He was diagnosed with hyperbilirubinemia on day 2 of life. His bilirubin was checked and graphed in the hospital by the nursing staff and physicians. A lactation consultant in the hospital assessed Noah's milk intake and his parent's milk production after the hyperbilirubinemia diagnosis. Noah was discharged to home on phototherapy. His parents were instructed to follow up with a home health service for phototherapy at home; to follow up with a lactation consultant to monitor Noah's weight gain, milk intake, and the parent's milk production; and to follow up with Noah's pediatric provider to monitor his bilirubin levels and weight gain.

Questions

1. How many different healthcare providers were involved in Noah's care?
2. What information did the hospital team utilize in their decision to discharge Noah with home phototherapy?
3. How might the outcome change if these interdisciplinary providers are not available?

🔍 CASE STUDY 2

Tanya gave birth to Alicia, a late preterm infant, at 36 weeks gestational age. Alicia, exclusively breastfed, was diagnosed with 10 percent weight loss on day 3 of life. Tanya reported pain with latch. The lactation consultant reported feeding difficulty, possibly related to a restriction of Alicia's tongue movement. An oral assessment by a family medicine

(continues)

🔍 CASE STUDY 2   *(continued)*

physician revealed ankyloglossia. Alicia was referred to a pediatric ear, nose, and throat physician for evaluation and frenotomy. Tanya's pain with latch resolved after the procedure, and Alicia demonstrated weight gain by the day of discharge. Tanya is primiparous, 17 years old, and will return to school. The WIC Food and Nutrition Service referred Tanya for additional lactation education and support and a free electric breast pump. Tanya was also referred to a home visiting nurse and community-based lactation consultant for follow-up after discharge.

Questions

1. How many different healthcare providers could potentially be involved in Tanya's and Alicia's care?
2. How did the interdisciplinary care approach impact the costs of care for Tanya's family?
3. How will the interdisciplinary care approach impact the breastfeeding outcomes for this family?

🔍 CASE STUDY 3

Delores was admitted to a hospital for a cholecystectomy (gall bladder removal). Delores is exclusively breastfeeding her second baby, Timothy, who is 4 months of age. Delores consults a lactation consultant on a community breastfeeding hotline about managing breastfeeding around the surgery. The general surgeon and anesthesiologist will consult with Delores's obstetric provider and lactation consultant about the safety of resuming breastfeeding or milk expression as soon as Delores is responsive after surgery. Delores was also informed of the hospital's policy to allow breastfeeding babies to stay in the room with their parent on general hospital units if the parent or another family member can care for the baby. The nursing staff will provide a hospital bassinet and bedding for Timothy. Delores is able to resume breastfeeding immediately after transfer from the recovery room to the hospital room.

Questions

1. What is likely to happen when breastfeeding parents need surgery or are admitted to general hospital units without the involvement of an interdisciplinary healthcare team?
2. What healthcare providers were involved in creating the environment in this situation?
3. What else could be done to ensure the same outcome for another breastfeeding parent in the future?

References

1. Brennan CW, Daly BJ. Patient acuity: a concept analysis. *J Adv Nurs.* 2009;65:1114-1126.
2. Mannel R. Essential leadership skills, part iii: fostering change through collaboration. *J Hum Lactation.* 2008;24(3):244-245.
3. World Health Organization. *Framework for Action on Interprofessional Education and Collaborative Care.* Geneva, Switerland: World Health Organization; 2010. http://www.who.int/hrh/resources/framework_action/en/. Accessed August 1, 2013.
4. Institute of Medicine. *Measuring the Impact of Interprofessional Education on Collaborative Practice and Patient Outcomes.* Washington, DC: National Academies Press; 2015.
5. Mannel R. Defining lactation acuity to improve patient safety and outcomes. *J Hum Lactation.* 2011;27(2):163-170.
6. Institute for Patient- and Family-Centered Care. Transforming health care through partnerships. What is patient and family centered care. Institute for Patient- and Family-Centered Care website. http://www.ipfcc.org/about/pfcc.html. Accessed March 16, 2018.
7. OneView. The eight principles of patient-centered care. From OneView website article. May 15, 2015. http://www.oneviewhealthcare .com/the-eight-principles-of-patient-centered-care/. Accessed March 16, 2018.
8. Institute of Medicine. *Crossing the Quality Chasm: A New Health System for the 21st Century.* Washington, DC: Institute of Medicine; 2001.
9. Beake S, Pellowe C, Dykes F, Schmied V, Bick D. A systematic review of structured compared with non-structured breastfeeding programmes to support the initiation and duration of exclusive and any breastfeeding in acute and primary health care settings. *Matern Child Health J.* 2012;4:141-161.
10. Chuang CH, Chang PJ, Chen YC, et al. Maternal return to work and breastfeeding: a population-based cohort study. *Int J Nurs Stud.* 2010;47(4):461-474.
11. Renfrew M, Craig D, Dyson L, et al. Breastfeeding promotion for infants in neonatal units: a systematic review and economic analysis. *Health Tech Assess.* 2009;13(40):1-170.
12. Wambach KA, Aaronson L, Breedlove G, Domian EW, Rojjanasrirat W, Yeh H-W. A randomized controlled trial of breastfeeding support and education for adolescent mothers. *West J Nurs Res.* 2011;33(4):486-505.
13. Karol S, Tah T, Kenon C, et al. Bringing Baby-Friendly to the Indian Health Service. *J Hum Lactation.* 2016;32(2):369-372.

14. Larsen JS, Hall EOC, Aagaard H. Shattered expectations: when mothers' confidence in breastfeeding is undermined—a metasynthesis. *Scand J Caring Sci.* 2008;22(4):653-661.

15. Mörelius E, Anderson GC. Neonatal nurses' beliefs about almost continuous parent–infant skin-to-skin contact in neonatal intensive care. *J Clin Nurs.* 2015;24(17-18):2620-2627.

16. Geddes DT. Discard the stereotype, strengthen the science, and experience success. *J Hum Lactation.* 2013;29(2):122-122.

17. Rollins NC, Bhandari N, Hajeebhoy N, et al. Why invest, and what it will take to improve breastfeeding practices? *Lancet.* 2016;387(10017):491-504.

18. Hansen K. The power of nutrition and the power of breastfeeding. *Breastfeed Med.* 2015;10(8):385-388.

19. Greiner AC, Knebel E, eds. *Health Professions Education: A Bridge to Quality.* Washington, DC: National Academies Press; 2003.

20. Frenk J, Chen L, Bhutta ZA, et al. Health professionals for a new century: transforming education to strengthen health systems in an interdependent world. *Lancet.* 2010;376(9756):1923-1958.

21. McGill Office of Interprofessional Education. Canadian Interprofessional Health Collaborative (CIHC) framework. McGill University website. https://www.mcgill.ca/ipeoffice/ipe-curriculum/cihc-framework. Published 2016. Accessed May 22, 2017.

22. Interprofessional Education Collaborative. *Core Competencies for Interprofessional Collaborative Practice: 2016 Update.* Washington, DC: Interprofessional Education Collaborative; 2016. https://nebula.wsimg.com/2f68a39520b03336b41038c370497473?AccessKeyId=DC06780E69ED19E2B3A5&disposition=0&alloworigin=1. Accessed March 6, 2018.

23. Reeves S, Perrier L, Goldman J, Freeth D, Zwarenstein M. Interprofessional education: effects on professional practice and healthcare outcomes (update). *Cochrane Database Sys Rev.* 2013;3:CD002213. doi:10.1002/14651858.CD002213.pub3.

24. Chisholm-Burns MA, Lee JK, Spivey CA, et al. US pharmacists' effect as team members on patient care: systematic review and meta-analyses. *Med Care.* 2010;48(10):923-933.

25. Hardee SG, Osborne KC, Njuguna N, et al. Interdisciplinary diabetes care: a new model for inpatient diabetes education. *Diabetes Spectrum.* 2015;28(4):276-282.

26. Willens D, Cripps R, Wilson A, Wolff K, Rothman R. Interdisciplinary team care for diabetic patients by primary care physicians, advanced practice nurses, and clinical pharmacists. *Clin Diabetes.* 2011;29(2):60-68.

27. Croke JM, El-Sayed S. Multidisciplinary management of cancer patients: chasing a shadow or real value? An overview of the literature. *Curr Oncol.* 2012;19(4):e232-e238.

28. Tremblay D, Roberge D, Touati N, Maunsell E, Berbiche D. Effects of interdisciplinary teamwork on patient-reported experience of cancer care. *BMC Health Serv Res.* 2017;17(1):217-218.

29. Pannick S, Davis R, Ashrafian H, et al. Effects of interdisciplinary team care interventions on general medical wards: a systematic review. *JAMA Int Med.* 2015;175(8):1288-1298.

30. Kouzes JM, Pozner BZ. *The Leadership Challenge.* 4th ed. San Francisco, CA: Jossey-Bass; 2007.

31. Patterson K, Grenny J, McMillan R, Switzer A. *Crucial Conversation: Tools for Talking When Stakes Are High.* 2nd ed. New York, NY: McGraw Hill Education; 2012.

32. Edwards RA, Colchamiro R, Tolan E, et al. Online continuing education for expanding clinicians' roles in breastfeeding support. *J Hum Lactation.* 2015;31(4):582-586.

33. Bardes CL. Defining "patient-centered medicine." *New Engl J Med.* 2012;366(9):782-783.

34. Morgan BE, Horn AR, Bergman NJ. Should neonates sleep alone? *Biol Psychiatry.* 2011;70(9):817-825.

35. Hörnell A, Lagström H, Lande B, Thorsdottir I. Breastfeeding, introduction of other foods and effects on health: a systematic literature review for the 5th Nordic nutrition recommendations. *Food Nutr Res.* 2013;57. doi:10.3402/fnr.v57i0.20823.

36. Bhandari N, Iqbal Kabir AKM, Adbus Salam M. Mainstreaming nutrition into maternal and child health programmes: scaling up of exclusive breast-feeding. *Matern Child Nutr.* 2008;4(1):5-23.

37. Pérez-Escamilla R, Martinez JL, Segura-Pérez S. Impact of the Baby-friendly Hospital Initiative on breastfeeding and child health outcomes: a systematic review. *Matern Child Nutr.* 2016;12(3):402-417.

38. Dodgson JE. What is a lactation professional? *J Hum Lactation.* 2016;32(4):592-594.

39. Edwards RA. Pharmacists as an underutilized resource for improving community-level support of breastfeeding. *J Hum Lactation.* 2014;30(1):14-19.

40. Lenell A, Friesen C, Hormuth L. Breastfeeding support in a community pharmacy. *J Hum Lactation.* 2015;31(4):577-581.

41. Cichero JAY, Nicholson TM, September C. Thickened milk for the management of feeding and swallowing issues in infants: a call for interdisciplinary professional guidelines. *J Hum Lactation.* 2013;29(2):132-135.

42. World Health Organization. *Postnatal Care for Mothers and Newborns.* Geneva Switzerland: World Health Organization; 2015. http://www.who.int/maternal_child_adolescent/publications/WHO-MCA-PNC-2014-Briefer_A4.pdf?ua=1. Accessed March 6, 2018.

43. World Health Organization. Global strategy for infant and young child feeding. WHO website. http://www.who.int/nutrition/topics/global_strategy_iycf/en/. Published 2003. Accessed August 11, 2017.

44. Carothers C, Gribble K. Infant and young child feeding in emergencies. *J Hum Lactation.* 2014;30(3):272-275.

45. World Health Organization. Baby-friendly Hospital Initiative. WHO website. http://www.who.int/nutrition/topics/bfhi/en/. Accessed January 8, 2018.

46. Baby-Friendly USA. *The Baby-Friendly Hospital Initiative: Guidelines and Evaluation Criteria for Facilities Seeking Baby-Friendly Designation.* Albany, NY: Baby-Friendly USA; 2016. https://www.babyfriendlyusa.org/get-started/the-guidelines-evaluation-criteria. Accessed March 9, 2018.

47. Benoit B, Semenic S. Barriers and facilitators to implementing the Baby-Friendly Hospital Initiative in neonatal intensive care units. *J Obs Gyn Neonat Nurs.* 2014;43(5):614-624.

48. Breastfeeding Committee for Canada. *The Baby-Friendly Initiative (BFI) in Canada.* Drayton Valley, Canada: Breastfeeding Committee for Canada; 2012. http://breastfeedingcanada.ca/documents/BFI_Status_report_2012_FINAL.pdf. Accessed November 26, 2016.

49. Baby-Friendly Initiative UK. *Guidance for Neonatal Units.* London, England: Baby-Friendly Initiative UK; 2015. https://www.unicef .org.uk/babyfriendly/wp-content/uploads/sites/2/2015/12/Guidance-for-neonatal-units.pdf. Accessed June 26, 2017.

50. International Lactation Consultant Association. The Neo-BFHI: the Baby-Friendly Hospital Initiative for neonatal wards. ILCA website. http://www.ilca.org/main/learning/resources/neo-bfhi. Published 2015. Accessed December 7, 2016.

51. World Health Organization, UNICEF. *Baby-Friendly Hospital Initiative: Revised, Updated and Expanded for Integrated Care.* Geneva, Switzerland: World Health Organization, UNICEF. http://www.who.int/nutrition/publications/infantfeeding/bfhi_trainingcourse/en/. Accessed March 9, 2018.

52. Witt AM, Smith S, Mason MJ, Flocke SA. Integrating routine lactation consultant support into a pediatric practice. *Breastfeed Med.* 2012;7(1):38-42.

Additional Resources

Collective Impact Forum. Breastfeeding Coalitions: Building a Grassroots to Treetops Movement for Change. http://www.collectiveimpactforum .org/initiatives/breastfeeding-coalitions-building-grassroots-treetops-movement-change.

Interprofessional Education Collaborative. *Core Competencies for Interprofessional Collaborative Practice: 2016 Update.* Washington, DC: Interprofessional Education Collaborative; 2016. https://nebula.wsimg.com/2f68a39520b03336b41038c370497473?AccessKeyId =DC06780E69ED19E2B3A5&disposition=0&alloworigin=1.

La Leche League International. http://www.llli.org.

UNICEF, World Health Organization. *Advocacy Strategy: Breastfeeding Advocacy Initiative.* New York, NY: UNICEF; 2015. https://www .unicef.org/nutrition/files/Breastfeeding_Advocacy_Strategy-2015.pdf.

United States Breastfeeding Committee. Coalitions Directory. http://www.usbreastfeeding.org/coalitions-directory.

U.S. Department of Agriculture. Women, Infants, and Children (WIC). https://www.fns.usda.gov/wic/women-infants-and-children-wic.

World Alliance for Breastfeeding Action. http://waba.org.my/.

Organizations for Interprofessional Education

American Interprofessional Health Collaborative. http://www.aihc-us.org.

Canadian Interprofessional Health Collaborative. www.cihc.ca.

Centre for the Advancement of Interprofessional Education. www.caipe.org.uk.

Journal of Interprofessional Care. https://www.caipe.org/resources/journal-of-interprofessional-care.

University of British Columbia. http://www.chd.ubc.ca.

University of Toronto Centre for Interprofessional Education. www.ipe.utoronto.ca.

University of Washington Center for Health Sciences Interprofessional Education Research and Practice. http://collaborate.uw.edu.

Index

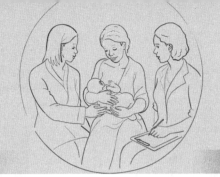

Note: Page numbers followed by *b*, *f*, or *t* indicate material in boxes, figures, or tables, respectively.